MULTIPLE SCLEROSIS 3

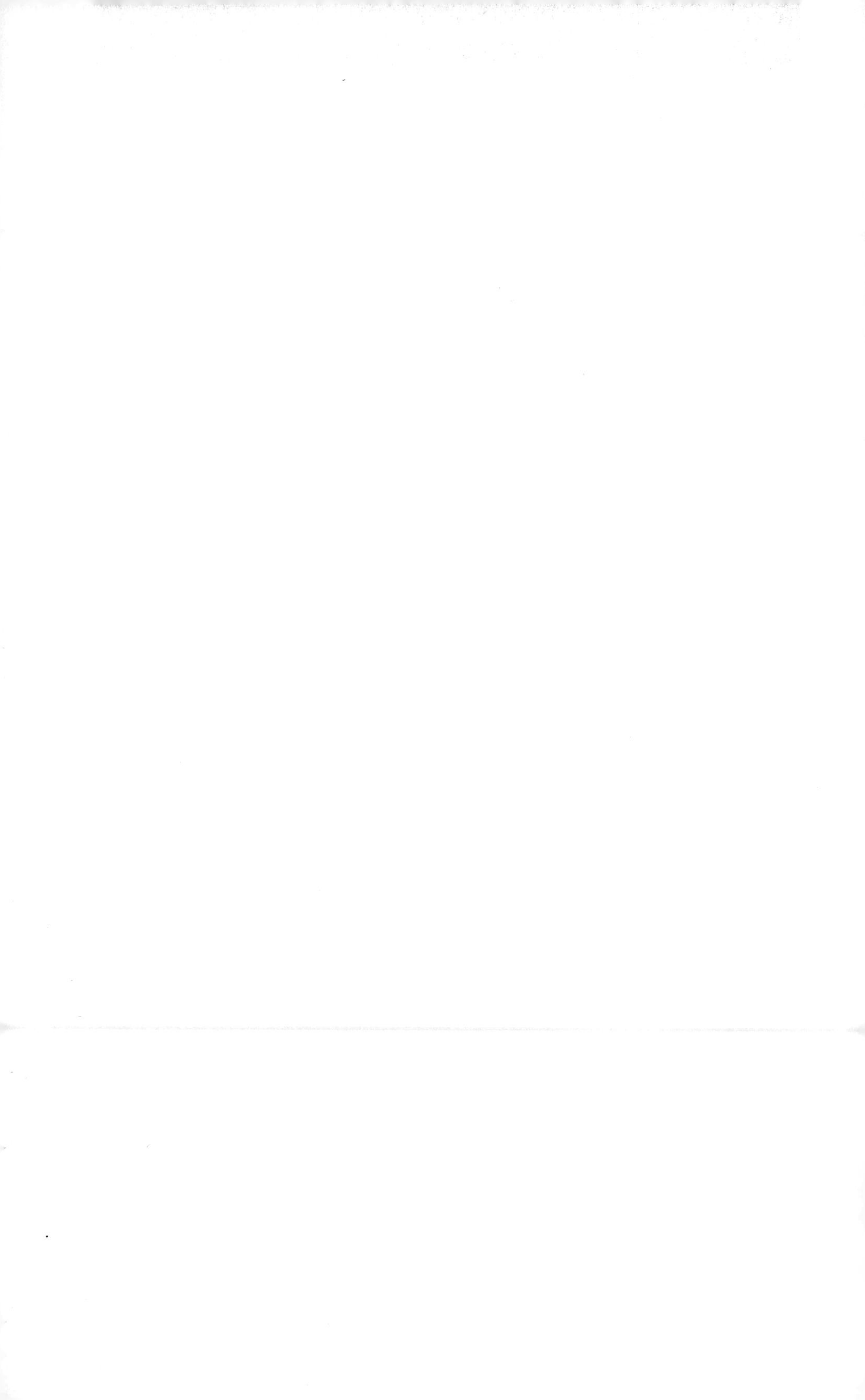

MULTIPLE SCLEROSIS 3

Edited by

CLAUDIA F. LUCCHINETTI, MD
Professor of Neurology
Chair, Division of Multiple Sclerosis and
Autoimmune Neurology
Mayo Clinic College of Medicine
Rochester, Minnesota, USA

REINHARD HOHLFELD, MD
Professor and Director
Institute for Clinical Neuroimmunology
Klinikum Grosshadern
Ludwig Maximilians University
Munich, Germany

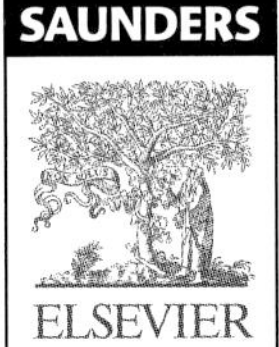

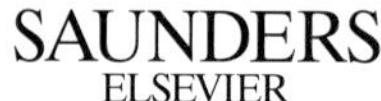

1600 John F. Kennedy Blvd.
Ste 1800
Philadelphia, PA 19103-2899

MULTIPLE SCLEROSIS 3 ISBN: 978-1-4160-6068-0

Notice

Knowledge and best practice in this field are constantly changing. As new research and experience broaden our knowledge, changes in practice, treatment, and drug therapy may become necessary or appropriate. Readers are advised to check the most current information provided (i) on procedures featured or (ii) by the manufacturer of each product to be administered, to verify the recommended dose or formula, the method and duration of administration, and contraindications. It is the responsibility of the practitioner, relying on his or her own experience and knowledge of the patient, to make diagnoses, to determine dosages and the best treatment for each individual patient, and to take all appropriate safety precautions. To the fullest extent of the law, neither the publisher nor the editors assume any liability for any injury and/or damage to persons or property arising out of or related to any use of the material contained in this book.

The Publisher

Library of Congress Cataloging-in-Publication Data
Multiple sclerosis 3 / [edited by] Claudia F. Lucchinetti, Reinhard Hohlfeld. — 1st ed.
p. cm. — (Blue books of neurology series; 35)
Includes bibliographical references and index
ISBN 978-1-4160-6068-0 (alk. paper)
1. Multiple sclerosis. I. Lucchinetti, Claudia F. II. Hohlfeld, R. (Reinhard) III. Title: Multiple sclerosis three. IV. Series: Blue books of neurology; 35.
[DNLM: 1. Multiple Sclerosis. W1 BU9749 v.35 2009 / WL 360 M96256 2009]

RC377.M8394 2009
616.8'34—dc22

2009007831

ISBN-13: 978-1-4160-6068-0

Acquisitions Editor: Adrianne Brigido
Developmental Editor: John Ingram
Project Manager: Hemamalini Rajendrababu
Design Direction: Steve Stave

Printed in China
Last digit is the print number: 9 8 7 6 5 4 3 2 1

BLUE BOOKS OF NEUROLOGY

1 **Clinical Neurophysiology**
ERIC STALBERG • ROBERT R. YOUNG

2 **Movement Disorders**
C. DAVID MARSDEN • STANLEY FAHN

3 **Cerebral Vascular Disease**
MICHAEL J.G. HARRISON • MARK L. DYKEN

4 **Peripheral Nerve Disorders**
ARTHUR K. ASBURY • R.W. GILLIATT

5 **The Epilepsies**
ROGER J. PORTER • PAOLO I. MORSELLI

6 **Multiple Sclerosis**
W. IAN McDONALD • DONALD H. SILBERBERG

7 **Movement Disorders 2**
C. DAVID MARSDEN • STANLEY FAHN

8 **Infections of the Nervous System**
PETER G.E. KENNEDY • RICHARD T. JOHNSON

9 **The Molecular Biology of Neurological Disease**
ROGER N. ROSENBERG • ANITA E. HARDING

10 **Pain Syndromes in Neurology**
HOWARD L. FIELDS

11 **Principles and Practice of Restorative Neurology**
ROBERT R. YOUNG • PAUL J. DELWAIDE

12 **Stroke: Populations, Cohorts, and Clinical Trials**
JACK P. WHISNANT

13 **Movement Disorders 3**
C. DAVID MARSDEN • STANLEY FAHN

14 **Mitochondrial Disorders in Neurology**
A.H.V. SCHAPIRA • SALVATORE DIMAURO

CONTENTS

CONTRIBUTING AUTHORS

NUHAD E. ABOU ZEID, MD

Department of Neurology
Mayo Clinic College of Medicine
Rochester, Minnesota

ALBERTO ASCHERIO, MD, DRPH

Department of Nutrition
Harvard School of Public Health
Boston, Massachusetts

BRENDA BANWELL, MD

Associate Professor of Paediatrics (Neurology)
Director, Pediatric Multiple Sclerosis Program
The Hospital for Sick Children
Toronto, Ontario, Canada

ANGELA BATES, MD

Fellow, Department of Neurology
University of Texas Southwestern Medical Center at Dallas
Dallas, Texas

TAMIR BEN-HUR, MD, PhD

Professor and Head, Department of Neurology
The Agnes Ginges Center for Human Neurogenetics
Hadassah–Hebrew University Medical Center
Jerusalem, Israel

ALLEN C. BOWLING, MD, PhD

Medical Director
Multiple Sclerosis Service
Colorado Neurological Institute
Clinical Associate Professor of Neurology
University of Colorado–Denver and Health Sciences Center
Englewood, Colorado

SCOTT L. DAVIS, PhD

Assistant Professor, Department of Neurology
University of Texas Southwestern Medical Center at Dallas
Dallas, Texas

PHILIP L. DE JAGER, MD

Instructor, Department of Neurology
Harvard Medical School
Division of Molecular Immunology
Center for Neurologic Diseases
Brigham & Women's Hospital
Boston, Massachusetts
Program in Medical and Population Genetics
Broad Institute of Harvard University and Massachusetts Institute of Technology
Cambridge, Massachusetts

RANJAN DUTTA, PhD

Department of Neuroscience
Lerner Research Institute
The Cleveland Clinic Foundation
Cleveland, Ohio

GILLES EDAN, MD

Department of Neurology
University Hospital of Rennes, Pontchaillou
Rennes, France

ELLIOT M. FROHMAN, MD, PhD

Professor, Departments of Neurology and Ophthalmology
University of Texas Southwestern Medical Center at Dallas
Dallas, Texas

TERESA C. FROHMAN, BA

Department of Neurology
University of Texas Southwestern Medical Center at Dallas
Dallas, Texas

RALF GOLD, MD

Professor and Chair, Department of Neurology
St. Josef-Hospital/Ruhr-University Bochum
Bochum, Germany

DAVID A. HAFLER, MD

Jack, Sadie, and David Breakstone Professor of Neurology
Harvard Medical School
Division of Molecular Immunology
Center for Neurologic Diseases
Brigham & Women's Hospital
Boston, Massachusetts
Program in Medical and Population Genetics
Broad Institute of Harvard University and Massachusetts Institute of Technology
Cambridge, Massachusetts

ANU JACOB, MD

Consultant Neurologist
The Walton Centre for Neurology and Neurosurgery
Liverpool, England, United Kingdom

ILIJAS JELČIĆ, MD

Center for Molecular Neurobiology
Institute for Neuroimmunology and Clinical Multiple Sclerosis Research
University Medical Centre Hamburg-Eppendorf
Hamburg, Germany

ADAM I. KAPLIN, MD

Assistant Professor, Departments of Psychiatry and Neurology
Johns Hopkins University School of Medicine
Baltimore, Maryland

DOUGLAS A. KERR, MD, PhD

Associate Professor, Neurology
Director, Johns Hopkins Transverse Myelitis Center
Johns Hopkins University School of Medicine
Baltimore, Maryland

CHRISTOPH KLEINSCHNITZ, MD

Department of Neurology
University of Würzburg
Würzburg, Germany

DANA E. KOZUBAL, BA

Department of Psychiatry
Johns Hopkins University School of Medicine
Baltimore
Maryland

GARY E. LEMACK, MD
Helen J. and Robert S. Strauss Professor in Urology
Department of Urology
University of Texas Southwestern Medical Center at Dallas
Dallas, Texas

RALF A. LINKER, MD
Department of Neurology
St. Josef-Hospital/Ruhr-University Bochum
Bochum, Germany

CLAUDIA F. LUCCHINETTI, MD
Professor of Neurology
Chair, Division of Multiple Sclerosis and Autoimmune Neurology
Mayo Clinic College of Medicine
Rochester, Minnesota, USA

JAMES J. MARRIOTT, MD, FRCPC
Clinical Fellow
St. Michael's Hospital
Toronto, Ontario, Canada

ROLAND MARTIN, MD
Professor
Institute for Neuroimmunology and Clinical Multiple Sclerosis Research
Center for Molecular Neurobiology Hamburg
University Medical Center Eppendorf
Hamburg, Germany

MARCELO MATIELLO, MD
Department of Neurology
Mayo Clinic
Rochester, Minnesota

NICO MELZER, MD
Department of Neurology
University of Würzburg
Würzburg, Germany

SVEN G. MEUTH, MD, PhD

Physician and Researcher
Neurology Clinic
Julius-Maximilians-University
Würzburg, Germany

SEAN P. MORRISSEY, MD

Department of Neurology
University Hospital, Pontchaillou
Rennes, France

KASSANDRA L. MUNGER, MSC

Department of Nutrition
Harvard School of Public Health
Boston, Massachusetts

PAUL W. O'CONNOR, MD, MSC, FRCPC

Division of Neurology
Director, MS Clinic and MS Research
St. Michael's Hospital
Professor of Medicine (Neurology)
University of Toronto
Toronto, Ontario, Canada

MARIA PIA AMATO, MD

Department of Neurology
University of Florence
Florence, Italy

ISTVAN PIRKO, MD

Associate Professor of Neurology
Director, Waddell Center for Multiple Sclerosis
University of Cincinnati
Cincinnati, Ohio

SEAN JOSEPH PITTOCK, MD

Associate Professor of Neurology
Departments of Neurology and Laboratory Medicine and Pathology
Mayo Clinic College of Medicine
Rochester, Minnesota

ALEXANDRA SCHRÖDER, MD

Department of Neurology
St. Josef-Hospital/Ruhr-University Bochum
Bochum, Germany

ANJALI SHAH, MD

Assistant Professor
Departments of Neurology and Physical Medicine and Rehabilitation
University of Texas Southwestern Medical Center at Dallas
Dallas, Texas

BRUCE D. TRAPP, PhD

Chairman
Department of Neuroscience
Lerner Research Institute
The Cleveland Clinic Foundation
Cleveland, Ohio

CARRILIN C. TRECKER, BA

Departments of Psychiatry and Neurology
Johns Hopkins University School of Medicine
Baltimore, Maryland

SUNITA VENKATESWARAN, MD, FRCPC

Department of Pediatrics
Children's Hospital of Western Ontario
University of Western Ontario
Toronto, Ontario, Canada

RHONDA VOSKUHL, MD

Professor of Neurology
Jack H. Skirball Chair for Multiple Sclerosis Research
Director, Multiple Sclerosis Program
University of California, Los Angeles
Los Angeles, California

BRIAN G. WEINSHENKER, MD, FRCP(C)

Professor of Neurology
Department of Neurology
Mayo Clinic
Rochester, Minnesota

HEINZ WIENDL, MD

Head, Clinical Research Group for Multiple Sclerosis and Neuroimmunology
Department of Neurology
University of Würzburg
Würzburg, Germany

DEAN M. WINGERCHUK, MD

Associate Professor of Neurology
Mayo Clinic Scottsdale
Scottsdale, Arizona

NATHAN P. YOUNG, MD

Department of Neurology
Mayo Clinic
Rochester, Minnesota

VALENTINA ZIPOLI, MD

Department of Neurology
University of Florence
Florence, Italy

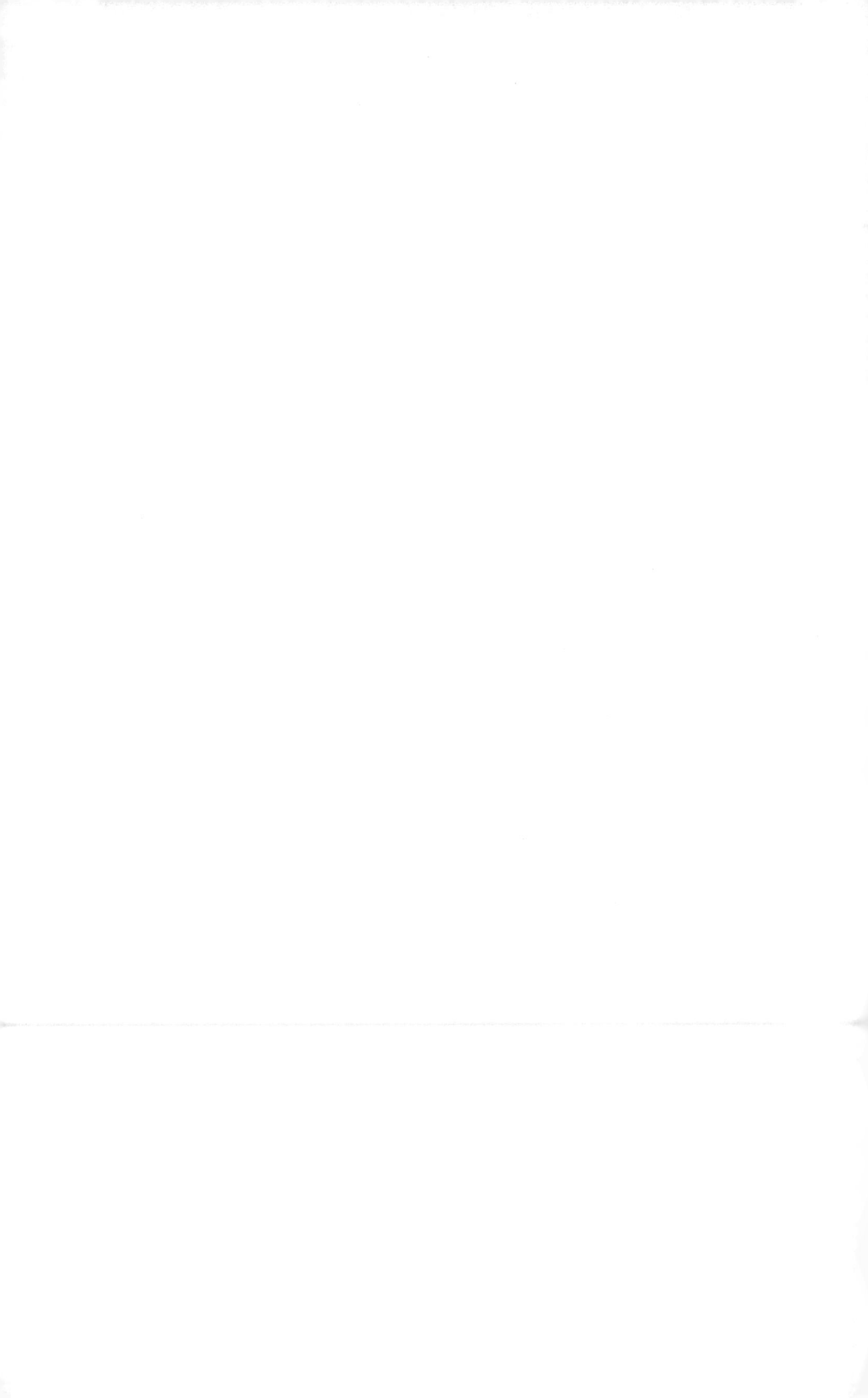

SERIES PREFACE

The *Blue Books of Neurology* have a long and distinguished lineage. Life began as the *Modem Trends in Neurology* series and continued with the monographs forming *BIMR Neurology*. The present series was first edited by David Marsden and Arthur Asbury, and saw the publication of 25 volumes over a period of 18 years.

The guiding principle of each volume, the topic of which is selected by the Series Editors, was that each should cover an area where there had been significant advances in research and that such progress had been translated to new or improved patient management.

This has been the guiding spirit behind each volume, and we expect it to continue. In effect, we emphasize basic, translational, and clinical research but principally to the extent that it changes our collective attitudes and practices in caring for those who are neurologically afflicted.

Tony Schapira took over as joint editor in 1999 following David's death, and together with Art oversaw the publication and preparation of a further 8 volumes. In 2005, Art Asbury ended his exceptional co-editorship after 25 years of distinguished contribution and Martin Samuels was asked to continue the co-editorship with Tony.

The current volumes represent the beginning of the next stage in the development of the Blue Books. The editors intend to build upon the excellent reputation established by the Series with a new and attractive visual style incorporating the same level of high-quality review. The ethos of the Series remains the same: up-to-date reviews of topic areas in which there have been important and exciting advances of relevance to the diagnosis and treatment of patients with neurological diseases. The intended audience remains those neurologists in training and those practicing clinicians in search of a contemporary, valuable, and interesting source of information.

ANTHONY H.V. SCHAPIRA
MARTIN A. SAMUELS
Series Editors

PREFACE

Multiple Sclerosis 3, volume 34 of the Blue Books of Neurology series, is dedicated to the memory of the late Ian W. McDonald, who edited *Multiple Sclerosis 1* with Donald H. Silberberg and *Multiple Sclerosis 2* with John H. Noseworthy. Prof. McDonald pioneered several key areas of multiple sclerosis (MS) research, including characterization of the physiology and morphology of demyelination and remyelination of the central nervous system (CNS). He developed new laboratory methods, such as evoked potentials, to supplement the clinical diagnosis of MS, and he was among the first to envision the enormous potential of magnetic resonance imaging for dissecting the complex problems of inflammatory brain disease. He applied brain imaging and spectroscopy to improve understanding of the pathogenesis of this disorder and to evaluate new therapies. Moreover, Ian McDonald took a leading position in formulating the consensus diagnostic criteria that have since come to bear his name.

Although the clinicopathologic hallmarks of MS are well recognized, the last decade has witnessed significant clinical and scientific advances that have led to improved diagnosis and treatment as well as new insights into the pathogenesis of this enigmatic disorder. We are confident that Prof. McDonald would be delighted to see how rapidly the field has continued to grow, and we are honored to have been invited to edit this volume. We have endeavored to provide a comprehensive, clinically relevant, up-to-date summary on MS and the heterogenous spectrum of CNS inflammatory demyelinating disorders, including clinically isolated syndromes, pediatric MS, transverse myelitis, acute disseminated encephalomyelitis, and neuromyelitis optica. Topics discussed include natural history, diagnosis, genetics, epidemiology, neuroimaging, pathogenesis, immunology, biomarkers, gender issues, and cognitive and mood disorders. A strong emphasis on treatment is also included, with a focus on current disease-modifying drugs, attack therapy, symptomatic therapy, complementary alternative approaches, management of aggressive MS, and future immunologic and neuroprotective or reparative strategies.

We would like to express our sincere gratitude to our distinguished coauthors who have given generously of their time and expertise. We also appreciate the support from the Elsevier editorial staff (Hemamalini Rajendrababu and Adrianne Brigido) throughout the development of this text.

CLAUDIA F. LUCCHINETTI, MD
REINHARD HOHLFELD, MD

1 Clinical Features and Natural History of Multiple Sclerosis: The Nature of the Beast

SEAN JOSEPH PITTOCK

For the practicing neurologist, knowledge of the natural history of multiple sclerosis (MS) that encompasses the overall course and prognosis is a prerequisite to the counseling of a patient who is given such a diagnosis. When confronted with the reality of MS for the first time, patients' first questions relate to long-term prognosis: What will happen to me? From a health research point of view, knowledge of the natural history of MS affects how we think about the pathophysiology of MS, guides therapeutic trial design, assists in health care economics and service provision, and provides a benchmark against which therapeutic trial efficacy can be compared.

Natural history data is best obtained from populations of patients that are representative of MS as a whole, such as all MS patients living within a well-defined geographic area. These population-based cohorts are more representative of the disease than hospital- or clinic-based cohorts, which tend to overrepresent more severe disability and may provide an overpessimistic view.

The natural history of MS is among the best studied chronic medical illnesses. Despite a wealth of information gained from large, population-based studies on clinical features predictive of future course and outcome, the ability to apply this knowledge to an individual patient to allow prediction or prognostication has been problematic.

This review focuses on recently published natural history studies, early clinical predictors of disability outcome and their application to an individual patient, the controversy surrounding the entity of benign MS, and some recent new approaches to data set analysis with emphasis on age at disability milestones rather than time to reach disability milestones.

Disability Progression: What Happens to Patients over Time?

The evolution of MS over time is well studied worldwide, and results are generally consistent among investigators, although some recent natural history studies from North America have suggested a better global prognosis.[1,2] It is important to note that these studies have relied heavily on measures of impairment, specifically the Expanded Disability Status Scale (EDSS) score, as an outcome measure.[3] The EDSS scores range from 0 (no disability) to 10 (death). Cutoff scores most commonly used in natural history studies include mild to moderate disability, with an EDSS score of 3 (e.g., mild paralysis) or EDSS 4 (limited walking ability but able to walk without aid or rest for > 500 m); EDSS 6, which indicates the need for a cane or unilateral support and ability to walk no more than 100 m without rest; and EDSS 8 (need for wheelchair) or EDSS 7 (ability to walk no more than 10 m without rest while leaning against a wall or holding onto furniture for support).

TIME FROM ONSET TO DISABILITY MILESTONES

Natural history studies have focused on the time from onset or diagnosis of the disease to the assignment of one of these EDSS scores; these data provide information regarding the rate of disability progression. If one considers population-based studies of MS in general, median time from onset of MS to EDSS 3 or EDSS 4 ranged from 6 to 23 years.[1,2,4-8] Median time from onset of disease to EDSS 6 was somewhat more consistent (because need for a cane is a more robust and reliable outcome measure) and varied between 16 and 28 years.[1,5-8] Time from onset to the need for a wheelchair ranged from 30 to 52 years for population-based cohorts.[1,5,8]

In a retrospective review of prospectively collected data from all 2837 patients, followed prospectively for 22,723 patient years, registered with one of the four MS clinics in British Columbia, 21% required a cane after 15 years of disease.[2] This frequency increased to 69% by 40 years after onset. At 30 and 40 years after onset, 14% and 22% of patients, respectively, required a wheelchair.

TIME FROM ONSET TO DISABILITY MILESTONES STRATIFIED BY MULTIPLE SCLEROSIS CLINICAL SUBGROUPS

The initial course has a significant impact on the time from onset to specific levels of disability. In 1996, a formal classification of MS disease subtypes was published that has become widely accepted.[9]

- Relapsing-remitting (RR): Clearly defined disease relapses with full recovery or with sequelae and residual deficit on recovery; periods between disease relapses characterized by a lack of disease progression
- Secondary progressive (SP): Initial RR disease course followed by progression with or without occasional relapses, minor remissions, and plateaus

- Primary progressive (PP): Disease progression from onset with occasional plateaus and temporary minor improvements allowed
- Progressive relapsing (PR): Progressive disease from onset with clear acute relapses, with or without full recovery; periods between relapses characterized by continuing progression. A more recent proposed classification is illustrated in Figure 1-1.[10]
- Another classification type used by some investigators is that of single-attack progressive (SAP) MS, in which there is a single "onset attack" followed later by a progressive course.[11]

In population-based studies, an RR onset is most frequent (95% in Olmsted County, Minnesota; 66% in London, Ontario; 87.6% in British Columbia; 85% in Lyon, France).[1,2,5,8] The frequency of conversion from RRMS to SPMS reported for the Ontario cohort increased with duration of disease (12% at 5 years, 41% at 10 years, 58% at 15 years, and 89% at >26 years).[8] Other studies have reported a lower frequency of conversion.[1,2] Frequencies of PPMS and PRMS (both of which are considered progressive from onset) vary from 9% to 19% and from 6% to 15%, respectively.[5,8]

Patients with an RR course take a longer time from onset to reach disability milestones than do patients with an initially progressive course (Fig. 1-2). Myhr and colleagues reported a 72% probability of not needing a cane after 15 years of disease for patients with RRMS, compared with only 10% for those with PPMS.[12] Similarly, RRMS patients had an 84% probability of not needing a wheelchair after 15 years, compared with 42% for those with PPMS. In the Olmsted County 2000 study, median time from onset to the need for a cane (see Fig. 1-2B) in patients who continued to have an RR course was 51 years, compared with 17.9 years for those with SPMS and 6.3 years for those with PPMS.[1] In the French population-based Lyon cohort, the median time from onset to need for a cane was

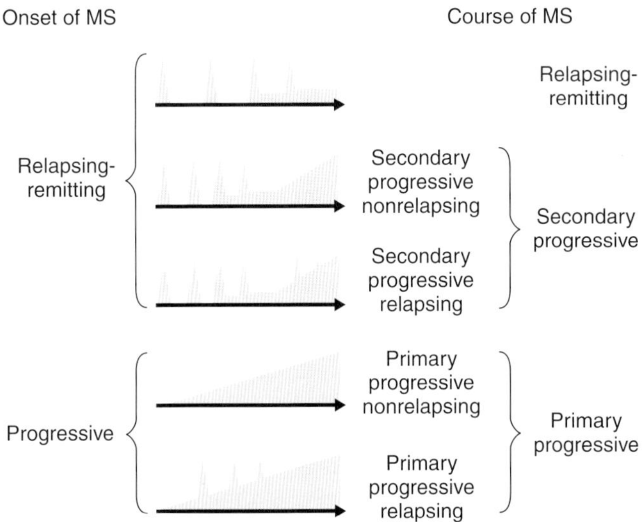

Figure 1–1 Proposed classification of the onset and course of multiple sclerosis (MS). (Reproduced from Confavreux C, Vukusic S: Natural history of multiple sclerosis: Implications for counselling and therapy. Curr Opin Neurol 2002;15:257-266, with permission of Lippincott Williams and Wilkins, online at http://www.lww.com.)

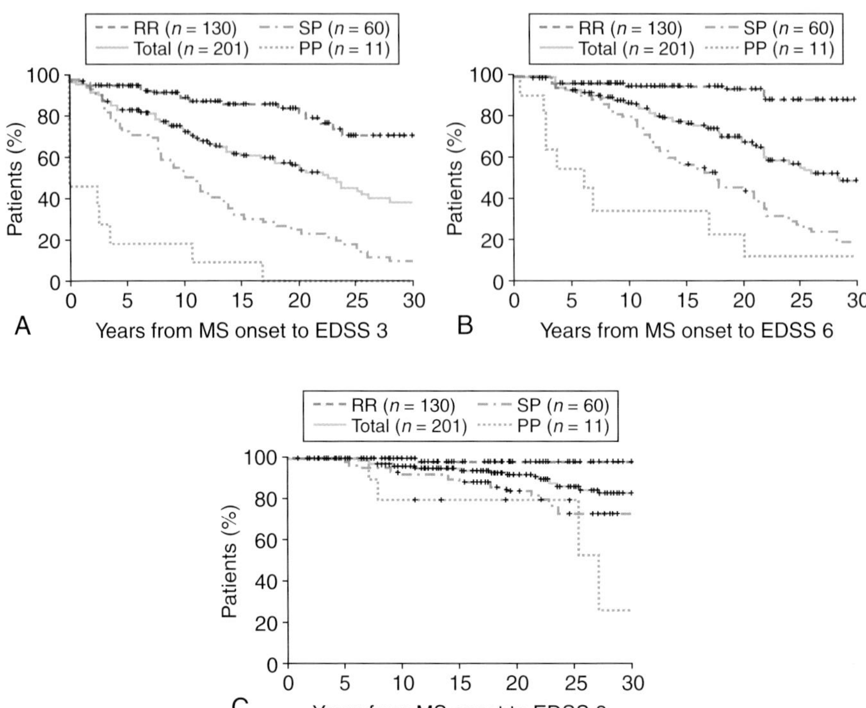

Figure 1–2 Time to Expanded Disability Status Scale (EDSS) score by multiple sclerosis (MS) subtype for the 2000 Olmsted County MS population. **A,** Years from MS onset to EDSS 3 (minimal disability but fully ambulatory). **B,** Years from MS onset to EDSS 6 (use of a cane). **C,** Years from MS onset to EDSS 8 (use of a wheelchair). RR refers to patients who continue to have a relapsing-remitting course and therefore excludes secondary progressive cases. PP, primary progressive; SP, secondary progressive. (Data from Pittock SJ, Mayr WT, McClelland RL, et al: Disability profile of MS did not change over 10 years in a population-based prevalence cohort. Neurology 2004;62:601-606.)

23 years for patients with an RR course, compared with 7 years for patients with a PP course.[5] In a recent natural history study of PPMS from British Columbia, Canada, progression of disability was slower than previously reported. The median time from onset to requiring a cane was 13.3 years; however, there was considerable variation. Although 25% of the patients had reached EDSS 6 after 7.3 years, another 25% did not require a cane after 25 years.[13]

What Affects Long-Term Disability Outcome?

A multitude of demographic and clinical variables including female gender, a younger age at onset, sensory symptoms or optic neuritis, and a monosymptomatic presentation at onset have been associated with a favorable course.[14-16] In contrast, prognostic variables associated with a poor outcome have included male gender; onset with motor, sphincter, or cerebellar features; poor recovery from initial or early attacks; higher attack rate in the first 5 years; and a progressive course.[8,14-16] These statistically significant associations have generally been reported in the context of univariate and, less frequently, multivariate analysis. Few predictors of outcome have been reported for PPMS.[13] Although individual factors are often statistically significant when considering large population-based cohorts, their clinical prognostic applicability to an individual MS patient is much less reliable. There is little doubt that the initial course from onset is the strongest clinical predictor of how quickly a patient will reach disability milestones.

CLINICAL RELAPSES

Disease-modifying agents (DMAs) have been shown in large, randomized controlled trials to reduce the relapse rate and to reduce the accrual of lesions identified on magnetic resonance imaging.[14,17-19] Whether they have a significant clinical benefit over the long term remains unclear. For RRMS, a central and highly controversial question is whether the frequency (and severity) of relapses influences disability progression in MS.[20,21] Reported relapse rates have differed among MS studies, with prospective assessments at close intervals yielding the highest and probably the most sensitive results.[20] A yearly relapse rate of 0.5 is probably a reasonable estimate in a population-based sample of patients with RRMS.[20]

In the Ontario study, 58% of 681 patients with RR disease had one attack during the first 2 years, 21% had two attacks, and only 20% had three or more attacks in the first 2 years of disease.[22] Natural history studies from Lyon, Ontario, and Turkey have shown a weak association between number of relapses in the first 2 to 5 years and long-term disability outcome, although causality has not been established.[5,6,16] Other studies failed to conclude that number of relapses in the first few years influences final outcome, and more recent, large natural history studies have provided convincing evidence of a dissociation between relapses and disability progression.[11,21,23,24] In fact, at the Jekyll Island conference on MS clinical trial outcome measures, relapse frequency was ranked 11th in terms of perceived importance in measuring therapeutic response in MS.[25]

The Lyon group reported that, once a detectable threshold of irreversible disability (EDSS 4) was reached, the disease entered a state of uniform progression that did not appear to be influenced by the presence or absence of superimposed relapses (Fig. 1-3).[21] Patients with a progressive course from onset reached irreversible disability much quicker than patients with an RR-onset course (median, 0.0 versus 11.4 years). However, once this point of irreversible disability was reached, the times to EDSS 6 (median, 5.7 versus 5.4 years) or EDSS 7 (median, 12.1 versus 12.0 years) were similar ($P > .70$) regardless of onset course.[21] In the Olmsted County population-based study, the time to development of a clinical threshold of disability (EDSS 3), whether 2, 5, or 10 years, did not affect the rate of further progression (Fig. 1-4).[1] Among patients with PPMS, the time course of progressive disability was not significantly influenced by the presence or absence of superimposed relapses (Fig. 1-5).[21] For patients with SPMS (initially RR), the median time from EDSS 4 to EDSS 6 was similar for 292 patients without and 191 patients with superimposed relapses (4.0 versus 4.4, respectively; $P = .68$; see Fig. 1-5).[21] Surprisingly, patients with superimposed relapses had a more favorable outcome than those without superimposed relapses, with a longer time from EDSS 4 to EDSS 7 (10 versus 7.8 years; $P = .04$). Similarly, superimposed relapses were

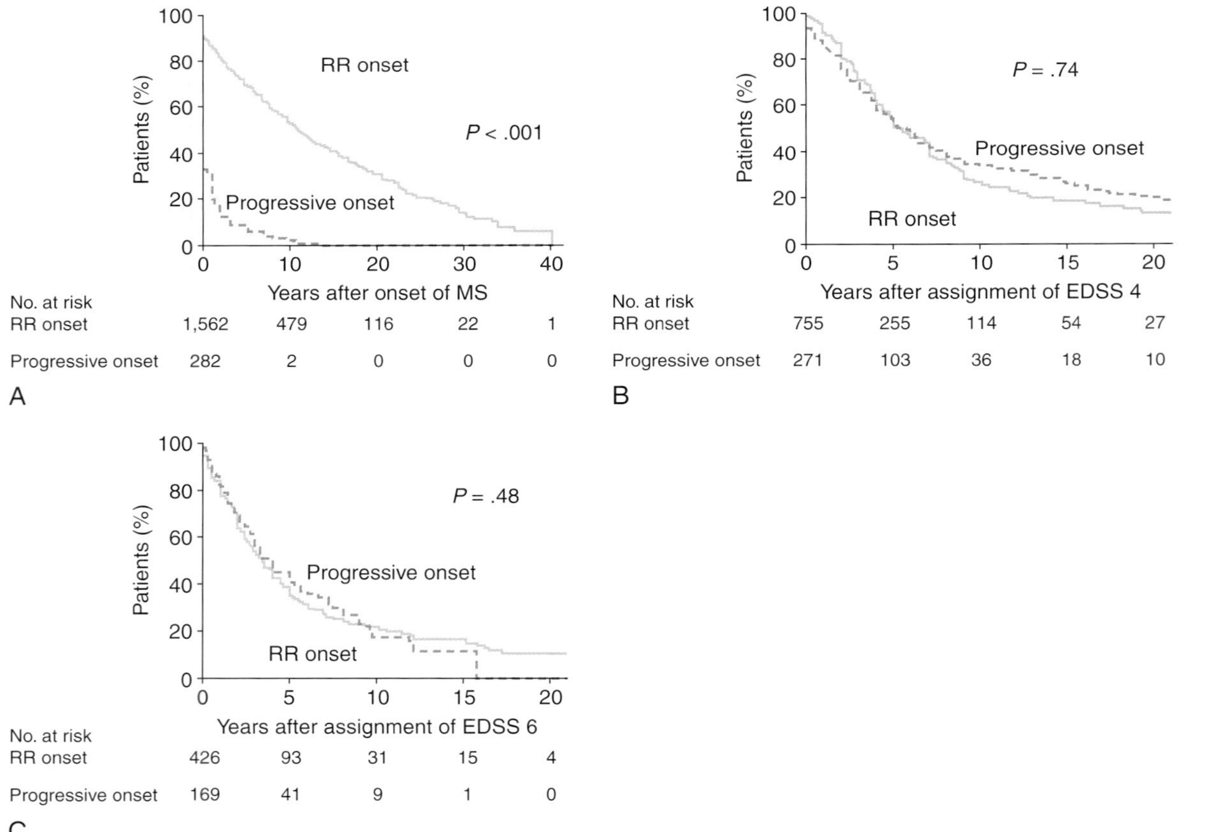

Figure 1–3 Irreversible disability, based on Expanded Disability Status Scale (EDSS) score, occurs sooner in patients with a progressive course from onset, compared with those with a relapsing-remitting (RR) course from onset, although, once irreversible disability has occurred, the time course of progressive disability is similar regardless of the initial course (relapsing or progressive). Kaplan–Meier estimates are shown for time from onset of multiple sclerosis to assignment of EDSS 4 **(A),** time from EDSS 4 to EDSS 6 **(B),** and time from EDSS 6 to EDSS 7 **(C)** among 1844 MS patients stratified by initial course. (Data from Confavreux C, Vukusic S, Moreau T, Adeleine P: Relapse, remission, and progression in multiple sclerosis. N Engl J Med 2000;343:1430-1438.)

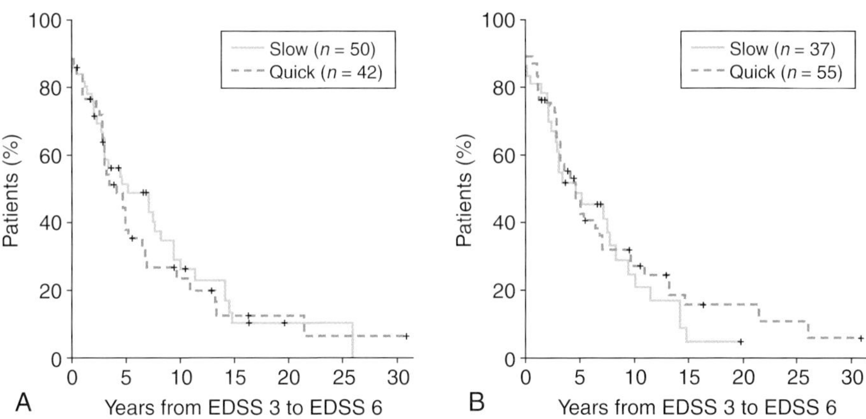

Figure 1–4 Initial rate of progression ("quick" versus "slow") from diagnosis to EDSS 3 as a predictor of further progression from Expanded Disability Status Scale (EDSS) 3 to EDSS 6. **A,** "Quick" progression is defined as progression from diagnosis to EDSS 3 within 2 years, "slow" progression as longer than 2 years (P = .57). **B,** "Quick" progression is within 5 years, and "slow" progression is longer than 5 years (P = .61). (Data from Pittock SJ, Mayr WT, McClelland RL, et al: Disability profile of MS did not change over 10 years in a population-based prevalence cohort. Neurology 2004;62:601-606.)

associated with a more favorable course and longer time from EDSS 6 to EDSS 7 (4.3 versus 2.6 years; P = .002), compared with no superimposed relapses.

Kremenchutzky and colleagues also showed that disability progression after one, multiple, or no relapses results in similar survival curves, suggesting that, once progression has begun, its rate is largely independent of factors that have preceded it (Fig. 1-6).[11]

Relapses and progression are the central clinical features of MS. Many in the field consider relapses to be the clinical product of an acute inflammatory focal lesion, whereas progression reflects a chronic diffuse degenerative process. The recent population-based studies from both Ontario, Canada, and Lyon, France, suggest a dissociation at the biologic level between the acute inflammatory process (relapse) and the progressive degenerative process (disability progression).[5,11,21,24]

Although DMAs may significantly reduce the clinical relapse rate, their potential benefits in terms of disability progression may be small. The most important outcome measure in treatment trials with early RRMS should be, first, prevention and, second, attenuation of the progressive course.[18] Patients who continue to have RR disease tend to do extremely well; in fact, it is only on entering the secondary progressive course of the disease that more rapid disability progression occurs.

In the study by Myhr and colleagues, the probability of entering a progressive course after 20 years of disease was 57.5% for patients with an RR onset.[12] Similarly, as previously discussed, 57.6% of patients with disease duration of 11 to 15 years in the Ontario relapsing-onset cohort developed a progressive course.[8] In the Olmsted County 2001 study, patients remaining in the RR group had a favorable course, with fewer than 25% reaching EDSS 3 after 20 years of disease (see Fig. 1-2).[1]

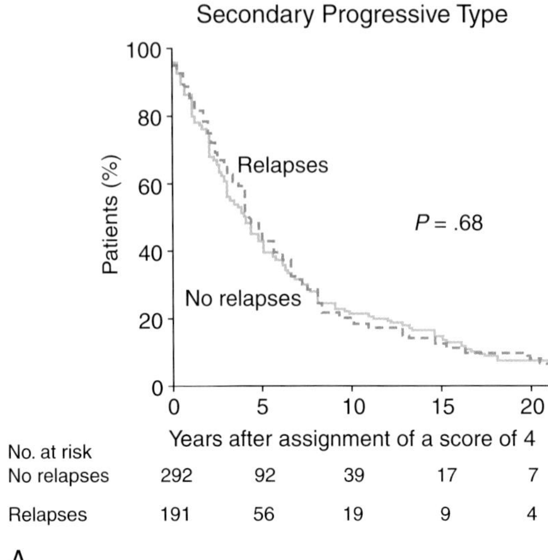

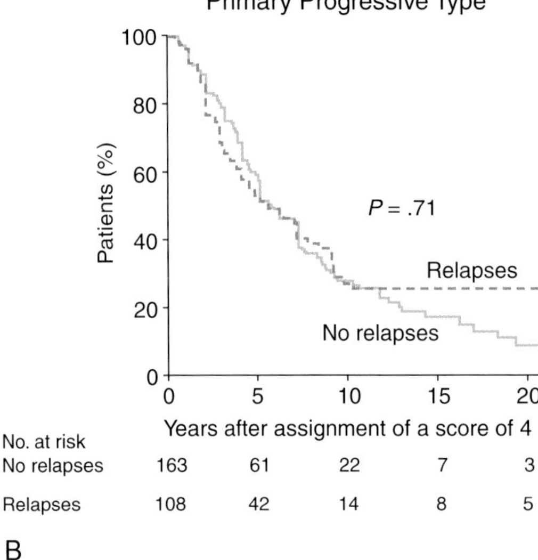

Figure 1–5 Among patients with primary or secondary progressive multiple sclerosis, the time course of progressive irreversible disability (from Expanded Disability Status Scale [EDSS] 4 to EDSS 6) was not significantly influenced by the presence or absence of superimposed relapses. Kaplan–Meier estimates of time from EDSS 4 to EDSS 6 are shown according to the presence or absence of superimposed relapses among 496 patients with secondary progressive disease (**A**) and 282 patients with progressive primary disease (**B**). (Data from Confavreux C, Vukusic S, Moreau T, Adeleine P: Relapse, remission, and progression in multiple sclerosis. N Engl J Med 2000;343:1430-1438.)

CLINICAL STATUS AT 5 AND 10 YEARS AS A PREDICTOR OF LONG-TERM OUTCOME

In 1977, Kurtzke and associates reported that the level of disability in a U.S. World War II MS cohort at 5 years from diagnosis was one of the best predictors of disability at 10 and 15 years.[26] Similarly, multiple groups have shown in multivariate analyses that a low EDSS score at 5 and 10 years is predictive of a benign course.[27-29] For PPMS, there are few predictors of disability progression. A recent

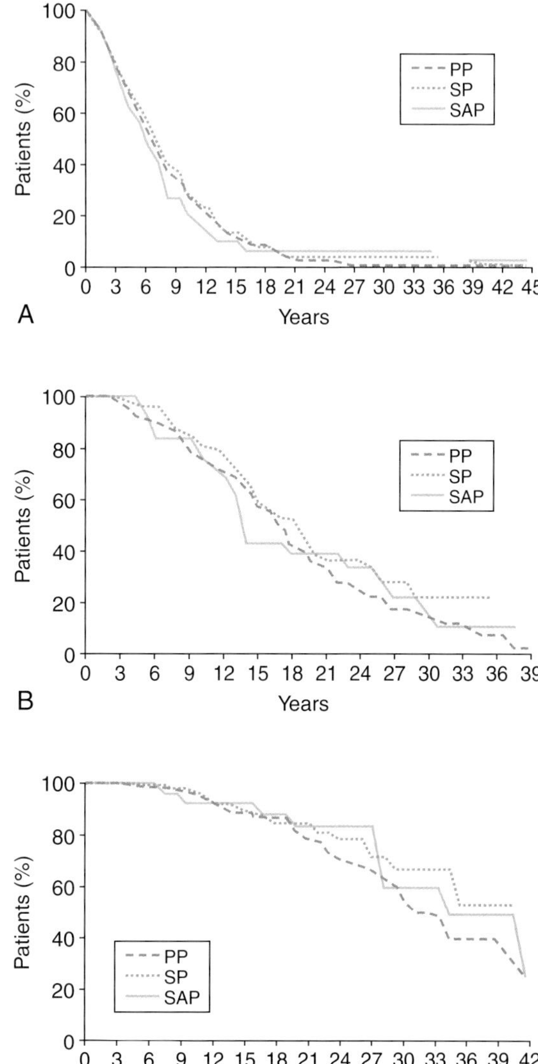

Figure 1–6 Progression after one, multiple, or no relapses results in similar survival curves, suggesting that, once progression has begun, its rate is largely independent of factors that have preceded it. Patients with single-attack progressive (SAP), secondary progressive (SP), and primary progressive (PP) multiple sclerosis are compared, showing time to Expanded Disability Status Scale (EDSS) 6 (**A**), EDSS 8 (**B**), and EDSS 10 (**C**) from onset of progressive disease. (Data from Kremenchutzky M, Rice GP, Baskerville J, et al: The natural history of multiple sclerosis: A geographically based study. 9: Observations on the progressive phase of the disease. Brain 2006;129:584-594.)

natural history study of 352 PPMS patients found that "sooner to cane, sooner to wheelchair" was the only predictor of longer-term outcome.[13]

AGE AT DISABILITY MILESTONES: A NOVEL APPROACH TO DATA ANALYSIS

Despite years of epidemiologic, histopathologic, and radiographic study, the underlying pathogenesis of MS remains poorly understood. How MS is initiated, how it changes over time, how it correlates with clinical course and symptoms and other markers of disease activity, and how it is affected by therapeutic interventions are all largely unknown.[30] The discovery of heterogeneity in demyelinating lesions has suggested that different mechanisms may be involved in MS pathogenesis.[31] It remains unclear whether the RR phase and the progressive phase of MS (see Fig. 1-1) are on an immunopathologic continuum or are distinctly different.

Previous studies of MS natural history have focused on time from onset or diagnosis of MS to specific disability milestones. They have paid little attention to the age at which patients reached these landmarks. Younger age at MS onset has been previously considered associated with a better prognosis, and older age at onset with a worse prognosis. Median age at onset for RRMS range in the late twenties to early thirties, whereas median age of onset for progressive MS is in the late thirties to early forties.[13]

Analysis of MS disability in regard to date of birth creates a unique perspective, reduces reliance on imprecise dates (for onset), and allows more accurate assessment of the age at which patients attained disability milestones. Recently, Confavreux and colleagues analyzed their natural history data in this novel way, with a focus on the age at which disability milestones were reached, rather than the time from onset to disability milestone.[23] They showed that, if one considers age at disability milestones, MS appears to have a very homogenous prognosis that is not influenced significantly by relapses or by the initial course of the disease (Fig. 1-7; Table 1-1).[23 32] These authors analyzed 1562 patients with an RR course and 282 with a progressive course at onset. Surprisingly, the age at assignment of a score of EDSS 7 was similar in both groups, despite the fact time from onset to EDSS 7 was much greater for the former group. For lower disability milestones (EDSS 4 and EDSS 6), patients with an RR onset were older than those with a progressive onset; the differences, although statistically significant, were very small (2.7 years for EDSS 4 and 2.3 years for EDSS 6), and there appeared to be overlap in the 95% confidence intervals of the median.[23]

Overall, the data suggest that the initial course of the disease, whether RR or progressive, does not appear to have substantial influence on the age at which disability milestones are reached in MS, providing further evidence that neurologic relapses have only a limited influence on development of disability over the long term. Tremlett and colleagues also showed that younger age at onset predicts a slower progression, but those patients who were older at onset were consistently older when reaching EDSS 6.[2,33] These authors suggested that younger age at MS onset should no longer be considered a good prognostic factor.[2]

The age at onset is different for patients with SP, PP, and SAP MS, but the age at which progression begins appears to be similar and is not dependent in any way on the number of previous relapses.[11] Although times from MS onset to disability landmarks are longer for patients with RRMS/SP and SAP MS than for PPMS, the times from irreversible disability (progressive phase) to disability landmarks are similar in all three groups (Tables 1-2 and 1-3; see Fig. 1-6).[11,21]

The authors of these recent papers suggested that the progressive phase of MS (which accounts for most of the time course of the disease and most of the disability) could be an age-dependent degenerative process independent of previous

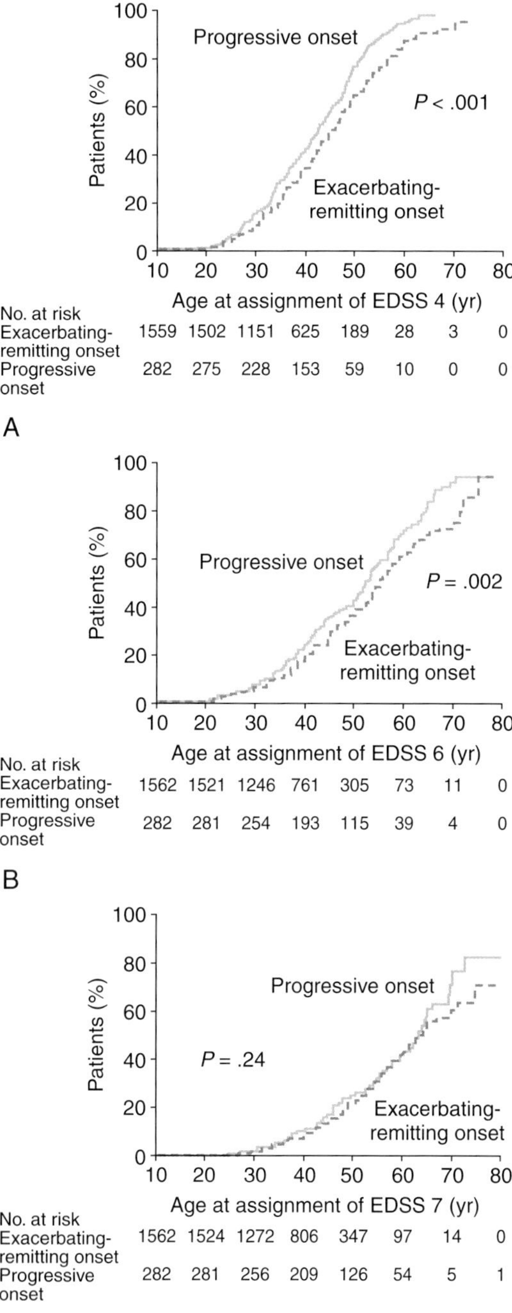

Figure 1–7 For the 1844 patients from the Lyon, France, population-based cohort, median ages at time of assignment of Expanded Disability Status Score (EDSS) 4, EDSS 6, and EDSS 7 were 44.3 years (95% confidence interval [CI], 43.3 to 45.2 years), 54.7 years (95% CI, 53.5 to 55.8 years), and 63.1 years (95% CI, 61.0 to 65.1 years), respectively. These results were essentially similar whether the initial course of multiple sclerosis was exacerbating-remitting or progressive. Kaplan–Meier estimates of the age of the patients at EDSS 4 (**A**), EDSS 6 (**B**), and EDSS 7 (**C**) are shown according to the initial course of multiple sclerosis. (Data from Confavreux C, Vukusic S: Age at disability milestones in multiple sclerosis. Brain 2006;129:595-605.)

TABLE 1–1 Comparative Demographic and Clinical Characteristics of Multiple Sclerosis Patients with a Progressive Initial Course and Patients with an Exacerbating Relapsing-Remitting (RR) Initial Course

Parameter	RR Onset (n = 1562)	Progressive Onset (n = 282)	Probability Value
Gender (% male)	34	43	.006
Age at onset (yr)	29.6	39.3	<.001
Time from onset to EDSS 6 (yr)	23.1	7.1	<.001
Time from onset to EDSS 7 (yr)	33.1	13.4	<.001
Time from EDSS 4 to EDSS 7 (yr)	12.1	12.0	.70
Age at EDSS 6 (yr)	55.3	53.0	.002
Age at EDSS 7 (yr)	62.8	63.1	.24

EDSS, Expanded Disability Status Scale score.

Data from Confavreux C, Vukusic S: Natural history of multiple sclerosis: A unifying concept. Brain 2006;129:606-616.

TABLE 1–2 Age at Onset of Disease and Age at Onset of Progression for Multiple Sclerosis Clinical Subgroups

Subgroup	Age at Onset (mean, yr)	Age at Onset of Progression (mean, yr)
Secondary progressive (SP)	29.8	39.4
Primary progressive (PP)	38.6	38.6
Single-attack progressive (SAP)	33.3	40.9

Data from Kremenchutzky M, Rice GP, Baskerville J, et al: The natural history of multiple sclerosis: A geographically based study. 9: Observations on the progressive phase of the disease. Brain 2006;129:584-594.

TABLE 1–3 Comparison of Patients with Secondary Progressive (SP), Single-Attack Progressive (SAP), and Primary Progressive (PP) Multiple Sclerosis: Time from Onset of Progressive Disease to EDSS 6, EDSS 8, and EDSS 10

Years to	SP	SAP	PP	Probability Value
EDSS 6	6.63	5.71	6.4	.08
EDSS 8	18.20	13.62	16.81	.47
EDSS 10	NA	32.96	31.24	.86

EDSS, Expanded Disability Status Scale score; NA, not applicable.

Data from Kremenchutzky M, Rice GP, Baskerville J, et al: The natural history of multiple sclerosis: A geographically based study. 9: Observations on the progressive phase of the disease. Brain 2006;129:584-594.

clinical relapses.[11,23] The aging-related mechanisms that may be accelerated in MS should provide potential additional therapeutic targets in acute recurrent inflammation and chronic neurodegeneration.[11,23] Figure 1-8 provides an illustrative interpretation of these recent data analyses.

Benign Multiple Sclerosis

DEFINITION

Controversy exists regarding the precise definition of "benign MS," mainly because not all patients fulfilling criteria for benign MS at one time point will remain benign at a later time point.[34] Although most studies suggest that about one third of patients have minimal disease progression with little or no disability after many decades of disease, there is a wide range of reported frequencies, 6% to 64%.[15] This wide range is the result of several factors, including definition used (more

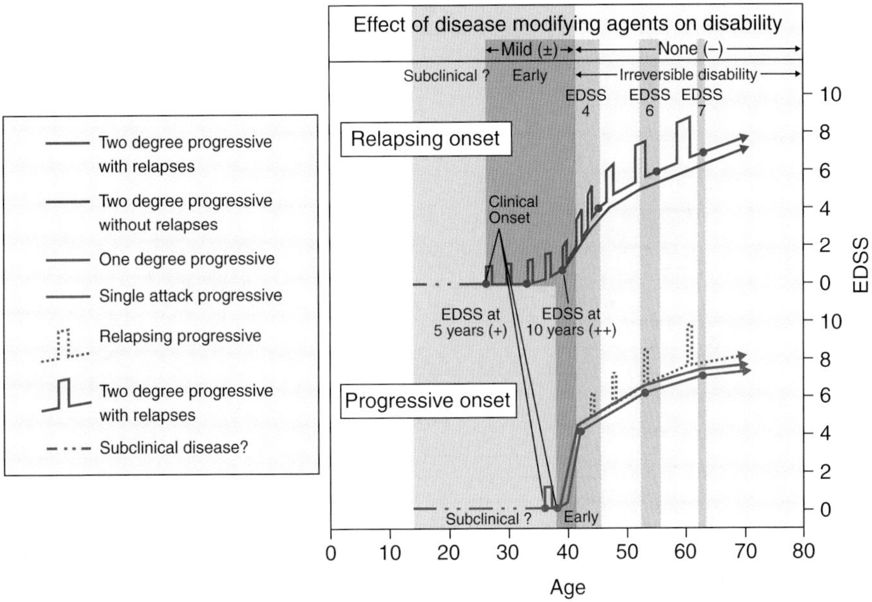

Figure 1–8 Schematic representation of the natural history of multiple sclerosis, incorporating recent natural history data from Lyon, France[15,17]; London, Ontario[18]; and Olmsted County, Minnesota.[1,23] The median age at which disability milestones Expanded Disability Status Score (EDSS) 3 (or 4), EDSS 6, and EDSS 7 (or 8) were reached are similar regardless of early course (relapsing or progressive). The majority of the clinical disease course falls within the progressive phase. Subclinical onset precedes clinical onset by an unknown length of time. Once a threshold of disability is reached (EDSS 3 or EDSS 4, termed "irreversible disability"), the median rate of further progression is similar for all clinical subtypes. The time of onset of the disease is unclear. EDSS scores at 5 and 10 years appear to be the best clinical predictors of long-term outcome. Although disease-modifying agents (DMAs) may have mild to moderate benefit (relapse rate reduction, delayed early disability) in the "early" course of the disease, there is no proven benefit once "irreversible disability" is reached.

conservative definitions lower the frequency) and type of population studied (hospital-based versus community-based).

The concept of benign MS was suggested in 1872 by Charcot when he wrote, "It is not rare to encounter complete remission which is hoped to be definitive."[35] In a study of 241 hospital-based patients monitored over a mean disease duration of 18.2 years, McAlpine reported that 26% of the patients, although not necessarily symptom free, could walk for more than 500 m without assistance and were unrestricted in regard to employment.[36] After the introduction of the EDSS score by John Kurtzke in 1983,[3] investigators began to define benign MS in terms of having a low disability score (EDSS 0 to EDSS 4) after a long disease duration (5 to 20 years). The most commonly used definition of benign MS is EDSS 3 after a disease duration of 10 or more years, although more conservative definitions have been suggested recently. The National Multiple Sclerosis Society of the United States performed a survey and arrived at the following consensus definition of benign MS: "fully functional in all neurologic systems 15 years after onset."[9] More recently, the definition "EDSS score of less than or equal to two for greater than or equal to ten years" was proposed based on a longitudinal follow-up study of benign MS in the Olmsted County MS population-based cohort (Fig. 1-9).[27] In that study, the prevalence of benign MS (EDSS ≤2 for >10 years) was 17%. If this figure is applied to the U.S. MS population as a whole, then approximately

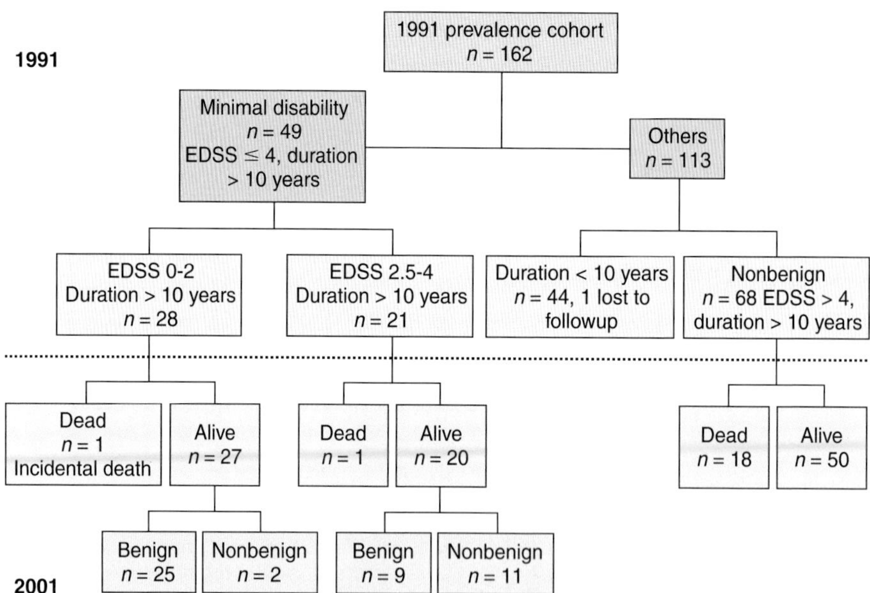

Figure 1–9 Patient profile of original 1991 Olmsted County multiple sclerosis prevalence cohort (*above broken line*) and 2001 data (*below broken line*). Benign MS in 2001 is defined as an Expanded Disability Status Scale (EDSS) score of 4 or lower and duration of MS longer than 20 years. Nonbenign is defined as an EDSS score higher than 4 and duration of MS longer than 20 years. (From Pittock SJ, McClelland RL, Mayr WT, et al: Clinical implications of benign multiple sclerosis: A 20-year population-based follow-up study. Ann Neurol 2004;56:303-306. © 2004 American Neurological Association. Reproduced with permission from John Wiley & Sons, Inc.)

36,000 patients in the United States have benign MS and probably would not benefit from potentially lifelong pharmacotherapy.[19] The difficulty arises in trying to identify these patients early in their disease course.

PREDICTING A BENIGN COURSE

Three recent papers have contributed to the literature on this subject and have supported Kurtzke's previous observation that the level of disability at 5 years is a reliable predictor of later outcome.[26] In the 2001 Olmsted County MS study, 93% of patients who had an EDSS of 2 or less after at least 10 years of disease duration in 1991 continued to have low levels of disability (EDSS ≤3) a decade later (Fig. 1-10).[27] In contrast, only 42% of patients with a moderate level of disability (EDSS 2.5 to EDSS 4.0) after 10 or more years of disease duration in 1991 continued to have low levels of disability (EDSS ≤3) in 2001 (see Fig. 1-10). Therefore, the lower the level of disability after 10 years, the more likely a patient is to remain with that low level of disability in the future. This study suggested a more conservative definition of benign MS: EDSS 2 or less after at least 10 years of disease duration.

In a much larger British Columbia MS cohort of 2204 patients, investigators reported that 68% of patients with an EDSS score of 2 or less after 10 years of disease remained benign with EDSS of 2 or less at the 20-year time point.[29]

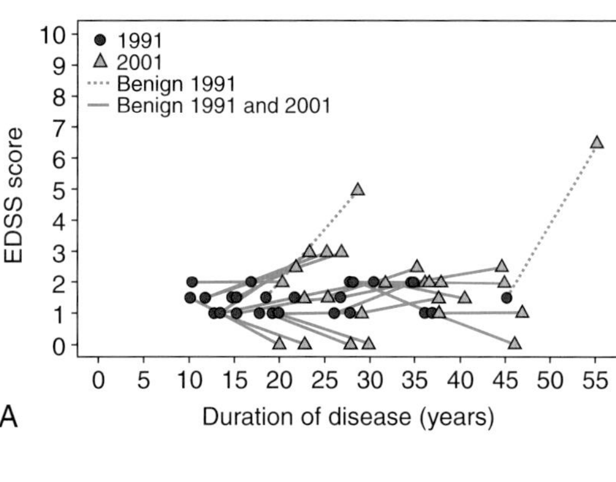

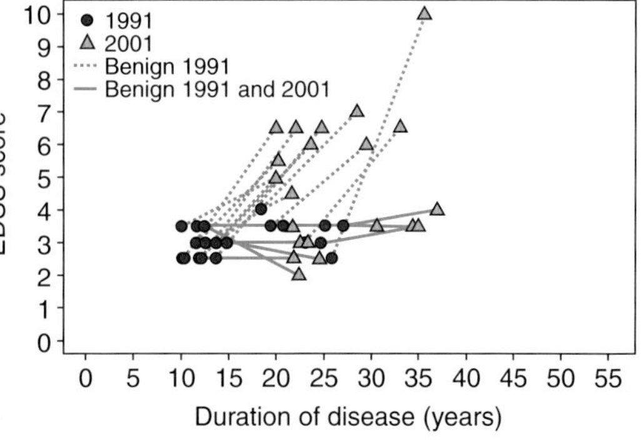

Figure 1–10 Change in Expanded Disability Status Scale (EDSS) score over 10 years versus duration of disease in 1991. Each line represents an individual patient. **A,** How are patients with minimal disability (EDSS ≤ 2 for ≥ 10 years) doing a further decade later? **B,** How are patients with moderate disability (EDSS 2.5 to EDSS 4 for ≥ 10 years) doing a further decade later? (From Pittock SJ, McClelland RL, Mayr WT, et al: Clinical implications of benign multiple sclerosis: A 20-year population-based follow-up study. Ann Neurol 2004;56:303-306, reproduced with permission.)

If a similar analysis is used for the Olmsted County Study, then 67% of patients would remain with EDSS of 2 or less after 20 or more years.[27]

Ramsaransing and De Keyser investigated a cohort of 496 patients who had had MS for at least 10 years. They found that 151 (30%) of these patients had an EDSS score of 3 or less and were considered to have benign MS[29]; 69% of these patients continued to have benign disease 10 years later. However, when a more conservative definition with cutoff of EDSS 2 after 10 years (as proposed by the Mayo Clinic group) was used, 84% still had benign disease at the 20-year time point.

In a multivariate regression analysis, an RR course, a low EDSS score at 5 years, and a low number of relapses during the first 5 years were predictive for benign MS at 10 years, in agreement with other previously published studies. Other variables such as gender, age at clinical onset, disease course, number of systems involved at onset, degree of recovery from first symptoms, and time between first and second relapse had no additional value in outcome prediction, again in line with most other studies.

Although the Olmsted County study focused on EDSS score at 10 years or more as a predictor of outcome at 20 years or more, a review of the data suggested that the 5-year time point may also be a robust and reliable cutoff point for outcome prediction. In a subgroup analysis of EDSS and number of relapses, Ramsaransing showed that patients with lower EDSS scores at 5 years had a high probability of remaining benign at the 10-year time point, but the probability of developing disability was somewhat dependent on the number of relapses in the first 5 years. Patients with EDSS 1 at 5 years but with two, three, or four relapses had an 85%, an 80%, and a 74% chance, respectively, of remaining benign at the 10-year time point. In contrast, patients with EDSS 3 at 5 years but with two, three, or four relapses had a 36%, a 28%, and a 22% chance of remaining benign at the 10-year time point. Patients with an EDSS score between 1 and 3 at 5 years had probabilities that were dependent on the frequency of relapses distributed between these two extremes.

In summary, the longer the duration of MS and the lower the disability level, the more likely a patient is to remain stable and not progress. The predictive power of this measure appears to be greatest after 10 years or longer, although there is some evidence that the 5-year cutoff point may have reasonable predictive value. However, it does not appear possible to accurately predict outcome within the first 5–6 years after onset of MS.

COGNITIVE OUTCOMES IN BENIGN MULTIPLE SCLEROSIS

Most studies on the natural history of MS, and particularly benign MS, have focused on physical impairment. Some researchers have argued appropriately that patients may remain well physically but have significant cognitive problems, and that current definitions of benign MS based on EDSS alone therefore overestimate its frequency.

A recent study examined cognitive, psychosocial, and social aspects of benign MS in 163 patients with an EDSS score of 3 or less after 15 or more years of disease duration.[37] Patients' cognitive performances were compared with those of 111 demographically matched, healthy controls. Cognitive impairment, significant fatigue, and depression were found in 45%, 49%, and 54% of patients, respectively. Using a more conservative definition of benign MS (EDSS ≤2 for

≥15 years), the frequency of cognitive impairment was 39%. This is lower than the frequency of 58.5% in patients who had an EDSS score between 2.5 and 3 after 15 or more years.

Though this study raised important concerns regarding the issue of nonambulatory disorders in benign MS, there were some significant limitations of the study that most likely overestimated the frequency of these problems in benign MS. First, the study was not population based and therefore was not likely to be representative of benign MS in the general population. Second, as the authors pointed out, patient "self-selection" probably contributed to the high frequencies of problems encountered, because patients with MS who are doing well physically but experiencing depression or cognitive problems are more likely to seek medical treatment and thus more likely to be attending a hospital-based clinic. Third, the high frequency of depression may be a significant confounder.

Population-based studies of nonambulatory impairments and clinical disability are needed to address this issue. Such studies can help better define the phenotypic variability in patients with MS and guide better patient selection for treatment trials and future genotype-to-phenotype analyses.

REFERENCES

1. Pittock SJ, Mayr WT, McClelland RL, et al: Disability profile of MS did not change over 10 years in a population-based prevalence cohort. Neurology 2004;62:601-606.
2. Tremlett H, Paty D, Devonshire V: Disability progression in multiple sclerosis is slower than previously reported. Neurology 2006;66:172-177.
3. Kurtzke JF: Rating neurologic impairment in multiple sclerosis: An expanded disability status scale (EDSS). Neurology 1983;33:1444-1452.
4. Confavreux C, Aimard G, Devic M: Course and prognosis of multiple sclerosis assessed by the computerized data processing of 349 patients. Brain 1980;103:281-300.
5. Confavreux C, Vukusic S, Adeleine P: Early clinical predictors and progression of irreversible disability in multiple sclerosis: An amnesic process. Brain 2003;126(Pt 4):770-782.
6. Kantarci O, Siva A, Eraksoy M, et al: Survival and predictors of disability in Turkish MS patients. Turkish Multiple Sclerosis Study Group (TUMSSG). Neurology 1998;51:765-772.
7. Runmarker B, Andersen O: Prognostic factors in a multiple sclerosis incidence cohort with twenty-five years of follow-up. Brain 1993;116(Pt 1):117-134.
8. Weinshenker BG, Bass B, Rice GP, et al: The natural history of multiple sclerosis: A geographically based study. I: Clinical course and disability. Brain 1989;112(Pt 1):133-146.
9. Lublin FD, Reingold SC: Defining the clinical course of multiple sclerosis: Results of an international survey. National Multiple Sclerosis Society (USA) Advisory Committee on Clinical Trials of New Agents in Multiple Sclerosis. Neurology 1996;46:907-911.
10. Confavreux C, Vukusic S: Natural history of multiple sclerosis: Implications for counselling and therapy. Curr Opin Neurol 2002;15:257-266.
11. Kremenchutzky M, Rice GP, Baskerville J, et al: The natural history of multiple sclerosis: A geographically based study. 9: Observations on the progressive phase of the disease. Brain 2006; 129(Pt 3):584-594.
12. Myhr KM, Riise T, Vedeler C, et al: Disability and prognosis in multiple sclerosis: Demographic and clinical variables important for the ability to walk and awarding of disability pension. Mult Scler 2001;7:59-65.
13. Tremlett H, Paty D, Devonshire V: The natural history of primary progressive MS in British Columbia, Canada. Neurology 2005;65:1919-1923.
14. Noseworthy JH, Lucchinetti C, Rodriguez M, Weinshenker BG: Multiple sclerosis. N Engl J Med 2000;343:938-952.
15. Ramsaransing GS, De Keyser J: Benign course in multiple sclerosis: A review. Acta Neurol Scand 2006;113:359-369.
16. Weinshenker BG, Bass B, Rice GP, et al: The natural history of multiple sclerosis: A geographically based study. 2: Predictive value of the early clinical course. Brain 1989;112(Pt 6):1419-1428.

17. Frohman EM, Havrdova E, Lublin F, et al: Most patients with multiple sclerosis or a clinically isolated demyelinating syndrome should be treated at the time of diagnosis. Arch Neurol 2006; 63:614-619.
18. Pittock SJ: Interferon beta in multiple sclerosis: How much BENEFIT? Lancet 2007;370:363-364.
19. Pittock SJ, Weinshenker BG, Noseworthy JH, et al: Not every patient with multiple sclerosis should be treated at time of diagnosis. Arch Neurol 2006;63:611-614.
20. Confavreux C: The natural history of MS. In Compston A, McDonald IR, Noseworthy J, et al (eds): McAlpine's Multiple Sclerosis, 4th ed. New York, Churchill Livingstone, 2005, pp 183-272.
21. Confavreux C, Vukusic S, Moreau T, Adeleine P: Relapses and progression of disability in multiple sclerosis. N Engl J Med 2000;343:1430-1438.
22. Ebers GC: Natural history of multiple sclerosis. In McDonald WI, Noseworthy JH (eds): Multiple Sclerosis, 2nd rev. ed. London, Butterworth-Heinemann, 2003, pp 21-32.
23. Confavreux C, Vukusic S: Age at disability milestones in multiple sclerosis. Brain 2006;129(Pt 3): 595-605.
24. Vukusic S, Confavreux C: Natural history of multiple sclerosis: Risk factors and prognostic indicators. Curr Opin Neurol 2007;20:269-274.
25. Noseworthy JH, Vandervoort MK, Hopkins M, Ebers GC: A referendum on clinical trial research in multiple sclerosis: The opinion of the participants at the Jekyll Island workshop. Neurology 1989;39:977-981.
26. Kurtzke JF, Beebe GW, Nagler B, et al: Studies on the natural history of multiple sclerosis: 8. Early prognostic features of the later course of the illness. J Chronic Dis 1977;30:819-830.
27. Pittock SJ, McClelland RL, Mayr WT, et al: Clinical implications of benign multiple sclerosis: A 20-year population-based follow-up study. Ann Neurol 2004;56:303-306.
28. Ramsaransing GS, De Keyser J: Predictive value of clinical characteristics for 'benign' multiple sclerosis. Eur J Neurol 2007;14:885-889.
29. Sayao AL, Devonshire V, Tremlett H: Longitudinal follow-up of "benign" multiple sclerosis at 20 years. Neurology 2007;68:496-500.
30. Pittock SJ, Lucchinetti CF: The pathology of MS: New insights and potential clinical applications. Neurologist 2007;13:45-56.
31. Lucchinetti C, Bruck W, Parisi J, et al: Heterogeneity of multiple sclerosis lesions: Implications for the pathogenesis of demyelination. Ann Neurol 2000;47:707-717.
32. Confavreux C, Vukusic S: Natural history of multiple sclerosis: A unifying concept. Brain 2006; 129(Pt 3):606-616.
33. Tremlett H, Devonshire V: Is late-onset multiple sclerosis associated with a worse outcome? Neurology 2006;67:954-959.
34. Pittock SJ, Rodriguez M: Benign multiple sclerosis: A distinct clinical entity with therapeutic implications. Curr Top Microbiol Immunol 2008;318:1-17
35. Charcot J: Leçons sur les maladies du système nerveux faites à La Salpetière. Paris, 1872.
36. McAlpine D: The benign form of multiple sclerosis: Results of a long-term study. Br Med J 1964; 2:1029-1032.
37. Amato MP, Zipoli V, Goretti B, et al: Benign multiple sclerosis: Cognitive, psychological and social aspects in a clinical cohort. J Neurol 2006;253:1054-1059.

2 Differential Diagnosis and Diagnostic Criteria for Multiple Sclerosis: Application and Pitfalls

PAUL W. O'CONNOR • JAMES J. MARRIOTT

One of the paradoxes of multiple sclerosis (MS) is that the diagnosis can be relatively routine in most circumstances but very challenging in other situations. The differentiation of MS from other inflammatory demyelinating conditions can be difficult, and there is debate about the precise phenotypic and pathologic distinctions between these disorders. Diagnostic complexity also arises because MS can (theoretically) cause any symptom or sign referable to the central nervous system (CNS), so the initial differential diagnoses in individual patients can be broad.

MS diagnostic criteria have evolved over time with an increasing use of paraclinical markers (especially magnetic resonance imaging [MRI]) to reach a definite diagnosis earlier in the disease course than a strict reliance on clinical features would allow. Despite these technological advancements, current criteria still rely on the key principles of MS diagnosis articulated in the middle of the 20th century: (1) demonstration of the cardinal characteristics of dissemination in space (DIS) and dissemination in time (DIT) and (2) the exclusion of alternative etiologies.

The first portion of this chapter outlines the development of the current diagnostic criteria for MS. The differentiation of MS from other CNS inflammatory demyelinating conditions is then addressed. Finally, the considerations involved in developing an appropriate, individualized differential diagnosis in a given patient are reviewed.

TABLE 2–1 Schumaker Criteria for the Diagnosis of Multiple Sclerosis

1. Objective signs attributable to CNS dysfunction
2. Historical or objective evidence of two or more areas of CNS involvement
3. Objective signs should be attributable to white matter involvement
4. One of these temporal patterns:
   a. Two or more relapses; each lasting ≥24 hr and separated by at least 1 mo
   b. Slow or stepwise progression ≥6 mo
5. Patients between 10 and 50 yr old
6. No better explanation for patient's symptoms and signs, preferably as determined by a neurologist

Adapted from Schumaker GA, Beebe GW, Kibler RF, et al: Problems of experimental trials of therapy in multiple sclerosis. Ann N Y Acad Sci 1965;122:552-568.

Multiple Sclerosis Diagnostic Criteria

Numerous different diagnostic criteria have been proposed over the years.[1-9] The criteria that Schumaker and colleagues[3] formulated in 1965 are summarized in Table 2-1. These criteria codified the essential components necessary for the diagnosis of MS. As shown in Table 2-1, the diagnosis is dependent on the demonstration of neurologic abnormalities referable to anatomically distinct regions of the CNS that develop in either a progressive or a relapsing-remitting pattern. The Schumaker definition of relapses—worsening symptoms lasting longer than 24 hours and separated by 1 month—is still used in practice and research protocols today. In contrast, the stated strict age cutoffs are now known to be inappropriate. In the modern era, MRI allows both pediatric and late-onset MS to be more easily differentiated from etiologies that are more common in these age groups.

In 1985, the recommendations arising from the Workshop on the Diagnosis of Multiple Sclerosis (commonly known as the Poser criteria)[6] supplanted previous criteria. The Poser criteria formed the basis for patient selection in the seminal trials of disease-modifying agents and have been used as the "gold standard" in the evaluation of newer criteria (discussed later). It has been demonstrated that the Poser requirements for "clinically definite" MS (CDMS) have an 87% sensitivity in comparison with postmortem histopathologic diagnosis.[10] As illustrated in Table 2-2, the Poser criteria are hierarchical and rely increasingly on paraclinical and cerebrospinal fluid (CSF) findings when fewer numbers of relapses and/or examination findings are present. In contrast to more recent criteria, historical symptom descriptions (provided that they suggest "typical" MS relapses) and subjective symptoms without objective signs can be used to make the diagnosis.

These criteria were also the first to incorporate the then-nascent modality of MRI into the diagnostic process, establishing the important concept that MRI is able to provide evidence for both DIS and DIT without any subjective or objective clinical change in the patient's condition. Understandably, given the state of MRI technology at that time, Poser and colleagues did not delve into the specific MRI findings that are useful in the diagnosis of MS. Rather, MRI was simply included along with computed tomography, hyperthermia testing, evoked potentials, and

TABLE 2–2 **Poser Criteria for the Diagnosis of Multiple Sclerosis**

Category	Attacks	Clinical Evidence	Paraclinical Evidence	CSF OB/IgG
A. Clinically Definite (CD)				
CDMS A1	2	2		
CDMS A2	2	1	1	
B. Laboratory-Supported Definite (LSD)				
LSDMS B1	2	1*	1*	+
LSDMS B2	1	2		+
LSDMS B3	1	1	1	+
C. Clinically Probable (CP)				
CPMS C1	2	1		
CPMS C2	1	2		
CPMS C3	1	1	1	
D. Laboratory-Supported Probable (LSP)				
LSPMS D1	2			+

OB/IgG, oligoclonal bands or increased immunoglobulin G.
*Either clinical or paraclinical evidence must be present.
Adapted from Poser CM, Paty DW, Scheinberg L et al: New diagnostic criteria for multiple sclerosis: Guidelines for research protocols. Ann Neurol 1983;13:227-231.

urodynamic evaluation in the category of "paraclinical evidence" that are useful in arriving at a diagnosis when the clinical examination is insufficiently revealing. Poser separated CSF evidence of intrathecal inflammatory activity from other paraclinical evaluations to allow for patients to be defined as having "laboratory-supported" definite or probable MS in situations in which the clinical and paraclinical features are insufficient to demonstrate DIS or DIT (see Table 2-2).

By classifying some patients as having either "laboratory supported" or "probable" MS (categories B, C, and D in Table 2-2), the committee aimed to create a sufficiently large population for research studies while also allowing such patients to be prospectively evaluated for conversion to CDMS. Conversely, as the criteria were developed to produce a homogenous patient population, all patients with progressive symptoms from onset were excluded from the scheme. Nevertheless, the authors acknowledged that such patients (now said to have primary progressive multiple sclerosis [PPMS]) could be considered "probable cases of MS."[6]

Various groups subsequently developed standardized criteria for MRI characteristics that support the diagnosis of MS.[11-14] These authors focused on "clinically isolated syndromes" (CIS), that is, identifying MRI features that predicted conversion to CDMS by Poser criteria.

These predictive MRI features were subsequently used to develop the most recent diagnostic criteria, known as the "McDonald criteria," which were initially published in 2001[7] and subsequently revised and adapted in 2005.[8] As shown in Tables 2-3 and 2-4, a hierarchical ranking is maintained, but the nuanced diagnostic categories of Poser are replaced with simply "MS," "not MS," and "possible MS." The last category defines patients who have an appropriate clinical presentation but whose workup is incomplete or not diagnostic. It is important to note

TABLE 2–3 McDonald Criteria of Diagnostic Certainty

Diagnosis	Features
Multiple sclerosis (MS)	1. MS diagnostic criteria fulfilled 2. No better explanation
Possible MS	Clinician suspicious that patient has MS but diagnostic criteria not completely fulfilled
Not MS	Another diagnosis is made that explains the clinical presentation

Adapted from Polman CH, Reingold SC, Edan G, et al: Diagnostic criteria for multiple sclerosis: 2005 Revisions to the "McDonald Criteria." Ann Neurol 2005;58:840-846.

that the authors intended for this category to include only patients where MS was felt to be a potential diagnosis, not a catchall diagnosis for vague symptoms of uncertain etiology. In contrast to the Poser criteria, objective evidence of neurologic dysfunction is required. A diagnosis cannot be based on subjective deficits (e.g., a subjective sensory level) or on remote episodes that are not accompanied by either historical documentation of neurologic signs or residual deficits. While useful for defining trial populations, expert clinicians can perhaps relax this requirement in specific patients.

In the original McDonald criteria, the authors used Barkhof MRI criteria,[13] as modified by Tintoré,[14] to define DIS. These criteria have been shown to be more sensitive and more specific than those of Paty[11] or Fazekas.[12] Although potentially cumbersome, the Barkhof/Tintoré criteria have the advantage of a high specificity by decreasing the chance that T2-weighted hyperintensities not secondary to demyelination (e.g., ischemia, unidentified bright objects) will be erroneously labeled as MS. The 2001 McDonald criteria for DIT were designed to prevent misdiagnosis of patients with acute disseminated encephalomyelitis (ADEM), who can develop new MRI lesions for up to 3 months after symptom onset without the development of new clinical deficits.

The original McDonald criteria were revised in 2005 in an effort to clarify and streamline the diagnostic process. The revised criteria keep the necessity of having objective evidence of clinical attacks or signs despite the authors' acknowledgement of situations in which clinicians get clear descriptions of typical symptoms such as trigeminal neuralgia or Lhermitte's phenomenon.[8] The Barkhof/Tintoré criteria for DIS remained unchanged, with the exception of an expanded role for spinal MRI (Table 2-5). It was felt that spinal lesions of a typical appearance (>3 mm in cross-section, <2 vertebral bodies in length) could be counted toward the total lesion load requirement of 9 and could also substitute for an infratentorial (but not a juxtacortical or periventricular) lesion. Furthermore, an enhancing spinal lesion could count toward the total of 2 required.

Of greater significance were the revisions to the somewhat cumbersome DIT criteria (Table 2-6). DIT confirmation can now be based on the development of a new T2 lesion at any time point after a "reference scan" performed at least 30 days after CIS onset. Otherwise, an enhancing lesion on a scan done at any time after 3 months from symptom onset can demonstrate DIT, provided the location does not correspond to the CIS symptoms.

TABLE 2–4 McDonald 2005 Criteria for the Diagnosis of Multiple Sclerosis (MS)

Clinical Presentation	Additional Data Needed for MS Diagnosis*
≥2 attacks; objective clinical evidence of ≥2 lesions	None (*but* caution if further investigations do not support the diagnosis)
≥2 attacks; objective clinical evidence of 1 lesion	Dissemination in space, demonstrated by • MRI *or* • ≥2 MRI-detected lesions consistent with MS plus positive CSF *or* Await further clinical attack implicating a different site
1 attack; objective clinical evidence of ≥2 lesions	Dissemination in time, demonstrated by • MRI *or* • Second clinical attack
1 attack; objective clinical evidence of 1 lesion (monosymptomatic presentation; CIS)	Dissemination in space, demonstrated by • MRI *or* • ≥2 MRI-detected lesions consistent with MS plus positive CSF *and* Dissemination in time, demonstrated by • MRI *or* • Second clinical attack
Insidious neurologic progression suggestive of MS†	1 yr of disease progression (retrospectively or prospectively determined) *and* Two of the following: • Positive brain MRI (9 T2 lesions or ≥4 T2 lesions with positive VEP) • Positive spinal cord MRI (2 focal T2 lesions) • Positive CSF

CIS, clinically isolated syndrome; CSF, cerebrospinal fluid; MRI, magnetic resonance imaging; VEP, visual evoked potential.

*MRI criteria for dissemination in space and time are outlined in Tables 2-5 and 2-6, respectively.

†The original McDonald criteria mandated that the CSF show oligoclonal bands or an elevated immunoglobulin G index.

Adapted from Polman CH, Reingold SC, Edan G, et al: Diagnostic criteria for multiple sclerosis: 2005 Revisions to the "McDonald Criteria." Ann Neurol 2005;58:840-846.

The 2005 panel also liberalized the diagnosis of PPMS by removing the absolute need for CSF demonstration of oligoclonal banding or elevated immunoglobulin G (IgG) index, while acknowledging that a clinician's "comfort" can be greatly increased with CSF positivity (Table 2-7).

Recently, Swanton and colleagues proposed further modifications to the McDonald criteria in an effort to increase diagnostic sensitivity in CIS patients.[9,15] Their criteria for DIS require at least one lesion in two of four anatomic areas derived from Barkhof/Tintoré (periventricular, juxtacortical, infratentorial, and spinal cord). DIT requires interval development of a new T2 hyperintense lesion

TABLE 2–5 McDonald Criteria for Dissemination in Space (DIS)

Original 2001 Criteria	Revised 2005 Criteria
Three of the following: • At least 1 gadolinium-enhancing lesion or 9 T2 hyperintense lesions if there is no gadolinium-enhancing lesion • At least 1 infratentorial lesion • At least 1 juxtacortical lesion • At least 3 periventricular lesions *(NOTE: 1 spinal cord lesion can substitute for one brain lesion.)*	Three of the following: • At least 1 gadolinium-enhancing lesion or 9 T2 hyperintense lesions if there is no gadolinium-enhancing lesion • At least 1 infratentorial lesion • At least 1 juxtacortical lesion • At least 3 periventricular lesions *(NOTE: A spinal cord lesion can be considered equivalent to a brain infratentorial lesion: an enhancing spinal cord lesion is considered to be equivalent to an enhancing brain lesion, and individual spinal cord lesions can contribute together with individual brain lesions to reach the required number of T2 lesions.)*

Adapted from Polman CH, Reingold SC, Edan G, et al: Diagnostic criteria for multiple sclerosis: 2005 Revisions to the "McDonald Criteria." Ann Neurol 2005;58:840-846.

TABLE 2–6 McDonald Criteria for Dissemination in Time (DIT)

Original 2001 Criteria	Revised 2005 Criteria
If the first scan occurs ≥3 mo after onset of the clinical event, the presence of a gadolinium-enhancing lesion is sufficient to demonstrate DIT, provided that it is not at the site implicated in the original clinical event. If there is no enhancing lesion at this time, a follow-up scan is required. The timing of this follow-up scan is not crucial, but 3 mo is recommended. A new T2 or gadolinium-enhancing lesion on the follow-up scan fulfills the criterion for DIT.	Two ways to show DIT: 1. Detection of gadolinium enhancement at least 3 mo after onset of the initial clinical event, if not at the site corresponding to the initial event 2. Detection of a new T2 lesion if it appears at any time compared with a reference scan done at least 30 days after onset of the initial clinical event
If first scan is performed <3 mo after onset of the clinical event, a second scan done ≥3 mo after the clinical event showing a new gadolinium-enhancing lesion provides sufficient evidence for DIT. If no enhancing lesion is seen on this second scan, a further scan not <3 mo after the first scan that shows a new T2 lesion or an enhancing lesion will suffice.	

Adapted from Polman CH, Reingold SC, Edan G, et al: Diagnostic criteria for multiple sclerosis: 2005 Revisions to the "McDonald Criteria." Ann Neurol 2005;58:840-846.

TABLE 2-7 **Diagnosis of Primary Progressive Multiple Sclerosis**

Original 2001 McDonald Criteria	Revised 2005 McDonald Criteria
1. Positive CSF *and* 2. Dissemination in space, demonstrated by • MRI evidence of ≥9 T2 brain lesions *or* ≥2 cord lesions *or* 4-8 brain lesions and 1 cord lesion *or* • Positive VEP with 4-8 MRI lesions *or* • Positive VEP with <4 brain lesions plus 1 cord lesion *and* 3. Dissemination in time, demonstrated by • MRI *or* • Continued progression for 1 year	1 yr of disease progression (retrospectively or prospectively determined) *plus* Two of the following: • Positive brain MRI (9 T2 lesions or ≥4 T2 lesions with positive VEP) • Positive spinal cord MRI (2 focal T2 lesions) • Positive CSF

CSF, cerebrospinal fluid; MRI, magnetic resonance imaging; VEP, visual evoked potential.
Adapted from Polman CH, Reingold SC, Edan G, et al: Diagnostic criteria for multiple sclerosis: 2005 Revisions to the "McDonald Criteria." Ann Neurol 2005;58:840-846.

comparing two scans done at least 3 months apart. In contrast to the McDonald criteria, the timing of the first scan with respect to symptom onset is not considered.

Two studies have retrospectively applied the 2001 McDonald criteria to prospectively collected serial MRI databases to assess their efficacy in predicting conversion to Poser-defined CDMS.[16,17] In a Spanish study that followed patients for 3 years, patients who met McDonald criteria at 12 months met Poser CDMS criteria by 3 years, with an accuracy of 80%, a sensitivity of 74%, and a specificity of 86%.[17] Similar findings were obtained in a British cohort, in which the sensitivity, specificity, and accuracy were all 83%.[16] All three of these new MRI-based criteria were recently retrospectively applied to a multicenter European CIS population using conversion to Poser CDMS as the gold standard.[7,15] As shown in Table 2-8, the Swanton criteria were the most sensitive and most accurate, although the original McDonald criteria were the most specific.

The original and revised McDonald and Swanton diagnostic criteria were all developed from assessing patients with clinical presentations suggestive of MS. Inappropriate extrapolation of these criteria to broader populations increases the possibility of mislabeling patients with MS. The higher sensitivity of the Swanton criteria (see Table 2-8) is associated with lower specificity for both the DIS and DIT components and demonstrates that relaxing the stringency of the Barkhof/Tintoré MRI criteria increases the risk of false-positive MS diagnoses. The criterion that "no better explanation" has to exist for the diagnosis of MS to be confirmed is paramount. However, the complexity of the differential diagnosis precludes use of a "cookbook" stepwise diagnostic algorithm to exclude alternative etiologies.

Although the McDonald criteria have been highly influential and have gained widespread acceptance within the neurology community, it is important to draw attention to certain issues that have been raised.[18] As discussed previously, the criteria make limited allowances for historical symptoms, and it is unclear whether afferent symptoms (visual, sensory) that are inherently subjective can be used to demonstrate "objective" DIS or DIT. The arbitrary definitions of attack length and interattack interval also create ambiguity in classifying both the recurrent and paroxysmal symptoms that are frequently seen in the MS population. Furthermore, in addressing paraclinical investigations, the McDonald criteria do not provide detailed considerations of the need to standardize technical aspects (e.g., MRI sequencing parameters, definition of oligoclonal banding). More recently, other groups have produced consensus-driven, expert opinion–based position papers addressing CSF analysis[19] and MRI sequencing.[20]

The remainder of this chapter addresses how to frame the differential diagnosis within the global term of "no better explanation." First, other CNS inflammatory demyelinating conditions within the MS spectrum are considered. Second, a framework for developing rational differentials based on the consideration of an individual patient's clinical phenotype is discussed.

TABLE 2–8 Comparison of the Three MRI-Based Diagnostic Criteria in Predicting Conversion to Clinically Definite MS (Poser)

	Sensitivity (%)	Specificity (%)	Accuracy (%)	PPV (%)	Positive LR	Negative LR
Overall Criteria (DIS and DIT)						
McDonald 2001	47.1	91.1	73.1	78.4	5.3	0.6
McDonald 2005	60.0	87.8	76.4	77.3	4.9	0.5
Swanton 2006	71.8	87.0	80.8	79.2	5.5	0.3
DIS criteria						
McDonald 2001	71.8	68.3	71.6	62.5	2.4	0.4
McDonald 2005	75.3	69.1	71.6	62.8	2.4	0.4
Swanton 2006	85.9	59.4	70.2	59.4	2.1	0.2
DIT criteria						
McDonald 2001	51.8	88.6	73.6	75.9	4.6	0.5
McDonald 2005	68.2	82.1	76.4	72.5	3.8	0.4
Swanton 2006	74.1	79.7	77.4	71.6	3.7	0.3
DIT on Follow-up Scan						
New gadolinium-enhancing lesion	49.4	89.4	73.1	76.4	4.7	0.6
New T2 lesion (all cases)	74.1	79.7	77.4	71.6	3.7	0.3
New T2 lesion and baseline scan ≥ 30 days after CIS onset	68.9	81.3	75.7	75.0	3.7	0.4

CIS, clinically isolated syndrome; LR, likelihood ratio; PPV, positive predictive value.

Adapted from Swanton JK, Rovira A, Tintoré M, et al: MRI criteria for multiple sclerosis in patients presenting with clinically isolated syndromes: A multicentre retrospective study. Lancet Neurol 2007;6:677-686.

Idiopathic Inflammatory Demyelinating Diseases

It has long been appreciated that inflammatory CNS demyelination is not synonymous with MS. However, the lack of a formal classification system as well as clinical, radiologic, or pathologic features that reliably differentiate among these MS-spectrum entities has hampered interpretation of the literature. The term "idiopathic inflammatory demyelinating diseases" (IIDDs) has been coined to encompass these related conditions (Table 2-9).[21,22]

It is unclear to what degree the various IIDD clinical phenotypes reflect fundamental pathophysiologic differences.[23] Conversely, it is unclear why some MS patients have ADEM-like (predominantly in pediatric MS) or tumefactive presentations before developing a more typical MS phenotype. This section focuses specifically on the differential diagnosis of the IIDDs. Neuromyelitis optica (NMO), transverse myelitis (TM), and ADEM are all discussed in detail in separate chapters in this volume.

NEUROMYELITIS OPTICA

The specific IIDD for which the distinction from MS has perhaps best been clarified is NMO or Devic's disease. Clinically, NMO is characterized by severe (often bilateral) relapses of optic neuritis and longitudinally extensive transverse myelitis (LETM).[24] Spinal plaques in MS tend to involve only a partial cross-section of the cord and usually extend for only one vertebral body in length. In contrast, spinal lesions in NMO extend longitudinally over multiple (three or more) vertebral bodies and are frequently associated with significant cord swelling.[24,25] The clinical tempo differs between the two conditions as well; in contrast to MS, "remission" is typically incomplete in NMO, and patients are left with significant permanent myelopathic syndromes (e.g., paraparesis, sphincter dysfunction) and/or visual loss.[26] Conversely, whereas NMO patients are left with significant disability as a result of relapses, it is unusual for such patients to transition into a progressive

TABLE 2–9 Idiopathic Inflammatory Demyelinating Diseases
Multiple sclerosis
Relapsing-remitting
Secondary progressive
Primary progressive/progressive relapsing
Multiple sclerosis variants (presumed)
Marburg variant
Tumefactive MS
Balo's concentric sclerosis
Acute disseminated encephalomyelitis (including acute hemorrhagic leukoencephalitis)
Optic neuritis (monophasic and recurrent)*
Transverse myelitis (monophasic and recurrent)*
Neuromyelitis optica

*Recurrent optic neuritis and longitudinally extensive transverse myelitis may be variants of neuromyelitis optica.

disease course.[27] The demographics of NMO also differ from those of MS. Whereas MS occurs primarily in patients of Northern European descent, NMO is more common in African- or Asian-descended populations.[24,28]

Based on a retrospective review of patients seen at the Mayo Clinic, diagnostic criteria for NMO were devised in 1999 and subsequently revised in 2006 (Table 2-10).[29,30] The revisions were prompted by two important developments. First, an autoantibody, termed NMO-IgG, was isolated from American NMO and Japanese "optic-spinal" MS patients.[31] This antibody recognizes aquaporin-4, an astrocytic endfoot water channel protein.[32] The sensitivity and specificity of NMO-IgG in distinguishing NMO from MS were reported as 73% and 91%, respectively.[31] Second, it was increasingly appreciated that NMO patients can have both MRI evidence and, less often, clinical evidence of spatial dissemination outside of the spinal cord and optic nerve.[33-35] Unlike the typical periventricular ovoid lesions seen in MS, cerebral lesions in NMO tend to involve the midline white and gray matter structures, including the thalamus and hypothalamus, and correspond to regions with high expression of aquaporin-4.[36]

Recently, the original and revised NMO diagnostic criteria were applied to a series of Italian and Spanish patients using the clinician's final diagnosis as the reference standard.[37] The authors reported the sensitivity and specificity of the original criteria as 94% and 25%, respectively. In contrast, the revised 2006 criteria had a sensitivity of 88% and a specificity of 84%. In addition, this study demonstrated NMO-IgG positivity in 27% of patients with TM, including two of four patients with recurrent LETM. One (14%) of the seven patients with recurrent optic neuritis also was positive for NMO-IgG.

Several issues have been raised concerning the NMO diagnostic criteria. It can be argued that it is circular logic to define a putative biomarker (in this case, NMO-IgG) by its association with a disorder (NMO) and then to subsequently use the same biomarker to define the disorder.[38] It is also not clear to what degree optic-spinal MS in Asian populations represents a variant of prototypic MS or a separate disease (NMO).[39,40] Some authors also define "Devic's phenotype" more broadly to encompass all disorders that can cause simultaneous or sequential myelitis and optic neuritis, including optic-spinal MS, NMO, and connective tissue diseases such as systemic lupus erythematosus (SLE).[41,42] Finally, as mentioned earlier, NMO-IgG positivity has been demonstrated in patients with isolated LETM and recurrent myelitis or optic neuritis, suggesting that these patients represent a *forme fruste* of NMO.[37,43]

TABLE 2–10 Proposed Diagnostic Criteria for Definite Neuromyelitis Optica (NMO)

Optic neuritis
Transverse myelitis
At least two of three supportive criteria:
- Contiguous spinal cord MRI lesion extending over ≥3 vertebral segments
- Brain MRI not meeting diagnostic criteria for multiple sclerosis
- NMO-IgG seropositive status

IgG, immunoglobulin G; MRI, magnetic resonance imaging.

Adapted from Wingerchuk DM, Lennon VA, Pittock SJ, et al: Revised diagnostic criteria for neuromyelitis optica. Neurology 2006;66:1485-1489.

ACUTE DISSEMINATED ENCEPHALOMYELITIS

ADEM is typically defined as a subacute, monophasic, postinfectious, or postvaccination syndrome characterized by multifocal neurologic deficits with concurrent encephalopathy or obtundation.[44] Although this is markedly different from the usual monofocal presentation of MS, there is sufficient clinical overlap to make differentiation between the two disorders impossible at initial presentation. Longitudinal observational studies in both children and adults show that between 30% and 35% of patients diagnosed with ADEM are subsequently reclassified as having MS.[45-47] The distinction between ADEM and MS is further complicated by the ill-defined entities "multiphasic disseminated encephalomyelitis" (MDEM) and "recurrent ADEM."[23,44] The latter is defined as a separate ADEM episode, distinct from and occurring after resolution of the primary event that is triggered by another immune challenge (e.g., another infection). MDEM describes patients who have either clinical or radiologic disease evolution during the primary event. As discussed earlier, the McDonald criteria for DIT were designed to exclude MDEM.[7]

Although no pathognomic features conclusively differentiate MS from ADEM, the subacute onset of severe multifocal neurologic symptoms with an associated alteration in consciousness favors the latter diagnosis. ADEM is more common in children, but it can occur at any age, and cases have been reported in the elderly.[48] Adult patients tend not to have either fever or headache as frequently as do patients in the pediatric population, and encephalopathy is less frequently observed in patients older than 10 years of age.[44,49] Among adult patients, 46% to 73% report a recent infection or vaccination[46,47]; however, such immunological challenges can also trigger MS relapses.

MRI can also be helpful in differentiating ADEM from MS. Indistinct lesion borders, gray matter involvement, and diffuse or multilesional enhancement all favor the radiologic diagnosis of ADEM over MS.[50] MRIs performed early in the disease course can be normal, so repeat imaging may be required. In contrast, evidence of disease chronicity (e.g., T1 hypointense "black holes," non-uniform lesion enhancement) suggests MS. The demonstration of blood products indicates the fulminant ADEM variant of acute hemorrhagic leukoencephalitis (AHLE).

Diagnostic criteria for ADEM have recently been proposed based on a multicenter, retrospective review of patients enrolled in the European Database for Multiple Sclerosis (EDMUS) (Table 2-11).[47] This was predominantly an adult population, although patients older than 15 years of age were included. The authors did not include patients with multiphasic ADEM (10% of the original 60 patients identified). The proposed criteria had a sensitivity of 83% and a specificity of 95% in distinguishing ADEM from MS, with a mean follow-up period of 3 years. It is unknown whether longer follow-up would increase the number of patients diagnosed with MS. These criteria require prospective validation.

VARIANTS OF MULTIPLE SCLEROSIS

The IIDD spectrum also includes Balo's concentric sclerosis (BCS), also called Balo's disease, and the tumefactive and Marburg variants of MS.[21,22,51] These rare conditions are all characterized by an acute and fulminating presentation and are typically considered to be variants of MS rather than distinct disorders. Cases with

TABLE 2–11 Proposed Diagnostic Criteria for Acute Disseminated Encephalomyelitis (ADEM)

Patients must have ≥ 2 of the following 3 criteria to be diagnosed with ADEM:

1. One or more clinical atypical symptoms of multiple sclerosis
   - Alteration of consciousness
   - Hypersomnia
   - Seizures
   - Cognitive impairment
   - Hemiplegia
   - Tetraplegia
   - Aphasia
   - Bilateral optic neuritis
2. Absence of oligoclonal bands in the cerebrospinal fluid
3. Gray matter involvement (basal ganglia or cortical lesions)

Adapted from de Seze J, Debouverie M, Zephir H, et al: Acute fulminant demyelinating disease: A descriptive study of 60 patients. Arch Neurol 2007;64:1426-1432.

similar clinical phenotypes have also been labeled differently in the literature, complicating the differentiation among these conditions.[50]

The Marburg variant (also referred to as acute MS or acute Marburg MS) was first described by Otto Marburg in 1906. This disorder typically follows a monophasic course, with the acute development of large, typically supratentorial, lesions with associated mass effect and edema.[51,52] Although some patients have been reported to survive with aggressive corticosteroid and/or immunosuppressive therapy, the Marburg variant usually is fulminant, and most patients die within months. Clinical differentiation from ADEM can be difficult, but pathologic evaluation of the Marburg variant demonstrates a more severe destruction of both myelin and underlying axons and associated significant necrosis.[51]

Tumefactive MS refers to the presentation of MS plaques as large, space-occupying mass lesions that clinically and radiologically mimic brain tumors.[51,53] Such lesions are typically supratentorial and cause hemiparesis, hemisensory loss, visual field deficits, decreased consciousness, and seizures. When tumefactive lesions occur in patients with established MS or when the initial presentation involves a symptomatic tumefactive lesion and concurrent "typical" periventricular, ovoid MS plaques, the diagnosis is easier to establish. Differentiation from a neoplastic process is more problematic if the initial presentation is with a solitary mass lesion. Advanced MRI techniques, including magnetic resonance spectroscopy and magnetic resonance perfusion, are useful in excluding tumor without resorting to biopsy.[50,51] In addition, the presence of an "open" ring of enhancement oriented toward the cortex suggests a demyelinating etiology.[54] Biopsy can confirm the demyelinating nature of the lesion, although the presence of Creuztfelt-Peters cells (astrocytes with fragmented nuclear inclusions) can be mistaken for mitotic glial cells.[55] One third of biopsies are inconclusive.[53] Patients with tumefactive presentations tend to subsequently follow a typical relapsing-remitting course, although monophasic cases have also been reported.

BCS is clinically similar to the Marburg and tumefactive variants, with an acute, severe phenotype involving severe neurologic compromise. Lesions in BCS are characterized by the pathognomic pathologic appearance of alternating bands of demyelination and myelination.[56] This pattern can also be seen on MRI, either with alternate hypointense/hyperintense bands on both T1- and T2-weighted sequences or with concentric rings of gadolinium enhancement.[57,58] As with the other acute MS variants, the ability to detect BCS antemortem through MRI has widened the clinical spectrum to include patients with a more favorable long-term prognosis. BCS patients can transition to a more typical RRMS course and Balo-type lesions can be seen on MRI alongside typical MS plaques.

The mechanism behind the concentric lamellae of demyelination and myelination in BCS is unknown.[59] It has been proposed that the myelinated rings are in fact areas of remyelination.[60] Alternatively, some mechanism might exist wherein progressive demyelination extending outward from the nidus is repeatedly halted, only to recur at a later point.[61] This might be due to diffusion of a protective molecule outward from an area of demyelination, which is able to prevent inflammatory demyelination within its radius of diffusion. Other authors have noted that demyelinated lamellae of Balo-type lesions show features suggestive of hypoxic damage and that the preserved lamellae show upregulation of molecules that protect against hypoxic-ischemic injury.[62] They suggest that alternating concentric regions of protective preconditioning may produce bands of preserved tissue in an expanding lesion.

Differential Diagnosis

In addition to the IIDDs discussed here, the differential diagnosis of MS is vast. One hundred separate conditions have been compiled that can mimic MS[63] and this figure is likely an underestimate. However, applying such a large differential on a routine basis is both impractical and unnecessary. Instead, consideration of the singular presentation of each patient permits a more rational consideration of only the relevant alternate diagnoses.

In CIS patients, for example, routine neurological history and examination allows for the formulation of a circumscribed differential based on the anatomic localization of the symptomatic lesion. Most relapsing onset patients present with brainstem or myelitic syndromes or optic neuritis (ON), each of which can usually be easily distinguished from potential MS "mimics."

ON is a clinical diagnosis that classically has no associated abnormality on funduscopic examination; hence the adage that "the patient and physician see nothing." On occasion, disc hyperemia is present but usually the fundus is normal because only the retrobulbar aspect of the optic nerve is inflamed. The patient complains of a subacute, usually unilateral, visual acuity or field defect and associated retro-orbital pain with eye movement.[64,65] Achromatopsia may be appreciated by the patient, or it may only be detected on formal testing. A relative afferent pupillary defect (RAPD) is apparent if acuity is sufficiently diminished. Like MS itself, ON has a large differential diagnosis (Table 2-12).[65-68] It can occur as an idiopathic, monophasic episode or as a manifestation of an IIDD. Patients with monophasic ON are typically male and tend to have a more severe phenotype, with no light perception in the affected eye, prominent papillitis, and retinal hemorrhages or exudates.[64] Approximately 20% to 25% of MS patients initially present with ON.[69] Recurrent, bilateral, sequential, or simultaneous ON should prompt consideration of NMO. ON can occur as a postinfectious or postvaccination event

TABLE 2–12 Differential Diagnosis of Optic Neuritis

Inflammatory Optic Neuritis

Idiopathic isolated optic neuritis
Idiopathic inflammatory demyelinating diseases (IIDDs)
  Multiple sclerosis
  Acute disseminated encephalomyelitis (ADEM)
  Neuromyelitis optica (NMO)
Parainfectious optic neuritis
  Viral: adenovirus, coxsackievirus, cytomegalovirus, Epstein-Barr virus, hepatitis A, hepatitis B, HIV, measles, mumps, herpes zoster, herpes simplex
  Bacterial: *Borrelia burgdorferi*, *Bartonella henselae*, *Treponema pallidum*, *Mycobacterium tuberculosis*
  Fungal: *Cryptococcus* spp., *Aspergillus* spp.
  Parasitic: *Toxoplasmosis gondii*, *Toxocara canis*, *Leptospira*
Systemic inflammatory disorders: sarcoid, SLE, Sjögren's disease, Behçet's disease
Postvaccination optic neuritis

Optic Neuropathies

Vascular
  Anterior ischemic optic neuropathy: giant cell arteritis, SLE, nonarteritic anterior ischemic optic neuropathy (atherosclerosis)
Posterior ischemic optic neuropathy (hypotension)
  Infectious: herpes zoster virus, cytomegalovirus, *T. pallidum*, *B. henselae*, *M. tuberculosis*, *T. gondii*, *T. canis*, *Cryptococcus* spp., *Aspergillus* spp.
Infiltrative/compressive
  Neoplastic: optic glioma, meningioma, hemangioma, metastases, lymphoma
  Nonneoplastic: sarcoid, SLE, inflammatory bowel disease
Hereditary: Leber's hereditary optic neuropathy, other mitochondrial disorders
Traumatic
Radiation-induced
Vitamin deficiency: B_1, B_6, B_{12}, niacin, folic acid
Toxic: methanol, ethanol, ethambutol, ethylene glycol, disulfiram, tobacco

Other Ophthalmologic Disorders

Anterior segment diseases: corneal trauma or inflammation, acute angle closure glaucoma
Retinal diseases: retinitis pigmentosa, cone-rod dystrophy, central serous retinopathy, cancer-associated retinopathy, melanoma-associated retinopathy, recoverin-associated retinopathy

HIV, human immunodeficiency virus; SLE, systemic lupus erythematosus.

similar to ADEM or as a manifestation of a systemic inflammatory disorder. It is important to distinguish optic neuritis from other optic neuropathies resulting from vascular, infectious, metabolic, mitochondrial, compressive, and/or neoplastic causes, as shown in Table 2-12.

Brainstem syndromes account for 10% of CIS presentations.[69] The most frequent is an intranuclear ophthalmoplegia (INO), which in a young adult is as close to a pathognomic sign as exists in MS. Nevertheless, cerebrovascular disease or, less commonly, a myriad of other neoplastic, infectious, or toxic/metabolic conditions can produce an INO. Isolated or multiple ocular motor and lower

TABLE 2–13 Criteria for Idiopathic Acute Transverse Myelitis

Inclusion Criteria	Exclusion Criteria
Development of sensory, motor, or autonomic dysfunction attributable to the spinal cord	History of previous radiation to the spine within the last 10 yr
Bilateral signs or symptoms (not necessarily symmetrical)	Clear arterial distribution of clinical deficit consistent with thrombosis of the anterior spinal artery
Clearly defined sensory level	Abnormal flow voids on the surface of the spinal cord consistent with AVM
Exclusion of extra-axial compressive causes by neuroimaging (MRI or myelography; CT of spine is not adequate)	Serologic or clinical evidence of connective tissue disease (e.g., sarcoidosis, Behçet's disease, Sjögren's syndrome, SLE, mixed connective tissue disorder)*
Inflammation within the spinal cord demonstrated by CSF pleocytosis *or* elevated IgG index *or* gadolinium enhancement. If no inflammatory criterion is met at symptom onset, repeat MRI and lumbar puncture evaluation 2-7 days after symptom onset may be used to meet criteria.	CNS manifestations of syphilis, Lyme disease, HIV, HTLV-1, *Mycoplasma*, other viral infection (e.g., HSV-1, HSV-2, VZV, EBV, CMV, HHV-6, enteroviruses)*
Progression to nadir between 4 hr and 21 days after onset of symptoms (if patient awakens with symptoms, symptoms must become more pronounced from point of awakening)	Brain MRI abnormalities suggestive of multiple sclerosis*
	History of clinically apparent optic neuritis*

*Patients who meet all the inclusion criteria and have evidence of a connective tissue disease could have "disease-associated acute transverse myelitis."

AVM, arteriovenous malformation; CNS, central nervous system; CMV, cytomegalovirus; CSF, cerebrospinal fluid; CT, computed tomography; EBV, Epstein-Barr virus; HHV, human herpesvirus; HIV, human immunodeficiency virus; HSV, herpes simplex virus; HTLV, human T-cell lymphotropic virus; IgG, immunoglobulin G; MRI, magnetic resonance imaging; SLE, systemic lupus erythematosus; VZV, varicella-zoster virus.

Adapted from Transverse Myelitis Consortium Working Group: Proposed diagnostic criteria and nosology of acute transverse myelitis. Neurology 2002;59:499-505.

cranial neuropathies can also be seen in MS, and, depending on the precise distribution, the differential diagnosis includes intrinsic brainstem mass lesions or infarcts; aneurysmal, neoplastic, inflammatory, or infectious peripheral nerve compression or infiltration; and meningeal disease.[70] Guillain-Barré syndrome also needs to be considered, especially if multiple cranial neuropathies are present, and myasthenia gravis can mimic isolated ocular motor nerve palsies and can even produce a "pseudo-INO."[71]

TM is the initial presentation in approximately one half of MS patients, but it can also occur as an isolated monophasic, idiopathic event, possibly due to postinfectious or postvaccination molecular mimicry or other immune dysregulation mechanisms.[69,72] Criteria proposed by the Transverse Myelitis Consortium working group in 2002 differentiate idiopathic TM from "disease-associated TM" occurring in the context of an IIDD, a systemic inflammatory disorder such as

TABLE 2–14 Differential Diagnosis of Chronic Myelopathies

Idiopathic inflammatory demyelinating diseases (IIDDs)
- Primary progressive multiple sclerosis (PPMS)

Infectious
- HIV myelopathy
- HTLV-1–associated myelopathy/tropical spastic paraparesis (HAM/TSP)
- *Treponema pallidum* (tabes dorsalis)
- Brucellosis
- Schistosomiasis
- *Borrelia burgdorferi*

Hereditary/degenerative
- Hereditary spastic paraparesis (autosomal recessive, autosomal dominant, X-linked)
- Friedrich's ataxia
- Adrenomyeloneuropathy
- Spinocerebellar ataxias
- Amyotrophic lateral sclerosis

Vascular
- CADASIL
- Dural arteriovenous malformation/fistula

Compression/structural
- Spondylosis
- Tumor
- Syrinx

Inflammatory
- Sarcoid
- Vasculitis
- Behçet's disease
- Sjögren's syndrome

Deficiency states
- Vitamin B_{12} (subacute combined degeneration)
- Copper

CADASIL, cerebral autosomal dominant arteriopathy with subcortical infarcts and leukoencephalopathy; HIV, human immunodeficiency virus; HTLV, human T-cell lymphotropic virus.

SLE, or a CNS infection (Table 2-13).[73] Clinically, TM occurring in the context of or heralding MS tends to produce patchy or incomplete deficits, in contrast to the severe myelopathies seen in NMO or SLE. It is, of course, imperative that TM be differentiated from other acute myelopathies.[73-75] Acute spinal cord compression due to an epidural abscess or hematoma, acute disc herniation, or less commonly an intraspinal tumor is a surgical emergency and necessitates spinal imaging. Spinal cord ischemia associated with an arteriovenous malformation or fistula, anterior spinal artery or watershed infarction can also mimic an inflammatory myelopathy. The flaccid, arreflexic myelopathy seen in acute severe myelopathies ("spinal shock") can also mimic Guillain-Barré syndrome.

PPMS typically presents as an insidiously worsening, spastic paraparesis, and the chronic time-course necessitates the development of a differential diagnosis different from that of acute TM (Table 2-14).[76,77] Less often, ataxic symptoms can predominate and should prompt consideration of autosomal or dominant hereditary ataxic syndromes or paraneoplastic disorders.

TABLE 2–15 Disorders that Can Cause Lesions Disseminated in Space or Time or Both

IIDDs	MS, NMO, ADEM, Recurrent Optic Neuritis, TM
Inflammatory	CNS vasculitis, neurosarcoidosis, SLE, Behçet's disease, Sjögren's disease, TTP, Wegener's granulomatosis, polyarteritis nodosa
Infectious	Mycoplasma, HIV, HTLV-1, herpes zoster, neurosyphilis, Lyme disease, PML, Whipple's disease
Neoplastic	Lymphoma, CNS metastases
Structural	Spondylosis, syringomyelia, Arnold-Chiari malformation
Metabolic	Vitamin B_{12} deficiency, porphyria
Hereditary/degenerative	Spinocerebellar degeneration, motor neuron disease, leukodystrophies, mitochondrial disease, hereditary spastic paraparesis, Fabry's disease, CADASIL, multisystem atrophy, Friedrich's ataxia
Vascular	Small-vessel disease, proximal embolic source, antiphospholipid syndrome, CADASIL
Other	Migraine with aura

ADEM, acute disseminated encephalomyelitis; CADASIL, cerebral autosomal dominant arteriopathy with subcortical infarcts and leukoencephalopathy; CNS, central nervous system; HIV, human immunodeficiency virus; HTLV, human T-cell lymphotropic virus; MS, multiple sclerosis; NMO, neuromyelitis optica; PML, progressive multifocal leukoencephalopathy; SLE, systemic lupus erythematosus; TM, transverse myelitis; TTP, thrombotic thrombocytopenic purpura.

In contrast to the typical monofocal CIS presentations discussed previously, patients who have clinical features indicative of multiple lesions require consideration of conditions that can cause DIT, DIS, or both. This list is quite broad, and an inexhaustive sampling is provided in Table 2-15.[63,68,78,79] Frequently, these conditions can be ruled either in or out of the differential with a careful history and examination supplemented by appropriate ancillary investigations. The breadth of the required laboratory, neurophysiological, and imaging investigations should be individualized. Most patients with typical clinical and imaging features do not need a large battery of tests to screen for mimics, and doing so is likely to result in a significant frequency of false-positive test results.

It must be acknowledged that in routine clinical practice, the majority of the conditions listed that mimic the DIS and DIT characteristics of inflammatory demyelination are infrequently encountered. Various studies have shown that most patients in MS referral centers who were not diagnosed with MS tended to receive a limited number of alternative diagnoses.[63,80,81] Frequent neurologic alternative diagnoses were migraines, cerebrovascular disease, and peripheral neuropathies. Commonly (30% to 75% of cases), these patients were diagnosed with a psychiatric disorder.[63,80,81]

It is also critical to watch for atypical features that, although not necessarily incompatible with MS, should at the least prompt consideration of alternative etiologies. These features have been labeled "red flags" by various authors and can include both the presence of characteristics not usually seen in MS (e.g., seizures or other cortical symptoms) and the absence of expected features (e.g., a normal cranial MRI).[25,63,82,83] Table 2-16 lists clinical features that are atypical for MS.

TABLE 2–16 Clinical Features that Are Atypical in Multiple Sclerosis

"Positive" Features
Seizures
Headache
Cortical syndromes (aphasia, apraxia)
Prominent early encephalopathy/dementia
Prominent early cerebral/cord atrophy
Fasciculations, lower motor neuron findings
Incidentally discovered white matter abnormalities on MRI
Strong family history (Mendelian pattern)
Systemic abnormalities
Pediatric or older-age onset
"Negative" Features
Normal examination (especially in long-standing cases)
No long tract abnormalities (especially in long-standing cases)
No sphincter dysfunction (especially in long-standing cases)
No fatigue
No dissemination in space/time
Static abnormalities
Normal cranial and/or spinal MRI
No increased IgG index or oligoclonal bands

IgG, immunoglobulin G; MRI, magnetic resonance imaging.

It is important to appreciate that such "red flags" do not rule out MS. Given the wide range of phenotypes seen in confirmed MS, it is not uncommon for individual patients to have some unusual clinical features. Rather, diagnostic uncertainty should increase with the number of atypical features present.[83]

In evaluating whether an atypical feature requires further investigation, it is necessary to consider the patient's temporal course. For example, whereas significant cognitive impairment is unusual early in the course of MS, this feature would not be "atypical" in a chronic patient with severe motor deficits. Conversely, the absence of typical findings (e.g., INO, hyperreflexia) is not unexpected in the early stages of MS but would be a "red flag" in a patient with long-standing symptoms. Similarly, although approximately 10% of patients with MS report a family history, a pedigree with numerous affected individuals should prompt consideration of an alternative hereditary diagnosis (e.g., cerebral autosomal dominant arteriopathy with subcortical infarcts and leukoencephalopathy [CADASIL], hereditary spastic paraparesis). MS typically affects patients in early adulthood, but it is being increasingly recognized in children as well as the elderly. Although presentation in a child or older adult does require consideration of other age-appropriate etiologies (e.g., ADEM or cerebrovascular disease, respectively), the possibility of MS cannot be discarded purely on the basis of age.

In 2006, an expert consensus statement was released that sought to formally expand the diagnostic role of MRI beyond its use in the McDonald criteria to identify characteristics that are sensitive and specific for MS.[25] The authors developed a list of imaging features that can act as "exclusion criteria" and are suggestive of alternative diagnoses (Table 2-17).

TABLE 2–17 MRI Features that Are Atypical for Multiple Sclerosis

MRI Feature	Alternative Diagnosis
Brain white matter	
Normal	NMO (absent or few lesions), ATM
Large lesions	AMS (confluent and perilesional edema), BCS (concentric whorls of alternating rings of enhancement), PACNS (with mass effect)
Symmetrically distributed lesions	ADEM, AFL
Poorly defined lesion margins	ADEM
Absent or rare Dawson fingers, corpus callosum and periventricular lesions	ADEM
Absent MRI activity at follow-up	ADEM
Lesions of the temporal pole, U fibers at vertex, external capsule, and insular regions	CADASIL
Multiple bilateral microhemorrhagic foci	CADASIL, small-vessel disease
Sparing of corpus callosum and cerebellum	CADASIL, small-vessel disease
Lesions in the center of the corpus callosum	Susac's syndrome
Hemorrhages	PACNS
Simultaneous enhancement of all lesions	ADEM, PACNS, sarcoidosis, infarcts, SID, PACNS, small-vessel disease
Punctiform parenchymal enhancement	PACNS, sarcoidosis, NBD
Predominance of lesions at cortical/subcortical junction	SID
Diffuse white matter involvement	NBD, encephalitis (HIVE), small-vessel disease, CADASIL
Cerebral venous sinus thrombosis	NBD
Large and infiltrating brainstem lesions	NBD
Anterior temporal and inferior frontal lobe involvement, associated with enhancement or mass effect	Encephalitis (HSE)
Isolated lesions with ring enhancement (often complete)	Abscesses
Mass effect	Abscesses
Multifocal, asymmetrical lesions starting in a juxtacortical location and progressively enlarging	PML
Large lesions with absent or rare mass effect	PML
Extensive and bilateral periventricular abnormalities in isolation	B_{12} deficiency, acquired copper deficiency
Cortical gray matter	
Cortical/subcortical lesions crossing vascular territories	MELAS

Table continued on following page

TABLE 2–17 MRI Features that Are Atypical for Multiple Sclerosis (Continued)

MRI Feature	Alternative Diagnosis
Prevalent involvement compared with white matter	Encephalitis
Infiltrating lesions that do not remain in gray or white matter boundaries	Abscesses
Deep gray matter	
Bilateral lesions	ADEM (at the gray–white-matter junction), CADASIL
Lacunar infarcts	CADASIL, small-vessel disease
T1 hyperintensity of the pulvinar	Fabry's disease
Multiple discrete lesions in the basal ganglia and thalamus	Susac's syndrome
Large and infiltrating basal ganglia lesions	NBD
Infiltrating lesions without respecting gray-matter or white-matter boundaries	Abscesses
T2-hyperintense lesions in the dentate nuclei	AFL (CTX)
Spinal cord	
Large and swelling lesions	NMO (with corresponding T1 hypointensity), ADEM, ATM, Sjögren's syndrome
Diffuse abnormalities in the posterior columns	B_{12} deficiency, acquired copper deficiency
Other	
No "occult" changes in the NAWM	NMO, Lyme disease, SID (except in NSLE)
Pontine lacunar infarcts	CADASIL, small-vessel disease
Dilation of Virchow-Robin spaces	HHC, PACNS
Diffuse lactate increase on brain magnetic resonance spectroscopy	MELAS
Meningeal enhancement	Susac's syndrome, PACNS, NBD, meningitis, Lyme disease, sarcoidosis
Hydrocephalus	Sarcoidosis
Absence of optic nerve lesions	PML
Regional atrophy	HHC (hippocampus and amygdala), NBD (brainstem)

ADEM, acute disseminated encephalomyelitis; AFL, adult forms of leukoencephalopathies; AMS, acute multiple sclerosis (Marburg type); ATM, acute transverse myelitis; BCS, Balo's concentric sclerosis; CADASIL, cerebral autosomal dominant arteriopathy with subcortical infarcts and leukoencephalopathy; CTX, cerebrotendinous xanthomatosis; HHC, hyperhomocysteinemia; HIVE, HIV encephalitis; HSE, herpes simplex encephalitis; MELAS, mitochondrial encephalopathy with lactic acidosis and stroke-like episodes; MRI, magnetic resonance imaging; NAWM, normal-appearing white matter; NBD, Behçet's disease with central nervous system involvement; NMO, neuromyelitis optica; NSLE, neuropsychiatric systemic lupus erythematosus; PACNS, primary angiitis of the central nervous system; PML, progressive multifocal leukoencephalopathy; SID, systemic immune-mediated diseases; SSP, subacute sclerosing panencephalitis.

Adapted from Chaury A, Yousry TA, Rovaris M, et al: MRI and the diagnosis of multiple sclerosis: Expanding the concept of "no better explanation." Lancet Neurol 2006;5:841-852.

Although the importance of MRI in allowing for both early and definitive diagnosis of MS cannot be overstated, it is important to acknowledge the danger of misinterpretation or overinterpretation of MRI findings. The pattern of abnormalities on MRI can suggest but cannot confirm the underlying etiological or pathological substrate. Between 5% and 10% of the population 20 to 40 years old have lesions consistent with small-vessel disease.[25] This is two orders of magnitude more common than MS. Migraineurs also have an increased incidence of punctuate white matter T2 hyperintensities, likely explaining why this is a common alternative diagnosis in MS referral centers.[81] Patients who are referred to such centers solely on the basis of nonspecific MRI findings without any history of typical MS symptoms frequently have an alternative diagnosis.[81]

Conclusion

MRI-based diagnostic criteria represent a profound advancement as they correspond to the modern pathophysiological conceptualization of MS as a disease in which immunologic dysregulation is associated with ongoing neurodegeneration. In relapsing MS, therefore, MRI lesion burden may be a more sensitive marker of disease activity than relapse rate, and allowing a definite MS diagnosis to be made earlier on the basis of MRI changes is intuitively attractive.

The majority of patients with typical clinical and paraclinical features of MS do indeed have MS and it is inappropriate to consider this disease as a diagnosis of exclusion. However, it is still imperative that neurologists appreciate the limitations of the current diagnostic criteria and avoid the numerous potential pitfalls that exist.

As the authors of the McDonald criteria acknowledged, such diagnostic schemes have the inherent limitation that they were both designed for and tested in patients in whom the assessing neurologist already has determined that there is a high “pre-test probability” for a diagnosis of MS. T2 hyperintensities may represent inflammatory demyelination, ischemic, metabolic, or other alternative etiologies or may even be within the normal spectrum. Clinicians must also avoid premature diagnosis in patients who have atypical features suggesting alternative diagnoses within the MS spectrum of IIDDs or other neurologic, systemic, or psychiatric disorders. An appropriate clinical presentation is still necessary for the diagnosis of MS.

REFERENCES

1. Allison RS, Millar JD: Prevalence and familial incidence of disseminated sclerosis. A report to the Northern Ireland Hospitals Authority on the results of a three-year study: Prevalence of Disseminated Sclerosis in Northern Ireland. Ulster Med J 1954;23(Suppl 2):5-27.
2. McAlpine D, Lumsden CE, Acheson ED: Multiple sclerosis: A reappraisal. Edinburgh, Churchill Livingstone, 1972.
3. Schumaker GA, Beebe GW, Kibler RF, et al: Problems of experimental trials of therapy in multiple sclerosis. Ann N Y Acad Sci 1965;122:552-568.
4. McDonald WI, Halliday AM: Diagnosis and classification of multiple sclerosis. Br Med Bull 1977; 33:4-9.
5. Rose AS, Ellison GW, Myers LW, Tourtellotte WW: Criteria for the clinical diagnosis of multiple sclerosis. Neurology 1976;26:20-22.
6. Poser CM, Paty DW, Scheinberg L et al: New diagnostic criteria for multiple sclerosis: Guidelines for research protocols. Ann Neurol 1983;13:227-231.

7. McDonald WI, Compston A, Edan G, et al: Recommended diagnostic criteria for multiple sclerosis: Guidelines from the International Panel on the Diagnosis of Multiple Sclerosis. Ann Neurol 2001;50:121-127.
8. Polman CH, Reingold SC, Edan G, et al: Diagnostic criteria for multiple sclerosis: 2005 Revisions to the "McDonald Criteria." Ann Neurol 2005;58:840-846.
9. Swanton JK, Fernando KT, Dalton CM, et al: Modification of MRI criteria for multiple sclerosis in patients with clinically isolated syndromes. J Neurol Neurosurg Psychiatry 2006;77:830-833.
10. Izquierdo G, Hauw J-J, Lyon-Caen O, et al: Value of multiple sclerosis diagnostic criteria: 70 Autopsy-confirmed cases. Arch Neurol 1985;42:848-850.
11. Paty DW, Oger JJ, Kastrukoff LF, et al: MRI in the diagnosis of MS: A prospective study with comparison of clinical evaluation, evoked potentials, oligoclonal banding and CT. Neurology 1988; 38:180-185.
12. Fazekas F, Offenbacher H, Fuchs S, et al: Criteria for an increased specificity of MRI interpretation in elderly subjects with suspected multiple sclerosis. Neurology 1988;38:1822-1825.
13. Barkhof F, Filippi M, Miller D, et al: Comparison of MRI criteria at first presentation to predict conversion to clinically definite multiple sclerosis. Brain 1997;120:2059-2069.
14. Tintoré M, Rovira A, Martínez MJ, et al: Isolated demyelinating syndromes: Comparison of different MR imaging criteria to predict conversion to clinically definite multiple sclerosis. Am J Neuroradiol 2000;21:702-706.
15. Swanton JK, Rovira A, Tintoré M, et al: MRI criteria for multiple sclerosis in patients presenting with clinically isolated syndromes: A multicentre retrospective study. Lancet Neurol 2007;6:677-686.
16. Dalton CM, Brex PA, Miszkiel KA, et al: Application of the new McDonald criteria to patients with clinically isolated syndromes suggestive of multiple sclerosis. Ann Neurol 2002;52:47-53.
17. Tintoré M, Rovira A, Rio J, et al: New diagnostic criteria for multiple sclerosis: Application in first demyelinating episode. Neurology 2003;60:27-30.
18. O'Connor P: Key issues in the diagnosis and treatment of multiple sclerosis: An overview. Neurology 2002;59:1-33.
19. Freedman MS, Thompson EJ, Deisenhammer F, et al: Recommended standard of cerebrospinal fluid analysis in the diagnosis of multiple sclerosis: A consensus statement. Arch Neurol 2005; 62:865-870.
20. Filippi M, Falini A, Arnold DL, et al: Magnetic resonance techniques for the in vivo assessment of multiple sclerosis pathology: Consensus report of the white matter study group. J Magn Reson Imaging 2005;21:669-675.
21. Weinshenker BG: The natural history of multiple sclerosis. Neurol Clin 1995;13:119-146.
22. Weinshenker BG, Lucchinetti CF: Acute leukoencephalopathies: Differential diagnosis and investigation. Neurologist 1998;4:148-166.
23. Wingerchuk DM, Lucchinetti CF: Comparative immunopathogenesis of acute disseminated encephalomyelitis, neuromyelitis optica, and multiple sclerosis. Curr Opin Neurol 2007;20:343-350.
24. Wingerchuk DM, Lennon VA, Lucchinetti CF, et al: The spectrum of neuromyelitis optica. Lancet Neurol 2007;6:805-815.
25. Chaury A, Yousry TA, Rovaris M, et al: MRI and the diagnosis of multiple sclerosis: Expanding the concept of "no better explanation." Lancet Neurol 2006;5:841-852.
26. Wingerchuk DM: Neuromyelitis optica: Current concepts. Front Biosci 2004; 9:834-840.
27. Wingerchuk DM, Pittock SJ, Lucchinetti CF, et al: A secondary progressive clinical course is uncommon in neuromyelitis optica. Neurology 2007;68:603-605.
28. Compston A: 'The marvellous harmony of the nervous parts': The origins of multiple sclerosis. Clin Med 2004;4:346-354.
29. Wingerchuk DM, Hogancamp WF, O'Brien PC, et al: The clinical course of neuromyelitis optica (Devic's syndrome). Neurology 1999;53:1107-1114.
30. Wingerchuk DM, Lennon VA, Pittock SJ, et al: Revised diagnostic criteria for neuromyelitis optica. Neurology 2006;66:1485-1489.
31. Lennon VA, Wingerchuk DM, Kryzer TJ, et al: A serum autoantibody marker of neuromyelitis optica: Distinction from multiple sclerosis. Lancet 2004;364:2106-2112.
32. Lennon VA, Kryzer TJ, Pittock SJ, et al: IgG marker of optic-spinal multiple sclerosis binds to the aquaporin-4 water channel. J Exp Med 2005;202:473-477.
33. Pittock SJ, Lennon VA, Kreche K, et al: Brain abnormalities in neuromyelitis optica. Arch Neurol 2006;63:390-396.
34. Chalumeau-Lemoine L, Chretien F, Gaelle Si Larbi A, et al: Devic disease with brainstem lesions. Arch Neurol 2006;63:591-593.

35. Hengstman GJD, Wesseling P, Frenken CWGM, et al: Neuromyelitis optica with clinical and histopathological involvement of the brain. Mult Scler 2007;13:679-682.
36. Pittock SJ, Weinshenker BG, Lucchinetti CF: Neuromyelitis optica brain lesions localized at sites of high aquaporin 4 expression. Arch Neurol 2006;63:964-968.
37. Saiz A, Zuliani L, Blanco Y, et al: Revised diagnostic criteria for neuromyelitis optica (NMO): Application in a series of suspected patients. J Neurol 2007;254:1233-1237.
38. Kikuchi S, Kukazawa T: "OSMS is NMO, but not MS": Confirmed by NMO-IgG? Lancet Neurol 2005;4:594-595.
39. Misu T, Fujihara K, Nakashima I: Pure optic-spinal form of multiple sclerosis in Japan. Brain 2002; 125:2460-2468.
40. Nakashima I, Fukazawa T, Ota K: Two subtypes of optic-spinal form of multiple sclerosis in Japan: Clinical and laboratory features. J Neurol 2007;254:488-492.
41. Scolding N: Devic's disease and autoantibodies. Lancet Neurol 2005;4:136-137.
42. Cree BAC, Goodin DS, Hauser SL: Neuromyelitis optica. Semin Neurol 2002;22:105-122.
43. Weinshenker BG, Wingerchuk DM, Vukusic S, et al: Neuromyelitis optica IgG predicts relapse after longitudinally extensive transverse myelitis. Ann Neurol 2006;59:566-569.
44. Menge T, Hemmer B, Nessler S, et al: Acute disseminated encephalomyelitis: An update. Arch Neurol 2005;62:1673-1680.
45. Banwell B, Ghezzi A, Bar-Or A, et al: Multiple sclerosis in children: Clinical diagnosis, therapeutic strategies, and future directions. Lancet Neurol 2007;6:887-902.
46. Schwarz S, Mohr A, Knauth M, et al: Acute disseminated encephalomyelitis: A follow-up study of 40 adult patients. Neurology 2001;56:1313-1318.
47. de Seze J, Debouverie M, Zephir H et al. Acute fulminant demyelinating disease: A descriptive study of 60 patients. Arch Neurol 2007;64:1426-1432.
48. Marchioni E, Marinou-Aktipi K, Uggetti C, et al: Effectiveness of intravenous immunoglobulin treatment in adult patients with steroid-resistant monophasic or recurrent acute disseminated encephalomyelitis. J Neurol 2002;249:100-104.
49. Menge T, Kiesseier BC, Nessler S: Acute disseminated encephalomyelitis: An acute hit against the brain. Curr Opin Neurol 2007;20:247-254.
50. Canellas AC, Gols AR, Izquierdo JR, et al: Idiopathic inflammatory-demyelinating diseases of the central nervous system. Neuroradiology 2007;49:393-409.
51. Pittock SJ, Lucchinetti CF: The pathology of MS: New insights and potential clinical applications. Neurologist 2007;13:45-56.
52. Capello E, Mancardi GL: Marburg type and Balo's concentric sclerosis: Rare and acute variants of multiple sclerosis. Neurol Sci 2004;25:S361-S363.
53. Comi G: Multiple sclerosis: Pseudotumoral forms. Neurol Sci 2004;25:S374-S379.
54. Masdeu JC, Moreira J, Trasi S, et al: The open ring: A new imaging sign in demyelinating disease. J Neuroimaging 1996;6:104-107.
55. Zagzag D, Miller DC, Kleinman GM, et al: Demyelinating disease versus tumor in surgical neuropathology: Clues to a correct pathological diagnosis. Am J Surg Pathol 1993;17:537-545.
56. Yao D-L, Webster HdeF, Hudson LD, et al: Concentric sclerosis (Balo): Morphometric and in situ hybridization study of lesions in six patients. Ann Neurol 1994;35:18-30.
57. Ng S-H, Ko S-F, Cheung Y-C, et al: MRI features of Balo's concentric sclerosis. Br J Radiol 1999; 72:400-403.
58. Karaarslan E, Altintas A, Senol U, et al: Balo's concentric sclerosis: Clinical and radiologic features of five cases. AJNR Am J Neuroradiol 2001;22:1362-1367.
59. Mowry EM, Woo JH, Ances BM: Technology insight: Can neuroimaging provide insights into the role of ischemia in Balo's concentric sclerosis? Nat Clin Pract Neurol 2007;3:341-348.
60. Moore GR, Neumann PE, Suzuki K, et al: Balo's concentric sclerosis: New observations on lesion development. Ann Neurol 1985;17:604-611.
61. Moore GRW, Berry K, Oger JJF, et al: Balo's concentric sclerosis: Surviving normal myelin in a patient with a relapsing-remitting course. Mult Scler 2001;7:375-382.
62. Stadelmann C, Ludwin S, Tabira T, et al: Tissue preconditioning may explain concentric lesions in Balo's type of multiple sclerosis. Brain 2005;128:979-987.
63. Rolak LA, Fleming JO: The differential diagnosis of multiple sclerosis. Neurologist 2007;13:57-72.
64. Balcer LJ: Optic neuritis. N Engl J Med 2006;354:1273-1280.
65. Boomer JA, Siatkowski RM: Optic neuritis in adults and children. Semin Ophthalmol 2003; 18:174-180.
66. Bianchi Marzoli S, Martinelli V: Optic neuritis: Differential diagnosis. Neurol Sci 2001;22:S52-S54.

67. Martinelli V, Bianchi Marzoli S: Non-demyelinating optic neuropathy: Clinical entities. Neurol Sci 2001;22:S55-S59.
68. Scolding N: The differential diagnosis of multiple sclerosis. J Neurol Neurosurg Psychiatry 2001; 71:ii9-ii15.
69. Miller D, Barkhof F, Montalban X: Clinically isolated syndromes suggestive of multiple sclerosis: Part I. Natural history, pathogenesis, diagnosis, and prognosis. Lancet Neurol 2005;4:281-288.
70. Brazis PW, Masdeu JC, Biller J: Localization in Clinical Neurology, 3rd ed. Boston, Little Brown, 1996.
71. Khanna S, Liao K, Kaminski HJ, et al: Ocular myasthenia revisited: Insights from pseudo-internuclear ophthalmoplegia. J Neurol 2007;254:1569-1574.
72. Pittock SJ, Lucchinetti CF: Inflammatory transverse myelitis: Evolving concepts. Curr Opin Neurol 2006;19:362-368.
73. Transverse Myelitis Consortium Working Group: Proposed diagnostic criteria and nosology of acute transverse myelitis. Neurology 2002;59:499-505.
74. Ghezzi A, Baldini SM, Zaffaroni M: Differential diagnosis of acute myelopathies. Neurol Sci 2001; 22:S60-S64.
75. Kaplin AI, Krishnan C, Deshpande DM: Diagnosis and management of acute myelopathies. Neurologist 2005;11:2-18.
76. Montalban X, Rio J: Primary progressive multiple sclerosis. Neurol Sci 2001;22:S41-S48.
77. Miller DH, Leary SM: Primary progressive multiple sclerosis. Lancet Neurol 2007;6:903-912.
78. Gasperini C: Differential diagnosis in multiple sclerosis. Neurol Sci 2001;22:S93-S97.
79. Trojano M, Paolicelli D: The differential diagnosis of multiple sclerosis: Classification and clinical features of relapsing and progressive neurological syndromes. Neurol Sci 2001;22:S98-S102.
80. Murray TJ, Murray SJ: Characteristics of patients found not to have multiple sclerosis. CMAJ 1984;131:336-337.
81. Carmosino MJ, Brousseau KN, Arciniegas DB, et al: Initial evaluations for multiple sclerosis in a university multiple sclerosis center. Arch Neurol 2005;62:585-590.
82. Rudick RA, Schiffer RB, Schwetz KM, et al: Multiple sclerosis: The problem of incorrect diagnosis. Arch Neurol 1986;43:578-583.
83. Herndon RM: Multiple sclerosis mimics. Adv Neurol 2006;98:161-166.

3 Uncovering the Genetic Architecture of Multiple Sclerosis

PHILIP L. DE JAGER • DAVID A. HAFLER

The sequencing of the human genome has heralded a new era in complex trait genetics in the study of susceptibility to human diseases. A convergence of (1) resources such as the HapMap, a catalogue of common genetic variation,[1] (2) novel high-throughput genotyping technologies, and (3) new statistical methods has enabled us,[2] for the first time, to powerfully explore the genetic architecture of common human diseases. Multiple sclerosis (MS) was among the first diseases to be successfully studied in this manner, as evidenced by the discovery of several susceptibility loci in 2007.[3-5] This success is a testament to a whole community's effort to come together to accomplish studies that no one group could perform by themselves.

Unlike other common neurologic diseases such as Alzheimer's disease or Parkinson's disease, no Mendelian form of MS has been described to date; there are no families in which mutations in a single locus or chromosomal region are responsible for the clinical manifestations of MS. Nonetheless, susceptibility to this chronic inflammatory demyelinating and neurodegenerative disorder of the central nervous system has a genetic component.[6] It is a genetically complex trait, meaning that a large number of loci with incomplete penetrance contribute to an individual's genetic risk of MS. In other words, a number of regions within the human genome have a modest effect on risk of MS, and only a subset of individuals who carry the risk-associated version of a specific susceptibility locus develop MS. The process by which genetic predisposition becomes expressed clinically is not known today but probably involves both stochastic events in the development and function of the immune system and an individual's history of environmental exposure to viruses, sunlight, and other factors.[7]

This chapter reviews the rapid progress that has occurred in the field of MS genetics and the repercussions of these findings on the broader community of researchers and clinicians involved in understanding MS and caring for patients with this disease. For the first time in more than 30 years, we have moved beyond the study of a single locus, the major histocompatibility complex (MHC), to identify and validate susceptibility loci elsewhere in the human genome. Here, we describe the first glimpse of the genetic architecture of MS, with interpretations of what current discoveries mean in terms of their impact on understanding disease pathophysiology. Whole genome association scans that are scheduled to conclude in 2008-2010 will increase the number of genotyped subjects more than 10-fold and provide a much more comprehensive assessment of genetic susceptibility to MS.

The MHC and Multiple Sclerosis Susceptibility

The association of the MHC and, more specifically, the human leukocyte antigen HLA-DR2 haplotype (now referred to as the HLA-DRB1*1501 haplotype) with susceptibility to MS was first noted[8] in 1972 and remains one of the most reproduced findings in MHC genetics.[9-16] In all of the linkage scans of families with MS performed to date, the MHC is the only one to have achieved genome-wide significance as an MS susceptibility locus both in a meta-analysis of linkage studies[14] and in a subsequent high-resolution linkage screen in MS.[15] Recently, coarse association studies of the MHC based on single nucleotide polymorphisms (SNPs) confirmed the preeminent role of the DRB1*1501 haplotype in MS in populations of European ancestry.[16,17] Indeed, populations with a high concentration of the DRB1*1501 haplotype, such as northern Scots, exhibit some of the highest known prevalence rates of MS.[18] Although its effect on susceptibility is relatively undisputed, correlation between the DRB1*1501 haplotype and disease course or severity remains inconclusive, with some studies suggesting an association with an earlier age at onset.[19-24]

Because of strong linkage disequilibrium within the MHC (and particularly in the regions that contain the MHC class II genes such as *HLA-DRB1*), it remains unclear whether the primary driver for the association between the MHC and MS is the DRB1*1501 allele or other alleles, such as DQB1*0602, that are generally inherited with DRB1*1501 as a single large block of DNA (reviewed in Harbo et al.[25]). The long-range linkage disequilibrium noted within the DRB1*1501–DQB1*0602 haplotype (that is, the strong correlation existing between other genetic markers and DRB1*1501 over long distances) and its strong effect on risk of disease (odds ratio [OR] = 2.7 for one copy of the allele[26]) hinders the identification of the causal allele. To date, the best evidence rests with HLA-DRB1*1501 itself, since Oksenberg and colleagues demonstrated the preeminent role of this allele over DQB1*0602 in African Americans with MS.[27] This observation has been supported by a similar analysis of rare subjects of European ancestry who had recombination events between these two alleles (De Jager, unpublished results).

The frequency and strong effect of the HLA-DRB1*1501 haplotype also makes evaluations of other associations in the MHC, even those several megabases away in the MHC class I region, challenging; it is uncertain whether many MHC class I associations to MS susceptibility are truly independent of the DRB1*1501 haplotype effect.[25] However, some evidence suggests that the DRB1*1501–DQB1*0602-associated *HLA-A3* allele may be an independent susceptibility signal in MS.[28] Investigators in the Netherlands have also reported an association with the microsatellite HLA-C1_3_2*35, which is independent of *DR2* but in strong linkage disequilibrium with *DR3*.[29] However, perhaps the best evidence for a second susceptibility locus within the MHC class I region was presented for the HLA-Cw05 allele in a large population of subjects of European descent with MS.[17] In this study, after all effects from *HLA-DRB1* were excluded, a residual association remained within the MHC class I region. Later, a sample of subjects with MS from the United States was analyzed and demonstrated the same association (De Jager, unpublished results). Overall, it is likely that one or more MHC class I susceptibility loci for MS exist; however, formally, these data have not yet reached a level of overwhelming or genome-wide statistical evidence, such as a *P* value of less than 5×10^{-8}. Additional sample collections will be needed to fully validate the existence of a second MHC susceptibility locus, one that is independent of the HLA-DRB1*1501 haplotype.

Whereas the HLA-DRB1*1501 haplotype plays a preeminent role in MS susceptibility, it is not the only *HLA-DRB1* allele to have a role: allelic heterogeneity at *HLA-DRB1* is well documented, and several other haplotypes also show association with MS, particularly in non-European populations.[22,30] In populations of European ancestry, haplotypes containing the HLA-DRB1*03 or HLA-DRB1*0103 alleles have evidence for making a modest contribution to increasing an individual's risk of MS.[17,22] Outside of northern Europe, the haplotype tagged by HLA-DRB1*1501 remains a risk haplotype for MS, particularly when one considers the typical disseminated forms of demyelinating disease captured by the MS diagnostic rubric.[31,32] In Japan, disseminated MS similar to that seen in Europeans may be associated with DRB1*1501, whereas the association of the DRB1*1501 haplotype with the optic-spinal MS variant fails to reach significance (reviewed by Kira[31]). Instead, optic-spinal MS may be associated with DPB1*0501 and DPB1*0301 in the Japanese population.[31,33] An association with the DR6 antigen in Japanese subjects has also been reported but without replication.[34] In the Turkish population, an association has been suggested with DR4.[35,36] The same haplotype has also been reported to be associated with susceptibility to MS in Mexican Mestizos[37] and in Mediterranean populations such as Sardinians (reviewed by Compston and Coles[38]). The geographically and historically unique Sardinian population actually displays both DR4 and DR3 associations in its subjects with MS.[39] Among African Americans, MS association has also been demonstrated with DRB1*0301 (DR3) and DRB1*1503 in addition to the expected DRB1*1501.[27] Therefore, a number of different *HLA-DRB1* alleles may have a role in increasing an individual's susceptibility to MS. To balance these effects, a number of other alleles have been implicated in protection from MS, including DR1, DR7, and DR11 at *HLA-DRB1* as well as the HLA-A*0201 allele in the MHC class I region.[28]

Aside from the class I and II genes, the MHC also contains other immunologically relevant genes, such as *TNF* and *NOTCH4*, that have been associated with MS, but these associations were shown to be secondary to that of DRB1*1501.[40] At least 10 small studies have shown no DRB1*1501-independent associations with microsatellites and SNPs in linkage disequilibrium with the *TNF* gene,[40] although one, as yet unreplicated, larger study suggested such an association in a Spanish population.[41] Overall, non-HLA genes have not been examined in great detail to date, and thorough investigations of the entire MHC in large samples are needed to obtain a more comprehensive picture of the important role of this large segment of the genome (>4 megabases) in MS susceptibility.

A Meta-analysis of MHC Studies in Multiple Sclerosis

As can be surmised from the previous section, the examination of the MHC until now has not been done in a coordinated manner. Limitations of sample collections and cost have driven investigators to examine their own subjects as best as they could, using genotyping technologies that are constantly evolving. This has made a clear overview of the role of the MHC in MS difficult to achieve. Nonetheless, Fernando et al.[42] were able to complete a meta-analysis of existing studies of the MHC in MS in 2008. As expected, the meta-analysis highlighted the preeminent role of the extended haplotype defined by HLA-DRB1*1501 and DQB1*0602 (Fig. 3-1). Whether typed as Dw2, DR2, DR15, or DRB1*1501, the presence of a 1501 allele of the *HLA-DRB1* gene is associated with an odds ratio greater than 2.0 for susceptibility to MS. Furthermore, two other ancestral haplotypes, DR3 and DR4, appear to enhance susceptibility to MS in this analysis, although their effect on disease is probably more modest than that of the DR2 haplotypes.

Although the evidence for its role in MS susceptibility is overwhelming, the MHC does not appear to have a significant effect on other phenotypes, such age at symptom onset and course of the disease. Therefore, triggering and progression of MS may well be distinct processes, with different collections of contributing alleles. Even in susceptibility, however, the functional consequences of the HLA-DRB1*1501 haplotype remain unclear. One possibility is that these

Meta Analysis: Multiple Sclerosis

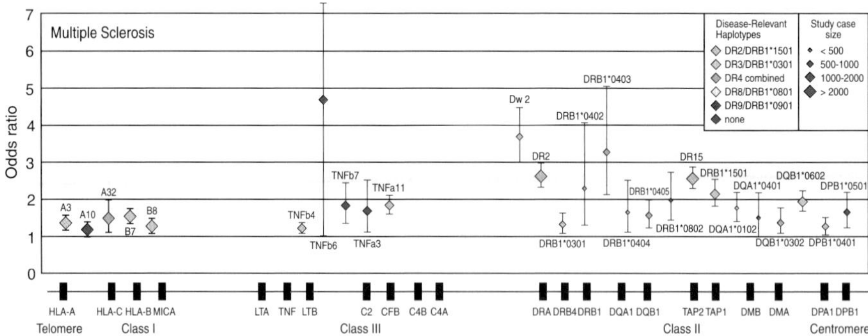

Figure 3–1 Major histocompatibility complex (MHC) susceptibility alleles identified by meta-analysis. An allele is considered to be associated with susceptibility if the lower confidence interval (CI) is greater than 1.0. Odds ratios with 95% CI for multiple sclerosis are shown at each locus. Beneath is a schematic representation of MHC class I, class III, and class II genes in genomic order but not to scale. Diamond size represents total number of cases included in meta-analysis for each allele. Diamond color reflects different disease-relevant ancestral haplotypes. (Courtesy of Christine Stevens, Dr. Michelle Fernando, and Dr. John Rioux.)

DRB1-containing antigen-presenting molecules may facilitate autoreactive activation of T cells. Indeed, antigen presentation by different *HLA-DRB1* alleles has been studied, and HLA-DRB1*1501 can generate reactivity to myelin basic protein (MBP 84-102)[43,44]; proteolipid protein (PLP 95-116, 184-199, and 190-206)[45,46]; and overlapping myelin oligodendrocyte glycoprotein (MOG) peptides.[47] However, at this point, the utility of these observations remains marginal, and non-MHC alleles may hold the key to new insights into immunologic dysfunction in MS.

Whole Genome Scan Methodology and Its Application in Multiple Sclerosis

By the end of the 1990s, it had become clear that the use of linkage studies exploring families with MS was an ineffective study design for finding susceptibility loci. Seminal theoretical modeling by Risch and Merikangas suggested that this study design was underpowered to discover variation affecting complex human traits; their prediction has since been proven correct in MS and many other diseases.[2] Even a very large linkage study with relatively dense genotyping provided no evidence of significant linkage between human genetic variation and MS susceptibility outside of the MHC.[15] Instead, a relatively simple association study design, such as a case-control study, was suggested as being theoretically powerful enough to identify even loci of modest effect on disease risk. The challenge was that such a study design requires very large numbers of subjects and very large numbers of genetic markers to achieve its goal. This realization was one of the main driving forces behind the establishment of the International Multiple Sclerosis Genetics Consortium (IMSGC), because no one group of investigators had the requisite combination of large subject population, large genotyping array, and analysis resources to tackle this project by itself. The need for analysis should not be underestimated, because the manipulation and examination of 500,000 or more SNPs in each of thousands of subjects has required the development of a whole family of new computational methods.

The novelty of these analyses and their size meant that there was little information on the robustness of the results. To address this issue, we decided to use an analysis method called transmission disequilibrium testing (TDT) that relies on the study of trio families (i.e., families consisting of a subject with MS and his or her biologic parents).[48] The primary statistic calculated in TDT relies on the fact that humans have two copies of each chromosome, so that a child has a 50/50 chance of inheriting any one chromosome or allele on that chromosome from a parent. The TDT simply calculates the likelihood or significance of an observed distortion of the inheritance of a single allele away from the expected 50/50 chance. This study design has the distinct advantage of being robust to population stratification, which is an unrecognized difference between a set of cases and the set of control subjects. Such cryptic differences may skew the analysis of an outcome of interest in a case-control study design. This form of robustness comes at a cost, however: the method's statistical power is somewhat less than that of a case-control study of similar size and also requires the genotyping of two parents instead of one control per affected subject, increasing the study's cost. With the completion of a host of genome-wide scans over the past year, it is now clear that population stratification can be estimated and accounted for using new statistical techniques, and this study design is now the preferred one for future studies of MS. In fact, we included a parallel case-control analysis comparing the subjects with MS from the trio families to unrelated healthy control subjects in our whole genome scan.[3]

Whereas the scale of the original MS whole genome scan is much greater than the prior generation of genetic analyses, the primary analysis is relatively simple, because the TDT is calculated for each of the 334,923 SNPs independently. Because of the number of SNPs tested, a small number of extreme *P* values ($<10^{-6}$) are expected to be observed by chance, and validation of these results is essential to discriminate statistical noise from true results. To avoid relying on any one method in selecting SNPs for replication, we used (1) the best results of the TDT analysis, (2) the best results of the case-control analysis, and (3) results that were more modest in their statistical evidence but occurred in genes and loci previously implicated in MS or autoimmune diseases. Replication data were successfully generated for 110 SNPs, and 34 of these had enhanced evidence of association to MS susceptibility at the conclusion of the replication analysis. These 34 SNPs can therefore be regarded as having survived a first round of validation, but, to be accepted as true susceptibility loci, they need to meet a stringent level of statistical significance, a *P* value of less than 5×10^{-8}. This threshold corrects for the fact that we are, in practice, testing approximately a million common genetic variations found in the human genome for association to disease susceptibility in MS.

Based on the results of our whole genome association scan and subsequent investigations, allelic variants in two loci and perhaps a third gene region have been associated with risk of developing MS. In the original IMSGC genome scan, one SNP outside of the MHC region met the predetermined threshold of genome-wide significance; this SNP (rs12722489) was found in a segment of the genome that contains the *IL2RA* and *RBM17* genes ("*IL2RA* locus"). At least one other group of investigators has confirmed this association in a large set of families with MS.[49] A second locus containing the *IL7R* and *CAPSL* genes nearly met the threshold of genome-wide significance in our screen. This locus had previously been associated with MS in candidate gene studies, and the combined evidence from all pertinent studies clearly marks it as another true susceptibility locus.[50] The other 32 SNPs that emerged so far from this first genome scan await further validation. Evidence for the role of *CD58* has been enhanced by genotyping of additional subjects, although it has yet to meet a threshold of genome-wide significance (De Jager et al.[51]). The combination of MHC region, *IL2RA*, and *IL7R* loci are estimated to account for not more than about 15% of the genetic susceptibility in MS; so many more such loci remain to be discovered. The current complement of susceptibility loci is shown in Figure 3-2.

Perhaps the most important result of the whole genome scan for MS susceptibility loci is that it was successful in identifying genetic variants that affect disease risk at a genome-wide level of statistical significance. We now know that this method works in MS, and therefore the issue simply becomes one of accumulating enough subjects to maximize the yield of the study design. Estimates vary, but it appears that approximately 10,000 subjects and an equivalent or greater number of control subjects is required for the study to be fully powered.[2] The IMSGC will have more than 15,000 subjects genotyped by the end of 2010, and this effort may allow the identification of additional susceptibility alleles of modest effect that are

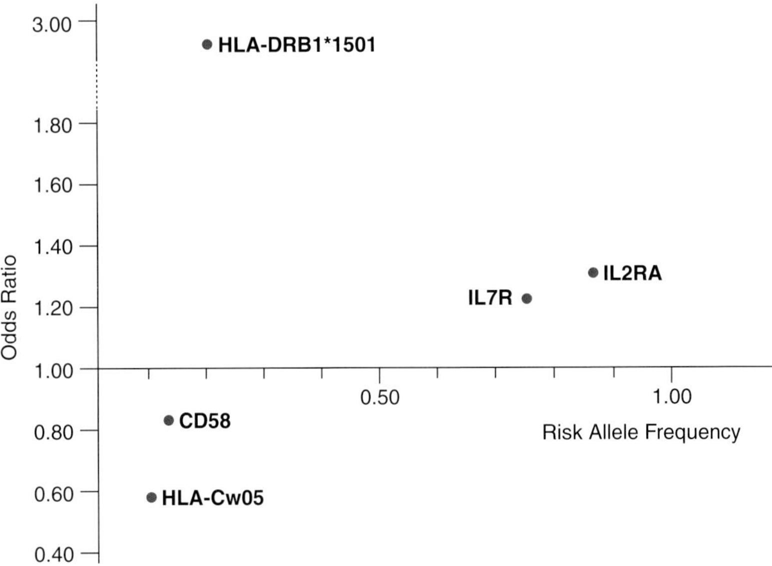

Figure 3–2 Multiple sclerosis (MS) susceptibility alleles determined by 2007. The HLA-DRB1*1501, IL2RA, and IL7R have been validated and have attained a genome-wide level of statistical significance. Two other alleles with substantial evidence of association to MS susceptibility, CD58 and HLA-Cw05, have been validated in at least one independent set of samples but have yet to attain a genome-wide level of statistical significance. The odds ratios and allele frequencies are based on published results from European populations.

relatively common in the general population. At that juncture, the genome-wide analysis of common genetic variants will probably reach a plateau in terms of statistical power, and the addition of further subjects will not have an appreciable effect on the likelihood of finding additional susceptibility loci. This will probably lead to a period of intense focus on the functional consequences of these susceptibility loci on immune and central nervous system function. The next phase of genome-wide searches for MS susceptibility loci will come with whole genome sequencing of each subject, within 5 to 10 years, once sequencing costs for whole genomes on a large scale becomes reasonable.

Genome Scan Results: What Do They Mean?

We now have two well-validated genetic loci that affect MS susceptibility, and there will soon be many more, but what does that mean practically? To be more specific, we have identified two genetic variants, one in the vicinity of the *IL2RA* gene and the other in the *IL7R* gene, that are found more commonly is subjects with MS than in healthy subjects. However, we do not yet know whether these genetic variants are the causal risk alleles or simply markers that are linked to causal alleles not yet discovered. The comprehensive characterization of each of these two loci will eventually answer this question and pinpoint the genetic lesion that affects an individual's risk of developing MS. Nonetheless, in these markers, we already have powerful tools with which to guide further investigation: These surrogate markers can be used to partition subjects in analyses exploring the role of these two loci in the immune function of healthy individuals and in studies investigating their utility in the diagnosis and management of MS.

It is worth emphasizing that the *IL2RA* and *IL7R* loci are associated with susceptibility to MS, meaning that they are implicated in the events that lead up to the initiation of an inflammatory demyelinating process within the central nervous system. Their role in the subsequent disease course is an important question to pursue as the functions of these loci are investigated. Some loci may affect both processes, but, as seen with HLA-DRB1*1501, an important role in disease susceptibility does not necessarily translate into an equally strong effect on the measures used to evaluate MS disease course. Both disease onset and disease course need to be targeted by genetic studies, and success in exploring the first phenotype argues strongly for the targeting of resources to study the genetic factors that affect disease severity.

Clinical end points are critical to ensure that results of genetic scans are meaningful in relation to efforts to improve patient care. However, these clinical end points are typically the culmination of the interactions of multiple different risk factors within an individual subject, and therefore they are far removed from a genetic lesion. This, in part, explains why any one risk allele has a relatively modest effect on disease susceptibility (OR of approximately 1.2 to 1.3 for *IL2RA* and *IL7R*, respectively). It is likely that these risk alleles have a much greater effect on more proximal events, such as transcription of RNA from DNA. In many cases, the effect of these alleles will be discernable in experiments of practical size that explore immune function and central nervous system function *in vivo*, *ex vivo*, and *in vitro*. Research in MS pathophysiology will clearly benefit from the identification of molecules and pathways that are implicated in MS susceptibility. Such experiments may allow the partitioning of MS subjects into subgroups that share pathophysiologic features, and it is possible such efforts may, in turn, identify subgroups of subjects within which a particular allele has a stronger effect.

One common misconception is that disease risk alleles of modest effect are not medically important. At one level, this is true, because the presence of a single such risk allele is not very informative for an individual patient. If, as in the case of the *IL2RA* allele, 98% of the general population of European descent has at least one copy of the allele that confers risk of MS, this information does not help much in a diagnostic algorithm when it is used by itself. The value of these genetic associations comes when they are considered together. We suspect that dozens of such alleles exist, and that researchers will soon be able to establish a gradient of genetic risk for MS within the general population. Placing an "at risk" individual, such as the child of a patient with MS, on this gradient may be informative in the future: It may help a clinician determine how aggressive a particular unaffected individual's monitoring should be and, ultimately, whether prophylactic treatment is indicated in a subset of "at risk" individuals who are genetically loaded and carry other meaningful features of disease susceptibility such as immunologic or radiologic biomarkers. In this way, genetic information may become useful at the individual level after a more comprehensive picture of the genetic lesions associated with MS is elucidated.

When considering the results of these genetic analyses, it is important to focus not just on the effects in an individual subject but also on the effects at the population level, where even modest influences on risk are meaningful if a risk factor is common. This is seen, for example, with cholesterol and cholesterol-lowering drugs and stroke.[52] An intervention targeting a genetic lesion could be meaningful at the population level, particularly if it synergizes with a different factor, such as an environmental risk.

Integrating Disease Risk

In the transition from gene discovery to the application of risk alleles in MS research and disease management, it will be important to integrate the various susceptibility factors for MS to determine the components of a useful biomarker-driven adjunct in a diagnostic algorithm for MS. Specifically, do existing biomarkers have enough information to meaningfully contribute to such an algorithm? In particular, the redundancy of known risk factors needs independent assessment before they are promoted to clinical use. We focused our initial investigation on integrating the role of the well-validated HLA-DRB1*1501 risk haplotype with that of exposure and response to Epstein-Barr virus (EBV). HLA-DRB1 serves as a co-receptor for EBV entry and may present microbial antigens that are similar to endogenous antigens and could generate cross-reactivity of T cells against myelin.[53,54] Thus, we assessed whether these genetic and environmental risk factors were independent of one another or whether EBV-associated risk of MS was dependent on the presence of HLA-DRB1*1501. Our analysis of subjects from the Nurse Health Studies suggests that the effects of these two risk factors are largely independent of one another and that their effect on disease risk is in fact synergistic.[55] As shown in Figure 3-3, a subject with both high titers of anti-EBNA1 (an EBV antigen) antibodies and one or more copies of HLA-DRB1*1501 has a nine-fold greater relative risk of developing MS than someone without the major MHC risk factor who has low antibody titers. This intriguing result needs to be validated in additional collections of subjects, but it already illustrates the path that we must follow to move forward with emerging genetic data.

The nine-fold difference in magnitude of risk in subjects stratified using HLA-DRB1*1501 and anti-EBNA1 titers suggests that they may be useful components of a diagnostic algorithm when used in conjunction with clinical findings and imaging or in settings where imaging may not be readily accessible. Adding additional variants, such as *IL2RA* and *IL7R*, would not enhance an algorithm much at this time, given their relatively modest effects in a single subject. However, with identification of the full complement of MS loci, it may be possible to explore their aggregate effect on disease risk more effectively. In particular, we may be able to define "highly genetically susceptible" classes of individuals, or perhaps individuals with multiple genetic lesions in a single pathway, who are particularly vulnerable to an environmental risk factor for MS.

Susceptibility to Autoimmunity

With the identification of multiple genetic risk factors for MS and other inflammatory autoimmune disorders, it is becoming clear that certain loci play a role in multiple diseases. It is likely that a set of loci affecting basic immunologic mechanisms (e.g., tolerance or regulation of inflammation) have nonspecific effects on

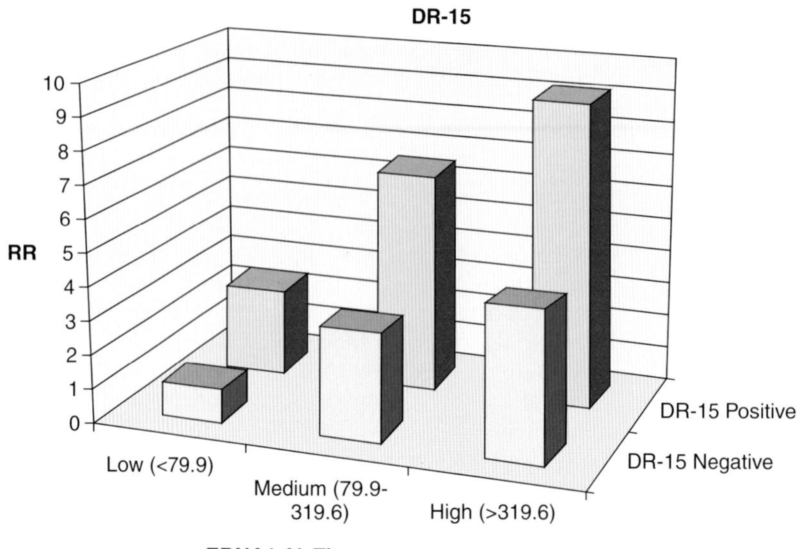

Figure 3–3 Synergistic effect of the HLA-DRB1*1501 (DR15) allele and antibody against the EBV-encoded nuclear antigen 1 (anti-EBNA1 Ab titer) in conferring risk of multiple sclerosis. The relative risk (RR) in comparison with the reference population of DR15-negative subjects with low titers is plotted. (Courtesy of Dr. Alberto Ascherio.)

reducing a threshold for an autoimmune reaction. The exact manifestation of such an autoimmune reaction is probably directed by the activity of disease-specific loci, such as insulin in type 1 diabetes mellitus,[56] and specific environmental triggers, such as smoking, which has a large effect on disease risk in anti-cyclic citrullinated peptide antibody positive (anti-CCP+) rheumatoid arthritis (RA).[57] The *PTPN22* locus is the prototypical example of a pan-autoimmune locus, with validated associations to RA, type 1 diabetes, and thyroiditis; more modest evidence supports a role in systemic lupus erythematosus as well.[58] All of these associations to the *PTPN22* locus are to the same allele that is overrepresented in the respective disease populations. However, the immune system appears to be more complex, because there is now robust evidence that this same allele is underrepresented in inflammatory bowel disease (M. Daly, personal communication). The idea of a balance in immune function that can be tipped toward different disease states depending on the exact genetic constitution and environmental history of an individual is not new but may now begin to be quantitated and modeled as a more comprehensive picture of genetic contributions to autoimmunity is obtained.

In the case of MS, as seen in Figure 3-4, the *IL2RA* locus and the *IL7R* locus may be shared with type 1 diabetes mellitus; more modest evidence exists for the *KIAA0350* locus (now called *CLEC16A*) in both diseases and for the *IL2RA* locus in RA.[3,59,60] However, as with *PTPN22*, the situation is not straightforward, because different alleles have different effects within the *IL2RA* locus. The strongest risk allele for type 1 diabetes has no effect on risk of MS; an independent risk allele within the same locus has a more modest effect on both diseases; and a third allele has opposing effects on each disease, Maier et al.[61] This allelic and

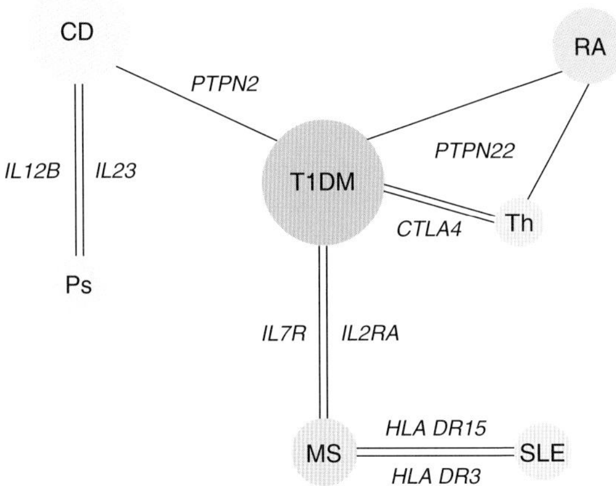

Figure 3–4 Shared susceptibility loci in autoimmune diseases. Each disease is connected to other diseases that share a locus of disease susceptibility at a genome-wide level of significance. The shared locus is listed next to the line that connects each disease pair. The diameter of each colored circle is proportional to the number of risk alleles discovered to date in each disease. On the left margin, a scale reports the number of samples tested using a genome-wide strategy in each disease. CD, Crohn's disease; MS, multiple sclerosis; Ps, psoriasis; RA, rheumatoid arthritis; SLE, systemic lupus erythematosus; T1DM, type 1 diabetes mellitus; Th, thyroiditis. (From data collected by Drs. Chris Cotsapas and Mark Daly.)

phenotypic heterogeneity within the *IL2RA* locus highlights the need for comprehensive and detailed characterization of each autoimmunity locus in each disease: The testing of a single risk allele for a given locus in each disease, as has been done with *PTPN22* for example, is insufficient to resolve the complexity of genetic susceptibility to MS or any other autoimmune disorder.

The greater prevalence of other autoimmune diseases in subjects with MS and their families has long been noted,[62] and it is now possible to dissect the genetic component of these associations. Such studies can give us a more broad-based picture of the dysfunctional immune system of people with MS, one that is integrated into a pan-autoimmune framework. This perspective will prove valuable not only in understanding the pathophysiology found in different individuals with MS but also in guiding the selection of treatments that affect the immune system. Once a drug has been validated in one autoimmune disease, such information could guide the early testing of other diseases or disease subsets that share some of the underlying genetic lesions affecting the targeted immune pathway.

The Impact and Role of Genetic Analysis in Multiple Sclerosis Research and Care

The year 2007 will remain a landmark for the field of genetics in MS, the year that non-MHC susceptibility loci and another MHC susceptibility locus in the vicinity of *HLA-C* were discovered, thus validating the strategy of integrated efforts by a community of researchers able to maximize sample size and access novel technologies effectively. This community effort has now expanded to include many other groups of investigators in an effort to accomplish a definitive and comprehensive assessment of association between susceptibility to MS and common genetic variation found in European populations. The method of this large-scale experiment has been validated, and further collaborative studies are planned. The results of these investigations and their associated evidence of functional consequences on immune function strongly suggest that researchers will have to take into account the genetic architecture of subjects with MS and of healthy control subjects as we move forward in managing the care of MS patients, executing clinical trials, and studying the *in vivo*, *ex vivo*, and *in vitro* characteristics of individuals with MS.

REFERENCES

1. International HapMap Consortium: A haplotype map of the human genome. Nature 2005;437: 1299-1320.
2. Risch N, Merikangas K: The future of genetic studies of complex human diseases. Science 1996;273:1516-1517.
3. International Multiple Sclerosis Genetics Consortium; Hafler DA, Compston A, Sawcer S, et al: Risk alleles for multiple sclerosis identified by a genomewide study. N Engl J Med 2007;357: 851-862.
4. Lundmark F, Duvefelt K, Iacobaeus E, et al: Variation in interleukin 7 receptor alpha chain (IL7R) influences risk of multiple sclerosis. Nat Genet 2007;39:1108-1113.
5. Gregory SG, Schmidt S, Seth P, et al: Interleukin 7 receptor alpha chain (IL7R) shows allelic and functional association with multiple sclerosis. Nat Genet 2007;39:1083-1091.
6. McElroy JP, Oksenberg JR: Multiple sclerosis genetics. Curr Top Microbiol Immunol 2008;318: 45-72.
7. Ascherio A, Munger K: Epidemiology of multiple sclerosis: From risk factors to prevention. Semin Neurol 2008;28:17-28.
8. Jersild C, Svejgaard A, Fog T: HL-A antigens and multiple sclerosis. Lancet 1972;1:1240-1241.
9. Winchester R, Ebers G, Fu SM, et al: B-cell alloantigen Ag 7a in multiple sclerosis. Lancet 1975;2:814.
10. Compston DA, Batchelor JR, McDonald WI: B-lymphocyte alloantigens associated with multiple sclerosis. Lancet 1976;2:1261-1265.
11. Olerup O, Hillert J: HLA class II-associated genetic susceptibility in multiple sclerosis: A critical evaluation. Tissue Antigens 1991;38:1-15.
12. Stewart GJ, Teutsch SM, Castle M, et al: HLA-DR, -DQA1 and -DQB1 associations in Australian multiple sclerosis patients. Eur J Immunogenet 1997;24:81-92.
13. Haines JL, Terwedow HA, Burgess K, et al: Linkage of the MHC to familial multiple sclerosis suggests genetic heterogeneity. The Multiple Sclerosis Genetics Group. Hum Mol Genet 1998;7: 1229-1234.
14. GAMES; Transatlantic Multiple Sclerosis Genetics Cooperative: A meta-analysis of whole genome linkage screens in multiple sclerosis. J Neuroimmunol 2003;143:39-46.
15. Sawcer S, Ban M, Marianian M, et al: A high-density screen for linkage in multiple sclerosis. Am J Hum Genet 2005;77:454-467.
16. Lincoln MR, Montpetit A, Cader MZ, et al: A predominant role for the HLA class II region in the association of the MHC region with multiple sclerosis. Nat Genet 2005;37:1108-1112.
17. Yeo TW, De Jager PL, Gregory SG, et al: A second major histocompatibility complex susceptibility locus for multiple sclerosis. Ann Neurol 2007;61:228-236.
18. Downie AW, Phadke JG: The chief scientist reports: Multiple sclerosis in North East Scotland. Health Bull (Edinb) 1984;42:151-156.
19. Weinshenker BG, Santrach P, Bissonet AS, et al: Major histocompatibility complex class II alleles and the course and outcome of MS: A population-based study. Neurology 1998;51:742-747.
20. Hensiek AE, Sawcer SJ, Feakes R, et al: HLA-DR 15 is associated with female sex and younger age at diagnosis in multiple sclerosis. J Neurol Neurosurg Psychiatry 2002;72:184-187.
21. Weatherby SJ, Thomson W, Pepper L, et al: HLA-DRB1 and disease outcome in multiple sclerosis. J Neurol 2001;248:304-310.
22. Barcellos LF, Sawcer S, Ramsay PP, et al: Heterogeneity at the HLA-DRB1 locus and risk for multiple sclerosis. Hum Mol Genet 2006;15:2813-2824.

23. Smestad C, Brynedal B, Jonasdottir G, et al: The impact of HLA-A and -DRB1 on age at onset, disease course and severity in Scandinavian multiple sclerosis patients. Eur J Neurol 2007;14:835-840.
24. DeLuca GC, Ramagopalan SV, Herrera BM, et al: An extremes of outcome strategy provides evidence that multiple sclerosis severity is determined by alleles at the HLA-DRB1 locus. Proc Natl Acad Sci U S A 2007;104:20896-20901.
25. Harbo HF, Lie BA, Sawcer S, et al: Genes in the HLA class I region may contribute to the HLA class II-associated genetic susceptibility to multiple sclerosis. Tissue Antigens 2004;63:237-247.
26. Barcellos LF, Oksenberg JR, Begovich AB, et al: HLA-DR2 dose effect on susceptibility to multiple sclerosis and influence on disease course. Am J Hum Genet 2003;72:710-716.
27. Oksenberg JR, Barcellos LF, Cree BA, et al: Mapping multiple sclerosis susceptibility to the HLA-DR locus in African Americans. Am J Hum Genet 2004;74:160-167.
28. Fogdell-Hahn A, Ligers A, Gronning M, et al: Multiple sclerosis: A modifying influence of HLA class I genes in an HLA class II associated autoimmune disease. Tissue Antigens 2000;55: 140-148.
29. de Jong BA, Huizinga TW, Zanelli E, et al: Evidence for additional genetic risk indicators of relapse-onset MS within the HLA region. Neurology 2002;59:549-555.
30. Noseworthy JH, Lucchinetti C, Rodriguez M, Weinshenker BG: Multiple sclerosis. N Engl J Med 2000;343:938-952.
31. Kira J: Multiple sclerosis in the Japanese population. Lancet Neurol 2003;2:117-127.
32. Brassat D, Salemi G, Barcellos LF, et al: The HLA locus and multiple sclerosis in Sicily. Neurology 2005;64:361-363.
33. Fukazawa T, Kikuchi S, Sasaki H, et al: Genomic HLA profiles of MS in Hokkaido, Japan: Important role of DPB1*0501 allele. J Neurol 2000;247:175-178.
34. Naito S, Kuroiwa Y, Itoyama T, et al: HLA and Japanese MS. Tissue Antigens 1978;12:19-24.
35. Saruhan-Direskeneli G, Esin S, Baykan-Kurt B, et al: HLA-DR and -DQ associations with multiple sclerosis in Turkey. Hum Immunol 1997;55:59-65.
36. Compston A: The genetic epidemiology of multiple sclerosis. Philos Trans R Soc Lond B Biol Sci 1999;354:1623-1634.
37. Alaez C, Corona T, Ruano L, et al: Mediterranean and Amerindian MHC class II alleles are associated with multiple sclerosis in Mexicans. Acta Neurol Scand 2005;112:317-322.
38. Compston A, Coles A: Multiple sclerosis. Lancet 2002;359:1221-1231.
39. Marrosu MG, Murru R, Murru MR, et al: Dissection of the HLA association with multiple sclerosis in the founder isolated population of Sardinia. Hum Mol Genet 2001;10:2907-2916.
40. Duvefelt K, Anderson M, Fogdell-Hahn A, Hillert J: A NOTCH4 association with multiple sclerosis is secondary to HLA-DR*1501. Tissue Antigens 2004;63:13-20.
41. Fernandez-Arquero M, Arroyo R, Rubio A, et al: Primary association of a TNF gene polymorphism with susceptibility to multiple sclerosis. Neurology 1999;53:1361-1363.
42. Fernando MM, Stevens CR, Walsh EC, et al. Defining the role of the MHC in autoimmunity: a review and pooled analysis. PLOS Genet 2008;4:e1000024.
43. Ota K, Matsui M, Milford EL, et al: T-cell recognition of an immunodominant myelin basic protein epitope in multiple sclerosis. Nature 1990;346:183-187.
44. Jingwu Z, Medaer R, Hashim GA, et al: Myelin basic protein-specific T lymphocytes in multiple sclerosis and controls: Precursor frequency, fine specificity, and cytotoxicity. Ann Neurol 1992;32:330-338.
45. Ohashi T, Yamamura T, Inobe J, et al: Analysis of proteolipid protein (PLP)-specific T cells in multiple sclerosis: Identification of PLP 95-116 as an HLA-DR2,w15-associated determinant. Int Immunol 1995;7:1771-1778.
46. Greer JM, Sobel RA, Sette A, et al: Immunogenic and encephalitogenic epitope clusters of myelin proteolipid protein. J Immunol 1996;156:371-319.
47. Wallstrom E, Khademi M, Andersson M, et al: Increased reactivity to myelin oligodendrocyte glycoprotein peptides and epitope mapping in HLA DR2(15)+ multiple sclerosis. Eur J Immunol 1998;28:3329-3335.
48. Spielman RS, Ewens WJ: The TDT and other family-based tests for linkage disequilibrium and association. Am J Hum Genet 1996;59:983-939.
49. Ramagopalan SV, Anderson C, Sadovnick AD, Ebers GC: Genomewide study of multiple sclerosis. N Engl J Med 2007;357:2199-2200; author reply 2200-2201.
50. Zhang Z, Duvefelt K, Svensson F, et al: Two genes encoding immune-regulatory molecules (LAG3 and IL7R) confer susceptibility to multiple sclerosis. Genes Immun 2005;6:145-152.
51. De Jager PL, Baecher-Allan C, Maier LM, et al. The role of the CD58 locus in multiple sclerosis. Proc Natl Acad Sci U S A, Feb 23, 2009.

52. Amarenco P, Goldstein LB, Szarek M, et al: Effects of intense low-density lipoprotein cholesterol reduction in patients with stroke or transient ischemic attack: The Stroke Prevention by Aggressive Reduction in Cholesterol Levels (SPARCL) trial. Stroke 2007;38:3198-3204.
53. Lang HL, Jacobsen H, Ikemizu S, et al: A functional and structural basis for TCR cross-reactivity in multiple sclerosis. Nat Immunol 2002;3:940-943.
54. Li Q, Spriggs MK, Kovats S, et al: Epstein-Barr virus uses HLA class II as a cofactor for infection of B lymphocytes. J Virol 1997;71:4657-4662.
55. De Jager PL, Simon KC, Munger KL, et al: Integrating risk factors. HLA-DRB1*1501 and Epstein-Barr virus in multiple sclerosis. Neurology 2008;70(13 Pt 2):1113-1118.
56. Bennett ST, Todd JA: Human type 1 diabetes and the insulin gene: Principles of mapping polygenes. Annu Rev Genet 1996;30:343-370.
57. Padyukov L, Silva C, Stolt P, et al: A gene-environment interaction between smoking and shared epitope genes in HLA-DR provides a high risk of seropositive rheumatoid arthritis. Arthritis Rheum 2004;50:3085-3092.
58. Wu H, Cantor RM, Graham DS, et al: Association analysis of the R620W polymorphism of protein tyrosine phosphatase PTPN22 in systemic lupus erythematosus families: Increased T allele frequency in systemic lupus erythematosus patients with autoimmune thyroid disease. Arthritis Rheum 2005;52:2396-2402.
59. Todd JA, Walker NM, Cooper JD, et al: Robust associations of four new chromosome regions from genome-wide analyses of type 1 diabetes. Nat Genet 2007;39:857-864.
60. Wellcome Trust Case Control Consortium: Genome-wide association study of 14,000 cases of seven common diseases and 3,000 shared controls. Nature 2007;447:661-678.
61. Maier LM, Lowe CE, Cooper J, et al. IL2RA genetic heterogeneity in multiple selerosis and type 1 diabetes susceptibility and soluble interleukin-2 receptor production. PLOS Genet, Jan 2009;5: e1000322.
62. Barcellos LF, Kamdar BB, Ramsay PP, et al: Clustering of autoimmune diseases in families with a high-risk for multiple sclerosis: A descriptive study. Lancet Neurol 2006;5:924-931.

4 Epidemiology of Multiple Sclerosis: Environmental Factors

ALBERTO ASCHERIO • KASSANDRA L. MUNGER

Epidemiology in Perspective

Epidemiology is the study of the distribution and determinants of disease frequency in human populations. By studying who is affected, where, and when, epidemiologists try to obtain clues about the causes of a disease, develop hypotheses, and design specific studies to test those hypotheses. At the core of epidemiology is the notion of "webs of causation"[1]; that is, the awareness that diseases are almost always the result of multiple contingencies, most often including several aspects of the environment as well as genetic predisposition, so that no single cause can be identified. Epidemiologists consider some aspect of the environment as "causally associated" with a disease if their modification results in a change in disease frequency. Well-known historical examples include the relations between poor sewage disposal and cholera, consumption of a diet deficient in thiamine and pellagra, and, more recently, prone sleep position and risk of sudden infant death. Evidence of causality and even disease prevention (e.g., reduction in infant deaths after implementation of the "back to sleep" campaign[2]) have often occurred without a complete understanding of the underlying biologic mechanisms. Indeed, reliance on the identification of biologic mechanisms as a *sine qua non* for establishing causality is probably unwise, because it may delay progress in disease prevention. On the other hand, knowledge of molecular mechanisms clearly strengthens the evidence for causality. Multiple, well-conducted epidemiologic investigations may lead to experimental studies, but experimental proof of causality is not uncommonly unfeasible, unethical, or unaffordable, and public health decisions need to rely primarily on observational data. Such has been the case, for example, with interventions to reduce lung cancer incidence by reducing exposure to tobacco smoke.

As discussed in this chapter, epidemiologic evidence points to three environmental risk factors—infection with the Epstein-Barr virus (EBV), low levels of vitamin D, and cigarette smoking—whose association with multiple sclerosis (MS) seems to satisfy in varying degrees most of the criteria that support causality, including temporality (i.e., the cause must precede the effect), strength, consistency, biologic gradient, and plausibility. None of these associations, however, has been tested experimentally in humans, and only one (vitamin D deficiency) is presently amenable to experimental interventions. This chapter also summarizes the evidence, albeit more sparse and inconsistent, linking other environmental factors to MS risk.

Descriptive Epidemiology of Multiple Sclerosis

For many years, it appeared that the "who, where, and when" of MS epidemiology was well understood. However, some aspects of MS epidemiology may be changing, notably the observations of an attenuation of the latitude gradient[3,4] and the increasing female-to-male ratio.[5] In this section, we discuss the "classic" view of MS epidemiology, some of which has been known for more than 50 years, and then some recent developments that may provide new clues to the etiology of MS.

CLASSIC VIEW

MS is the most common neurologic disease in young adults. Incidence rates are low in childhood and adolescence (<6/100,000/year) high in the middle to late twenties and early thirties (11 to 18/100,000/year in high-risk populations), and gradually decline thereafter, with rates less than 9/100,000/year among those older than 45 years of age.[3,6] Women are approximately twice as likely as men to develop MS,[7,8] and the lifetime risk among white women is about 1 in 200.[3,9] MS exhibits a worldwide latitude gradient, with high prevalence and incidence in Northern Europe,[7] Canada,[10,11] the northern United States,[3,12,13] and southern Australia[14] and decreasing prevalence and incidence in regions closer to the equator.[15] Exceptions to the latitude gradient exist and include a lower than expected prevalence in Japan[16] and higher than expected prevalence and incidence in the Mediterranean islands of Sardinia and Sicily.[7] Kurtzke[17] summarized the early descriptive studies by depicting areas of high (≥30/100,000), medium (5 to 29/100,000), and low (<5/100,000) prevalence of MS; we have updated his figures with more recent prevalence estimates[7,16,18-24] (Fig. 4-1). A more comprehensive review of MS incidence and prevalence worldwide was published in 2005.[18] It is important to note that differences in estimated incidence across countries or time periods can result from differences in study design, case ascertainment, or diagnostic criteria, rather than from real changes in disease occurrence. Differences in prevalence are even more difficult to interpret, because they may reflect increased survival or earlier diagnosis, both of which can occur even if the incidence is the same.[25] In spite of these limitations, the collective data do support a higher risk of MS at higher latitudes, both north and south of the equator.

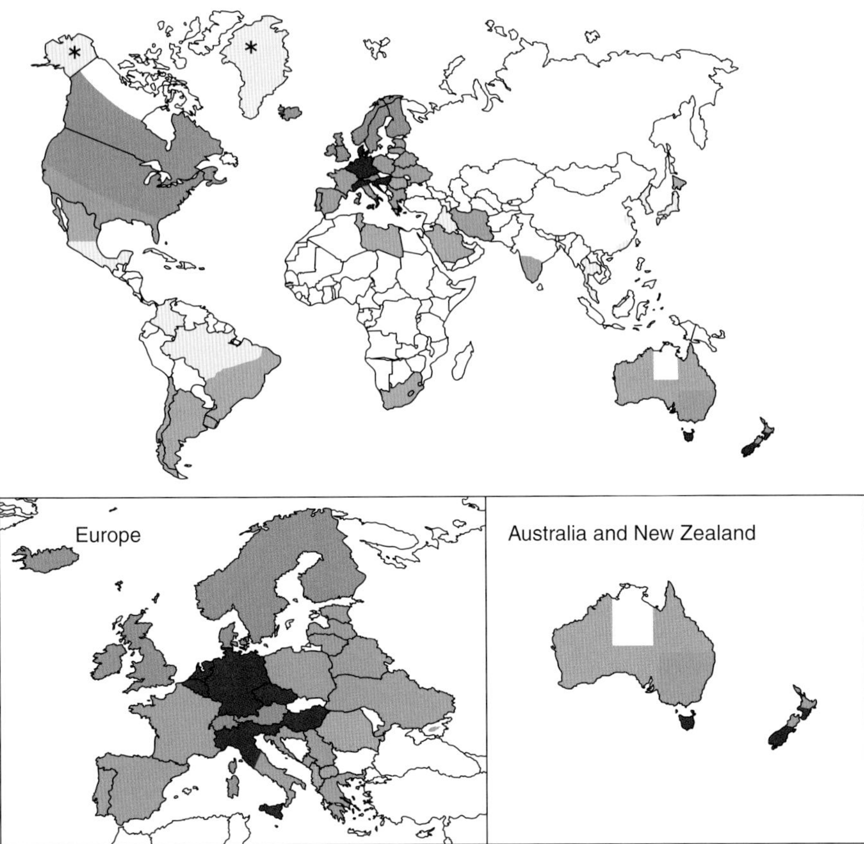

Figure 4–1 Worldwide prevalence estimates of multiple sclerosis. Blue, more than 90 cases per 100,000 population; purple, 60 to 89/100,000; green, 30 to 59/100,000; orange, 5 to 29/100,000; yellow, fewer than 5/100,000; white, insufficient data. An asterisk indicates that data for that region or country are older and should be interpreted cautiously.

The existence of the latitude gradient alone is not enough to support an environmental component, because it could be explained by genetic differences.[18,26] However, studies of MS incidence and prevalence among migrant populations also support a role for environmental factors. These studies have limitations, in that migrants may be different from nonmigrants in socioeconomic and health status, may not utilize local health care resources, and therefore they may be less likely to be diagnosed; in addition, enumeration of the immigrant population for disease statistics may be difficult or impossible.[25,27] Nevertheless, migrant studies on MS collectively support a decreased prevalence of MS among those who migrate from high- to low-risk areas, particularly if the migration occurs before 15 years of age.[27] Moreover, one study found a decreased prevalence of MS in all age groups among immigrants from Europe to Australia, suggesting that the protective effect may extend into adulthood as well.[28] Studies within the United States have also supported a decreased risk of MS among migrants from northern (>41° to 42° N), high-risk parts of the country to southern (<37° N), low-risk regions.[29,30] The study of U.S. veterans[30] is particularly compelling because of its large sample size and rigorous design. In this study, Kurtzke observed that individuals who were born in the northern United States but migrated to the southern part of the country before joining the military had a 50% reduced risk of MS compared with those who did not migrate (Fig. 4-2).

Fewer studies have been conducted among migrants from low- to high-risk areas. In general, these studies have found that a low risk of MS is retained after migration, but that the offspring of migrants have a higher risk of MS, similar to that in the host country.[27,31-35] In the U.S. veterans study,[30] individuals who were born in the southern part of the country and migrated to northern states before entering the military had a 20% increased risk of MS, and those migrating from the middle tier of states to northern regions had a 31% increased risk (see Fig. 4-2). More recently, in a study conducted in the French West Indies (a low-risk area), an increased risk of MS was found among individuals who had moved to France (a high-risk area) and then returned to the West Indies. The increase in risk was greatest among those who migrated to France before the age of 15 years.[36]

RECENT DEVELOPMENTS

The incidence of MS appears to have been relatively stable over the past 50 years in several high-risk areas, including Denmark[6] and the northern United States,[37] but there is some evidence that MS may be increasing in Japan[16] and in parts of Southern Europe, most notably in Sardinia.[38] Interestingly, the island of Malta has continued to experience low, stable rates of MS[39] despite its proximity to Sardinia and Sicily and a high frequency of the MS-associated HLA-DRB1*1501 allele.[40] There is also evidence of an increased female-to-male ratio in MS incidence. In Canada, the

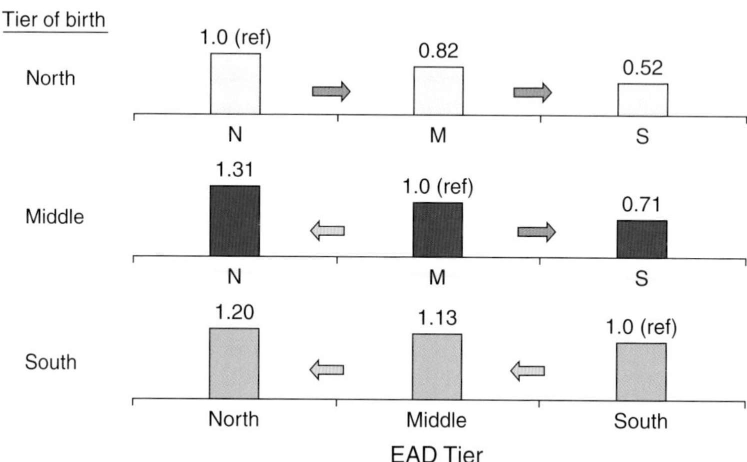

Figure 4–2 Relative risk for multiple sclerosis among white male veterans of World War II or the Korean conflict, by tier of residence at birth and at entry into active duty (EAD). Data are for coterminous United States only. *P* values for no change in birthplace risk are as follows: All, .0003; North, .003; Middle, .002; and South, .57. Adapted from Kurtzke, Beebe, and Norman. Epidemiology of multiple sclerosis in US veterans: III: Migration and the risk of MS. Neurology 1985;35:672-678.

female-to-male ratio apparently has increased from approximately 2:1 among individuals born in the 1930s and 1940s to approximately 3:1 among those born in the 1970s.[5] This change is strongly correlated with, and could be at least in part explained by, a sharp increase in the female-to-male ratio in smoking behavior (unpublished data), because smoking is a strong risk factor for MS (see later discussion).

An attenuation of the latitude gradient was observed independently in a population of U.S. nurses[3] and in U.S. military veterans.[4] Among nurses born between 1920 and 1946 and among veterans of World War II or the Korean conflict, those living in the northern tier of states (>41° to 42° N) had a greater than threefold increased risk of MS compared to those in the southern tier (<37° N). Among Vietnam and Gulf War veterans, however, this gradient was attenuated to less than twofold, and among nurses born between 1947 and 1964 it completely disappeared (Fig. 4-3). Because the methods used to determine rates of MS in the early and later cohorts were the same, and because the individuals in the cohorts had similar socioeconomic status[3] or access to health care,[4] this attenuation was unlikely to be due to artifact. A change of this magnitude over such a short period of time argues for an environmental, rather than a genetic, explanation of the latitude gradient; as discussed later, this environmental factor may involve changes in patterns of infection or sun exposure, or both. Further, the attenuation was probably caused by an increase in MS incidence in the southern United States, because incidence rates in the northern states, based at least on data from the longitudinal study in Olmsted County, Minnesota, seem to have remained relatively stable.[37] An attenuation of the latitude gradient in Europe has also been observed; however, no systematic studies have assessed this gradient within the same population over

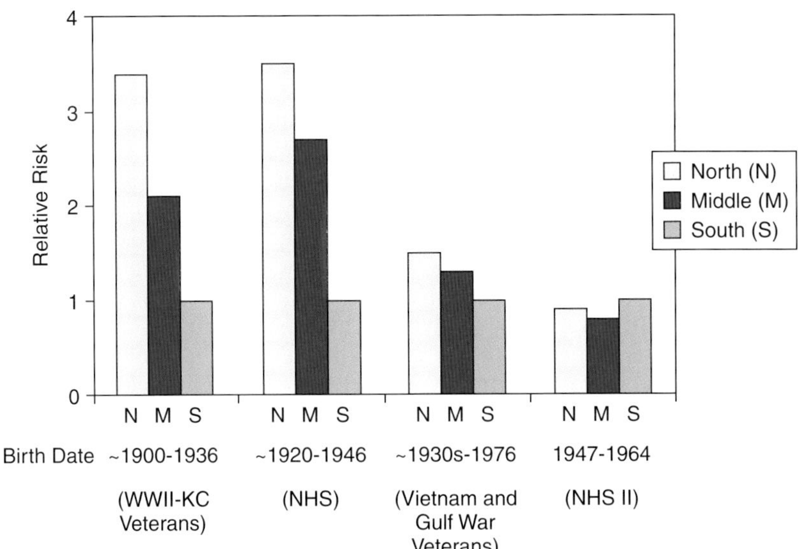

Figure 4–3 Relative risk for multiple sclerosis by latitude at birth in different birth cohorts of U.S. white women. KC, Korean conflict; NHS, Nurses Health Study; NHSII, Nurses Health Study II; WWII, World War II. Adapted from Hernan et al. Neurology 1999;53:1711-1718 and Wallin et al. Ann Neurol 2001;55:65-71.

time, and the attenuation therefore may be due to improved study methodology and case ascertainment, particularly within the United Kingdom.[18]

Infection and Multiple Sclerosis

The possibility of an infectious cause was considered early in MS history, and numerous viruses and bacteria were, at different times, implicated as likely etiologic agents. The results of early studies, based on microscopic examination of pathologic material and attempts to transmit the disease to animals, often were null or spuriously positive because of contamination and could not be replicated. Later, numerous serologic studies were conducted, often demonstrating significantly elevated antibody titers against several viruses in MS patients compared with healthy controls, but these differences were probably an epiphenomenon of the immune activation rather than being of etiologic significance.[41] In part as a consequence of these investigations, many researchers became skeptical about the existence of an infectious agent causing MS, and this skepticism persists today.

Epidemiologic clues to the hypothetical role of infection in MS are complex and often seem to point in opposite directions. On the one hand, results of family studies, including investigations of half-siblings, adopted children, and spouses of individuals with MS, support a strong genetic component as the leading explanation of MS clustering within families and provide little evidence of person-to-person transmission.[42] On the other, there are well-documented, albeit controversial,[43] reports of epidemics of MS, most notably in the Faroe Islands,[44] that are most easily explained by the introduction and transmission of an infectious agent. To reconcile these findings, it has been postulated that MS is a rare complication of a common infection, with the disease occurring in genetically or otherwise predisposed individuals. In this scenario, the epidemics would be a consequence of the introduction of the MS-causing agent for the first time in remote, previously naïve populations.[45] Two hypotheses as to the nature of this infection have been proposed: (1) the responsible microorganism is more common in areas of high MS prevalence (the "prevalence" hypothesis), and (2) the MS-causing agent is ubiquitous and more easily transmitted in areas of low MS prevalence, where infection occurs predominantly in infancy, when it would be less harmful and more likely to confer protective immunity. The latter proposal is called the "poliomyelitis" hypothesis, by analogy with the epidemiology of poliomyelitis before vaccination.[46] The poliomyelitis hypothesis is also consistent with the higher prevalence of MS in communities with better hygiene,[47] in individuals with higher education,[48,49] and in those with late age at infection with common viruses,[50] as well as the general lack of increase in MS incidence among individuals migrating from low- to high-prevalence areas.[27] However, the poliomyelitis hypothesis cannot explain the reduced risk of MS among migrants from high- to low-risk areas and, in fact, would predict an *increase* in MS risk in this circumstance, whereas the prevalence hypothesis is consistent with the observations.

Failure to identify a specific microbe as the cause of MS, despite evidence that is consistent with some role for infection in at least modulating MS risk, has strengthened support for a third, more general, "hygiene" hypothesis, according to which exposure to multiple infections in childhood primes the immune responses later in life toward a less inflammatory and a less autoimmunogenic profile.[51] The hygiene hypothesis can explain all the features of MS epidemiology that are explained by the original formulation of the poliomyelitis hypothesis. In addition, the protective effect of migration from high- to low-MS areas, which is paradoxical under the poliomyelitis hypothesis, could be beneficial because of increased exposure of migrants to parasitic and other infections in the low-risk area. At the population level, prevalence of MS is positively correlated with high levels of hygiene, as measured, for example, by prevalence of intestinal parasites.[52] The improving hygienic conditions in southern Europe in the last few decades could explain the increased prevalence of MS reported in multiple surveys (although whether there was a true increase in MS incidence remains unsettled).[7] It is also interesting that infection with intestinal helminths, which is highly prevalent in developing countries, had been reported to cause an immune deviation with attenuation of helper T-cell 1 cellular immune responses and remission of MS.[53] Finally, the hygiene hypothesis provides a convincing explanation for the observations that infectious mononucleosis (IM) is associated with an increased risk of MS (relative risk [RR] = 2.3; $P < .00000001$)[54] and that the epidemiology of IM is strikingly similar to that of MS (Table 4-1).[55] Because IM is common in individuals who are first infected with EBV in adolescence or adulthood[56] but rare when EBV infection occurs in childhood, it is a strong marker of age at EBV infection, which is itself strongly correlated with socioeconomic development across populations and with socioeconomic status within populations.[57] An exception to this pattern is seen in Asia, where EBV infection occurs uniformly early in life and IM is thus rare. It is noteworthy that the incidence of MS remains relatively low in Asian countries, including Japan, despite the fast industrialization and reduction of infectious diseases,[58] although there is evidence that the incidence may be increasing in Japan.[16]

According to the hygiene hypothesis, the association between IM and MS risk does not reflect a causal effect of EBV but rather the indirect manifestation of a common cause; that is, both MS and IM are the result of high hygiene and a resulting low burden of infection during childhood. An important prediction of this hypothesis is that MS risk will be high among individuals reared in a highly hygienic environment, even if they do not happen to be infected with EBV later in life, whereas,

TABLE 4–1 Similarities between Multiple Sclerosis (MS) and Infectious Mononucleosis (IM) Epidemiology

Parameter	MS	IM
Age at peak incidence (yr)	25-34	15-24
Age at onset	F < M	F < M
Geography:		
Extremely rare in the tropics	+++	+++
Latitude gradient within temperate regions	+++	+++
Rare in Japan	+++	+++
Rare in Inuits	++	++
Positive association with SES	+	++
Incidence in blacks < whites	+	++
Incidence in Asians < whites	++	++

+++, Strong evidence; ++, moderate evidence; +, weak evidence; F, female; M, male; SES, socioeconomic status.

if EBV has a causal role in MS, individuals who are not infected with EBV would have a low risk of MS.[59] The data on this point are unequivocal: individuals who are not infected with EBV, even though they have the same hygienic upbringing as those with IM, have an extremely low risk of MS (odds ratio [OR] from meta-analysis = 0.06; $P < .00000001$) (Table 4-2). The contrast could not be sharper or more consistent: MS risk among individuals who are not infected with EBV is at least 10-fold lower than that of individuals who are EBV-positive, and 20-fold lower than that of individuals with a history of IM.[59] Because studies in pediatric MS[60,61] rule out a common genetic resistance to MS and EBV infection,[59] we can conclude either that EBV itself or some other factor closely related to EBV is a strong causal risk factor for MS or that MS itself strongly predisposes to EBV infection.

Temporality is the only truly necessary criteria for causality. The association between EBV infection and MS is strong and consistent across multiple studies in different populations, and there is to some extent a biologic gradient (higher risk associated with severity of infection, as indicated by history of IM). Until recently, all studies on MS and infection used a cross-sectional design and could not completely rule out the possibility that EBV infection was a consequence rather than a cause of MS. However, the results of four longitudinal serologic studies have now been published (Table 4-3).[62-65] The most consistent finding across these studies is that, among individuals who will develop MS, there is an elevation of serum antibodies against the EBV nuclear antigen 1 (EBNA1) that precedes the onset of MS symptoms by many years. The presence of anti-EBNA1 antibodies is a marker of past infection with EBV, because titers typically rise only weeks after the acute infection. Further, there is no evidence in clinical studies of acute primary EBV infection in individuals with MS.[66] Taken together, these results indicate that MS is a consequence rather than a cause of EBV infection.

Until recently, EBV had not been found in MS lesions,[67,68] and therefore the link between EBV and MS was postulated to be mediated by indirect mechanisms. The leading hypothesis was that the immune response to EBV infection in genetically susceptible individuals cross-reacts with myelin antigens (molecular mimicry). The discovery that MS patients have an increased frequency and broadened specificity of CD4-positive T cells recognizing EBNA1[69] and the identification of two EBV peptides (one of which is from EBNA1) as targets of the immune response in the cerebrospinal fluid of MS patients[70] provided support to the molecular mimicry theory. Other proposed hypotheses included the activation of superantigens,[71] an increased expression of alpha B-crystallin,[72] and infection of autoreactive B lymphocytes.[73]

However, in a recent, rigorous pathologic study,[74] large numbers of EBV-infected B cells were found in the brain of most of MS patients. These cells were more numerous in areas with active inflammatory infiltrates, where cytotoxic CD8-positive T cells displaying an activated phenotype were seen contiguous to the EBV-infected cells. Alone, these pathologic findings provide only suggestive evidence for a causal role of EBV in MS, because the infiltration of EBV-infected B cells could be secondary to the inflammatory process that is the hallmark of MS, but their convergence with the epidemiologic evidence described earlier[59] is so striking that noncausal explanations become improbable. However, independent replication of these findings is needed before any conclusion can be drawn. The strong increase in MS risk after EBV infection and (if confirmed) the presence of EBV in MS lesions suggest that antiviral drugs or a vaccine against EBV could contribute to MS treatment and prevention. Although antiviral drugs have been

TABLE 4–2 Odds Ratio (OR) of Multiple Sclerosis (MS) in Epstein-Barr Virus (EBV) Seronegative Versus Seropositive Subjects

Study	Ref. No.	*EBV Status* Cases +	Cases −	Controls +	Controls −	OR of MS for Seronegativity	Exact 95% CI
Sumaya et al., 1980	186	155	2	76	5	0.2	0.02-1.24
Bray et al., 1983	187	309	4	363	43	0.11	0.03-0.31
Larsen et al., 1985	188	93	0	78	15	0	0-0.05
Sumaya et al., 1985	189	104	0	99	5	0	0-1.07
Shirodaria et al., 1987	190	26	0	24	2	0	0-5.29
Ferrante et al., 1987	191	29	1	31	11	0.1	0-0.76
Munch et al., 1997	192	137	1	124	14	0.06	0-0.44
Myhr et al., 1998	193	144	0	162	8	0	0-0.67
Wagner et al., 2000	194	107	0	153	10	0	0-0.66
Ascherio et al., 2001	62	143	1	269	18	0.1	0-0.68
Haahr et al., 2004	195	153	0	50	3	0	0-0.82
Sundstrom et al., 2004	63	234	0	693	9	0	0-1.5
Ponsonby et al., 2005	196	136	0	252	9	0	0-0.96
Total		1770	9	2374	152	OR_{MH} = 0.06	0.03-0.13[†]

OR_{MH}, Mantel-Haenszel odds ratio.

*Confidence interval calculated as described in Mehta CR, Patel NR, Gray R: Computing an exact confidence interval for the common odds ratio in several 2 x 2 contingency tables. J Am Stat Assoc 1985;78:969-973.

†Cornfield confidence interval; $P < .000000001$.

From Ascherio A, Munger KL: Environmental risk factors for multiple sclerosis: Part I. The role of infection. Ann Neurol 2007;61:288-299.

tried in the past for MS treatment with borderline results,[75-77] none of the treatment regimens used was sufficiently effective against latent EBV infection.

Several aspects of MS epidemiology cannot be explained by EBV infection, indicating that other factors must contribute.[59] Genes are clearly important, and it is of interest that the association between anti-EBNA1 titers and MS risk has been found in both HLA-DRB1*1501–positive and HLA-DRB1*1501–negative individuals.[78] Variations in EBV strains could also play a role, although evidence in support of this hypothesis remains limited.[79,80] Many other infectious agents have been hypothesized to be related to MS, mostly because of pathologic studies or their role in animal models. Recent candidates include *Chlamydia pneumoniae*,[81-84] human herpesvirus 6,[85-87] retroviruses,[88,89] and coronaviruses,[90] but there are no convincing epidemiologic studies linking these infections to

TABLE 4–3 Comparison of Four Prospective Case-Control Studies of Immunoglobulin G Antibodies against Epstein-Barr Virus (EBV) and Risk of Multiple Sclerosis (MS)

Study	Population	No. Cases/ Controls	% Females	Age at MS Onset (Median [Range])	Time from Blood Collection to MS Onset, Yr (Median [Range])	RR (95% CI)†	
						EBNA1	VCA
Ascherio, 2001	Nurses' Health Study	18/36	100	52 (39-66)	1.9 (<1-6.5)	2.7 (1.0-7.2)	1.6 (0.7-3.7)
Sundström, 2004	Västerbotten County, Sweden	73/219	67	34 (22-65)	NA (<1->15)	4.5 (1.9-11)	0.86 (0.38-2.0)
Levin, 2005	U.S. Army	83/166	35	27 (18-41)*	4 (<1-11)*	3.0 (1.2-7.3)	1.3 (0.6-2.9)
DeLorenze, 2006	Kaiser Permanente, northern California	42/79	86	45 (24-69)	15 (<1-32)	1.8 (1.1-2.9)	1.2 (0.66-2.4)

EBNA1, EBV nuclear antigen 1; NA, not applicable; RR, relative risk; VCA, viral capsid antigen.

*Mean (range).

†For the Ascheno, Levin, and DeLorenze studies, reported RR is for a fourfold increase in antibody titers; for Sundström, RR is for "high" vs "low" activity to EBV antigen.

Data from Munger K, Ascherio A: Risk factors in the development of multiple sclerosis. Expert Rev Clin Immunol 2007;3:739-748, Future Drugs Ltd.

MS risk. Noninfectious factors may also be important, and prominent among them are vitamin D and cigarette smoking.

Sunlight Exposure and Vitamin D

One of the strongest correlates of latitude is the duration and intensity of sunlight, which in ecologic studies is inversely correlated with MS prevalence.[92-94] Because exposure to sunlight is for most people the major source of vitamin D,[95] average levels of vitamin D also display a strong latitude gradient. Ultraviolet B (UV-B) radiation (290 to 320 nm) converts cutaneous 7-dehydrocholesterol to previtamin D_3. Previtamin D_3 spontaneously isomerizes to vitamin D_3, which is then hydroxylated to $25(OH)D_3$ (25-hydroxyvitamin D_3), the main circulating form of the vitamin, and then to $1,25(OH)_2D_3$ (1,25-dihydroxyvitamin D_3), the biologically active hormone.[95] However, during the winter months at latitudes greater than 42° N (e.g., Boston, MA), even prolonged sun exposure is insufficient to generate vitamin D,[96] and levels decline.[97,98] Use of supplements or high consumption of fatty fish (a good source of vitamin D) or vitamin D–fortified foods (mostly milk in the United States) may partially compensate for this decline, but few people consume large enough amounts of vitamin D, and seasonal deficiency is common. A link between vitamin D deficiency and MS was proposed more than 30 years ago as a possible explanation of the latitude gradient and of the lower prevalence of MS in fishing communities with high levels of fish intake[99]; however, the immunomodulatory effects of vitamin D were not known, and the hypothesis did not generate much interest at the time. After the discovery that the vitamin D receptor is expressed in several cells in the immune system and is a potent immunomodulator,[100] a series of experiments revealed a protective role of $1,25(OH)_2D_3$ in several autoimmune conditions and in transplant rejection.[100] The effects in experimental autoimmune encephalomyelitis, an animal model of MS, were particularly striking: injection of $1,25(OH)_2D_3$ was found to completely prevent the clinical and pathologic signs of disease,[101,102] whereas vitamin D deficiency accelerated the disease onset.[102,103]

With vitamin D deficiency becoming a biologically plausible risk factor for MS, several epidemiologic studies were conducted to determine whether exposure to sunlight or vitamin D intake is associated with MS risk. The main results of these studies are shown in Table 4-4, and their strengths and limitations are discussed in the following paragraphs.

ECOLOGIC STUDIES

As mentioned earlier, the results of ecologic studies support an inverse association between sunlight exposure and MS risk. However, because people living in the same area share many characteristics other than the level of sunlight, the consensus is that evidence from these studies is weak.

DATABASE/LINKAGE ANALYSES

In an exploratory investigation based on death certificates, working outdoors was associated with a significantly lower MS mortality in areas of high, but not low, sunlight.[104] In a separate study in the United Kingdom, the skin cancer rate,

TABLE 4–4 Summary of Studies on Sun Exposure, Vitamin D, and Risk of Multiple Sclerosis (MS)

Author and Year	Population	No. Cases and Controls	Exposure	Main Results
Ecologic Studies				
Acheson et al., 1960	U.S. military veterans	556 MS cases	Average annual hours of sunshine	Correlation with MS prevalence: –0.73
			Average December solar radiation	Correlation with MS prevalence: –0.80
Leibowitz et al., 1967	Immigrants to Israel	—	Average annual hours of sunshine	Correlation with MS prevalence: –0.88
van der Mei et al., 2001	Australia	—	Ambient ultraviolet radiation	Correlation with MS prevalence: –0.91
Database/Linkage Analyses				
Freedman et al., 2000	United States	4,282 MS deaths; 115,195 deaths from other noncancer causes	Residential sun exposure	High vs low exposure: OR = 0.53 (95% CI, 0.48-0.57)
			Occupational sun exposure	Outdoor vs indoor occupation: OR = 0.74 (95% CI, 0.61-0.89)
Goldacre et al., 2004	Oxford region, England	5,004 cases; 432,091 non-cases	Skin cancer diagnosis in MS patients	Rate ratio = 0.49 (95% CI, 0.24-0.91)
Case-Control Studies				
Antonovsky et al., 1965	Israel	241 cases, 964 controls	≥2 hr outdoors daily in summer as youngster	89% cases vs 82% controls (P = .02)
			>5 hr outdoors daily in summer	63% cases vs 55% controls (P = .05)
Cendrowski et al., 1969	Western Poland	300 cases, 300 controls	Average time spent outdoors daily in summer before age 15 yr	No significant differences between cases and controls

TABLE 4–4 Summary of Studies on Sun Exposure, Vitamin D, and Risk of Multiple Sclerosis (MS)

Author and Year	Population	No. Cases and Controls	Exposure	Main Results
van der Mei et al., 2003	Tasmania, Australia	136 cases, 272 controls	≥2 hr sun exposure daily in summer ages 6-10 yr	OR = 0.50 (95% CI, 0.24-1.02)
			≥1 hr sun exposure daily in winter ages 6-10 yr	OR = 0.47 (95% CI, 0.26-0.84)
			Actinic damage to skin	More vs less: OR = 0.32 (95% CI, 0.11-0.88)
Kampman et al., 2007	Northern Norway	152 cases, 402 controls	Time spent outdoors in summer ages 16-20 yr	OR = 0.55 (95% CI, 0.39-0.78)
			Consumption of boiled/fried fish ≥ 3 times/week	OR = 0.55 (95% CI, 0.33-0.92)
Islam et al., 2007	North American twins	79 disease- and exposure-discordant monozygotic twin pairs	Sun-exposure index determined by seasonal/temperature-related outdoor exposure, sun exposure–related activities, and participation in team sports	For every 1 unit increase in the sun-exposure index (i.e., greater sun exposure), OR = 0.75 (95% CI, 0.62-0.90)
Munter et al., 2004	Nurses' Health Study, Nurses' Health Study II	173 cases	Total dietary intake of vitamin D	Top vs bottom quintile of intake: Rate ratio = 0.67 (95% CI, 0.40-1.12)
			Vitamin D intake from supplements	≥400 IU/day vs none: Rate ratio = 0.59 (95% CI, 0.38-0.91)
Munger et al., 2006	Active-duty U.S. military personnel	257 cases, 514 controls	Serum levels of 25(OH)D	Top vs bottom quintile of 25(OH)D in whites: OR = 0.38 (95% CI, 0.19-0.75)

CI, confidence interval; OR, odds ratio.
Data from Munger K, Ascherio A: Risk factors in the development of multiple sclerosis. Expert Rev Clin Immunol 2007;3:739-748, Future Drugs Ltd.

a marker of sunlight exposure, was found to be about 50% lower than expected among individuals with MS (P = .03).[106] Although the results of these investigations are consistent with a protective effect of UV light exposure, they could also represent "reverse causation" (i.e., individuals with MS could reduce their exposure to sunlight after disease onset).

CASE-CONTROL STUDIES

The results of case-control studies comparing history of sun exposure in childhood (presumed to be a critical period, mostly from the results of studies in migrants) between MS cases and controls have been conflicting. The results of one study were contrary to a protective effect of vitamin D,[106] and no association between sun exposure in childhood and MS risk was found in another.[107] In contrast, results consistent with a protective effect of sun exposure were reported in a study in Tasmania in which information on time spent in the sun was complemented by measurement of skin actinic damage, a biomarker of UV light exposure,[108] as well as an investigation in Norway[109] and a study of monozygotic twins in the United States.[110] In the Norway study, an inverse association was also found between consumption of fish and MS risk. Selection and recall biases are potential problems in case-control studies, but recall bias cannot explain the inverse association observed in Tasmania with actinic damage,[108] and selection bias is unlikely in the twin study.

LONGITUDINAL STUDIES

The strongest evidence relating vitamin D levels to MS risk has been provided by two longitudinal studies, one based on assessment of dietary vitamin D intake, and one on serum levels of 25(OH)D. The relation between vitamin D intake and MS risk was studied in more than 200,000 women in the Nurses' Health Study and Nurses' Health Study II cohorts.[111] Dietary vitamin D intake was assessed from comprehensive and previously validated semiquantitative food frequency questionnaires administered every 4 years during the follow-up of the cohorts.[112,113] Total vitamin D intake at baseline was inversely associated with risk of MS: the age-adjusted pooled relative risk (RR) comparing the highest with the lowest quintile of consumption was 0.67 (95% confidence interval [CI], 0.40 to 1.12; P for trend = .03). Intake of 400 IU/day of vitamin D from supplements only was associated with a 40% lower risk of MS. These RRs did not materially change after further adjustment for pack-years of smoking and latitude at birth. Confounding by other micronutrients cannot be excluded, but adjustments for them in the analyses did not change the results.

Because dietary vitamin D is only one component contributing to total vitamin D status (the other being sun exposure), a determination of whether serum levels of vitamin D are associated with MS risk in healthy individuals would strengthen the evidence in favor of a causal role for vitamin D. The serum level of 25(OH)D is a marker of vitamin D status and bioavailability; therefore, if vitamin D is protective, high serum levels of 25(OH)D would be expected to predict a lower risk of MS in healthy individuals. This question was recently addressed in a collaborative, prospective case-control study using the Department of Defense Serum Repository (DoDSR).[114] The study included 257 military personnel with confirmed MS and at least two serum samples collected before the onset of MS symptoms. Risk of MS was 51% lower among white individuals with 25(OH)D levels of 100 nmol/L or higher, compared with those levels lower than 75 nmol/L, and the reduction in MS risk associated with 25(OH)D levels ≥ 100 nmol/L compared with those levels < 100nmol/L was considerably stronger before the age of 20 years (16 to 19 years) than at ages 20 or older.

An important question concerning vitamin D and MS is the age intervals during which vitamin D may be important. The results of migration studies suggest that more pronounced changes in MS risk are likely to occur among individuals who migrate in childhood. The age of 15 years, chosen as an arbitrary cutoff point in early studies, is usually quoted in the literature, but the reality is that data are insufficient to identify a meaningful threshold above which migration would not alter MS risk,[27] and in at least one study a reduction in risk was also observed among individuals who migrated as adults.[115] The results of the case-control study in Tasmania suggest that exposure to sunlight is mostly protective in childhood.[108] Further, vitamin D exposure in utero has been proposed as a possible explanation for the peak in MS incidence among individuals born in May (whose mothers were not pregnant during the summer, when UV light levels are higher) and the dip among those born in November, according to recent data from Canada and Sweden.[116] On the other hand, the results of the longitudinal studies support a protective effect of vitamin D also later in life. Both the lower risk of MS among women taking vitamin D supplements[111] and the lower risk among men and women with higher levels of 25(OH)D[114] would be difficult to explain by a protective effect of vitamin D solely in utero or during childhood. Therefore, it seems likely that, if vitamin D effectively protects against MS, levels during early adult life are also important.

Overall, the epidemiologic evidence of a causal association between vitamin D and MS is strong but not compelling, mainly because there are few studies based on prospective measurement of levels of exposure to sunlight, vitamin D intake, or serum 25(OH)D concentration. However, the public health implications of a possible causal association are enormous. If vitamin D reduces the risk of MS, supplementation in adolescents and young adults could be used effectively for prevention. Based on studies among individuals with low sun exposure, supplements providing between 1000 and 4000 IU/day of vitamin D would increase serum 25(OH)D to the optimal levels.[117-120] There is an urgent need to conduct further longitudinal studies, preferably in a large, randomized controlled clinical trial assessing whether vitamin D supplementation in the general population prevents MS. The trial would have to be very large, because MS is a rare disease, but the sample size could be reduced by oversampling individuals who are at high risk, such as those with first-degree relatives who have MS. Alternative study designs might include national or multinational studies based on randomization of school districts or other suitable units.

Cigarette Smoking

Cigarette smoking was found to increase the risk of MS in some[121,122] but not all[123,124] case-control studies. A cross-sectional survey of the general population in Hordaland County, Norway, found an increased risk of MS in ever-smokers compared with never-smokers (RR = 1.8; 95% CI, 1.1 to 2.9).[125] Four prospective studies on smoking and MS have been conducted. Among 17,000 British women in the Oxford Family Planning Association Study, those who smoked 15 or more cigarettes per day were compared with never-smokers and had an 80% increased risk of MS (RR = 1.8; 95% CI, 0.8 to 3.6).[126] A total of 46,000 women from across the United Kingdom were enrolled in the Royal College of General Practitioners' Oral Contraception Study, which found that women smoking 15 or more cigarettes per day had a 40% increased risk of MS (RR = 1.4; 95% CI, 0.9 to 2.2), compared with never-smokers.[127] The Nurses' Health Study and Nurses' Health Study II cohorts included more than 200,000 U.S. women; those who smoked 25 or more pack-years had a 70% increased risk (RR = 1.7; 95% CI, 1.2 to 2.4; $P < .01$) compared with never-smokers.[128] In a prospective case-control study in the General Practice Research Database, which included both men and women, ever-smokers had a 30% increased risk of MS, compared with never-smokers (RR = 1.3; 95% CI, 1.0 to 1.7).[129] The suggestion of an increased risk of MS among smokers was consistent across all four studies, and pooled estimates of the relative risk were highly statistically significant when never-smokers were compared with past and current smokers (Fig. 4-4A) or with moderate and heavy smokers (see Fig. 4-4B). Additional support for a role of smoking includes a twofold increase in risk of pediatric MS among children exposed to parental smoking[130] and an increased risk of transition to secondary progressive MS among individuals with relapsing-remitting MS[129]; however, the latter finding was not confirmed in a recent investigation.[131]

Biologic mechanisms for smoking and increased risk of MS could be neurotoxic,[132] immunomodulatory,[133,134] or vascular (i.e., increased permeability of the blood–brain barrier), or they could involve increased frequency and duration of respiratory infections,[135] which may then contribute to increased MS risk. Smoking also appears to increase the risk of other autoimmune diseases, including rheumatoid arthritis[136-140] and systemic lupus erythematosus,[141] arguing for a more general effect of cigarette smoking on autoimmunity.

Other Possible Risk Factors

DIET

Although several foods or nutrients were found to be related to be MS risk in ecologic or case-control studies, the results overall were inconsistent and unconvincing. In ecologic studies, positive correlations were found between MS and intake of animal fat[142-144] and saturated fat,[144] as well as consumption of meat,[145] milk, and butter,[143,146] and inverse correlations were found with intake of fat from fish[143,145] and nuts[143] (sources of polyunsaturated fat). An increased risk of MS with increasing animal or saturated fat intake and a protective effect of increasing polyunsaturated fat intake were also reported in a case-control study,[147] but otherwise the results of case-control studies have largely not supported an association between increased MS risk and milk or meat consumption,[121,147-150] or decreased risk and consumption of sources of polyunsaturated fat such as fish or nuts.[121,147] However, in a recent study in Norway,[109] fish consumption 3 or more times per week among individuals living at latitudes between 66° and 71° N was inversely related to MS risk. Other results have included an inverse association of risk with

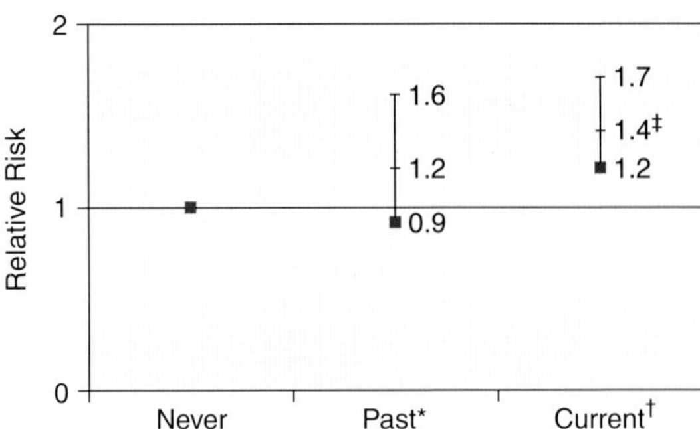

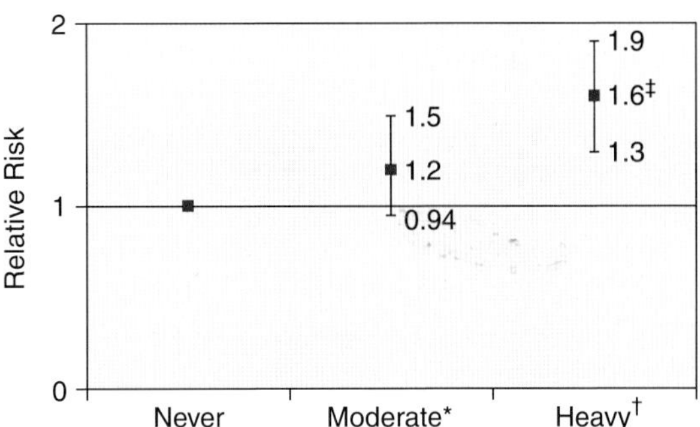

Figure 4–4 A, Relative risk of multiple sclerosis (MS) by smoking status. (*Past smoking not available for Thorogood and Hannaford. Br J Obstet Gynecol 1998;105:1296-1299; †1-14 or ≥ 15 cigarettes/day for Villard-Mackintosh and Vessey. Contraception 1993;47:161-168 and Thorogood and Hannaford. Br J Obstet Gynaecol 1998;105:1296-1299). **B,** Relative risk of MS by duration/frequency of smoking. (‡1-9 pack-years for Hernán et al. Am J Epidemiol 2001;154:69-74; ≥15 cigarettes/day for Villard-Mackintosh and Vessey and Thorogood et al.; not available for Hernán et al 2005 Brain 2005;128:1461-1465. Villard-Mackintosh and Vessey. Contraception 1993;47:161-168 and Thorogood and Hannaford. Br J Obstet Gynaecol 1998;105:1296-1299. 10-24 and ≥ 25 pack-years for Hernán et al. 2001 Am J Epidemiol 2001;154:69-74; ≥15 cigarettes/day for Villard-Mackintosh and Vessey Contraception 1993;47:161-168 and Thorogood and Hannaford. Br J Obstet Gynecol 1998;105:1296-1299; not available for Hernán et al. Brain 2005;128:1461-1465. (From Ascherio A, Munger KL: Environmental risk factors for multiple sclerosis: Part II. Noninfectious factors. Ann Neurol 2007;61:504-513.)

intake of vitamin C and juice,[147] but no association with other antioxidant vitamins[147] or with fruits and vegetables[121,123,147,151] has been reported.

It is important to note that ecologic studies are prone to be confounding and in general provide only very weak evidence of the potential effects of diet on disease risk. Retrospective case-control studies are also prone to bias due to both control selection and differential recall. The latter effect is particularly problematic, because even a modest difference in diet recall between cases and controls can cause a large bias in relative risk estimates.[152] This problem is compounded in MS by changes in diet that may occur in the early clinical or preclinical phases of the disease. Therefore, although these studies have been important in drawing attention to several aspects of diet as potentially important risk factors for MS, their results, whether in favor or against an hypothetical association, should be interpreted extremely cautiously. Understanding of the relation between diet and MS will require the conduct of large longitudinal investigations, with repeated assessment of diet using rigorous and validated methods and possibly measurements of biomarkers of nutrient intakes. So far, the only prospective studies of diet and MS were those conducted among women in the two Nurses' Health Study cohorts. In this population, neither animal fat nor saturated fat was associated with MS risk, but there was a suggestion of an inverse association with intake of the n-3 polyunsaturated fat linolenic acid.[153] There were also no significant associations between intakes of dairy products, fish, meat,[153] vitamins C or E, carotenoids, or fruits and vegetables and MS risk.[154] However, participants in these studies were already 25 to 55 years of age at time of recruitment, and therefore they shed little light on the possible effect of diet earlier in life and MS risk.

Studies have also examined whether intake of polyunsaturated fats affects MS progression. N-3 polyunsaturated fat supplementation in doses ranging from 2.85 to 3.90 g/day administered for periods of 6 to 24 months did not have significant effects on disability levels in two randomized controlled trials that included a total of 339 patients with relapsing-remitting MS,[155,156] although trends were in favor of the supplemented groups in both studies. Results of three randomized controlled trials examining the effects of n-6 polyunsaturated fat supplementation (17 to 20 g/day for 24 to 30 months) on MS progression, including a total of 279 patients with relapsing-remitting MS,[157-159] and a meta-analysis of these studies[160] suggested that supplementation may reduce the severity and duration of relapses.

In summary, there is no compelling evidence that dietary factors other than vitamin D play a causal role in MS, but neither can such a role be excluded, particularly for diet during adolescence or childhood, which may be important periods in the etiology of MS.

SEX HORMONES

Estrogen has been hypothesized to protect against MS, because in high levels it appears to promote the non-inflammatory type 2 immune response, rather than the pro-inflammatory type 1 response predominately seen in MS, and because during pregnancy, when estrogen levels are high, women with MS experience fewer relapses than during the puerperium.[161] In prospective studies,[126,127,162,163] neither oral contraceptive use, parity, nor age at first birth[162] was associated with MS risk. A decreased risk of MS during pregnancy followed by an increased risk during the first 6 months after delivery was shown in a study based on a general practice database in the United Kingdom.[163] In the same study, recent use of oral contraceptives was also associated with a reduced risk.[163] Collectively, these studies suggest that short-term exposure to estrogen may be protective against MS, but that this protection is transient.

HEPATITIS B VACCINE

Concerns that the hepatitis B vaccine may increase the risk of MS were raised after widespread administration of the vaccine in France,[164] but the results of most studies have not supported a causal association. Studies in the United States conducted among subjects included in a health care database,[165] among nurses,[166] and among participants in three health maintenance organizations[167] found no association between hepatitis B vaccination and risk of MS. Further, in studies of children and adolescents, no association was found between hepatitis B vaccination and MS risk[168] or risk of conversion to MS among children with a first demyelinating event.[170] However, a case-control study conducted in the General Practice Research Database in the United Kingdom did find a threefold increased risk associated with receipt of the vaccine within 3 years before MS onset,[170] and a French case-control study reported a nonsignificant increased risk of MS among individuals with clinically isolated syndrome after vaccination.[171] Among individuals with MS, the vaccine does not appear to increase the risk of relapses.[172] Overall, there is no convincing evidence that hepatitis B vaccination increases MS risk.

OTHER FACTORS

Other environmental factors have been associated with MS, but the available evidence is sparse, and the relevance of these factors to MS etiology remains uncertain. An *increased* risk of MS has been reported in relation to exposure to organic solvents,[173-177] physical trauma,[178] and psychological stress from the loss of a child (bereavement),[179] whereas a decreased risk has been observed for use of penicillin[180] and antihistamines,[181] high levels of serum uric acid,[182-184] and tetanus toxoid vaccination.[185]

REFERENCES

1. MacMahon B, Trichopolous D: Epidemiology: Principles and methods, 2nd ed. Boston: Little Brown, 1996.
2. Dwyer T, Ponsonby AL, Blizzard L, et al: The contribution of changes in the prevalence of prone sleeping position to the decline in sudden infant death syndrome in Tasmania. JAMA 1995; 273:783-789.
3. Hernan MA, Olek MJ, Ascherio A: Geographic variation of MS incidence in two prospective studies of US women. Neurology 1999;53:1711-1718.
4. Wallin MT, Page WF, Kurtzke JF: Multiple sclerosis in US veterans of the Vietnam era and later military service: Race, sex, and geography. Ann Neurol 2001;55:65-71.
5. Orton SM, Herrera BM, Yee IM, et al: Sex ratio of multiple sclerosis in Canada: A longitudinal study. Lancet Neurol 2006;5:932-936.
6. Koch-Henriksen N: The Danish Multiple Sclerosis Registry: A 50-year follow-up. Mult Scler 1999;5:293-296.
7. Pugliatti M, Rosati G, Carton H, et al: The epidemiology of multiple sclerosis in Europe. Eur J Neurol 2006;13:700-722.
8. Kurtzke JF, Beebe GW, Norman JE Jr: Epidemiology of multiple sclerosis in U.S. veterans: I. Race, sex, and geographic distribution. Neurology 1979;29:1228-1235.
9. Koch-Henriksen N, Hyllested K: Epidemiology of multiple sclerosis: Incidence and prevalence rates in Denmark 1948-64 based on the Danish Multiple Sclerosis Registry. Acta Neurol Scand 1988;78:369-380.
10. Kurland LT: The frequency and geographic distribution of multiple sclerosis as indicated by mortality statistics and morbidity surveys in the United States and Canada. Am J Hyg 1952; 55:457-476.
11. Stazio A, Paddison RM, Kurland LT: Multiple sclerosis in New Orleans, Louisiana, and Winnipeg, Manitoba, Canada: Follow-up of a previous survey in New Orleans, and comparison between the patient populations in the two communities. J Chron Dis 1967;20:311-332.
12. Visscher BR, Detels R, Coulson AH, et al: Latitude, migration, and the prevalence of multiple sclerosis. Am J Epidemiol 1977;106:470-475.
13. Baum HM, Rothschild BB: The incidence and prevalence of reported multiple sclerosis. Ann Neurol 1981;10:420-428.

14. Miller DH, Hammond SR, McLeod JG, et al: Multiple sclerosis in Australia and New Zealand: Are the determinants genetic or environmental? J Neurol Neurosurg Psychiatry 1990;53:903-905.
15. Kurtzke JF: MS epidemiology world wide: One view of current status. Acta Neurol Scand Suppl 1995;161:23-33.
16. Kira J: Multiple sclerosis in the Japanese population. Lancet Neurol 2003;2:117-127.
17. Kurtzke JF: Epidemiologic evidence for multiple sclerosis as an infection. Clin Microbiol Rev 1993;6:382-427.
18. Compston A, Confavreux C: The distribution of multiple sclerosis. In Compston A, McDonald IR, Noseworthy J, et al (eds): McAlpine's Multiple Sclerosis, 4th ed. Philadelphia, Churchill Livingstone Elsevier, 2005, pp 71-111.
19. Cardoso E, Fukuda T, Pereira J, et al: Clinical and epidemiological profile of multiple sclerosis in a reference center in the State of Bahia, Brazil. Arq Neuropsiquiatr 2006;64:727-730.
20. Corona T, Roman GC: Multiple sclerosis in Latin America. Neuroepidemiology 2006;26:1-3.
21. Bhigjee AI, Moodley K, Ramkissoon K: Multiple sclerosis in KwaZulu Natal, South Africa: An epidemiological and clinical study. Mult Scler 2007;13:1095-1099.
22. Williamson DM, Henry JP, Schiffer R, Wagner L: Prevalence of multiple sclerosis in 19 Texas counties, 1998-2000. J Environ Health 2007;69:41-45.
23. Mayr WT, Pittock SJ, McClelland RL, et al: Incidence and prevalence of multiple sclerosis in Olmsted County, Minnesota, 1985-2000. Neurology 2003;61:1373-1377.
24. Saadatnia M, Etemadifar M, Maghzi AH: Multiple sclerosis in Isfahan, Iran. Int Rev Neurobiol 2007;79C:357-375.
25. Ascherio A, Munger KL: Multiple sclerosis. In Nelson LM, Tanner CM, Van Den Eeden SK, McGuire VM (eds): Neuroepidemiology: From Principles to Practice. Oxford, Oxford University Press, 2004, pp 188-222.
26. Poser CM: The dissemination of multiple sclerosis: A Viking saga? A historical essay. Ann Neurol 1994;36 (Suppl 2):S231-S243.
27. Gale CR, Martyn CN: Migrant studies in multiple sclerosis. Prog Neurobiol 1995;47:425-448.
28. Hammond SR, English DR, McLeod JG: The age-range of risk of developing multiple sclerosis: Evidence from a migrant population in Australia. Brain 2000;123(Pt 5):968-974.
29. Detels R, Visscher BR, Haile RW, et al: Multiple sclerosis and age at migration. Am J Epidemiol 1978;108:386-393.
30. Kurtzke JF, Beebe GW, Norman JE: Epidemiology of multiple sclerosis in US veterans: III. Migration and the risk of MS. Neurology 1985;35:672-678.
31. Dean G, McLoughlin H, Brady R, et al: Multiple sclerosis among immigrants in Greater London. BMJ 1976;1:861-864.
32. Dean G, Brady R, McLoughlin H, et al: Motor neurone disease and multiple sclerosis among immigrants to Britain. Br J Prev Soc Med 1977;31:141-147.
33. Elian M, Dean G: Motor neuron disease and multiple sclerosis among immigrants to England from the Indian subcontinent, the Caribbean, and East and West Africa. J Neurol Neurosurg Psychiatry 1993;56:454-457.
34. Elian M, Dean G: Multiple sclerosis among the United Kingdom-born children of immigrants from the West Indies. J Neurol Neurosurg Psychiatry 1987;50:327-332.
35. Elian M, Nightingale S, Dean G: Multiple sclerosis among United Kingdom-born children of immigrants from the Indian subcontinent, Africa and the West Indies. J Neurol Neurosurg Psychiatry 1990;53:906-911.
36. Cabre P, Signate A, Olindo S, et al: Role of return migration in the emergence of multiple sclerosis in the French West Indies. Brain 2005;128:2899-2910.
37. Mayr WT, Pittock SJ, McClelland RL, et al: Incidence and prevalence of multiple sclerosis in Olmsted County, Minnesota, 1985-2000. Neurology 2003;61:1373-1377.
38. Pugliatti M, Sotgiu S, Solinas G, et al: Multiple sclerosis prevalence among Sardinians: Further evidence against the latitude gradient theory. Neurol Sci 2001;22:163-165.
39. Dean G, Elian M, de Bono AG, et al: Multiple sclerosis in Malta in 1999: An update. J Neurol Neurosurg Psychiatry 2002;73:256-260.
40. Dean G, Yeo TW, Goris A, et al: HLA-DRB1 and multiple sclerosis in Malta. Neurology 2008;70:101-105.
41. Johnson RT: The possible viral etiology of multiple sclerosis. Adv Neurol 1975;13:1-46.
42. Dyment DA, Ebers GC, Sadovnick AD: Genetics of multiple sclerosis. Lancet Neurol 2004;3:104-110.
43. Poser CM, Hiberd PL, Benedikz J, Gudmundsson G: Analysis of the 'epidemic' of multiple sclerosis in the Faroe Islands. Neuroepidemiology 1988;7:168-180.

44. Kurtzke JF, Hyllested K: Multiple sclerosis in the Faroe Islands: I. Clinical and epidemiological features. Ann Neurol 1979;5:6-21.
45. Kurtzke JF, Heltberg A: Multiple sclerosis in the Faroe Islands: An epitome. J Clin Epidemiol 2001;54:1-22.
46. Poskanzer DC, Schapira K, Miller H: Multiple sclerosis and poliomyelitis. Lancet 1963;2: 917-921.
47. Leibowitz U, Antonovsky A, Medalie JM, et al: Epidemiological study of multiple sclerosis in Israel: II. Multiple sclerosis and level of sanitation. J Neurol Neurosurg Psychiatry 1966;29:60-68.
48. Hammond SR, McLeod JG, Macaskill P, English DR: Multiple sclerosis in Australia: Socioeconomic factors. J Neurol Neurosurg Psychiatry 1996;61:311-313.
49. Kurtzke JF, Page WF: Epidemiology of multiple sclerosis in US veterans: VII. Risk factors for MS. Neurology 1997;48:204-213.
50. Granieri E, Casetta I. Part III: Selected reviews. Common childhood and adolescent infections and multiple sclerosis. Neurology 1997;49(Suppl 2):S42-S54.
51. Bach JF: The effect of infections on susceptibility to autoimmune and allergic diseases. N Engl J Med 2002;347:911-920.
52. Fleming J, Fabry Z: The hygiene hypothesis and multiple sclerosis. Ann Neurol 2007;61:85-89.
53. Correale J, Farez M: Association between parasite infection and immune responses in multiple sclerosis. Ann Neurol 2007;61:97-108.
54. Thacker EL, Mirzaei F, Ascherio A: Infectious mononucleosis and risk for multiple sclerosis: A meta-analysis. Ann Neurol 2006;59:499-503.
55. Warner HB, Carp RI: Multiple sclerosis and Epstein-Barr virus [letter]. Lancet 1981;2:1290.
56. Rickinson AB, Kieff E: Epstein-Barr virus. In Knipe DM, Howley PM, Griffin DE, et al (eds): Fields Virology, 5th ed. Philadelphia, Wolters Kluwer Health/Lippincott Williams & Wilkins, 2007, pp 2655-2700.
57. Niederman JC, Evans AS: Epstein-Barr virus. In Evans AS, Kaslow RA (eds): Viral infections of humans: Epidemiology and control, 4th ed. New York, Plenum, 1997, pp 253-283.
58. Houzen H, Niino M, Kikuchi S, et al: The prevalence and clinical characteristics of MS in northern Japan. J Neurol Sci 2003;211:49-53.
59. Ascherio A, Munger KL: Environmental risk factors for multiple sclerosis: Part I. The role of infection. Ann Neurol 2007;61:288-299.
60. Alotaibi S, Kennedy J, Tellier R, et al: Epstein-Barr virus in pediatric multiple sclerosis. JAMA 2004;291:1875-1879.
61. Pohl D, Krone B, Rostasy K, et al: High seroprevalence of Epstein-Barr virus in children with multiple sclerosis. Neurology 2006;67:2063-2065.
62. Ascherio A, Munger KL, Lennette ET, et al: Epstein-barr virus antibodies and risk of multiple sclerosis: A prospective study. JAMA 2001;286:3083-3088.
63. Sundstrom P, Juto P, Wadell G, et al: An altered immune response to Epstein-Barr virus in multiple sclerosis: A prospective study. Neurology 2004;62:2277-2282.
64. Levin LI, Munger KL, Rubertone MV, et al: Temporal relationship between elevation of Epstein Barr virus antibody titers and initial onset of neurological symptoms in multiple sclerosis. JAMA 2005;293:2496-2500.
65. DeLorenze GN, Munger KL, Lennette E, et al: Epstein-Barr virus and multiple sclerosis: Evidence of association from a prospective study with long-term follow-up. Arch Neurol 2006;63:839-844.
66. Wandinger K, Jabs W, Siekhaus A, et al: Association between clinical disease activity and Epstein-Barr virus reactivation in MS. Neurology 2000;55:178-184.
67. Hilton DA, Love S, Fletcher A, Pringle JH: Absence of Epstein-Barr virus RNA in multiple sclerosis as assessed by in situ hybridisation. J Neurol Neurosurg Psychiatry 1994;57:975-976.
68. Morré SA, van Beek J, De Groot CJ, et al: Is Epstein-Barr virus present in the CNS of patients with MS? Neurology 2001;56:692.
69. Lunemann JD, Edwards N, Muraro PA, et al: Increased frequency and broadened specificity of latent EBV nuclear antigen-1-specific T cells in multiple sclerosis. Brain 2006;129:1493-1506.
70. Cepok S, Zhou D, Srivastava R, et al: Identification of Epstein-Barr virus proteins as putative targets of the immune response in multiple sclerosis. J Clin Invest 2005;115:1352-1360.
71. Sutkowski N, Palkama T, Ciurli C, et al: An Epstein-Barr virus-associated superantigen. J Exp Med 1996;184:971-980.
72. van Sechel AC, Bajramovic JJ, van Stipdonk MJ, et al: EBV-induced expression and HLA-DR-restricted presentation by human B cells of alpha B-crystallin, a candidate autoantigen in multiple sclerosis. J Immunol 1999;162:129-135.

73. Pender MP: Infection of autoreactive B lymphocytes with EBV, causing chronic autoimmune diseases. Trends Immunol 2003;24:584-588.
74. Serafini B, Rosicarelli B, Franciotta D, et al: Dysregulated Epstein-Barr virus infection in the multiple sclerosis brain. J Exp Med 2007;204:2899-2912.
75. Lycke J, Svennerholm B, Hjelmquist E, et al: Acyclovir treatment of relapsing-remitting multiple sclerosis: A randomized, placebo-controlled, double-blind study. J Neurol 1996;243:214-224.
76. Bech E, Lycke J, Gadeberg P, et al: A randomized, double-blind, placebo-controlled MRI study of anti-herpes virus therapy in MS. Neurology 2002;58:31-36.
77. Friedman JE, Zabriskie JB, Plank C, et al: A randomized clinical trial of valacyclovir in multiple sclerosis. Mult Scler 2005;11:286-295.
78. De Jager PL, Simon KC, Munger KL, et al: Integrating risk factors: HLA-DRB1*1501 and Epstein-Barr virus in multiple sclerosis. Neurology 2008;70(13 Pt 2):1113-1118.
79. Munch M, Hvas J, Christensen T, et al: A single subtype of Epstein-Barr virus in members of multiple sclerosis clusters. Acta Neurol Scand 1998;98:395-399.
80. Lindsey JW, Patel S, Zou J: Epstein-Barr virus genotypes in multiple sclerosis. Acta Neurol Scand 2008;117:141-144.
81. Sriram S, Mitchell W, Stratton C: Multiple sclerosis associated with *Chlamydia pneumoniae* infection of the CNS. Neurology 1998;50:571-572.
82. Derfuss T, Gurkov R, Bergh FT, et al: Intrathecal antibody production against *Chlamydia pneumoniae* in multiple sclerosis is part of a polyspecific immune response. Brain 2001;124:1325-1335.
83. Munger KL, Peeling RW, Hernan MA, et al: Infection with *Chlamydia pneumoniae* and risk of multiple sclerosis. Epidemiology 2003;14:141-147.
84. Bagos PG, Nikolopoulos G, Ioannidis A: *Chlamydia pneumoniae* infection and the risk of multiple sclerosis: A meta-analysis. Mult Scler 2006;12:397-411.
85. Knox KK, Brewer JH, Henry JM, et al: Human herpesvirus 6 and multiple sclerosis: Systemic active infections in patients with early disease. Clin Infect Dis 2000;31:894-903.
86. Derfuss T, Hohlfeld R, Meinl E: Intrathecal antibody (IgG) production against human herpesvirus type 6 occurs in about 20% of multiple sclerosis patients and might be linked to a polyspecific B-cell response. J Neurol 2005;252:986-971.
87. Alvarez-Lafuente R, De Las Heras V, Bartolome M, et al: Human herpesvirus 6 and multiple sclerosis: A one-year follow-up study. Brain Pathol 2006;16:20-27.
88. Haahr S, Sommerlund M, Christensen T, et al: A putative new retrovirus associated with multiple sclerosis and the possible involvement of the Epstein-Barr virus in this disease. Ann N Y Acad Sci 1994;724:148-156.
89. Koch-Henriksen N, Rasmussen S, Stenager E, Madsen M: The Danish Multiple Sclerosis Registry: History, data collection and validity. Dan Med Bull 2001;48:91-94.
90. Jacomy H, Fragoso G, Almazan G, et al: Human coronavirus OC43 infection induces chronic encephalitis leading to disabilities in BALB/C mice. Virology 2006;349:335-346.
91. Acheson ED, Bachrach CA, Wright FM: Some comments on the relationship of the distribution of multiple sclerosis to latitude, solar radiation, and other variables. Acta Psychiatr Scand 1960;147:132-147.
92. Sutherland JM, Tyrer JH, Eadie MJ: The prevalence of multiple sclerosis in Australia. Brain 1962;85:146-164.
93. Leibowitz U, Sharon D, Alter M: Geographical considerations in multiple sclerosis. Brain 1967;90:871-886.
94. van der Mei IA, Ponsonby AL, Blizzard L, Dwyer T: Regional variation in multiple sclerosis prevalence in Australia and its association with ambient ultraviolet radiation. Neuroepidemiology 2001;20:168-174.
95. Holick MF: Sunlight and vitamin D for bone health and prevention of autoimmune diseases, cancers, and cardiovascular disease. Am J Clin Nutr 2004;80:1678S-1688S.
96. Webb AR, Kline L, Holick MF: Influence of season and latitude on the cutaneous synthesis of vitamin D3: Exposure to winter sunlight in Boston and Edmonton will not promote vitamin D3 synthesis in human skin. J Clin Endocrinol Metab 1988;67:373-378.
97. McKenna MJ, Freaney R, Byrne P, et al: Safety and efficacy of increasing wintertime vitamin D and calcium intake by milk fortification. Q J Med 1995;88:895-898.
98. Rockell JE, Skeaff CM, Williams SM, Green TJ: Serum 25-hydroxyvitamin D concentrations of New Zealanders aged 15 years and older. Osteoporos Int 2006;17:1382-1389.
99. Goldberg P: Multiple sclerosis: Vitamin D and calcium as environmental determinants of prevalence: A viewpoint. Part 1: Sunlight, dietary factors and epidemiology. Intern J Environ Studies 1974;6:19-27.

100. Hayes CE, Nashold FE, Spach KM, Pedersen LB: The immonological functions of the vitamin D endocrine system. Cell Mol Biol 2003;49:277-300.
101. Lemire JM, Archer DC: 1,25-Dihydroxyvitamin D3 prevents the in vivo induction of murine experimental autoimmune encephalomyelitis. J Clin Invest 1991;87:1103-1107.
102. Cantorna MT, Hayes CE, DeLuca HF: 1,25-Dihydroxyvitamin D3 reversibly blocks the progression of relapsing encephalomyelitis: A model of multiple sclerosis. Proc Natl Acad Sci U S A 1996;93:7861-7864.
103. Garcion E, Sindji L, Nataf S, et al: Treatment of experimental autoimmune encephalomyelitis in rat by 1,25-dihydroxyvitamin D(3) leads to early effects within the central nervous system. Acta Neuropathol (Berl) 2003;105:438-448.
104. Freedman DM, Dosemeci M, Alavanja MC: Mortality from multiple sclerosis and exposure to residential and occupational solar radiation: A case-control study based on death certificates. Occup Environ Med 2000;57:418-421.
105. Goldacre MJ, Seagroatt V, Yeates D, Acheson ED: Skin cancer in people with multiple sclerosis: A record linkage study. J Epidemiol Community Health 2004;58:142-144.
106. Antonovsky A, Leibowitz U, Smith HA, et al: Epidemiologic study of multiple sclerosis in Israel: I. An overall review of methods and findings. Arch Neurol 1965;13:183-193.
107. Cendrowski W, Wender M, Dominik W, et al: Epidemiological study of multiple sclerosis in Western Poland. Eur Neurol 1969;2:90-108.
108. van der Mei IAF, Ponsonby AL, Dwyer T, et al: Past exposure to sun, skin phenotype and risk of multiple sclerosis: A case-control study. BMJ 2003;327:316-321.
109. Kampman MT, Wilsgaard T, Mellgren SI: Outdoor activities and diet in childhood and adolescence relate to MS risk above the Arctic Circle. J Neurol 2007;254:471-477.
110. Islam T, Gauderman WJ, Cozen W, Mack TM: Childhood sun exposure influences risk of multiple sclerosis in monozygotic twins. Neurology 2007;69:381-388.
111. Munger KL, Zhang SM, O'Reilly E, et al: Vitamin D intake and incidence of multiple sclerosis. Neurology 2004;62:60-65.
112. Willett WC, Sampson L, Browne ML, et al: The use of a self-administered questionnaire to assess diet four years in the past. Am J Epidemiol 1988;127:188-199.
113. Salvini S, Hunter D, Sampson L, et al: Food-based validation of a dietary questionnaire: The effects of week-to-week variation in food consumption. Int J Epidemiol 1989;18:858-867.
114. Munger KL, Levin LI, Hollis BW, et al: Serum 25-hydroxyvitamin D levels and risk of multiple sclerosis. JAMA 2006;296:2832-2838.
115. Hammond SR, English DR, McLeod JG: The age-range of risk of developing multiple sclerosis: Evidence from a migrant population in Australia. Brain 2000;123:968-974.
116. Willer CJ, Dyment DA, Sadovnick AD, et al: Timing of birth and risk of multiple sclerosis: Population based study. BMJ 2005;330:120.
117. Hollis BW: Circulating 25-hydroxyvitamin D levels indicative of vitamin D sufficiency: Implications for establishing a new effective dietary intake recommendation for vitamin D. J Nutr 2005;135:317-322.
118. Dawson-Hughes B, Heaney RP, Holick MF, et al: Estimates of optimal vitamin D status. Osteoporos Int 2005;16:713-716.
119. Vieth R: Vitamin D supplementation, 25-hydroxyvitamin D concentrations, and safety. Am J Clin Nutr 1999;69:842-856.
120. Heaney RP, Davies KM, Chen TC, et al: Human serum 25-hydroxycholecalciferol response to extended oral dosing with cholecalciferol. Am J Clin Nutr 2003;77:204-210.
121. Antonovsky A, Leibowitz U, Smith HA, et al: Epidemiologic study of multiple sclerosis in Israel. Arch Neurol 1965;13:183-193.
122. Ghadirian P, Dadgostar B, Azani R, Maisonneuve P: A case-control study of the association between socio-demographic, lifestyle and medical history factors and multiple sclerosis. Can J Public Health 2001;92:281-285.
123. Warren SA, Warren KG, Greenhill S, Paterson M: How multiple sclerosis is related to animal illness, stress and diabetes. Can Med Assoc J 1982;126:377-385.
124. Casetta I, Granieri E, Malagù S, et al: Environmental risk factors and multiple sclerosis: A community-based, case-control study in the province of Ferrara, Italy. Neuroepidemiology 1994;13:120-128.
125. Riise T, Nortvedt MW, Ascherio A: Smoking is a risk factor for multiple sclerosis. Neurology 2003;61:1122-1124.
126. Villard-Mackintosh L, Vessey MP: Oral contraceptives and reproductive factors in multiple sclerosis incidence. Contraception 1993;47:161-168.

127. Thorogood M, Hannaford PC: The influence of oral contraceptives on the risk of mulitple sclerosis. Br J Obstet Gynaecol 1998;105:1296-1299.
128. Hernán MA, Olek MJ, Ascherio A: Cigarette smoking and incidence of multiple sclerosis. Am J Epidemiol 2001;154:69-74.
129. Hernan MA, Jick SS, Logroscino G, et al: Cigarette smoking and the progression of multiple sclerosis. Brain 2005;128:1461-1465.
130. Mikaeloff Y, Caridade G, Tardieu M, Suissa S: Parental smoking at home and the risk of childhood-onset multiple sclerosis in children. Brain 2007;130:2589-2595.
131. Koch M, van Harten A, Uyttenboogaart M, De Keyser J: Cigarette smoking and progression in multiple sclerosis. Neurology 2007;69:1515-1520.
132. Smith ADM, Duckett S, Waters AH: Neuropathological changes in chronic cyanide intoxication. Nature 1963;200:179-181.
133. Sopori ML, Kozak W: Immunomodulatory effects of cigarette smoke. J Neuroimmunol 1998;83:148-156.
134. Francus T, Klein RF, Staiano-Coico L, et al: Effects of tobacco glycoprotein (TGP) on the immune system: II. TGP stimulates the proliferation of human T cells and the differentiation of human B cells into Ig secreting cells. J Immunol 1988;140:1823-1829.
135. Graham NM: The epidemiology of acute respiratory infections in children and adults: A global perspective. Epidemiol Rev 1990;12:149-178.
136. Vessey MP, Villard-Mackintosh L, Yeates D: Oral contraceptives, cigarette smoking and other factors in relation to arthritis. Contraception 1987;35:457-464.
137. Hernandez Avila M, Liang MH, Willett WC, et al: Reproductive factors, smoking, and the risk for rheumatoid arthritis. Epidemiology 1990;1:285-291.
138. Voigt LF, Koepsell TD, Nelson JL, et al: Smoking, obesity, alcohol consumption, and the risk of rheumatoid arthritis. Epidemiology 1994;5:525-532.
139. Silman AJ, Newman J, MacGregor AJ: Cigarette smoking increases the risk of rheumatoid arthritis: Results from a nationwide study of disease-discordant twins. Arthritis Rheum 1996;39:732-735.
140. Heliovaara M, Aho K, Aromaa A, et al: Smoking and risk of rheumatoid arthritis. J Rheumatol 1993;20:1830-1835.
141. Hardy CJ, Palmer BP, Muir KR, et al: Smoking history, alcohol consumption, and systemic lupus erythematosus: A case-control study. Ann Rheum Dis 1998;57:451-455.
142. Alter M, Yamoor M, Harshe M: Multiple sclerosis and nutrition. Arch Neurol 1974;31:267-272.
143. Agranoff BW, Goldberg D: Diet and the geographical distribution of multiple sclerosis. Lancet 1974;2:1061-1066.
144. Esparza ML, Sasaki S, Kesteloot H: Nutrition, latitude, and multiple sclerosis mortality: An ecologic study. Am J Epidemiol 1995;142:733-737.
145. Lauer K: The risk of multiple sclerosis in the U.S.A. in relation to sociogeographic features: A factor-analytic study. J Clin Epidemiol 1994;47:43-48.
146. Malosse D, Perron H, Sasco A, Seigneurin JM: Correlation between milk and dairy product consumption and multiple sclerosis prevalence: A worldwide study. Neuroepidemiology 1992;11:304-312.
147. Ghadirian P, Jain M, Ducic S, et al: Nutritional factors in the aetiology of multiple sclerosis: A case-control study in Montreal, Canada. Int J Epidemiol 1998;27:845-852.
148. Westlund KB, Kurland LT: Studies on multiple sclerosis in Winnipeg, Manitoba, and New Orleans, Louisiana: II. A controlled investigation of factors in the life history of the Winnipeg patients. Am J Hyg 1953;57:397-407.
149. Cendrowski W, Wender M, Dominik W, et al: Epidemiological study of multiple sclerosis in western Poland. Eur Neurol 1969;2:90-108.
150. Butcher PJ: Milk consumption and multiple sclerosis–an etiological hypothesis. Med Hypotheses 1986;19:169-178.
151. Berr C, Puel J, Clanet M, et al: Risk factors in multiple sclerosis: A population-based case-control study in Hautes-Pyrenees, France. Acta Neurol Scand 1989;80:46-50.
152. Willett WC: Nutritional Epidemiology, 2nd ed. New York, Oxford University Press, 1998.
153. Zhang SM, Willett WC, Hernan MA, et al: Dietary fat in relation to risk of multiple sclerosis among two large cohorts of women. Am J Epidemiol 2000;152:1056-1064.
154. Zhang SM, Hernán MA, Olek MJ, et al: Intakes of carotenoids, vitamin C, and vitamin E and MS risk among two large cohorts of women. Neurology 2001;57:75-80.
155. Bates D, Cartlidge NEF, French JM, et al: A double-blind controlled trial of long chain n-3 polyunsaturated fatty acids in the treatment of multiple sclerosis. J Neurol Neurosurg Psychiatry 1989;52:18-22.

156. Weinstock-Guttman B, Baier M, Park Y, et al: Low fat dietary intervention with omega-3 fatty acid supplementation in multiple sclerosis patients. Prostaglandins Leukot Essent Fatty Acids 2005;73:397-404.
157. Millar JHD, Zilkha KJ, Langman MJS, et al: Double-blind trial of linoleate supplementation of the diet in multiple sclerosis. BMJ 1973;1:765-768.
158. Bates D, Fawcett PRW, Shaw DA, Weightman D: Polyunsaturated fatty acids in treatment of acute remitting multiple sclerosis. BMJ 1978;2:1390-1391.
159. Paty DW, Cousin HK, Read S, Adlakha K: Linoleic acid in multiple sclerosis: Failure to show any therapeutic benefit. Acta Neurol Scand 1978;58:53-58.
160. Dworkin RH, Bates D, Millar JHD, Paty DW: Linoleic acid and multiple sclerosis: A reanalysis of three double-blind trials. Neurology 1984;34:1441-1445.
161. Confavreux C, Hutchinson M, Hours MM, et al: Rate of pregnancy-related relapse in multiple sclerosis: Pregnancy in multiple sclerosis group. N Engl J Med 1998;339:285-291.
162. Hernán MA, Hohol MJ, Olek MJ, et al: Oral contraceptives and the incidence of multiple sclerosis. Neurology 2000;55:848-854.
163. Alonso A, Jick SS, Olek MJ, et al: Recent use of oral contraceptives and the risk of multiple sclerosis. Arch Neurol 2005;62:1362-1365.
164. Marshall E: A shadow falls on hepatitis B vaccination effort. Science 1998;281:630-631.
165. Zipp F, Weil JG, Einhaupl KM: No increase in demyelinating diseases after hepatitis B vaccination. Nat Med 1999;5:964-965.
166. Ascherio A, Zhang SM, Hernan MA, et al: Hepatitis B vaccination and the risk of multiple sclerosis. N Engl J Med 2001;344:327-332.
167. DeStefano F, Verstraeten T, Jackson LA, et al: Vaccinations and risk of central nervous system demyelinating diseases in adults. Arch Neurol 2003;60:504-509.
168. Sadovnick AD, Scheifele DW: School-based hepatitis B vaccination programme and adolescent multiple sclerosis. Lancet 2000;355:549-550.
169. Mikaeloff Y, Caridade G, Assi S, et al: Hepatitis B vaccine and risk of relapse after a first childhood episode of CNS inflammatory demyelination. Brain 2007;130:1105-1110.
170. Hernan MA, Jick SS, Olek MJ, Jick H: Recombinant hepatitis B vaccine and the risk of multiple sclerosis: A prospective study. Neurology 2004;63:838-842.
171. Touze E, Fourrier A, Rue-Fenouche C, et al: Hepatitis B vaccination and first central nervous system demyelinating event: A case-control study. Neuroepidemiology 2002;21:180-186.
172. Confavreux C, Suissa S, Saddier P, et al: Vaccinations and the risk of relapse in multiple sclerosis. Vaccines in Multiple Sclerosis Study Group. N Engl J Med 2001;344:319-326.
173. Landtblom AM, Flodin U, Soderfeldt B, et al: Organic solvents and multiple sclerosis: A synthesis of the current evidence. Epidemiology 1996;7:429-433.
174. Landtblom AM: Exposure to organic solvents and multiple sclerosis. Neurology 1997;49: S70-S74.
175. Mortensen JT, Bronnum-Hansen H, Rasmussen K: Multiple sclerosis and organic solvents. Epidemiology 1998;9:168-171.
176. Riise T, Moen BE, Kyvik KR: Organic solvents and the risk of multiple sclerosis. Epidemiology 2002;13:718-720.
177. Landtblom AM, Tondel M, Hjalmarsson P, et al: The risk for multiple sclerosis in female nurse anaesthetists: A register based study. Occup Environ Med 2006;63:387-389.
178. Goodin DS, Ebers GC, Johnson KP, et al: The relationship of MS to physical trauma and psychological stress: Report of the Therapeutics and Technology Assessment Subcommittee of the American Academy of Neurology. Neurology 1999;52:1737-1745.
179. Li J, Johansen C, Bronnum-Hansen H, et al: The risk of multiple sclerosis in bereaved parents: A nationwide cohort study in Denmark. Neurology 2004;62:726-729.
180. Alonso A, Jick SS, Jick H, Hernan MA: Antibiotic use and risk of multiple sclerosis. Am J Epidemiol 2006;163:997-1002.
181. Alonso A, Jick SS, Hernan MA: Allergy, histamine 1 receptor blockers, and the risk of multiple sclerosis. Neurology 2006;66:572-575.
182. Drulovic J, Dujmovic I, Stojsavljevic N, et al: Uric acid levels in sera from patients with multiple sclerosis. J Neurol 2001;248:121-126.
183. Rentzos M, Nikolaou C, Anagnostouli M, et al: Serum uric acid and multiple sclerosis. Clin Neurol Neurosurg 2006;108:527-531.
184. Peng F, Zhang B, Zhong X, et al: Serum uric acid levels of patients with multiple sclerosis and other neurological diseases. Mult Scler 2008;14:188-196.

185. Hernan MA, Alonso A, Hernandez-Diaz S: Tetanus vaccination and risk of multiple sclerosis: A systematic review. Neurology 2006;67:212-215.
186. Sumaya CV, Myers LW, Ellison GW: Epstein-Barr virus antibodies in multiple sclerosis. Arch Neurol 1980;37:94-96.
187. Bray PF, Bloomer LC, Salmon VC, et al: Epstein-Barr virus infection and antibody synthesis in patients with multiple sclerosis. Arch Neurol 1983;40:406-408.
188. Larsen PD, Bloomer LC, Bray PF: Epstein-Barr nuclear antigen and viral capsid antigen antibody titers in multiple sclerosis. Neurology 1985;35:435-438.
189. Sumaya CV, Myers LW, Ellison GW, Ench Y: Increased prevalence and titer of Epstein-Barr virus antibodies in patients with multiple sclerosis. Ann Neurol 1985;17:371-377.
190. Shirodaria PV, Haire M, Fleming E, et al: Viral antibody titers: Comparison in patients with multiple sclerosis and rheumatoid arthritis. Arch Neurol 1987;44:1237-1241.
191. Ferrante P, Castellani P, Barbi M, Bergamini F: The Italian Cooperative Multiple Sclerosis case-control study: Preliminary results on viral antibodies. Ital J Neurol Sci 1987(Suppl 6):45-50.
192. Munch M, Hvas J, Christensen T, et al: The implications of Epstein-Barr virus in multiple sclerosis: A review. Acta Neurol Scand 1997;169(Suppl):59-64.
193. Myhr K-M, Riise T, Barrett-Connor E, et al: Altered antibody pattern to Epstein-Barr virus but not to other herpesviruses in multiple sclerosis: A population based case-control study from western Norway. J Neurol Neurosurg Psychiatry 1998;64:539-542.
194. Wagner HJ, Hennig H, Jabs WJ, et al: Altered prevalence and reactivity of anti-Epstein-Barr virus antibodies in patients with multiple sclerosis. Viral Immunol 2000;13:497-502.
195. Haahr S, Plesner AM, Vestergaard BF, Hollsberg P: A role of late Epstein-Barr virus infection in multiple sclerosis. Acta Neurol Scand 2004;109:270-275.
196. Ponsonby AL, van der Mei I, Dwyer T, et al: Exposure to infant siblings during early life and risk of multiple sclerosis. JAMA 2005;293:463-469.

5 Advances in Multiple Sclerosis Imaging

ISTVAN PIRKO

Magnetic resonance imaging (MRI) has become a very important tool in the diagnosis and management of several neurologic conditions. MRI allows for high-resolution in vivo imaging of the central nervous system (CNS) in previously unprecedented detail. Nobel Prizes were awarded for the development of clinical MRI to Dr. Paul C. Lauterbur and Sir Peter Mansfield in 2003. Earlier, five individual Nobel Prizes highlighted the discovery of nuclear magnetic resonance—the physical principle behind MRI—and related scientific accomplishments.These discoveries have truly reshaped the field of medicine and biomedical sciences.

Over the past 2 decades, MRI has revolutionized the diagnosis and management of leukoencephalopathies, including that of multiple sclerosis (MS).[1] MRI-based disease markers have been incorporated in the currently used diagnostic criteria of MS, including the 2001 McDonald criteria,[2] and their recent modifications by Polman and colleagues.[3] In addition, MRI-derived measures are the best-known predictors for conversion to MS after a clinically isolated demyelinating syndrome (CIS), as has been demonstrated in the Optic Neuritis Treatment Trial cohort, the National Hospital cohort,[4] and other smaller studies. MRI findings constitute an important cornerstone in the diagnostic criteria of neuromyelitis optica (NMO), and MRI-based disease markers will most likely clarify the poorly defined entity of acute disseminated encephalomyelitis (ADEM).

At present, more than 5000 scientific papers investigating the role of MRI in MS have been published. Almost a quarter of these were published in the last 2 years, and 70% in the last 10 years, demonstrating the accelerated pace of MRI research in MS. MRI-based outcome measures are also frequently used in clinical trials, not only as a surrogate markers but often as primary outcome measures, especially in phase 0, I, and II trials of novel therapeutics. This is related to the increased sensitivity of MRI to inflammatory disease activity when compared with clinical markers.

Despite the advances, even the most sophisticated MRI techniques represent only an extension in the diagnostic armamentarium of the practicing neurologist and are not meant to replace clinical judgment. Moreover, several aspects of MS remain elusive to the routinely used standard MRI techniques, such as changes occurring to normal-appearing white and gray matter (NAWM and NAGM)—yet such changes clearly contribute to the development of disability in MS. In general, conventional MRI measures show, at most, a moderate correlation with disability, whereas measures of atrophy and advanced techniques capturing changes in normal-appearing brain tissue (NABT) may correlate better with the clinical outcome.[5]

This chapter discusses the significance of the widely available standard MRI techniques and reviews advanced MRI methods that are currently utilized primarily in research studies, some of which may become important in everyday clinical practice in the near future. In addition, the role of MRI findings in two important idiopathic inflammatory demyelinating diseases, NMO and ADEM, is discussed, and a new imaging modality, optical coherence tomography (OCT) and its role in MS research and future clinical trials are described.

Physics of Magnetic Resonance Imaging

A full review of MRI physics is beyond the scope of this text and is not necessary for the application of imaging findings; however, a few key points are important to understand. In clinical practice, MRI refers to ^{1}H-MRI, which means that a proton distribution map of the targeted tissue is acquired and analyzed. The studied protons occur most abundantly in water. The various "weighting" modalities (based on the longitudinal [T1] and transverse [T2] relaxation times, proton density, diffusion, susceptibility, and so on) refer to different physical properties in the molecular environment of the studied water molecules. Because the signal is generated at the molecular level, pathologic processes can be captured with great sensitivity. However, different mechanisms of tissue damage may result in similar signal changes from the standpoint of MRI detectability. Therefore, the specificity of MRI findings is relatively poor. A good example is the T2-hyperintense lesion, which may represent a large number of tissue processes including edema, axonal loss, demyelination, gliosis, infarcts, neoplasm, remyelination, infection, or other conditions. This poor specificity may be overcome by a rational combination of a variety of acquisition and post-processing techniques; by the inclusion of specific lesion descriptors (e.g., size, location, contour, edge profile) and relationship to other brain structures; and by the use of advanced MRI pulse sequences.

High-Field-Strength Magnetic Resonance Imaging

In the last few years, systems with higher field strengths, including 3 Tesla or greater, have become available at a growing number of centers. Higher field strength results in higher signal-to-noise ratio, which allows for higher-resolution acquisition in less time by reducing the need for oversampling, as well as better contrast-to-noise ratio in some studies. However, the relaxation properties are different at higher field strength, and susceptibility-based artifacts are much more pronounced.

Conventional Magnetic Resonance Imaging Techniques

T2-WEIGHTED STUDIES

The detection of MS lesions on T2-weighted MRI is the classic method of visualizing MS plaques in vivo (Fig. 5-1). T2-weighted images are highly sensitive for disease activity and lesion formation over time.[6] However, they show very poor specificity to the disease process at the tissue level, because not only demyelination but also inflammation, edema, cell infiltration, remyelination, Wallerian degeneration, axonal

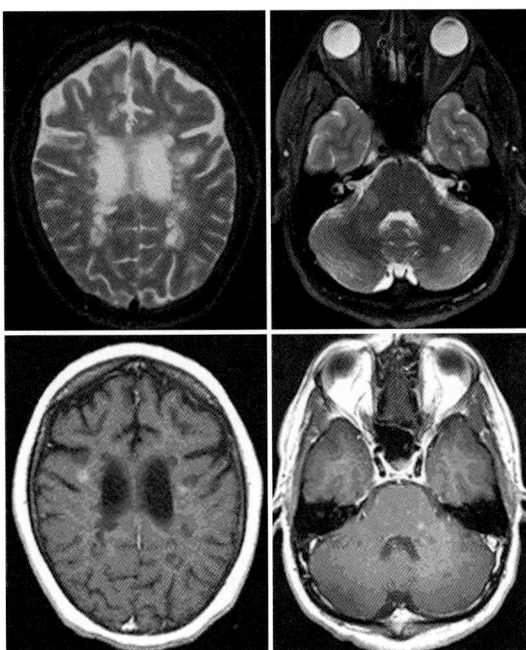

Figure 5–1 Conventional imaging of a case of relapsing-remitting multiple sclerosis. *Top row:* T2-weighted scans. *Bottom row:* Gadolinium-enhanced T1-weighted scans. Note the numerous periventricular, juxtacortical, and posterior fossa lesions, including pontine, brachium pontis, and cerebellar lesions. Contrast enhancement is seen in numerous lesions. This represents an unusually active case from the standpoint of inflammatory new lesion formation.

loss, ischemic changes, neoplasms, infection, and other conditions appear hyperintense on these scans. T2-weighted images are acquired using a variety of spin-echo or fast spin-echo–based techniques. Fast spin-echo or rapid acquisition relaxation enhancement (RARE) techniques have become the studies of choice, because they are much faster yet just as sensitive as the lengthy conventional spin-echo studies. The commonly used FLAIR images (discussed later) are also T2 weighted.

The location of T2-weighted hyperintense lesions is of great importance, because they help differentiate MS from other diseases. For this reason, lesion location has been incorporated into the current diagnostic criteria of MS.[2,3] The most common location is the periventricular white matter, where most patients have lesions. T2-hyperintense lesions are also commonly seen in the corpus callosum; on sagittal T2-weighted images, the typical "Dawson's fingers" configuration is often detectable.[7,8] Other important locations include the juxtacortical (immediate subcortical) areas and infratentorial areas, including the spinal cord,[9] brainstem, and cerebellum,[10] where lesions are often adjacent to spaces filled with cerebrospinal fluid (CSF). However, individual lesions may be seen virtually anywhere in the white matter.

In contrast to MS lesions, nonspecific small-vessel ischemic changes tend to spare the U-fibers, and lesions typically are not detected in the periventricular areas. Such lesions are rarely seen infratentorially, especially rarely in the spinal cord.

MS lesions seen on T2-weighted MRI can be multifocal or, as the disease advances, confluent. The number and total volume of T2-weighted lesions tend to increase with time. However, in advanced cases of secondary progressive MS, one may see a reduction in the number and the total volume of T2 lesions: This is related to the confluence of chronic lesions, an important but previously less recognized feature of late-stage MS. Due to prominent CNS atrophy at this stage, the overall brain volume and the white matter volume are reduced, and there is a consequential reduction in the overall volume of T2-weighted lesions. This is another explanation for the poor correlation between lesion load on T2-weighted imaging and overall disability: disability tends to increase despite the reduction of lesion load in these advanced cases.

To increase the sensitivity of lesion detection on T2-weighted MRI, several methodologic considerations have been proposed, including the following[11-13]:

1. Smaller slice thickness—for routine clinical use, slices of 4 to 5 mm may be sufficient, but for more accurate research studies, smaller slices are desirable.
2. Three-dimensional acquisition techniques with isometric resolution as small as 1 mm—this also helps eliminate potentially "lost lesions," which were relatively common with older techniques due to different positioning, different slice thickness, and different gap sizes.
3. Higher field strength—with the increasing availability of 3-Tesla clinical systems, one can expect 24% to 40% increased detectability of T2-weighted lesions.

As noted earlier, the correlation between T2-weighted measures and clinical evolution is only modest, except in subjects with early relapsing-remitting disease (RRMS).[14-16] There are many reasons for this "MRI-clinical paradox." The correlation appears stronger if only corticospinal tract lesions are considered, so part of the explanation relates simply to lesion location. However, other factors contribute just as importantly, including disregard of lesions in the cord, which are almost always symptomatic, as opposed to brain lesions, which are often clinically silent.

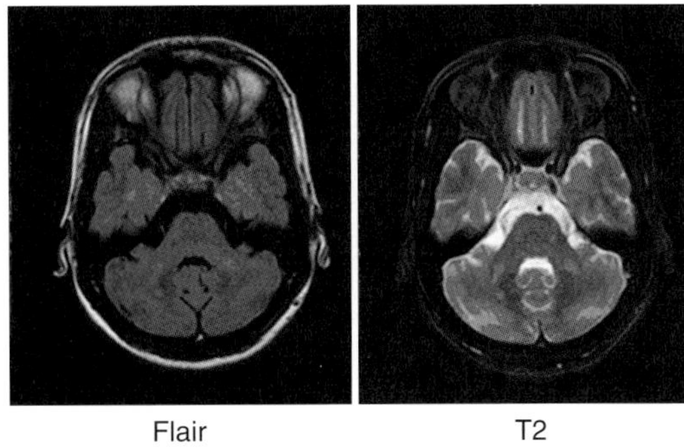

Figure 5–2 Comparison of fluid-attenuated inversion recovery (FLAIR) and T2-weighted magnetic resonance images in relapsing-remitting multiple sclerosis. Note the numerous T2-hyperintense lesions in the posterior fossa, including the cerebellar hemispheres, brachium pontis, and the pons itself. FLAIR images have much lower sensitivity to detect changes in the posterior fossa.

In addition, T2-weighted MRI disregards pathology in NAWM and NAGM areas, which clearly contributes to the overall pathology of MS and to disability.[14-16]

Although cortical and deep gray matter lesions are only infrequently detected on conventional MRI, MS has a very substantial gray matter involvement.[17] The commonly used T2-weighted sequences are inherently insensitive to cortical demyelination and to MS-related gray matter changes.

Fluid-attenuated inversion recovery (FLAIR) images are also T2 weighted in terms of their signal characteristics. They are acquired with the use of an additional inversion recovery pulse that is designed to minimize signal arising from unbound water (in this case, the CSF). FLAIR has increased sensitivity for cerebral hemispheric lesions, especially juxtacortical ones,[18] as well as cortical lesions. It reduces the difficulty of separating periventricular hyperintense lesions from CSF. For these reasons, many clinicians prefer FLAIR imaging as a screening tool for demyelinating diseases. However, FLAIR images are significantly less sensitive to infratentorial lesions, including brainstem, cerebellar, and spinal cord lesions; these are very common locations for MS lesions, and lesions in these locations are almost always symptomatic[19,20] (Fig. 5-2).

For cortical lesion detection, a newer technique, called double inversion recovery (DIR) imaging, has been reported to have much higher sensitivity, although it still captures only a fraction of the cortical plaques when compared to histologic analysis[21] (Fig. 5-3).

T2 Hyperintensities of the Cord

Part of the reason for the MRI-clinical paradox is that cord lesions are often ignored by practicing neurologists. The significance of cord involvement is underlined in the new diagnostic criteria of MS.[2,3] Cord lesions are best visualized on T2-weighted or proton density scans, and longitudinally they rarely exceed 1 spinal cord segment. This is in strong contrast with cord lesions of NMO (also known as Devic's disease), which are longitudinally extensive over 3 or more cord segments (see later discussion). Axial cord images commonly show involvement of less than half (usually one quarter to one third) of the cord area on axial cut, with white and often gray matter involvement. Short tau inversion recovery (STIR) imaging is also often used in the detection of cord lesions and may have better sensitivity.[22] STIR sequences also provide fat suppression, which results in increased

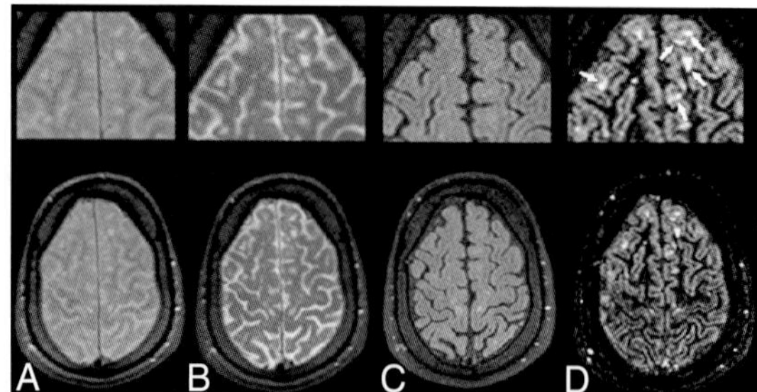

Figure 5–3 Double inversion recovery (DIR) imaging, showing intracortical and juxtacortical lesions in multiple sclerosis (MS). Top row shows zoomed views of axial magnetic resonance imaging scans presented in the bottom row. Proton density–weighted (**A**) and T2-weighted (**B**) images show hyperintense cortical and juxtacortical lesions. **C,** Multislab three-dimensional fluid-attenuated inversion recovery (FLAIR) image shows only a subset of the lesions. **D,** Multislab DIR image allows for superior depiction of MS lesions in and next to the cortex *(arrows)* and a better distinction between intracortical and mixed cortical/juxtacortical white matter lesions. (From Pirko I, Lucchinetti CF, Sriram S, Bakshi R: Gray matter involvement in multiple sclerosis. Neurology 2007;68: 634-642, with permission from Lippincott Williams & Wilkins, online at http://www.lww.com.)

sensitivity—not just in cord imaging but also in the imaging of optic nerves. Optic neuritis is a common CIS that may be the first manifestation of MS.[23,24]

Because the cord is almost never involved in small-vessel ischemic changes, cord imaging can increase the diagnostic certainty for a true demyelinating disease, and it can also help distinguish between CNS involvement of MS and that of other autoimmune or inflammatory diseases. In a recent study by Bot and associates, 92% of MS patients but only 6% of those with other immune-mediated diseases had cord lesions; 100% and 56%, respectively, had brain lesions.[25] In progressive forms of MS, and especially in primary progressive multiple sclerosis (PPMS), in which myelopathy-related symptoms predominate in the clinical picture, cord atrophy and increasing cord lesion load may be the only MRI manifestations of the disease.

T2 Hypointensities

A newer finding in MS is that hypointensities in the thalamus, deep gray nuclei, and cortical gray matter may be seen on standard T2-weighted images, as reported extensively by Bakshi and others.[26-30] The presence of such lesions appears to be associated with increased likelihood for cognitive problems, fatigue, brain atrophy, disability, and T2 lesion load. This MRI finding, along with that of T1 hypointensities (discussed later), may alert the clinician to a potentially more disabling disease course in individual cases. The finding most likely represents pathologic iron deposition, although this has not yet been proved conclusively. The changes may also be caused by other processes that result in susceptibility artifacts, including the presence of free radicals. Newer imaging techniques, including susceptibility-weighted imaging (SWI),[31] allow for easier quantification and advanced visualization of this finding. So far, this has been reported only in abstract form in MS patients (Fig. 5-4).

Proton density–weighted studies are often acquired in the same setting as the T2-weighted images, using dual-echo sequences: the image with the longer echo time is the T2-weighted image. These studies offer better lesion–tissue contrast,

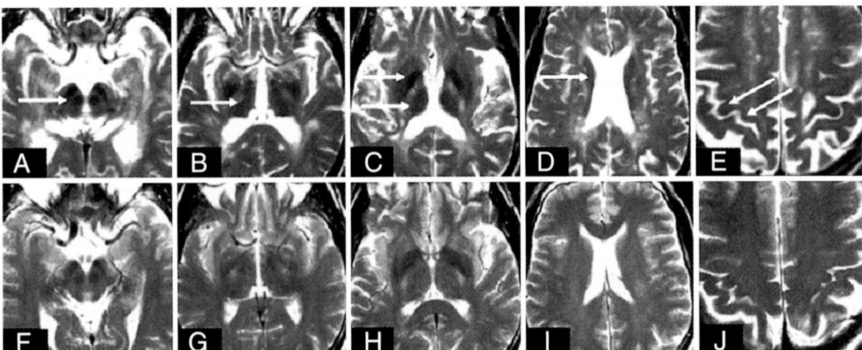

Figure 5–4 T2 hypointensities and brain atrophy in multiple sclerosis (MS). Fast spin-echo T2-weighted images are shown of a 43-year-old man with relapsing-remitting MS, a disease duration of 4 years, mild to moderate physical disability, and an Expanded Disability Status Scale score of 3.5 (**A** through **E**), compared with images of an age-matched healthy subject (**F** through **J**). In the MS patient, note the bilateral hypointensity of various gray matter areas *(arrows)*, including the red nucleus in **A**, the thalamus and lentiform nucleus in **B** and **C**, the caudate in **D**, and the rolandic cortex in **E**. The patient also has brain atrophy (note prominence of ventricular and subarachnoid spaces compared with the control). The T2 hypointensity most likely represents pathologic iron deposition. (From Pirko I, Lucchinetti CF, Sriram S, Bakshi R: Gray matter involvement in multiple sclerosis. Neurology 2007;68:634-642, with permission from Lippincott Williams & Wilkins, online at http://www.lww.com.)

including better differentiation of periventricular lesions. Unlike FLAIR, proton density scans are not hampered by poor sensitivity to infratentorial lesions. Overall, they are one of the most informative standard sequences in evaluating demyelinating diseases.

GADOLINIUM ENHANCEMENT ON T1-WEIGHTED STUDIES

Gadolinium is a rare earth metal that is used as the "gold standard" contrast material in MRI studies. It provides positive contrast (hyperintensity on T1-weighted images; see Fig. 5-1), as opposed to the iron-based negative contrast materials (hypointensity on gradient echo-based $T2^*$-weighted images, susceptibility effects). Although native gadolinium is highly toxic to living organisms, chelated forms are stable and are unlikely to exhibit toxicity. It must be noted that cases of nephrogenic systemic fibrosis and nephrogenic fibrosing dermopathy as a result of gadolinium administration have recently emerged. The incidence is higher with double- or triple-dose administration. To date, no such cases have been reported among patients with normal renal function. There also appear to be differences among the various gadolinium-based contrast agents in the incidence of this potentially serious adverse effect. The website of the International Society for Magnetic Resonance in Medicine provides continued updates regarding this topic (available at http://www.ismrm.org [accessed October 2008]).

In routine clinical imaging with gadolinium, the dose and the delay between administration and scanning are important determinants of overall sensitivity. The recommended standard dose is 0.1 mmol/kg, and a scanning delay of 5 to 10 minutes after administration is advisable. Gadolinium enhancement usually accompanies the formation of new lesions. Of note, most gadolinium-enhancing lesions in the brain will not result in new clinically detectable relapses: these scans are 5 to 10 times more sensitive to inflammatory activity than clinical observation alone.[32] This is the main reason for using post-contrast enhancing lesion load as an outcome measure in phase 0, I, and II clinical trials of new MS therapies. Although they efficiently capture inflammatory disease activity, gadolinium-enhancing lesions do not correlate well with disability on longitudinal studies: The mean number of enhancing lesions in the first 6 months after diagnosis of MS showed a weak correlation with disability 1 and 2 years later.[33] However, the presence of gadolinium-enhancing lesions is a strong predictor of subsequent relapses and can be considered a marker of an active inflammatory stage in MS. This observation is important, because it is this active stage that is addressed by the currently available immunomodulators. Therefore, practicing clinicians often utilize gadolinium-enhancing scans as an important decision-making tool in starting or upgrading immunomodulatory therapies.

The introduction of gadolinium-enhanced scanning was a very important step in the diagnosis and monitoring of MS lesion formation.[32,34-37] As mentioned earlier, gadolinium enhancement is considered the earliest sign of new lesion formation on conventional MRI.[38] The enhancement typically lasts for 4 to 6 weeks or less.[35,39] It is rarely detectable beyond 2 to 3 months, and if enhancement lasts longer than that, alternative diagnoses should be considered (e.g., neurosarcoidosis, neoplasms). In secondary progressive disease (SPMS), especially in patients who no longer have superimposed relapses, gadolinium enhancement becomes a very rare phenomenon.[40-41] In PPMS, as few as 5% of the cases exhibit gadolinium enhancement.[42] However, in the first 5 years of PPMS, up to 40% may demonstrate-enhancing lesions.[43]

There are methods to increase the sensitivity of post-gadolinium scans:

1. Higher dose—triple-dose gadolinium results in a 120% increase in sensitivity
2. Longer scanning delay—delays of 10 or 20 minutes may result in better detection than the standard 2- to 5-minute delays
3. A sensitizing magnetization transfer pulse[44]—in this setting, this can be considered "background noise reduction" and can greatly increase detectability
4. Higher field strength[11,13]
5. Acquisition of thinner slices or volume acquisition with small isometric voxel sizes
6. Post-processing methods that subtract the pre-contrast scan from the post-contrast scan after co-registration

Gadolinium-enhancing lesions may appear homogenously enhancing, ring enhancing, or open ring enhancing[32,34-37] (in which case the opening is often toward the cortex[45,46]). Open ring-enhancing lesions may be more specific for demyelinating lesions in general. Ring-enhancing lesions are typically larger, may exhibit a shorter duration of enhancement,[47] and have a lower apparent diffusion coefficient (ADC)[48] and magnetization transfer ratio (MTR)[49]; in some cases, they may predict the evolution of lesions to T1 black holes and may be associated with a higher likelihood for brain atrophy[50] (see later discussions of these topics). However, in the largest biopsy-proven cohort of demyelinating diseases, no such association was found between ring-enhancing lesions and increased risk for disability. Of note, ring-enhancing lesions are often seen with other conditions, including gliomas, metastases, and abscesses. Larger ring-enhancing lesions often

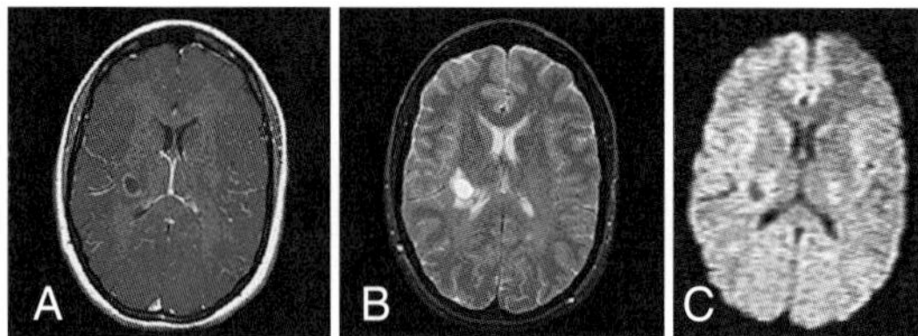

Figure 5–5 Ring enhancement and T2-hypointense rim in multiple sclerosis (MS) lesions. **A,** Large MS lesion with ring enhancement on T1-weighted post-gadolinium image. **B,** The lesion demonstrates a peripheral hypointense rim and is homogeneous centrally on T2-weighted magnetic resonance imaging. **C,** Diffusion-weighted imaging shows a mixed, although mostly dark, signal. (With kind permission from Springer Science+Business Media. Schwartz KM, Erickson BJ, Lucchinetti C: Pattern of T2 hypointensity associated with ring-enhancing brain lesions can help to differentiate pathology. Neuroradiology 2006;48:143-149.)

demonstrate a T2-hypointense border in the form of a rim or arc when they are caused by inflammatory demyelination; this may help in distinguishing demyelinating lesions from those associated with other etiologies[51] (Fig. 5-5).

Gadolinium enhancement is often considered a "passive process" signifying areas of damage to the blood–brain barrier. However, there is experimental evidence that areas of gadolinium enhancement are associated with vesicular transportation of gadolinium into endothelial cells, and subsequent deposition to the perivascular space, in the context of otherwise intact interendothelial junctions. The process of gadolinium uptake can also be pharmacologically inhibited in animal models. Therefore, it appears that endothelial cells may metabolically regulate gadolinium enhancement under certain conditions, including inflammation.[52] Of note, gadolinium enhancement does not always accompany the formation of new lesions, and preexisting lesions may enlarge without evidence for enhancement.

Novel Contrast Mechanisms

In addition to a positive contrast material such as gadolinium, negative contrast materials are increasingly used in MS-related MRI research. These materials are detected as hypointensities on $T2^*$-weighted images. The most prominent examples are the superparamagnetic ultrasmall iron oxide particles (USPIOs), which in their native form are picked up by monocytes and macrophages and can be utilized for imaging of active inflammation. USPIOs can also be functionalized, for example with antibodies or F(ab) fragments, which enables imaging of virtually any cell type with specific surface markers in animal models.[53,54] USPIOs have been used for macrophage imaging in human cases of MS.[55] The presence of USPIOs does not show full overlap with gadolinium-enhancing lesions. Some lesions may show gadolinium enhancement only, others combined uptake of gadolinium and USPIO, and yet others only USPIO uptake.[55] This demonstrates that gadolinium enhancement is not capable of detecting all inflammatory activity in the brain and that gadolinium uptake may represent an active process that does not always accompany all forms of CNS inflammation.

In a study comparing the enhancement pattern of a novel negatively charged USPIO particle with the longitudinal pattern of gadolinium enhancement in MS, 19 patients with relapsing-remitting disease were monitored monthly by gadolinium-enhanced MRI[56] (Fig. 5-6). When new enhancing lesions were detected,

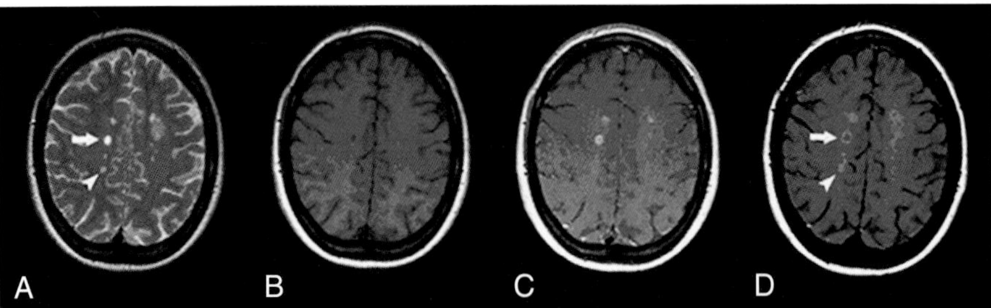

Figure 5–6 Comparative analysis of gadolinium enhancement and enhancement with negatively charged ultrasmall iron oxide particles (USPIOs). **A,** T2-weighted images show multiple sclerosis lesions. **B,** Pre-gadolinium T1-weighted images show T1 black holes. **C,** Some lesions enhance with standard gadolinium–diethylenetriamine penta-acetic acid (Gd-DTPA) contrast material. **D,** Post-USPIO images show a Gd-DTPA-positive, USPIO ring-enhancing lesion *(arrow)* and a Gd-DTPA–negative, focally USPIO-positive lesion *(arrowhead)*. The image in **D** illustrates that USPIOs may reveal more enhancing lesions than Gd-DTPA and that different enhancement patterns may be observed within the same patient with the use of USPIOs. (From Vellinga MM, Oude Engberink RD, Seewann A, et al: Pluriformity of inflammation in multiple sclerosis shown by ultra-small iron oxide particle enhancement. Brain 2008;131:800-807, by permission of Oxford University Press.)

USPIO contrast imaging was also performed with a 24-hour scanning delay. (For USPIO-based contrast materials, a long scanning delay is needed, because cellular uptake of the contrast material and tissue infiltration of the labeled cells take time.) As in earlier studies in an MS model,[53] USPIO enhancement was observed as hyperintensity on T1-weighted images. In 14 patients with disease activity, 188 USPIO-positive lesions were seen, 144 of which were gadolinium negative. At the same time, only 59 gadolinium-positive lesions were seen in these patients, 15 of which were USPIO negative. The patterns of USPIO enhancement included (a) focal or (b) ring-like enhancement and (c) return to isointensity of a previously hypointense lesion. This last pattern was most frequently observed in lesions that were only transiently hypointense, as demonstrated on follow-up scans. USPIO ring-enhancing lesions were less likely to evolve into T1 black holes, a finding that may be related to a more active tissue restorative process in such lesions. In 4% of the cases, USPIO enhancement preceded gadolinium enhancement by as much as 1 month. USPIO enhancement remained visible longer than gadolinium enhancement in one third of the cases, and in a few cases it persisted for up to 3 months.[56]

Future studies using a combination of contrast materials are likely to further clarify the role and significance of the various contrast-enhancing mechanisms and enhancement patterns, signifying the interindividual and, potentially, the intraindividual pluriformity of inflammation in CNS demyelinating diseases.

T1 Hypointensities and "T1 Black Holes"

A subset of T2-weighted lesions are identifiable as hypointensities on T1-weighted scans.[57] This may represent an early, transient stage in lesion formation,[50,58] thought to be caused by focal edema accompanying the inflammatory infiltrate in emerging lesions. Whereas the majority of acute T1 hypointensities resolve,[59,60] approximately 30% of MS patients also develop persistent T1 hypointensities, commonly referred to as "T1 black holes."[61] These areas are thought to represent more severe tissue loss, including axonal damage.[62,63] In contrast to T2-hyperintense lesion load, the persistent T1-weighted hypointense lesion load correlates well with chronic disability.[5] Therefore, the presence of T1 black holes on MRI is considered a worrisome finding by most MS clinicians (see Fig. 5-6B).

Classically, T1 black holes were thought to be confined to the cerebral white matter; however, similar abnormalities, likely of the same origin and significance, have been recently reported in the spinal cord as well.[64] In an MRI-histology correlational study of unfixed postmortem brains of MS patients,[62] the degree of hypointensity correlated best with axonal density. Correlation between matrix destruction and hypointensity showed a trend but did not reach significance. The observation that T1 hypointensities probably represent severe tissue damage, including axonal and neuronal loss, was also confirmed in a large-scale histology-based study by Bitsch and colleagues.[63] T1 black holes were found to have a low MTR, which is also indicative of structural loss.[65] In MRS studies, early acute T1 black hole formations showed an increased choline peak,[66] indicative of active membrane turnover or cell infiltration in the newly forming lesions; even at this stage, the axonal marker *N*-acetylaspartate (NAA) can be decreased.[67] The hallmark of chronic T1 black holes is decreased NAA.[68] The significance of chronic T1 black holes in human MS is related to their strong correlation with disability.[69-71] Recently, a novel animal model of this MRI finding was published and may allow for the identification of immune mechanisms responsible for this severe form of tissue damage in MS.[72]

Spontaneous T1 Hyperintensities

Another interesting finding that is newly reported—so far by one group only—is the presence of spontaneous hyperintensities on conventional spin-echo–based T1-weighted studies[73] (Fig. 5-7). They are more common in SPMS but can also be seen in RRMS. They manifest as hyperintense perilesional rims (two thirds of lesions) or as homogenous hyperintensities (one third of lesions). T1 hyperintensities are reported to have good correlation with disability and brain atrophy measures, but not with disease duration. If confirmed in future larger scale studies, this finding may become an important biomarker for a more disabling disease course.

The Role of Magnetic Resonance Imaging in the Diagnostic Criteria of Multiple Sclerosis

The diagnostic criteria for MS have undergone significant changes over the last few years. The most important of these was the addition of MRI-based paraclinical markers to the criteria. This clarifies the role of this diagnostic modality in establishing the diagnosis and allows for earlier diagnosis of MS by establishing "dissemination in time and space" criteria based not only on clinical grounds but also on imaging. In addition, MRI criteria for PPMS were established. The original McDonald criteria[2] were proposed in 2001 and modified by Polman and coworkers[3] in 2005 (Table 5-1). The current criteria for dissemination in space outline the importance of lesion location (juxtacortical, periventricular, infratentorial); compared with the 2001 version, these criteria emphasize the important role of

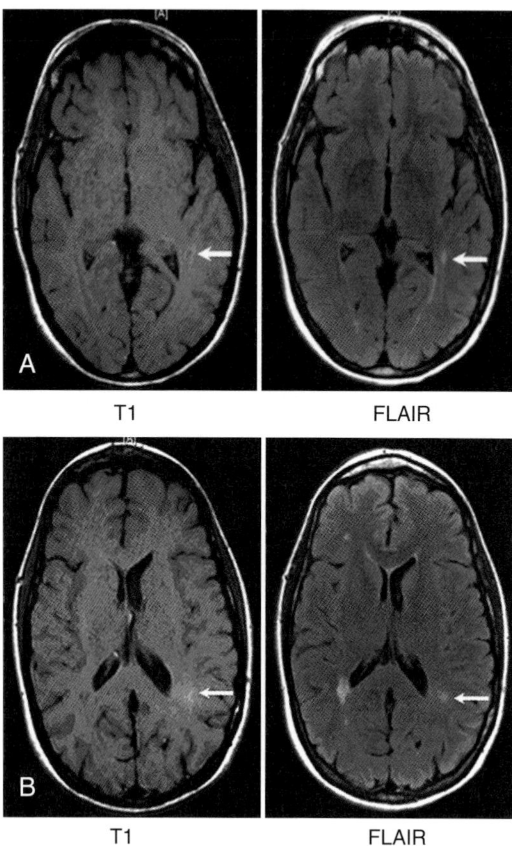

Figure 5–7 Spontaneous T1 hyperintensities in multiple sclerosis. Note the relationship of the T1-hyperintense lesions on non-contrast spin-echo T1 images to the hyperintensities visible on fluid-attenuated inversion recovery (FLAIR) images *(arrows)*. **A,** Perilesional T1 hyperintensity. **B,** Homogenous T1 hyperintensity. The finding is thought to be associated with a more disabling disease course, but this has not yet been prospectively validated in a large cohort. (Courtesy of Rohit Bakshi, MD, Associate Professor of Neurology, Harvard Medical School, Brigham and Woman Hospital, Partners MS Center.)

TABLE 5–1 The 2005 Magnetic Resonance Imaging Criteria in the Diagnosis of Multiple Sclerosis*

Criteria for dissemination in space—three of the following must be present:
1. At least one gadolinium-enhancing lesion, or nine T2-hyperintense lesions if there is no gadolinium-enhancing lesion
2. At least one infratentorial lesion
3. At least one juxtacortical lesion
4. At least three periventricular lesions

Criteria for dissemination in time—one of the following must be present:
1. Detection of gadolinium enhancement at least 3 months after the onset of the initial clinical event, and not at the site corresponding to the initial event
2. Detection of a *new* T2 lesion if it appears at any time compared with a reference scan done at least 30 days after the onset of the initial clinical event

*Notes about the role of spinal cord lesions: (a) a spinal cord lesion may be considered equivalent to a brain infratentorial lesion; (b) an enhancing spinal cord lesion is considered to be equivalent to an enhancing brain lesion; (c) individual spinal cord lesions can contribute, together with individual brain lesions, to reach the required number of T2 lesions.

cord lesions. A cord lesion can be considered equivalent to a brain infratentorial lesion; an enhancing cord lesion is considered equivalent to an enhancing brain lesion and can be counted *twice* (once as enhancing, and once as an infratentorial lesion). Cord lesions can contribute, together with brain lesions, to reach the required number of T2 lesions. The criteria for dissemination in time was simplified in the 2005 modification and now includes (1) detection of gadolinium enhancement at least 3 months after the initial event, at a different site than the initial lesion, or (2) the detection of a new T2 lesion if it appears at any time compared with a reference scan done at least 30 days after the onset of the initial clinical event.

PPMS often shows a cord-predominant MRI picture and a paucity of enhancing lesions compared to RRMS cases. The 2005 MRI criteria for PPMS include only two features: (1) positive brain MRI, which in this case is defined as nine or more T2-hyperintense lesions, or four or more T2-hyperintense lesions if the visual evoked potential (VEP) is positive; and (2) positive cord MRI, defined as two or more T2 lesions. Of note, only one criterion needs to be met if the CSF is positive, which in this case is defined as the presence of oligoclonal bands or immunoglobulin G (IgG) index elevation, or both.

Even though considerable attention was given to the development of these MRI criteria, their specificity is still relatively low, and other diseases of the CNS may meet these criteria. Overall, MS remains a clinical diagnosis, wherein data derived from the history, clinical examination, laboratory and MRI findings all contribute to making the proper diagnosis, and none of these components is sufficient alone.

RED FLAGS IN MISDIAGNOSING MULTIPLE SCLEROSIS ON MRI

Although MRI clearly plays an important role in the diagnosis of MS, its lack of specificity, coupled with its high sensitivity to a wide array of tissue pathology, easily gives rise to false interpretation of scans. In the hands of experienced clinicians who understand that MRI is no substitute for a careful and detailed history and examination, this usually does not represent a major problem. However, several CNS diseases have MRI "signatures" that can be mistaken for MS, and even the clinical features may be consistent with that of an inflammatory demyelinating disease, yet the actual diagnosis is different from MS. These scenarios obviously have important ramifications from the standpoint of prognosis and therapy. A workshop of the European Magnetic Resonance Network in Multiple Sclerosis (MAGNIMS) was held in 2005 with the intention of defining a set of MRI "red flags," derived from evidence-based findings and "educated guesses."[74] For example, T1-hypointense and T2-hyperintense lesions in the spinal cord that are more than 3 vertebral segments in length should prompt a thorough evaluation for NMO; likewise, the preferential involvement of temporal poles and external capsule should suggest cerebral autosomal dominant arteriopathy with subcortical infarcts and leukoencephalopathy (CADASIL), whereas nonspecific white matter lesions, dilated Virchow-Robin spaces with hippocampal and amygdala atrophy, may suggest hyperhomocysteinemia. Table 5-2 summarizes the identified sets of MRI features that are suggestive of specific etiologies. The presence of these specific features in the proper clinical setting should trigger a targeted workup of the affected patient.

TABLE 5–2 Red Flags for MRI Misdiagnosis of Multiple Sclerosis

MRI Finding	Disease
Brain White Matter	
Normal	NMO (absent or few lesions), ATM
Large lesions	AMS (sometimes confluent and perilesional edema), BCS (concentric whorls of alternating rings of enhancement), PACNS (with mass effect)
Symmetrically distributed lesions	ADEM, AFL
Poorly defined lesion margins	ADEM
Absent or rare Dawson fingers, corpus callosum and periventricular lesions	ADEM
Absent MRI activity at follow-up	ADEM
T2-hyperintensity of the temporal pole, U-fibers at the vertex, external capsule,and insular regions	CADASIL
Multiple bilateral microhaemorrhagic foci	CADASIL, SVD
Frequent sparing of corpus callosum and cerebellum	CADASIL, SVD
Lesions in the centre of corpus callosum, sparing the periphery	Susac's syndrome
Haemorrhages	PACNS
Simultaneous enhancement of all lesions	ADEM, PACNS, sarcoidosis
Infarcts	SID, PACNS, SVD
Punctiform parenchymal enhancement	PACNS, sarcoidosis, NBD
Predominance of lesions at the cortical/ subcortical junction	SID
Diffuse while matter involvement	NBD, encephalitis (HIVE), SVD, CADASIL
Cerebral venous sinus thrombosis	NBD
Large and infiltrating brainstem lesions	NBD
Anterior temporal and inferior frontal lobe involvement, associated with enhancement or mass effect	Encephalitis (HSE)
Isolated lesions with ring enhancement (often complete)	Abscesses
Mass effect	Abscesses
Multifocal, asymmetrical lesions starting in a juxtacortical location and progressively enlarging	PML
Large lesions with absent or rare mass effect	PML
Extensive and bilateral periventricular abnormalities in isolation	B12D, ACD
Cortical Gray Matter	
Cortical/subcortical lesions crossing vascular territories	MELAS
Prevalent involvement compared with white matter	Encephalitis

TABLE 5–2 Red Flags for MRI Misdiagnosis of Multiple Sclerosis (Continued)

MRI Finding	Disease
Infiltrating lesions that do not remain in gray or white matter boundaries	Abscesses
Deep Gray Matter	
Bilateral lesions	ADEM (at the gray-white-matter junction), CADASIL
Lacunar infarcts	CADASIL, SVD
T1 hyperintensity of the pulvinar	FD
Multiple discrete lesions in the basal ganglia and thalamus	Susac's syndrome
Large and infiltrating basal ganglia lesions	NBD
Infiltrating lesions without respecting gray-matter or white-matter boundaries	Abscesses
T2-hyperintense lesions in the dentate nuclei	AFL (CTX)
Spinal Cord	
Large and swelling lesions	NMO (with corresponding T1 hypointensity), ADEM, ATM, Sjögren's syndrome
Diffuse abnormalities in the posterior columns	B12D, ACD
Other	
No "occult" changes in the NAWN	NMO, Lyme disease, SID (except in NSLE)
Pontine lacunar infarcts	CADASIL, SVD
Dilation of Virchow-Robin spaces	HHC, PACNS
Diffuse lactate increase on brain MRS	MELAS
Meningeal enhancement	Susac's syndrome, PACNS, NBD, meningitis, Lyme disease, sarcoidosis
Hydrocephalus	Sarcoidosis
Absence of optic-nerve lesions	PML
Regional atrophy	HHC (hippocampus and amygdala), NBD (brainstem)

ACD, acquired copper deficiency; ADEM, acute disseminated encephalomyelitis; AFL, adult forms of leukoencephalopathies; AMS, acute multiple sclerosis (Marburg type); ATM, acute transverse myelitis; B12D, vitamin B_{12} deficiency; BCS, Balo's concentric sclerosis; CADASIL, cerebral autosomal dominant arteriopathy with subcortical infarcts and leukoencephalopathy; CTX, cerebrotendinous xanthomatosis; FD, Fabry's disease; HHC, hyperhomocysteinemia; HIVE, HIV encephalitis; HSE, herpes simplex encephalitis; MELAS, mitochondrial encephalopathy with lactic acidosis and stroke-like episodes; MRI, magnetic resonance imaging; MRS, magnetic resonance spectroscopy; NAWM, normal-appearing white matter; NBD, Behçet's disease with CNS involvement; NMO, neuromyelitis optica; NSLE, neuropsychiatric systemic lupus erythematosus; PACNS, primary angiitis of the central nervous system; PML, progressive multifocal leukoencephalopathy; SID, systemic immune-mediated diseases; SSP, subacute sclerosing panencephalitis; SVD, small-vessel disease.

(From Chrail A, Yousry TA, Rovaris M, et al: MRI and the diagnosis of multiple sclerosis: Expanding the concept of "no better explanation." Lancet Neurol 2006;5:841-852.)

THE ROLE OF MRI IN THE PROGNOSIS OF CLINICALLY ISOLATED DEMYELINATING SYNDROMES

The first presentation of MS commonly includes subacute onset of a well-defined demyelinating syndrome, such as optic neuritis, transverse myelitis, or isolated brainstem/cerebellar syndromes. In these patients, brain MRI plays a critically important role in clarifying the risk for conversion to MS. The best known predictor for conversion is the number of lesions on the initial scan. The best known study of this kind is the National Hospital series from London, UK[4,15,75-77] (Fig. 5-8). The findings of this group were very similar to those of the Optic Neuritis Study Group and other smaller series. The 1-year conversion rate to MS in those patients with abnormal MRI scans was 30%, and no patients from the normal scan group had converted to MS at this early time point. At 5 years, 65% of those with abnormal scans had converted to MS, compared with 3% of those with normal MRIs. At 10 years, the figures were 83% and 11%, respectively, and at 14 years, they were 88% and 19%. The rate of conversion at 20 years was 82% for those with an abnormal MRI but only 21% for those with a normal scan. The reason for the somewhat fluctuating percentages is that the availability of patients and follow-up scans was different at the various study time points.[4] As is evident from these data, the majority of conversions to MS occurred during the first few years after the initial demyelinating event. Those who converted after having an unsuggestive MRI at presentation also had milder disease. From the standpoint of risk for conversion, it did not matter whether the demyelinating syndrome was ON, transverse myelitis, or an isolated brainstem or cerebellar syndrome.

It is also important to look at these data from the standpoint of the development of disability in the converters. A 2008 study addressed these issues using the 20-year data.[4] Among those patients who developed MS, a concurrent correlation of change in T2 lesion volume with change in Expanded Disability Status Scale (EDSS) score was most evident in the first 5 years. The estimated rate of lesion growth over the duration of the study was 0.80 cm^3/year in those who remained with RRMS and 2.89 cm^3/year in those who developed SPMS; the difference was statistically significant. The study established that lesion volume and its change at earlier time points are correlated with disability after 20 years. Lesion volume increased for at least 20 years in relapse-onset MS, and the rate of lesion growth

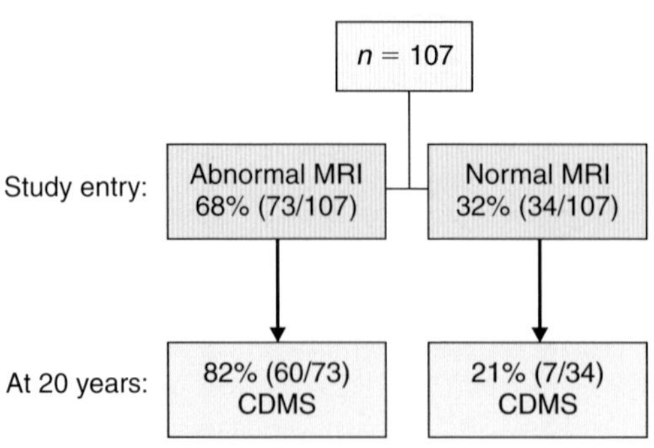

Figure 5–8 Risk for conversion to multiple sclerosis in clinically isolated demyelinating syndromes. Twenty-year follow-up of the National Hospital (UK) clinically isolated demyelinating syndrome (CIS) cohort. CDMS, clinically defined multiple sclerosis; MRI, magnetic resonance imaging.

was more than three times higher in those who developed SPMS than in those who remained with RRMS.

"PRECLINICAL MULTIPLE SCLEROSIS": INCIDENTAL MRI FINDINGS SUGGESTIVE OF MULTIPLE SCLEROSIS

An interesting scenario arises when MRI findings suggestive of MS-like changes are seen in the context of a workup for an unrelated complaint (e.g., headache, head injury). In such cases, often labeled preclinical MS, it is imperative that the workup include screening for potential MS mimics. This is especially important because in these cases the workup, by definition, was not initiated in the context of a CIS or MS-like presentation. Regarding prognostication in preclinical MS, a 5-year retrospective study of 30 patients with a normal neurologic examination whose MRI fulfilled the Barkhof/Tintoré criteria was recently reported.[78] The mean time for the second brain MRI was 6 months. Twenty-three (77%) of the 30 patients had temporal-spatial dissemination, and 11 patients (37%) had clinical conversion. The mean time between first brain MRI and CIS was 2.3 years. Although these numbers may appear higher than the usually quoted risk for conversion in CIS, it should be noted that most of these patients had multiple lesions on their scans, which in itself suggests higher risk for conversion. Also, the Queen Square series utilized the Poser "clinically definite" MS (CDMS) criteria and not the Barkhof/Tintoré criteria for establishing conversion to MS (see Chapter 2). In addition, the retrospective nature of this study may also hinder the ability to establish a valid conversion rate.

The Role of Magnetic Resonance Imaging in Treatment Decisions

As discussed earlier, MRI is the single most important prognostic factor when assessing the likelihood for conversion to MS. CIS patients with a high risk for conversion can be treated early, especially if the overall disability risk profile also appears high. A watchful "wait and see" approach is recommended for those cases in which the risk for conversion is low overall. The "dissemination in time" criteria provide good guidelines about how soon to perform a repeat MRI in cases of watchful waiting. However, it should be noted that the longer one waits, the more likely it is that MRI conversion will occur, so a wait of longer than 3 months for the repeat scan may be acceptable in individual cases. Overall, treatment decisions should always be individualized and based on a mutual agreement between the treating physician and the educated patient. Providing sufficient information and making decisions together with the patient is imperative. This can be very time-consuming, but in complex diseases such as MS the agreement and trust between patient and physician is one of the key components of appropriate patient care. One must also keep in mind that not every MS case is universally disabling, and benign MS is a well-recognized entity.[79] It is beyond the scope of this chapter to list the pros and cons of early or universal treatment of MS compared with the approach of watchful waiting and intervention when needed. Several excellent reviews have addressed these issues.[80-82]

MRI also plays an important part in treatment monitoring, and it can provide helpful guidance in determining treatment failure. In general, the currently available disease-modifying agents (DMAs) best address the active inflammatory stage of MS (e.g., gadolinium-enhancing new lesion formation by MRI). If a non-treated patient develops such lesions, especially if multiple such lesions are seen, treatment initiation becomes imperative. If increased inflammatory activity is seen in a patient already undergoing treatment, an upgrade to a stronger form of immunomodulation may be needed (e.g., from low-dose interferons or glatiramer acetate to high-dose interferons). Mitoxantrone and natalizumab are best used in those patients who fail to stabilize on conventional injectable DMAs from the standpoint of an MRI-detectable inflammatory profile. In progressive forms of MS, the currently available immunomodulatory therapies are largely ineffective. In the low proportion of SPMS cases with evidence for inflammatory activity on MRI, standard DMAs may provide some help. Advanced MRI can also clarify progression by the gradual worsening of low NAA levels, worsening atrophy on MRI volumetry, and changes in NAWM. However, despite the ability to identify these changes, the currently available DMAs are unable to meaningfully address the progressive neurodegenerative component of MS.

Advanced Magnetic Resonance Imaging Techniques

The techniques discussed in this section are important tools in MS research and are increasingly being applied in routine clinical practice, especially at larger centers. In MS research, these techniques have helped clarify several previously poorly understood features of this complex disease.

MAGNETIZATION TRANSFER IMAGING

Magnetization transfer imaging (MTI) is a newer modality first performed in MS patients by Dousset and colleagues.[83] MTI is especially suited to studying the influence of large macromolecules, including myelin, on their environment. Biologically important macromolecules have very short T2 relaxation times and cannot easily be studied with conventional MRI. Using special pulse sequences, one can saturate these macromolecular spins, and some of this saturated magnetization can then transfer to liquid protons as a result of the constant interaction between them and the large molecules. This results in reduced signal intensity from the mobile (small molecular) protons and serves as the basis of MTI.

MTI is a sensitive measure of disease progression in nonlesional areas, such as the NAWM and NAGM.[84-88] Changes in these areas are detectable very early in MS, and they correlate at least moderately with future disability.[87-89] However, despite this early detectability, the presence of such abnormalities does not increase the risk of conversion to clinically definite MS, according to a recently completed international longitudinal study of CIS patients. The validity of this observation may have been hampered by the relatively short follow-up interval, but it is intriguing that, despite the presence of seemingly diffuse abnormalities, patients might not develop CDMS for years.[90]

In contrast to MS and CIS, the NAWM shows no abnormalities on MTI in patients with ADEM. Therefore, MTI may be an important tool in distinguishing between MS and ADEM cases, although this observation requires further validation.[91]

MTI can also be used in the study of individual lesions. The magnetization transfer ratio or MTR, a parameter derived from images acquired with or without the magnetization transfer pulse, can be helpful in characterizing demyelination and remyelination.[92,93] MTR is lower in MS lesions than in nonspecific small-vessel lesions.[94,95] MTR may normalize as part of the normal lesion evolution,[96,97] or it may remain decreased.[97-99] This illustrates the sensitivity of this measure to detect tissue repair and remyelination, which may have a growing significance as therapeutic agents directed at enhancing remyelination enter early clinical trials.

In addition to its use in brain imaging, MTI of the spinal cord has been reported.[100] MTI-derived measures of cord pathology can be especially important as biomarkers for progressive forms of MS, in which the progression and level of disability show poor correlation with conventional MRI measures.

DIFFUSION-WEIGHTED IMAGING

Diffusion-weighted imaging (DWI) and diffusion tensor imaging (DTI) have allowed insight into the molecular movement of water in the studied tissues of interest. In general, DWI of the brain takes advantage of the spatial orientation of myelinated fibers and the restriction of water movement they cause: water diffuses much more easily in directions parallel with the fibers than perpendicular to the fibers. Monitoring of changes in free and restricted diffusion of water can identify various pathologic processes including stroke, ischemia, brain tumors, and white matter diseases. Several parameters have been used to numerically describe the tissue processes captured by DWI. One of the most important measures is the apparent diffusion coefficient (ADC), a measure of the random displacement of water in a particular direction of interest. In general, the ADC of brain structures is lower than that of free water due to diffusion-limiting membranes, myelinated axons, and the overall directional organization of CNS tissue, especially in the white matter. A direction-independent measure of diffusion is the mean diffusivity index (D), also known as directionally averaged ADC. D is the average of the ADCs measured in three orthogonal directions. Mean diffusivity is lower in structurally organized and higher in directionally disorganized tissue segments. In NABT, increases in D and ADC have been observed in MS patients, consistent with subtle tissue damage.[101,102] The D and ADC tend to be higher in lesions than in NAWM and are especially high in acute lesions. It has also been observed that subtle increases in D values predate the appearance of gadolinium-enhancing lesions by a few weeks and therefore may represent one of the earliest signs of focal tissue abnormalities leading to lesion formation.[103]

DTI studies can investigate the actual directional predominance of water movements, and, as such, they can identify the directions of fiber tracts and allow for very detailed tractography. In MS, a decrease in fractional anisotropy (FA), one of the DTI-derived measures, is often reported.[104-107] For practical purposes, FA can be considered a measure of how organized or how directionally restricted the tissue architecture is from the standpoint of water diffusion. Higher FA values represent higher orders of tissue organization. In the normal CNS, white matter areas always have a higher FA than gray matter areas, especially where there are coherently organized parallel fiber bundles. The FA is lower in areas of relatively incoherent organization, for example, where fiber bundles cross. Because FA is highest in organized tissue areas, a decrease in FA can sensitively detect abnormalities in white matter areas; however, FA is relatively insensitive to gray matter pathology. FA is decreased in gadolinium-enhancing lesions compared to nonenhancing ones.[108] Higher mean diffusivity and lower FA can be seen in lesions compared to NAWM, and these abnormalities are most prominent in lesions with the most extensive tissue damage, such as T1 hypointensities.[108-111]

PERFUSION-WEIGHTED IMAGING

Perfusion-weighted imaging is relatively rarely performed in the routine setting. It can be considered a form of functional imaging, because it investigates a dynamic process of perfusion of contrast material with very rapid acquisition sequences. A perfusion MRI method that allows for measurements of cerebral blood flow (CBF) and cerebral blood volume (CBV) is dynamic susceptibility contrast imaging. It consists of repeated and very rapid scanning of the brain utilizing ultrafast echoplanar imaging (EPI) sequences that generate $T2^*$-weighted image sets of the brain while gadolinium contrast is being injected in a synchronized fashion. Studies using this technique have revealed decreased perfusion in NAWM areas of PPMS and RRMS patients and reduced perfusion of gray matter areas in progressive cases.[112,113] The reduction was greater in PPMS, especially in the periventricular NAWM areas and in deep gray nuclei. Increased perfusion can be seen in the white matter in RRMS and SPMS,[112] especially before gadolinium enhancement becomes detectable in newly-forming lesions.[114,115] Reduced CBF is commonly seen in T1 black holes.[116]

In a study correlating cognitive changes with perfusion MRI measures, decreased CBF and CBV were found in gray matter structures as well as in the NAWM.[117] Another study reported good association between fatigue and deep gray matter hypoperfusion; in addition, there was lower perfusion in these structures in patients with PPMS compared with RRMS.[118] Experimental perfusion-based techniques are also important in the differential diagnosis of mass-like lesions, as discussed later in this chapter (Fig. 5-9).

T1 AND T2 RELAXOMETRY

The numerical measurement and mapping of T1 and T2 relaxation times in voxels of interest, including entire slices, has become possible.[119-122] Both T1 and T2 relaxometry often show increased relaxation times in lesional areas. Such metrics may aid in understanding the extent of severe tissue damage in lesions. T2 relaxation measurements allow for T2 component analysis, which can distinguishing areas of demyelination and remyelination. One of the most promising T2 relaxometry–based techniques is the myelin water fraction (MWF) measurement, which is derived from the short T2 component of multiecho T2 relaxometry experiments. Ex vivo MWF measurements showed excellent correlation with myelin stains[123] in MS and other demyelinating disorders. Monitoring of MWF changes is possible, although whole brain scanning with this technique is technically challenging. The long T2 component also appears to have unique significance: lesions with a long T2 component can be detected in a subset of patients. These lesions also exhibit increased water content (WC), higher T1, reduced MTR, and decreased MWF.

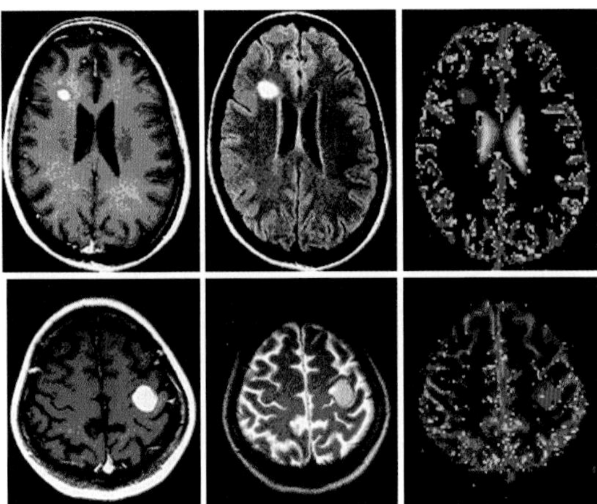

Figure 5–9 Relative cerebral blood volume (rCBV) map of a tumefactive demyelinating lesion *(top row)* versus a glioblastoma *(bottom row)*. T1-weighted gadolinium-enhanced images are shown on the left, fluid-attenuated inversion recovery (FLAIR) images in the middle column, and the rCBV maps on the right. rCBV is a perfusion-based method that enables differentiation of intracranial masses. The rCBV map of the glioblastoma case clearly shows increased blood volume, whereas the tumefactive demyelinating case shows no increase in blood volume. (From Cha S, Pierce S, Knopp EA, et al: Dynamic contrast-enhanced T2*-weighted MR imaging of tumefactive demyelinating lesions. Am J Neuroradiol 2001;22:1109-1116.)

Subjects with long T2 lesions had a significantly longer disease duration than subjects without this lesion subtype, so these may represent chronic, burnt-out lesions. Extracellular water is likely to be the origin of the long T2 component.[124]

MAGNETIC RESONANCE SPECTROSCOPY

MRS allows insight into the chemical composition of a studied voxel or voxels of interest (Fig. 5-10). Studied nuclei include protons (^{1}H) most commonly; phosphorus (^{31}P) is also occasionally studied, but this requires special hardware (a separate coil tuned to the frequency of ^{31}P at the given field strength). MRS is commonly done on single voxels; it can also be done on entire slices (chemical shift imaging), or MRS measures describing the entire brain can be derived. The spatial resolution of MRS is usually orders of magnitude lower than that of standard magnetic resonance imaging; voxel sizes in human MRS are rarely lower than 1 mL. MRS markers help characterize both demyelinating and axonal/neuronal pathologies in the studied areas of interest and also can detect inflammation, cell infiltration, and changes related to ischemia.[97,125,126] In areas of active inflammation, the choline, lactate, and lipid peaks are often increased. Choline peak increase is considered a cell membrane turnover marker, and its elevation may accompany immune cell infiltration, demyelination and remyelination, and gliosis. Areas of axonal and neuronal damage may reveal a relative decrease of NAA. Although NAA decrease has been thought to represent a "static" end point, it is becoming clear that NAA decrease is suggestive of a metabolic abnormality and not necessarily irreversible loss of axons and neurons. Selective serotonin reuptake inhibitors have been shown to result in increased NAA concentration in the CNS of MS patients; similar observations have been made in neurodegenerative diseases and

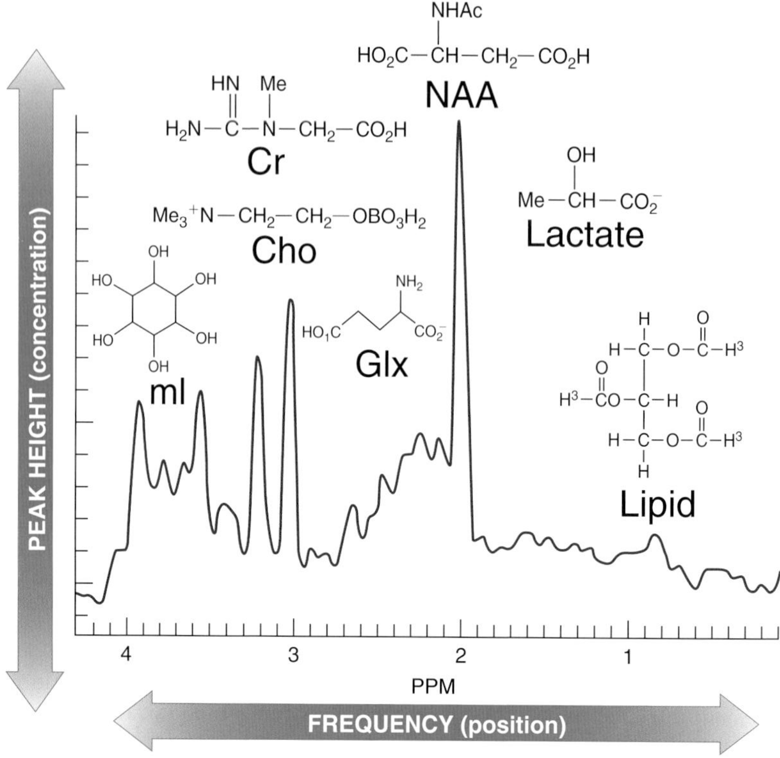

Figure 5–10 Typical proton magnetic resonance spectroscopy (^{1}H MRS) of a brain voxel, showing the spectrum of brain along with molecular assignment of resonances. The normal ^{1}H MRS spectrum is dominated by an N-acetylaspartate (NAA) resonance. To the left of NAA, peaks of glutamate/glutamine (Glx), creatine (Cr)/phosphocreatine, choline (Cho)-containing phospholipids, and *myo*-inositol (mI) are seen. On the right of the NAA peak are the lactate and free lipid peaks. In multiple sclerosis, abnormal findings often include a decrease in the NAA peak (indicative of axonal dysfunction/pathology) and an increase in the Cho peak (indicative of cell infiltration, inflammation, demyelination) or inositol (indicative of gliosis). In acute lesions, elevation of free lipids may also be seen. (From Narayana PA: Magnetic resonance spectroscopy in the monitoring of multiple sclerosis. J Neuroimaging 2005;15:46S-57S.)

animal models.[127] In addition, if NAA decrease truly represented the magnitude of axonal or neuronal loss, it would be expected to show reasonably good correlation with brain atrophy, which was not the case in a well-designed and well-performed MRS and brain volumetry correlational study in PPMS; it also did not show good correlation with lesion load.[128] Some of the controversies related to what NAA decrease really represents are related to the frequent use of relative measures, such as NAA/creatine or NAA/choline ratios, as opposed to true quantitative spectroscopy. Such techniques are gaining more recognition in MS research. A quantitative MRS study of NAWM reported that the reason for a nonlesional NAA/creatine decrease was not NAA decrease but creatine increase when compared to controls. The same study also found absolute increases in choline and myoinositol in NAWM.[129]

The function of NAA in axons and neurons remains unclear. The classic interpretation is that NAA is an osmotic regulator in neurons and axons. Although it probably does play such role, it seems unusual to have high concentrations of a metabolite present in billions of cells just for this reason. An interesting alternative hypothesis suggests that NAA may serve as a glutamate reservoir and may be converted into glutamate in a set of reactions that is energetically favorable, producing reduced nicotinamide adenine dinucleotide (NADH). Glutamate is not only needed for neuronal function and survival but also is utilized by astrocytes and oligodendrocytes, and NADH may serve as an additional energy reservoir for these metabolically active cells.[130]

Myoinositol has been proposed as a glial proliferation marker.[131,132] The excitatory neurotransmitters glutamate/glutamine have detectable peaks on MRS.[129,133] Cortical and deep gray matter changes may also be detected on MRS.[131,134,135] In CIS, ^{1}H MRS of a parietal white matter area conducted at 3 Tesla showed a decrease in total NAA concentration regardless of the presence or absence of dissemination in space, suggesting diffuse axonal/neuronal dysfunction in this patient population.[136]

PHOSPHORUS MAGNETIC RESONANCE SPECTROSCOPY

Phosphorous spectroscopy in commonly used for in vivo studies of energy metabolites. Because the phosphorous concentration in the CNS is orders of magnitude lower than that of protons, ^{31}P MRS voxels need to be much larger than ^{1}H MRS voxels to achieve acceptable signal-to-noise ratios. One of the most challenging parts of standard ^{1}H MRS acquisition is water suppression, because the water concentration is significantly higher than that of any other ^{1}H MRS–detectable metabolites, and the large water peak would not allow visualization of other components of the spectrum. In phosphorus spectroscopy, water suppression is not needed; this simplifies the acquisition and post-processing of such spectra.

Localized ^{31}P MRS revealed increased creatine phosphate levels in MS brains, suggestive of a low metabolic state of the brain. The increase correlated with the severity of the disability and was greater in patients with a progressive course. No clear abnormalities regarding phosphomonoesters, phosphodiesters, inorganic phosphate, or β-adenosine triphosphate were detected, and, similarly, the pH values (which are easily detectable with ^{31}P MRS) were not different between cases and controls.[137] A study of one patient showed changes contradicting these findings: reduced levels of phosphocreatine relative to adenosine triphosphate (ATP) and an increase in the phosphodiester (PDE) peak were demonstrated.[138] In a study utilizing both ^{1}H and ^{31}P MRS, white matter lesions and NAWM showed reduced NAA/creatine ratio and total ^{31}P peak integrals. In NAWM, total creatine and phosphocreatine were significantly increased compared to controls. These results suggest reduced neuronal/axonal functional integrity and altered phospholipid metabolites consistent with energy metabolism abnormalities in the NAWM and MS lesions.[139] A ^{31}P MRS study investigating lesions and NAWM found phospholipid broad component reduction, indicating of lowered phospholipid concentration in MS patients compared to controls.[140]

^{31}P MRS studies conducted on cardiac and skeletal muscle of MS patients revealed a pattern reminiscent of changes related to mitochondrial abnormalities.[141,142] The explanation of this finding, reported by two independent groups, is unclear at this time.

Although ^{31}P studies have not yet revealed a clear picture, the increased availability of higher-field-strength systems, more advanced coil designs, and much more powerful post-processing algorithms is likely to generate a new wave of ^{31}P MRS studies in the near future.

Overall, MRS markers show moderate to strong correlation with disability, may detect changes in NABT, and may be best utilized in the differential diagnosis of large T2-hyperintense lesions of unclear origin (see later discussion).

VOLUMETRIC MRI AND MEASURES OF BRAIN AND CORD ATROPHY

In addition measures of lesional pathology and markers of tissue damage in NABT, MRI also captures the overall tissue loss that appears to accompany all forms, but especially the progressive varieties, of MS. Several recent reviews have addressed this important aspect of MS[143-147] (see Fig. 5-4). In general, atrophy, especially cortical atrophy, may progress over a relatively short period of time. Atrophy becomes very prominent in the progressive stage of the disease, with ongoing disability, even when gadolinium enhancement is no longer detectable.[148-152] Atrophy-based MRI measures show a better correlation with disability than do standard lesion load measures.[5] CNS atrophy in MS includes both gray and white matter atrophy, and it remains debated which one predominates, but gray matter atrophy appears to dominate in more recent studies.[17,153] It is also likely that the predominant component is stage dependent: early on, cortical atrophy may predominate, whereas in advanced cases, especially in SPMS, white matter atrophy may become very significant. Atrophy-based measures can also be applied in therapeutic trials of novel medications.[148] Several publications reported progressive gray matter atrophy in the early years of MS.[154-156] This appears to contradict the dogma that gray matter involvement is always secondary to white matter damage. To fully appreciate early atrophy, especially cortical atrophy, advanced volumetric MRI techniques are needed, although the central and cortical atrophy of long-standing disease can be seen easily on standard scans.

Several volumetric post-processing techniques are available, including automated and semiautomated methods. The comparison of strengths and weaknesses is beyond the scope of this chapter. Volumetric measures of atrophy and of total lesion load are likely to find their way into clinical practice soon, because the major manufacturers of MRI scanners plan to add automatically generated volumetric measures to their platforms.

The Role of MRI in the Diagnosis of Tumefactive Demyelinating Lesions

A small subset of CIS patients present with unusually large or tumefactive lesions. These lesions are often mistaken for neoplasms, metastatic lesions, or even abscesses. Biopsies are not uncommon in the evaluation of these mass-like lesions; sometimes even repeated biopsies are needed for proper diagnosis. Such lesions are one of the common reasons for referrals to tertiary centers. It is very important to make the correct diagnosis, because irradiation of an MS lesion is not advisable: it leads to increased inflammatory activity and significant clinical worsening. A few features can help distinguish these lesions from neoplasms even on conventional MRI scans.

The presence of T2-hypointense rims or arcs and open ring enhancement may be suggestive of demyelination. However, hypointense rims and arcs can also be seen in neoplasms (especially gliomas and metastases) and in abscesses. In the largest study of ring-enhancing lesions conducted at the Mayo Clinic, 54% of tumefactive MS lesions had T2-hypointense borders, with 57% showing rims and 43% arcs. The hypointense borders are thought to correspond with the location of macrophages in these lesions. Almost all MS lesions are homogenously hyperintense centrally on T2-weighted scans. On diffusion-weighted images, abscesses were the most likely to show high signal; MS lesions were inconsistent from this standpoint.[51]

MRS of tumefactive MS lesions often shows elevated choline, lactate, and lipid peaks and a decreased NAA peak. However, these findings are not specific for a demyelinating lesion, because low-grade neoplasms may have exactly the same spectrum. An MRS signature that fails to show any change over several months may be more suggestive of a neoplasm than a demyelinating lesion, although this idea has not been validated in larger cohorts.[157] Case reports of increased glutamate and glutamine peaks in tumefactive demyelination also have not been confirmed in larger cohorts.

By a rational combination of advanced MRI techniques, including analysis of the enhancement pattern, DWI, and perfusion-based techniques such as relative cerebral blood flow (rCBV) and rCBF maps may allow for the early and effective identification of tumefactive demyelinating lesions without biopsy (see Fig. 5-9).

According to a recently proposed algorithm for the evaluation of intracranial masses (Fig. 5-11), contrast-enhancing mass-like lesions, if their diffusion is facilitated over 1.1/100 mm^2/ADC and their perfusion-weighted studies show an rCBV of 1.75 or less, are likely to be tumefactive lesions or abscesses. If the masses do not enhance but show a choline/NAA elevation of 2.2 or greater and an rCBV of 1.75 or less, they are also likely to be tumefactive lesions or abscesses. To distinguish between the two, clinical history and CSF findings may be helpful.[158]

Magnetic Resonance Imaging of Neuromyelitis Optica

Devic's disease (NMO) is the only inflammatory demyelinating disease with an identified serum marker, the NMO-IgG.[159,160] It is possible that NMO-IgG is actually pathogenic and not just a biomarker.[161] The fact that it is on astrocytes and not oligodendrocytes or on the myelin sheath is both surprising and very significant from the standpoint of new research directions in demyelinating conditions.

It is important to differentiate NMO from MS, because NMO responds poorly to standard MS DMAs but shows reasonable response to stronger immunosuppressive medications, especially those that modify B-cell function or decrease antibody production, or both. In the last few years, carefully designed diagnostic criteria were proposed, modified, and then simplified.[162,163] MRI findings play a critical role in the criteria, including the presence of a longitudinally extensive cord lesion over at least 3 spinal cord segments, which is almost pathognomic for this condition (Fig. 5-12). Of note, optic nerve lesions also have a tendency to be longitudinally extensive in this condition, and they often cross the optic chiasm, a feature that is unusual in MS-related optic neuritis. The cord lesions often appear

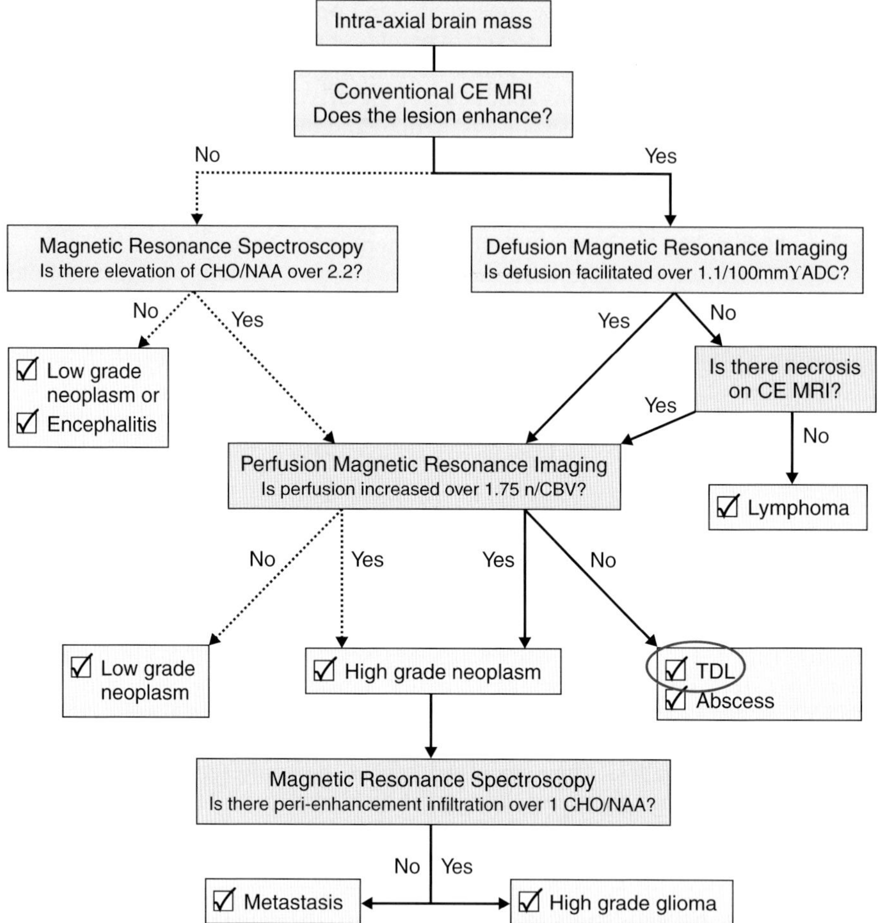

Figure 5–11 Algorithm for the evaluation of intra-axial brain masses utilizing advanced magnetic resonance imaging measures. The flow chart describes a possible method for differentiating low-grade gliomas, metastatic lesions, and abscesses from tumefactive multiple sclerosis (MS) lesions. To date, the method has not been validated in a large, histologically proven MS cohort. ADC, apparent diffusion coefficient; CE MRI, contrast-enhanced magnetic resonance imaging; CHO/NAA, choline/*N*-acetylaspartate ratio; rCBV, ??; TDL, tumefactive demyelinating lesion. (From Al-Okaili RN, Krejza J, Woo JH, et al: Intraaxial brain masses: MR imaging-based diagnostic strategy--initial experience. Radiology 2007;243:539-550.)

to have a mass effect ("swollen cord" appearance) and not uncommonly are mistaken for cord infarcts or tumors. In contrast to MS, NMO cord lesions on axial scans tend to involve more than half of the cord, including gray and white matter areas alike, and they most often involve central cord areas.

Whereas the earlier diagnostic criteria did not allow for brain lesions, the new criteria incorporate brain lesions that "do not meet criteria for MS." Nonspecific brain lesions are detectable in up to 60% of NMO cases. MS-like lesions may be seen in up to 10%, and 8% have unusual diencephalon and brainstem lesions,

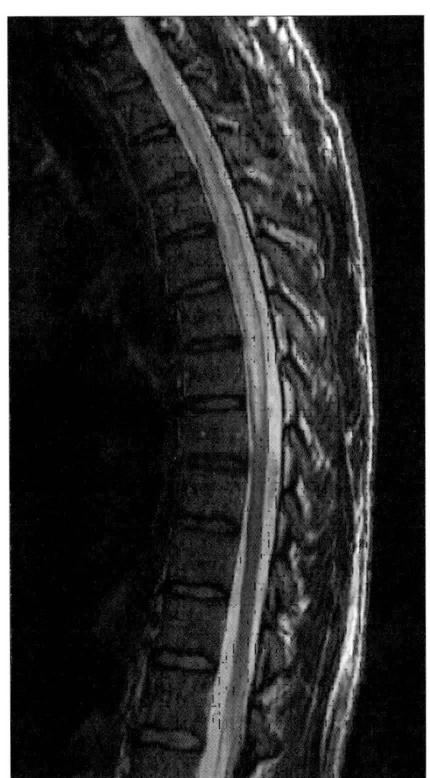

Figure 5–12 Neuromyelitis optica (NMO) lesion in the thoracic cord. Note the longitudinally extensive T2 hyperintensity over atleast seven spinal cord segments. This is characteristic of NMO, and longitudinally extensive lesions of three or more segments are part of the proposed NMO criteria.

which may include the hypothalamus and areas adjacent to the fourth ventricle. Interestingly, these brain areas have high density of aquaporin-4, the antigen recognized by NMO-IgG.[164,165] NAWM abnormalities, as detected on diffusion tensor imaging, can be seen in NMO but are much more restricted and appear to involve only the corticospinal tract and the optic radiation.[166] In an MT-based study, no NABT abnormalities were detected in NMO patients.[167] These studies strongly suggest that there is no "diffuse" NAWM involvement in NMO. Because of this, the fractional anisotropy and mean diffusivity of the corpus callosum may also aid in differentiating the two conditions.[168]

Acute Disseminated Encephalomyelitis

ADEM remains a relatively poorly defined entity among the idiopathic inflammatory demyelinating diseases. It is usually seen in children as a one-time postinfectious demyelinating condition that follows the trigger event by 2 to 4 weeks. It is almost always associated with encephalopathy, pyramidal signs, hemiplegia, spinal cord involvement, seizures, and aphasia; less commonly, optic neuritis or other cranial neuropathies are also seen.[169] Relapsing forms have been described, especially in children. However, it is important to realize that lesions of ADEM, although they may be numerous, tend to be in the same stage of lesion formation, include both white and gray matter structures, and do not always show gadolinium enhancement at presentation. In general, they show unusually good resolution compared with MS lesions. The lesions are best detected on T2-weighted and FLAIR images; they are multiple, often large, and patchy. Whereas the white matter lesions are asymmetrical and random in distribution, gray matter lesions tend to be symmetrical and often involve the thalamus and basal ganglia. A recent attempt to classify ADEM[169] proposed four patterns of cerebral involvement to describe the MRI findings: (1) ADEM with small lesions (<5 mm); (2) ADEM with large, confluent, or tumefactive lesions, with frequent extensive perilesional edema and mass effect; (3) ADEM with additional symmetrical bithalamic involvement; and (4) acute hemorrhagic encephalomyelitis (AHEM), in which T2 hypointensities are detected within the T2-hyperintense areas, suggesting the presence of blood or blood degradation products (Fig. 5-13). It is unclear whether all of these patterns truly represent ADEM rather than childhood manifestations of MS or other leukoencephalopathies. Until a histologically proven cohort of ADEM is assembled and appropriately studied, it is unlikely that the MRI findings or any other feature of this disease can be sufficiently clarified. In contrast to MS, advanced MRI markers of NABT tend not to show any abnormalities in ADEM. In ADEM cases, diverse changes have been reported on advanced MRI studies, including increased, decreased, or unchanged diffusion coefficients and reduced or normal perfusion. A recent international study of ADEM proposed three diagnostic criteria: atypical clinical symptoms for MS, absence of oligoclonal bands, and gray matter involvement.[169] These criteria have yet to be evaluated in a prospective cohort of ADEM cases and are likely to be modified in the future.

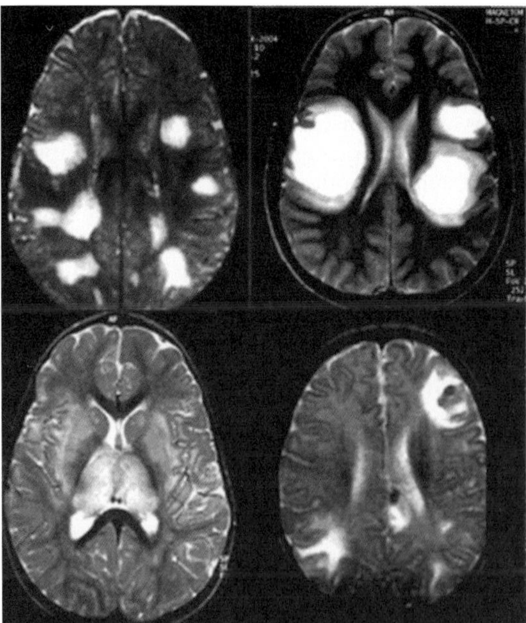

Figure 5–13 Proposed magnetic resonance imaging classification of acute disseminated encephalomyelitis (ADEM). *Left upper image:* ADEM with regular lesions. *Right upper image:* ADEM with tumefactive lesions. *Left lower image:* ADEM with bithalamic involvement. *Right lower image:* Acute hemorrhagic encephalomyelitis (AHLE or AHEM). Note that the proposed classification system has not been prospectively validated in a large cohort. (From Tenembaum S, Chitnis T, Ness J, Hahn JS: Acute disseminated encephalomyelitis. Neurology 2007;68:S23-S36, with permission from Lippincott Williams & Wilkins, online at http://www.lww.com.)

Non–MRI-Based Advanced Imaging Techniques: Optical Coherence Tomography

One of the main issues in MS research is how to influence the slow, progressive stage of the disease, which remains largely elusive to currently available disease-modifying therapies. There is growing evidence that the progressive stage of MS is characterized not only by ongoing demyelination but by progressive axonal and/or neuronal dysfunction and loss. To characterize this process, advanced MRI techniques such as MRS or diffusion- or MT-based methods may offer some insight; however, several technical issues hinder the universal applicability of these techniques. OCT is a new diagnostic modality that has emerged in MS research. OCT enables the investigation of retinal layer nerve fibers in vivo and in previously unprecedented detail. This allows the indirect study of processes leading to axonal and neuronal loss in the CNS. Technically, OCT is based on the principle of echo time delay of back-scattered infrared light from the retina. The tissue density–dependent reflections of infrared light provide the information that is used in the numeric characterization of tissue thickness and tissue volume. The resulting images allow for detailed differentiation of the major retinal layers, to a resolution of about 3 μm with high-resolution OCT. Figure 5-14 shows an example of OCT-derived measurements.

Intuitively, OCT would be able to capture pathology in the eyes that is related to optic neuritis. However, OCT is also capable of measuring MS-related axonal loss independently of optic neuritis.[171] Additionally, in unilateral optic neuritis, the noninvolved eye also shows changes on OCT.

For practical purposes, OCT provides two main measures: retinal nerve fiber layer thickness (RNFLT), which can be reported as a mean value or as values

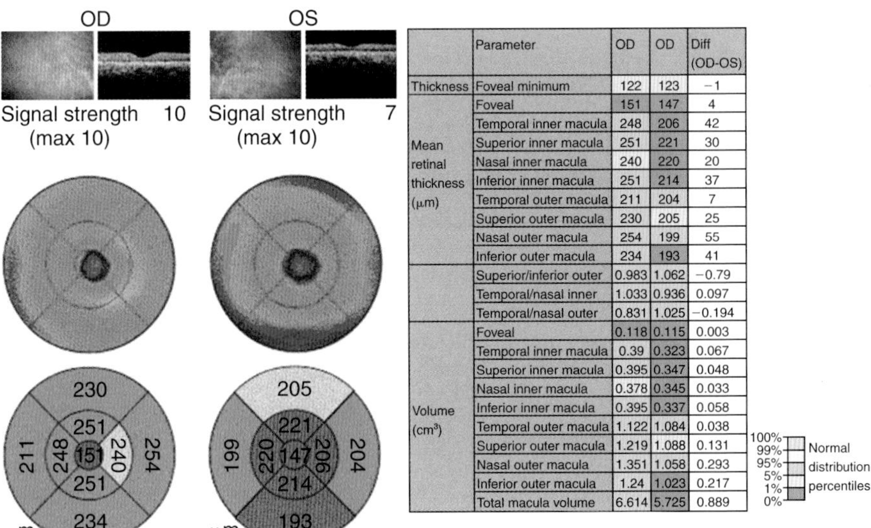

	Parameter	OD	OD	Diff (OD-OS)
Thickness	Foveal minimum	122	123	−1
Mean retinal thickness (μm)	Foveal	151	147	4
	Temporal inner macula	248	206	42
	Superior inner macula	251	221	30
	Nasal inner macula	240	220	20
	Inferior inner macula	251	214	37
	Temporal outer macula	211	204	7
	Superior outer macula	230	205	25
	Nasal outer macula	254	199	55
	Inferior outer macula	234	193	41
	Superior/inferior outer	0.983	1.062	−0.79
	Temporal/nasal inner	1.033	0.936	0.097
	Temporal/nasal outer	0.831	1.025	−0.194
Volume (cm³)	Foveal	0.118	0.115	0.003
	Temporal inner macula	0.39	0.323	0.067
	Superior inner macula	0.395	0.347	0.048
	Nasal inner macula	0.378	0.345	0.033
	Inferior inner macula	0.395	0.337	0.058
	Temporal outer macula	1.122	1.084	0.038
	Superior outer macula	1.219	1.088	0.131
	Nasal outer macula	1.351	1.058	0.293
	Inferior outer macula	1.24	1.023	0.217
	Total macula volume	6.614	5.725	0.889

Figure 5–14 Example of optical coherence tomography (OCT)-derived measures in a patient with remote (>2 years) optic neuritis. Mean retinal thickness maps and data in the table are color-coded using the percentile rank scale on the far right.

specific to quadrants, and macular volume (MV). In several studies, the temporal RNFLT appeared to be most affected in MS. Mean RNFLT and MV were found to be significantly reduced in SPMS, but not in PPMS, in a recent study.[172] Temporal RNFLT loss was also significant in PPMS cases compared with controls. In SPMS cases, a significant reduction in RNFLT and MV was seen in eyes not affected by optic neuritis. This association was not seen in PPMS. RNFLT and MV decrease also correlated well with measures of visual acuity in SPMS cases.[172]

In a study of 39 MS patients without visual symptoms, only temporal RNFLT showed significant reduction compared with controls. VEP-derived markers showed no correlation with RNFLT. This illustrates that, although VEP is very sensitive to the demyelinating pathology, RNFLT and OCT are sensitive to axonal and neuronal loss; therefore, they measure different components of MS pathology.[173]

In a study analyzing OCT-detectable differences among MS subtypes, decreased RNFLT values were demonstrated in RRMS (94.4 μm, $P < .001$), PPMS (88.9 μm, $P < .01$), and SPMS (81.8 μm, $P < .0001$) compared with controls. There were significant differences in RNFLT within quadrants of peripapillary retina when relapsing and progressive MS subtypes were compared. MV was decreased in MS eyes affected by optic neuritis (6.2 mm^3, $P < .0001$) and in subjects with SPMS (6.2 mm^3, $P < .05$) compared with controls (6.8 mm^3). Decreased RNFLT was found in optic neuritis–affected eyes (84.2 μm, $P < .0001$), in unaffected fellow eyes (93.9 μm, $P < .01$), and in eyes of MS patients with no history of optic neuritis (95.9 μm, $P < .05$), compared with controls (102.7 μm).[174]

In a study investigating the relationships between volumetric MRI and OCT-derived markers, a strong association was found between normalized brain volume and average RNFLT ($P < .001$, $r = .77$). T2-hyperintense lesion volume ($P = .002$, $r = -0.76$) and normalized white matter volume ($P = .005$, partial $r = .68$) were also significantly associated with average RNFLT. There were trends toward association with T1-hypointense lesion volume ($P = .041$) and normalized gray matter volume ($P = .067$). There was a negative correlation between average RNFLT and the EDSS score ($P = .02$).[175]

In the coming years, OCT is likely to become an important biomarker in clinical trials addressing progressive forms of MS and in trials of novel therapeutics attempting to influence neuronal or axonal loss in MS. Expert panel opinions already call for the standardization and more universal application of this technique in clinical trials.[176]

Conclusions

MRI of the CNS has become the single most important paraclinical marker of demyelinating diseases. MRI findings have been incorporated in the diagnostic criteria of MS and other demyelinating conditions. MRI-based markers are routinely used in the diagnosis and differential diagnosis of white matter diseases. MRI is also important in clarifying the prognosis of first-time MS-like presentations. It provides a very useful aid to therapy monitoring and planning in MS. Advanced MRI and MRS techniques have revolutionized the understanding of demyelinating diseases. In MS, they shed new light on disease activity in normal-appearing areas, and they clarify the importance of gray matter pathology and cortical and diffuse atrophy.

It is expected that additional new techniques will emerge in the coming years and that some of the advanced MRI techniques will gradually find their way into everyday clinical practice. OCT is expected to play an important part in assessing axonal and neuronal damage in all forms of MS, and it may be a useful outcome measure in clinical trials addressing repair and neuroprotection. Despite the great advances that sophisticated methods have brought to the field of clinical neuroimmunology, one must remember the relative lack of specificity of standard MRI techniques. Demyelinating diseases have complex diagnostic criteria and cannot be diagnosed based on neuroimaging findings alone. At the same time, some of the most significant milestones in MS research of the last few decades were related to advances in neuroimaging. The use of MRI and OCT as a research and clinical diagnostic tool will continue to evolve and reshape the field of experimental and clinical neuroimmunology.

REFERENCES

1. Noseworthy JH, Lucchinetti C, Rodriguez M, Weinshenker BG: Multiple sclerosis. N Engl J Med 2000;343:938-952.
2. McDonald WI, Compston A, Edan G, et al: Recommended diagnostic criteria for multiple sclerosis: Guidelines from the International Panel on the diagnosis of multiple sclerosis. Ann Neurol 2001;50:121-127.
3. Polman CH, Reingold SC, Edan G, et al: Diagnostic criteria for multiple sclerosis: 2005 Revisions to the "McDonald Criteria." Ann Neurol 2005;58:840-846.
4. Fisniku LK, Brex PA, Altmann DR, et al: Disability and T2 MRI lesions: A 20-year follow-up of patients with relapse onset of multiple sclerosis. Brain 2008;131:808-817.
5. Zivadinov R, Leist TP: Clinical-magnetic resonance imaging correlations in multiple sclerosis. J Neuroimaging 2005;15:10S-21S.
6. Paty DW, Li DK: Interferon beta-1b is effective in relapsing-remitting multiple sclerosis: II. MRI analysis results of a multicenter, randomized, double-blind, placebo-controlled trial. UBC MS/MRI Study Group and the IFNB Multiple Sclerosis Study Group. Neurology 1993;43:662-667.
7. Gean-Marton AD, Vezina LG, Marton KI, et al: Abnormal corpus callosum: A sensitive and specific indicator of multiple sclerosis. Radiology 1991;180:215-221.
8. Offenbacher H, Fazekas F, Schmidt R, et al: Assessment of MRI criteria for a diagnosis of MS. Neurology 1993;43:905-909.
9. Miller DH, Ormerod IE, McDonald WI, et al: The early risk of multiple sclerosis after optic neuritis. J Neurol Neurosurg Psychiatry 1988;51:1569-1571.
10. Barkhof F, Filippi M, Miller DH, et al: Comparison of MRI criteria at first presentation to predict conversion to clinically definite multiple sclerosis. Brain 1997;120(Pt 11):2059-2069.
11. Erskine MK, Cook LL, Riddle KE, et al: Resolution-dependent estimates of multiple sclerosis lesion loads. Can J Neurol Sci 2005;32:205-212.
12. Keiper MD, Grossman RI, Hirsch JA, et al: MR identification of white matter abnormalities in multiple sclerosis: A comparison between 1.5 T and 4 T. AJNR Am J Neuroradiol 1998;19:1489-1493.
13. Sicotte NL, Voskuhl RR, Bouvier S, et al: Comparison of multiple sclerosis lesions at 1.5 and 3.0 Tesla. Invest Radiol 2003;38:423-427.
14. Molyneux PD, Filippi M, Barkhof F, et al: Correlations between monthly enhanced MRI lesion rate and changes in T2 lesion volume in multiple sclerosis. Ann Neurol 1998;43:332-339.
15. O'Riordan JI, Thompson AJ, Kingsley DP, et al: The prognostic value of brain MRI in clinically isolated syndromes of the CNS: A 10-year follow-up. Brain 1998;121(Pt 3):495-503.
16. Sailer M, O'Riordan JI, Thompson AJ, et al: Quantitative MRI in patients with clinically isolated syndromes suggestive of demyelination. Neurology 1999;52:599-606.
17. Pirko I, Lucchinetti CF, Sriram S, Bakshi R: Gray matter involvement in multiple sclerosis. Neurology 2007;68:634-642.
18. Filippi M, Yousry T, Baratti C, et al: Quantitative assessment of MRI lesion load in multiple sclerosis: A comparison of conventional spin-echo with fast fluid-attenuated inversion recovery. Brain 1996;119;(Pt 4):1349-1355.
19. Stevenson VL, Gawne-Cain ML, Barker GJ, et al: Imaging of the spinal cord and brain in multiple sclerosis: A comparative study between fast FLAIR and fast spin echo. J Neurol 1997;244:119-124.

20. Gawne-Cain ML, O'Riordan JI, Thompson AJ, et al: Multiple sclerosis lesion detection in the brain: A comparison of fast fluid-attenuated inversion recovery and conventional T2-weighted dual spin echo. Neurology 1997;49:364-370.
21. Geurts JJ, Pouwels PJ, Uitdehaag BM, et al: Intracortical lesions in multiple sclerosis: Improved detection with 3D double inversion-recovery MR imaging. Radiology 2005;236:254-260.
22. Bot JC, Barkhof F, Lycklama ANGJ, et al: Comparison of a conventional cardiac-triggered dual spin-echo and a fast STIR sequence in detection of spinal cord lesions in multiple sclerosis. Eur Radiol 2000;10:753-758.
23. Moseley IF, Miller DH, Gass A: The contribution of magnetic resonance imaging to the assessment of optic nerve and spinal cord involvement in multiple sclerosis. J Neurol Neurosurg Psychiatry 1998;64(Suppl 1):S15-S20.
24. Campi A, Pontesilli S, Gerevini S, Scotti G: Comparison of MRI pulse sequences for investigation of lesions of the cervical spinal cord. Neuroradiology 2000;42:669-675.
25. Bot JC, Barkhof F, Lycklama ANGJ, et al: Differentiation of multiple sclerosis from other inflammatory disorders and cerebrovascular disease: Value of spinal MR imaging. Radiology 2002;223:46-56.
26. Grimaud J, Millar J, Thorpe JW, et al: Signal intensity on MRI of basal ganglia in multiple sclerosis. J Neurol Neurosurg Psychiatry 1995;59:306-308.
27. Bakshi R, Dmochowski J, Shaikh ZA, Jacobs L: Gray matter T2 hypointensity is related to plaques and atrophy in the brains of multiple sclerosis patients. J Neurol Sci 2001;185:19-26.
28. Tjoa CW, Benedict RH, Weinstock-Guttman B, et al: MRI T2 hypointensity of the dentate nucleus is related to ambulatory impairment in multiple sclerosis. J Neurol Sci 2005;234:17-24.
29. Bakshi R, Benedict RH, Bermel RA, et al: T2 hypointensity in the deep gray matter of patients with multiple sclerosis: A quantitative magnetic resonance imaging study. Arch Neurol 2002;59:62-68.
30. Bermel RA, Puli SR, Rudick RA, et al: Prediction of longitudinal brain atrophy in multiple sclerosis by gray matter magnetic resonance imaging T2 hypointensity. Arch Neurol 2005;62: 1371-1376.
31. Haacke EM, Ayaz M, Khan A, et al: Establishing a baseline phase behavior in magnetic resonance imaging to determine normal vs. abnormal iron content in the brain. J Magn Reson Imaging 2007;26:256-264.
32. Thompson AJ, Miller D, Youl B, et al: Serial gadolinium-enhanced MRI in relapsing/remitting multiple sclerosis of varying disease duration. Neurology 1992;42:60-63.
33. Kappos L, Moeri D, Radue EW, et al: Predictive value of gadolinium-enhanced magnetic resonance imaging for relapse rate and changes in disability or impairment in multiple sclerosis: A meta-analysis. Gadolinium MRI Meta-analysis Group. Lancet 1999;353:964-969.
34. Thorpe JW, Kidd D, Moseley IF, et al: Serial gadolinium-enhanced MRI of the brain and spinal cord in early relapsing-remitting multiple sclerosis. Neurology 1996;46:373-378.
35. Miller DH, Rudge P, Johnson G, et al: Serial gadolinium enhanced magnetic resonance imaging in multiple sclerosis. Brain 1988;111(Pt 4):927-939.
36. Grossman RI, Braffman BH, Brorson JR, et al: Multiple sclerosis: Serial study of gadolinium-enhanced MR imaging. Radiology 1988;169:117-122.
37. Grossman RI, Gonzalez-Scarano F, Atlas SW, et al: Multiple sclerosis: Gadolinium enhancement in MR imaging. Radiology 1986;161:721-725.
38. Kermode AG, Thompson AJ, Tofts P, et al: Breakdown of the blood-brain barrier precedes symptoms and other MRI signs of new lesions in multiple sclerosis: Pathogenetic and clinical implications. Brain 1990;113(Pt 5):1477-1489.
39. Cotton F, Weiner HL, Jolesz FA, Guttmann CR: MRI contrast uptake in new lesions in relapsing-remitting MS followed at weekly intervals. Neurology 2003;60:640-646.
40. Kidd D, Thorpe JW, Kendall BE, et al: MRI dynamics of brain and spinal cord in progressive multiple sclerosis. J Neurol Neurosurg Psychiatry 1996;60:15-19.
41. Tubridy N, Coles AJ, Molyneux P, et al: Secondary progressive multiple sclerosis: The relationship between short-term MRI activity and clinical features. Brain 1998;121(Pt 2):225-231.
42. Thompson AJ, Kermode AG, Wicks D, et al: Major differences in the dynamics of primary and secondary progressive multiple sclerosis. Ann Neurol 1991;29:53-62.
43. Ingle GT, Sastre-Garriga J, Miller DH, Thompson AJ: Is inflammation important in early PPMS? A longitudinal MRI study. J Neurol Neurosurg Psychiatry 2005;76:1255-1258.
44. Silver N, Lai M, Symms M, et al: Serial gadolinium-enhanced and magnetization transfer imaging to investigate the relationship between the duration of blood-brain barrier disruption and extent of demyelination in new multiple sclerosis lesions. J Neurol 1999;246:728-730.

45. Masdeu JC, Moreira J, Trasi S, et al: The open ring: A new imaging sign in demyelinating disease. J Neuroimaging 1996;6:104-107.
46. Masdeu JC, Quinto C, Olivera C, et al: Open-ring imaging sign: Highly specific for atypical brain demyelination. Neurology 2000;54:1427-1433.
47. Minneboo A, Uitdehaag BM, Ader HJ, et al: Patterns of enhancing lesion evolution in multiple sclerosis are uniform within patients. Neurology 2005;65:56-61.
48. Leist TP, Gobbini MI, Frank JA, McFarland HF: Enhancing magnetic resonance imaging lesions and cerebral atrophy in patients with relapsing multiple sclerosis. Arch Neurol 2001;58: 57-60.
49. Morgen K, Jeffries NO, Stone R, et al: Ring-enchancement in multiple sclerosis: Marker of disease severity. Mult Scler 2001;7:167-171.
50. Bagnato F, Jeffries N, Richert ND, et al: Evolution of T1 black holes in patients with multiple sclerosis imaged monthly for 4 years. Brain 2003;126:1782-1789.
51. Schwartz KM, Erickson BJ, Lucchinetti C: Pattern of T2 hypointensity associated with ring-enhancing brain lesions can help to differentiate pathology. Neuroradiology 2006;48:143-149.
52. Hawkins CP, Munro PM, Landon DN, McDonald WI: Metabolically dependent blood-brain barrier breakdown in chronic relapsing experimental allergic encephalomyelitis. Acta Neuropathol (Berl) 1992;83:630-635.
53. Pirko I, Johnson A, Ciric B, et al: In vivo magnetic resonance imaging of immune cells in the central nervous system with superparamagnetic antibodies. FASEB J 2004;18:179-182.
54. Pirko I, Fricke ST, Johnson AJ, et al: Magnetic resonance imaging, microscopy, and spectroscopy of the central nervous system in experimental animals. NeuroRx 2005;2:250-264.
55. Dousset V, Brochet B, Deloire MS, et al: MR imaging of relapsing multiple sclerosis patients using ultra-small-particle iron oxide and compared with gadolinium. AJNR Am J Neuroradiol 2006;27:1000-1005.
56. Vellinga MM, Oude Engberink RD, Seewann A, et al: Pluriformity of inflammation in multiple sclerosis shown by ultra-small iron oxide particle enhancement. Brain 2008;131:800-807.
57. Uhlenbrock D, Sehlen S: The value of T1-weighted images in the differentiation between MS, white matter lesions, and subcortical arteriosclerotic encephalopathy (SAE). Neuroradiology 1989;31:203-212.
58. Levesque I, Sled JG, Narayanan S, et al: The role of edema and demyelination in chronic T1 black holes: A quantitative magnetization transfer study. J Magn Reson Imaging 2005;21:103-110.
59. Brex PA, Molyneux PD, Smiddy P, et al: The effect of IFNbeta-1b on the evolution of enhancing lesions in secondary progressive MS. Neurology 2001;57:2185-2190.
60. Losseff NA, Miller DH, Kidd D, Thompson AJ: The predictive value of gadolinium enhancement for long term disability in relapsing-remitting multiple sclerosis: Preliminary results. Mult Scler 2001;7:23-25.
61. van Waesberghe JH, Kamphorst W, De Groot CJ, et al: Axonal loss in multiple sclerosis lesions: Magnetic resonance imaging insights into substrates of disability. Ann Neurol 1999;46:747-754.
62. van Walderveen MA, Kamphorst W, Scheltens P, et al: Histopathologic correlate of hypointense lesions on T1-weighted spin-echo MRI in multiple sclerosis. Neurology 1998;50:1282-1288.
63. Bitsch A, Kuhlmann T, Stadelmann C, et al: A longitudinal MRI study of histopathologically defined hypointense multiple sclerosis lesions. Ann Neurol 2001;49:793-796.
64. Losseff NA, Wang L, Miller DH, Thompson AJ: T1 hypointensity of the spinal cord in multiple sclerosis. J Neurol 2001;248:517-521.
65. Hiehle JF Jr., Grossman RI, Ramer KN, et al: Magnetization transfer effects in MR-detected multiple sclerosis lesions: Comparison with gadolinium-enhanced spin-echo images and nonenhanced T1-weighted images. AJNR Am J Neuroradiol 1995;16:69-77.
66. Simone IL, Tortorella C, Federico F, et al: Axonal damage in multiple sclerosis plaques: A combined magnetic resonance imaging and 1H-magnetic resonance spectroscopy study. J Neurol Sci 2001;182:143-150.
67. Li BS, Regal J, Soher BJ, et al: Brain metabolite profiles of T1-hypointense lesions in relapsing-remitting multiple sclerosis. AJNR Am J Neuroradiol 2003;24:68-74.
68. Brex PA, Parker GJ, Leary SM, et al: Lesion heterogeneity in multiple sclerosis: A study of the relations between appearances on T1 weighted images, T1 relaxation times, and metabolite concentrations. J Neurol Neurosurg Psychiatry 2000;68:627-632.
69. van Walderveen MA, Lycklama ANGJ, Ader HJ, et al: Hypointense lesions on T1-weighted spin-echo magnetic resonance imaging: Relation to clinical characteristics in subgroups of patients with multiple sclerosis. Arch Neurol 2001;58:76-81.

70. van Walderveen MA, Barkhof F, Hommes OR, et al: Correlating MRI and clinical disease activity in multiple sclerosis: Relevance of hypointense lesions on short-TR/short-TE (T1-weighted) spin-echo images. Neurology 1995;45:1684-1690.
71. Truyen L, van Waesberghe JH, van Walderveen MA, et al: Accumulation of hypointense lesions ("black holes") on T1 spin-echo MRI correlates with disease progression in multiple sclerosis. Neurology 1996;47:1469-1476.
72. Pirko I, Nolan TK, Holland SK, Johnson AJ: Multiple sclerosis: Pathogenesis and MR imaging features of T1 hypointensities in murine model. Radiology 2008;246:790-795.
73. Janardhan V, Suri S, Bakshi R: Multiple sclerosis: Hyperintense lesions in the brain on nonenhanced T1-weighted MR images evidenced as areas of T1 shortening. Radiology 2007;244:823-831.
74. Charil A, Yousry TA, Rovaris M, et al: MRI and the diagnosis of multiple sclerosis: Expanding the concept of "no better explanation." Lancet Neurol 2006;5:841-852.
75. Morrissey SP, Miller DH, Kendall BE, et al: The significance of brain magnetic resonance imaging abnormalities at presentation with clinically isolated syndromes suggestive of multiple sclerosis: A 5-year follow-up study. Brain 1993;116(Pt 1):135-146.
76. Brex PA, Ciccarelli O, O'Riordan JI, et al: A longitudinal study of abnormalities on MRI and disability from multiple sclerosis. N Engl J Med 2002;346:158-164.
77. Chard DT, Brex PA, Ciccarelli O, et al: The longitudinal relation between brain lesion load and atrophy in multiple sclerosis: A 14 year follow up study. J Neurol Neurosurg Psychiatry 2003;74:1551-1554.
78. Lebrun C, Bensa C, Debouverie M, et al: Unexpected multiple sclerosis: Follow-up of 30 patients with magnetic resonance imaging and clinical conversion profile. J Neurol Neurosurg Psychiatry 2008;792):195-198.
79. Pittock SJ, McClelland RL, Mayr WT, et al: Clinical implications of benign multiple sclerosis: A 20-year population-based follow-up study. Ann Neurol 2004;56:303-306.
80. Pittock SJ, Weinshenker BG, Noseworthy JH, et al: Not every patient with multiple sclerosis should be treated at time of diagnosis. Arch Neurol 2006;63:611-614.
81. Wingerchuk DM: Current evidence and therapeutic strategies for multiple sclerosis. Semin Neurol 2008;28:56-68.
82. Frohman EM, Havrdova E, Lublin F, et al: Most patients with multiple sclerosis or a clinically isolated demyelinating syndrome should be treated at the time of diagnosis. Arch Neurol 2006;63:614-619.
83. Dousset V, Grossman RI, Ramer KN, et al: Experimental allergic encephalomyelitis and multiple sclerosis: Lesion characterization with magnetization transfer imaging. Radiology 1992;182:483-491.
84. Filippi M, Iannucci G, Tortorella C, et al: Comparison of MS clinical phenotypes using conventional and magnetization transfer MRI. Neurology 1999;52:588-594.
85. Chen JT, Collins DL, Freedman MS, et al: Local magnetization transfer ratio signal inhomogeneity is related to subsequent change in MTR in lesions and normal-appearing white-matter of multiple sclerosis patients. Neuroimage 2005;25:1272-1278.
86. Laule C, Vavasour IM, Whittall KP, et al: Evolution of focal and diffuse magnetisation transfer abnormalities in multiple sclerosis. J Neurol 2003;250:924-931.
87. Rovaris M, Agosta F, Sormani MP, et al: Conventional and magnetization transfer MRI predictors of clinical multiple sclerosis evolution: A medium-term follow-up study. Brain 2003;126:2323-2332.
88. Santos AC, Narayanan S, de Stefano N, et al: Magnetization transfer can predict clinical evolution in patients with multiple sclerosis. J Neurol 2002;249:662-668.
89. Traboulsee A, Dehmeshki J, Brex PA, et al: Normal-appearing brain tissue MTR histograms in clinically isolated syndromes suggestive of MS. Neurology 2002;59:126-128.
90. Rocca MA, Agosta F, Sormani MP, et al: A three-year, multi-parametric MRI study in patients at presentation with CIS. J Neurol 2008;255:683-691.
91. Inglese M, Salvi F, Iannucci G, et al: Magnetization transfer and diffusion tensor MR imaging of acute disseminated encephalomyelitis. AJNR Am J Neuroradiol 2002;23:267-272.
92. Barkhof F, Bruck W, De Groot CJ, et al: Remyelinated lesions in multiple sclerosis: Magnetic resonance image appearance. Arch Neurol 2003;60:1073-1081.
93. Schmierer K, Scaravilli F, Altmann DR, et al: Magnetization transfer ratio and myelin in postmortem multiple sclerosis brain. Ann Neurol 2004;56:407-415.
94. Gass A, Barker GJ, Kidd D, et al: Correlation of magnetization transfer ratio with clinical disability in multiple sclerosis. Ann Neurol 1994;36:62-67.

95. Rovaris M, Viti B, Ciboddo G, et al: Brain involvement in systemic immune mediated diseases: Magnetic resonance and magnetisation transfer imaging study. J Neurol Neurosurg Psychiatry 2000;68:170-177.
96. Filippi M, Rocca MA: Magnetization transfer magnetic resonance imaging in the assessment of neurological diseases. J Neuroimaging 2004;14:303-313.
97. Inglese M, Grossman RI, Filippi M: Magnetic resonance imaging monitoring of multiple sclerosis lesion evolution. J Neuroimaging 2005;15:22S-29S.
98. Dousset V, Gayou A, Brochet B, Caille JM: Early structural changes in acute MS lesions assessed by serial magnetization transfer studies. Neurology 1998;51:1150-1155.
99. Oreja-Guevara C, Charil A, Caputo D, et al: Magnetization transfer magnetic resonance imaging and clinical changes in patients with relapsing-remitting multiple sclerosis. Arch Neurol 2006;63:736-740.
100. Bot JC, Blezer EL, Kamphorst W, et al: The spinal cord in multiple sclerosis: Relationship of high-spatial-resolution quantitative MR imaging findings to histopathologic results. Radiology 2004;233:531-540.
101. Cercignani M, Bozzali M, Iannucci G, et al: Magnetisation transfer ratio and mean diffusivity of normal appearing white and grey matter from patients with multiple sclerosis. J Neurol Neurosurg Psychiatry 2001;70:311-317.
102. Cercignani M, Inglese M, Pagani E, et al: Mean diffusivity and fractional anisotropy histograms of patients with multiple sclerosis. AJNR Am J Neuroradiol 2001;22:952-958.
103. Rocca MA, Cercignani M, Iannucci G, et al: Weekly diffusion-weighted imaging of normal-appearing white matter in MS. Neurology 2000;55:882-884.
104. Griffin CM, Chard DT, Ciccarelli O, et al: Diffusion tensor imaging in early relapsing-remitting multiple sclerosis. Mult Scler 2001;7:290-297.
105. Ciccarelli O, Werring DJ, Wheeler-Kingshott CA, et al: Investigation of MS normal-appearing brain using diffusion tensor MRI with clinical correlations. Neurology 2001;56:926-933.
106. Ciccarelli O, Parker GJ, Toosy AT, et al: From diffusion tractography to quantitative white matter tract measures: A reproducibility study. Neuroimage 2003;18:348-359.
107. Ciccarelli O, Toosy AT, Hickman SJ, et al: Optic radiation changes after optic neuritis detected by tractography-based group mapping. Hum Brain Mapp 2005;25:308-316.
108. Werring DJ, Clark CA, Barker GJ, et al: Diffusion tensor imaging of lesions and normal-appearing white matter in multiple sclerosis. Neurology 1999;52:1626-1632.
109. Filippi M, Cercignani M, Inglese M, et al: Diffusion tensor magnetic resonance imaging in multiple sclerosis. Neurology 2001;56:304-311.
110. Rovaris M, Gass A, Bammer R, et al: Diffusion MRI in multiple sclerosis. Neurology 2005;65:1526-1532.
111. Rovaris M, Filippi M: Diffusion tensor MRI in multiple sclerosis. J Neuroimaging 2007;17(Suppl 1):27S-30S.
112. Rashid W, Parkes LM, Ingle GT, et al: Abnormalities of cerebral perfusion in multiple sclerosis. J Neurol Neurosurg Psychiatry 2004;75:1288-1293.
113. Adhya S, Johnson G, Herbert J, et al: Pattern of hemodynamic impairment in multiple sclerosis: Dynamic susceptibility contrast perfusion MR imaging at 3.0 T. Neuroimage 2006;33:1029-1035.
114. Wuerfel J, Paul F, Zipp F: Cerebral blood perfusion changes in multiple sclerosis. J Neurol Sci 2007;259:16-20.
115. Wuerfel J, Bellmann-Strobl J, Brunecker P, et al: Changes in cerebral perfusion precede plaque formation in multiple sclerosis: A longitudinal perfusion MRI study. Brain 2004;127:111-119.
116. Haselhorst R, Kappos L, Bilecen D, et al: Dynamic susceptibility contrast MR imaging of plaque development in multiple sclerosis: Application of an extended blood-brain barrier leakage correction. J Magn Reson Imaging 2000;11:495-505.
117. Inglese M, Adhya S, Johnson G, et al: Perfusion magnetic resonance imaging correlates of neuropsychological impairment in multiple sclerosis. J Cereb Blood Flow Metab 2008;28:164-171.
118. Inglese M, Park SJ, Johnson G, et al: Deep gray matter perfusion in multiple sclerosis: Dynamic susceptibility contrast perfusion magnetic resonance imaging at 3 T. Arch Neurol 2007;64:196-202.
119. Moore GR, Leung E, MacKay AL, et al: A pathology-MRI study of the short-T2 component in formalin-fixed multiple sclerosis brain. Neurology 2000;55:1506-1510.
120. Davies GR, Hadjiprocopis A, Altmann DR, et al: Normal-appearing grey and white matter T1 abnormality in early relapsing-remitting multiple sclerosis: A longitudinal study. Mult Scler 2007;13:169-177.

121. Griffin CM, Dehmeshki J, Chard DT, et al: T1 histograms of normal-appearing brain tissue are abnormal in early relapsing-remitting multiple sclerosis. Mult Scler 2002;8:211-216.
122. Griffin CM, Parker GJ, Barker GJ, et al: MTR and T1 provide complementary information in MS NAWM, but not in lesions. Mult Scler 2000;6:327-331.
123. Laule C, Leung E, Lis DK, et al: Myelin water imaging in multiple sclerosis: Quantitative correlations with histopathology. Mult Scler 2006;12:747-753.
124. Laule C, Vavasour IM, Kolind SH, et al: Long T2 water in multiple sclerosis: What else can we learn from multi-echo T2 relaxation?. J Neurol 2007;254:1579-1587.
125. Narayana PA: Magnetic resonance spectroscopy in the monitoring of multiple sclerosis. J Neuroimaging 2005;15:46S-57S.
126. Tartaglia MC, Arnold DL: The role of MRS and fMRI in multiple sclerosis. Adv Neurol 2006;98:185-202.
127. Mostert JP, Sijens PE, Oudkerk M, De Keyser J: Fluoxetine increases cerebral white matter NAA/Cr ratio in patients with multiple sclerosis. Neurosci Lett 2006;402:22-24.
128. Rovaris M, Gallo A, Falini A, et al: Axonal injury and overall tissue loss are not related in primary progressive multiple sclerosis. Arch Neurol 2005;62:898-902.
129. Vrenken H, Barkhof F, Uitdehaag BM, et al: MR spectroscopic evidence for glial increase but not for neuro-axonal damage in MS normal-appearing white matter. Magn Reson Med 2005;53:256-266.
130. Clark JF, Doepke A, Filosa JA, et al: N-acetylaspartate as a reservoir for glutamate. Med Hypotheses 2006;67:506-512.
131. Geurts JJ, Reuling IE, Vrenken H, et al: MR spectroscopic evidence for thalamic and hippocampal, but not cortical, damage in multiple sclerosis. Magn Reson Med 2006;55:478-483.
132. Narayanan S, Francis SJ, Sled JG, et al: Axonal injury in the cerebral normal-appearing white matter of patients with multiple sclerosis is related to concurrent demyelination in lesions but not to concurrent demyelination in normal-appearing white matter. Neuroimage 2006;29:637-642.
133. Srinivasan R, Sailasuta N, Hurd R, et al: Evidence of elevated glutamate in multiple sclerosis using magnetic resonance spectroscopy at 3 T. Brain 2005;128:1016-1025.
134. Adalsteinsson E, Langer-Gould A, Homer RJ, et al: Gray matter N-acetyl aspartate deficits in secondary progressive but not relapsing-remitting multiple sclerosis. AJNR Am J Neuroradiol 2003;24:1941-1945.
135. Inglese M, Ge Y, Filippi M, et al: Indirect evidence for early widespread gray matter involvement in relapsing-remitting multiple sclerosis. Neuroimage 2004;21:1825-1829.
136. Wattjes MP, Harzheim M, Lutterbey GG, et al: High field MR imaging and (1)H-MR spectroscopy in clinically isolated syndromes suggestive of multiple sclerosis: Correlation between metabolic alterations and diagnostic MR imaging criteria. J Neurol 2008;255:56-63.
137. Minderhoud JM, Mooyaart EL, Kamman RL, et al: In vivo phosphorus magnetic resonance spectroscopy in multiple sclerosis. Arch Neurol 1992;49:161-165.
138. Cadoux-Hudson TA, Kermode A, Rajagopalan B, et al: Biochemical changes within a multiple sclerosis plaque in vivo. J Neurol Neurosurg Psychiatry 1991;54:1004-1006.
139. Husted CA, Goodin DS, Hugg JW, et al: Biochemical alterations in multiple sclerosis lesions and normal-appearing white matter detected by in vivo 31P and 1H spectroscopic imaging. Ann Neurol 1994;36:157-165.
140. Husted CA, Matson GB, Adams DA, et al: In vivo detection of myelin phospholipids in multiple sclerosis with phosphorus magnetic resonance spectroscopic imaging. Ann Neurol 1994;36:239-241.
141. Beer M, Sandstede J, Weilbach F, et al: Cardiac metabolism and function in patients with multiple sclerosis: A combined 31P-MR-spectroscopy and MRI study. Rofo 2001;173:399-404.
142. Argov Z, De Stefano N, Arnold DL: Muscle high-energy phosphates in central nervous system disorders: The phosphorus MRS experience. Ital J Neurol Sci 1997;18:353-357.
143. Zivadinov R, Bakshi R: Role of MRI in multiple sclerosis: II. Brain and spinal cord atrophy. Front Biosci 2004;9:647-664.
144. Kutzelnigg A, Lassmann H: Cortical lesions and brain atrophy in MS. J Neurol Sci 2005;233:55-59.
145. Bermel RA, Bakshi R: The measurement and clinical relevance of brain atrophy in multiple sclerosis. Lancet Neurol 2006;5:158-170.
146. De Stefano N, Battaglini M, Smith SM: Measuring brain atrophy in multiple sclerosis. J Neuroimaging 2007;17;(Suppl 1):10S-15S.
147. Simon JH: Brain atrophy in multiple sclerosis: What we know and would like to know. Mult Scler 2006;12:679-687.
148. Miller DH, Barkhof F, Frank JA, et al: Measurement of atrophy in multiple sclerosis: Pathological basis, methodological aspects and clinical relevance. Brain 2002;125:1676-1695.

149. Losseff NA, Wang L, Lai HM, et al: Progressive cerebral atrophy in multiple sclerosis: A serial MRI study. Brain 1996;119(Pt 6):2009-2019.
150. Fox NC, Jenkins R, Leary SM, et al: Progressive cerebral atrophy in MS: A serial study using registered, volumetric MRI. Neurology 2000;54:807-812.
151. Jasperse B, Valsasina P, Neacsu V, et al: Intercenter agreement of brain atrophy measurement in multiple sclerosis patients using manually-edited SIENA and SIENAX. J Magn Reson Imaging 2007;26:881-885.
152. Anderson VM, Fernando KT, Davies GR, et al: Cerebral atrophy measurement in clinically isolated syndromes and relapsing remitting multiple sclerosis: A comparison of registration-based methods. J Neuroimaging 2007;17:61-68.
153. Zivadinov R, Cox JL: Neuroimaging in multiple sclerosis. Int Rev Neurobiol 2007;79:449-474.
154. Tiberio M, Chard DT, Altmann DR, et al: Gray and white matter volume changes in early RRMS: A 2-year longitudinal study. Neurology 2005;64:1001-1007.
155. Sastre-Garriga J, Ingle GT, Chard DT, et al: Grey and white matter atrophy in early clinical stages of primary progressive multiple sclerosis. Neuroimage 2004;22:353-359.
156. Sastre-Garriga J, Ingle GT, Chard DT, et al: Grey and white matter volume changes in early primary progressive multiple sclerosis: A longitudinal study. Brain 2005;128:1454-1460.
157. Butteriss DJ, Ismail A, Ellison DW, Birchall D: Use of serial proton magnetic resonance spectroscopy to differentiate low grade glioma from tumefactive plaque in a patient with multiple sclerosis. Br J Radiol 2003;76:662-665.
158. Al-Okaili RN, Krejza J, Woo JH, et al: Intraaxial brain masses: MR imaging-based diagnostic strategy—Initial experience. Radiology 2007;243:539-550.
159. Lennon VA, Wingerchuk DM, Kryzer TJ, et al: A serum autoantibody marker of neuromyelitis optica: Distinction from multiple sclerosis. Lancet 2004;364:2106-2112.
160. Lennon VA, Kryzer TJ, Pittock SJ, et al: IgG marker of optic-spinal multiple sclerosis binds to the aquaporin-4 water channel. J Exp Med 2005;202:473-477.
161. Hinson SR, Pittock SJ, Lucchinetti CF, et al: Pathogenic potential of IgG binding to water channel extracellular domain in neuromyelitis optica. Neurology 2007;69:2221-2231.
162. Wingerchuk DM, Lennon VA, Pittock SJ, et al: Revised diagnostic criteria for neuromyelitis optica. Neurology 2006;66:1485-1489.
163. Wingerchuk DM, Hogancamp WF, O'Brien PC, Weinshenker BG: The clinical course of neuromyelitis optica (Devic's syndrome). Neurology 1999;53:1107-1114.
164. Pittock SJ, Weinshenker BG, Lucchinetti CF, et al: Neuromyelitis optica brain lesions localized at sites of high aquaporin 4 expression. Arch Neurol 2006;63:964-968.
165. Pittock SJ, Lennon VA, Krecke K, et al: Brain abnormalities in neuromyelitis optica. Arch Neurol 2006;63:390-396.
166. Yu C, Lin F, Li K, et al: Pathogenesis of normal-appearing white matter damage in neuromyelitis optica: Diffusion-tensor MR imaging. Radiology 2008;246:222-228.
167. Filippi M, Rocca MA, Moiola L, et al: MRI and magnetization transfer imaging changes in the brain and cervical cord of patients with Devic's neuromyelitis optica. Neurology 1999;53:1705-1710.
168. Yu CS, Zhu CZ, Li KC, et al: Relapsing neuromyelitis optica and relapsing-remitting multiple sclerosis: Differentiation at diffusion-tensor MR imaging of corpus callosum. Radiology 2007;244:249-256.
169. Tenembaum S, Chitnis T, Ness J, Hahn JS: Acute disseminated encephalomyelitis. Neurology 2007;68:S23-S36.
170. de Seze J, Debouverie M, Zephir H, et al: Acute fulminant demyelinating disease: A descriptive study of 60 patients. Arch Neurol 2007;64:1426-1432.
171. Albrecht P, Frohlich R, Hartung HP, et al: Optical coherence tomography measures axonal loss in multiple sclerosis independently of optic neuritis. J Neurol 2007;254:1595-1596.
172. Henderson AP, Trip SA, Schlottmann PG, et al: An investigation of the retinal nerve fibre layer in progressive multiple sclerosis using optical coherence tomography. Brain 2008;131:277-287.
173. Gundogan FC, Demirkaya S, Sobaci G: Is optical coherence tomography really a new biomarker candidate in multiple sclerosis? A structural and functional evaluation. Invest Ophthalmol Vis Sci 2007;48:5773-5781.
174. Pulicken M, Gordon-Lipkin E, Balcer LJ, et al: Optical coherence tomography and disease subtype in multiple sclerosis. Neurology 2007;69:2085-2092.
175. Grazioli E, Zivadinov R, Weinstock-Guttman B, et al: Retinal nerve fiber layer thickness is associated with brain MRI outcomes in multiple sclerosis. J Neurol Sci 2008;268:12-17.
176. Sergott RC, Frohman E, Glanzman R, Al-Sabbagh A: The role of optical coherence tomography in multiple sclerosis: Expert panel consensus. J Neurol Sci 2007;263:3-14.

6 Biomarkers in Multiple Sclerosis

ILIJAS JELČIĆ • ROLAND MARTIN

Multiple sclerosis (MS) is considered to be a complex genetic disease, and environmental factors probably contribute to disease induction and expression.[1] Several processes such as inflammation, demyelination, axonal damage, and disturbed regeneration of central nervous system (CNS) tissue contribute sequentially or simultaneously to its pathophysiology, to different extents in different patients. These varying degrees of contribution account for the broad heterogeneity in clinical phenotypes of the disease, as well as its prognosis and response to therapies. Ideally, a therapeutic strategy in MS includes a personalized set of therapeutic compounds targeting the disease-relevant processes. Therefore, as with other polygenetic and multifactorial diseases, there is an urgent need for biomarkers that reflect the various contributors to disease. Such biomarkers would be invaluable for (1) the diagnosis and stratification of MS subcategories, (2) prediction of disease courses, (3) individually tailored therapeutic regimens and improved prognosis for treatment success, and (4) the evaluation of novel therapeutics. A recently detected biomarker, immunoglobulin G (IgG) antibodies directed to aquaporin-4, is a first and robust example for defining an MS subcategory, neuromyelitis optica (NMO). Pharmacogenetics has also opened new ways to the personalization of treatment; for example, genetic variants of multidrug-resistance proteins influence the intracellular uptake of mitoxantrone,[2] and baseline interferon (IFN) signatures determine in advance the responsiveness to treatment with interferon-beta.[3] Nevertheless, these and many others potential biomarkers still warrant further validation and are far from being in routine clinical use.

Ideal biomarkers (1) should mirror the underlying pathophysiologic processes in MS in an unbiased way, (2) should be highly sensitive and specific, (3) should be validated for sensitivity and specificity as well as variability and reproducibility in independent studies from different laboratories, (4) should be collected in a minimally invasive manner, and (5) should offer an economic and simple monitoring tool in trials of novel therapeutics as well as in daily patient management.[4] So far, none of the putative biomarkers meets these conditions. In addition, the search for biomarkers in MS is constrained by the fact that samples from the target organ, the CNS, cannot be easily collected and that blood and cerebrospinal fluid (CSF) samples only to some degree reflect CNS local disease processes. Most of the putative biomarkers that have been identified to date are derived from whole blood and serum specimens and focus on the autoimmune component of the disease. More recently, there have been studies on putative markers in the CSF, some of which appear to reflect neurodegenerative processes of the disease. Novel technologies, most notably in the fields of genomics and proteomics, are expected to greatly enhance the establishment of true biomarkers. The approval of immunomodulatory drugs renders placebo-controlled trials increasingly difficult in terms of ethics. For this reason, trials of novel therapeutics in the future will more often be performed as add-on studies. Such trials are expected to show smaller treatment effects beyond the approved therapeutics, and, as a consequence, the sample size, duration, and costs of trials are expected to rise. Therefore, biomarkers will be of increasing interest for both preclinical assessment and phase I/II evaluation of drugs.

This chapter summarizes important findings in the field of biomarkers related to diagnosis, prognosis, activity, and treatment effect in MS; however, an exhaustive compilation of the existing data is beyond the scope of this text.

Definitions of Biomarkers

In recent years, the scientific literature has rapidly grown, and the terms "biomarker," "clinical biomarker," and "surrogate marker" have been used interchangeably and loosely, generating confusion with regard to their definition. The Biomarkers Definitions Working Group attempted to clarify this ambiguous terminology and proposed the following standard definitions, which are used throughout this chapter[5]:

- *Biologic marker:* a characteristic that is objectively measured and evaluated as an indicator of normal biologic processes, pathogenic processes, or pharmacologic responses to a therapeutic intervention
- *Clinical end point:* a clinically meaningful measure of how a patient feels, functions, or survives (e.g., the clinical exacerbation rate in patients with MS or the accumulation of irreversible disability)

- *Surrogate end point:* a biomarker that is intended to substitute for a clinical end point. A surrogate end point is expected to predict clinical benefit (or harm, or lack of benefit or harm) on the basis of epidemiologic, therapeutic, pathophysiologic, or other scientific evidence. The use of the term "surrogate marker" is discouraged, because it suggests that the substitution is for a marker rather than for a clinical end point.

Thus, surrogate end points are a subset of biomarkers. Surrogate end points should provide information about the efficacy or the clinical prognosis of a therapy in a significantly shorter time than that needed to follow the clinical end point. They can be essential to allow health authorities to accelerate marketing approval of novel therapeutic approaches. In MS, no such surrogate end point is able to sufficiently substitute for a clinical end point at this time. However, magnetic resonance imaging (MRI) is the method most widely used for diagnostic purposes and to track the activity and progression of disease in MS patients,[6-8] and it has emerged as the best-studied biomarker candidate in MS. MRI imaging is covered in Chapter 5; here, we summarize the data on biomarkers other than imaging that are indicative of immunologic alterations and neurodegenerative processes and discuss new, sensitive, high-throughput technologies.

Biomarkers Related to Diagnosis and Prognosis

OLIGOCLONAL BANDS AND ANTIBODIES

Currently, the only biomarker apart from MRI that is accepted in the diagnosis of MS is the detection of CSF oligoclonal bands (OCB), which are immunoglobulins separated by isoelectric focusing (IEF). Six decades after their discovery,[9] the precise origin and meaning of OCB are not yet understood, but their presence is strongly associated with MS. OCB are also found in infectious and inflammatory neurologic diseases such as Lyme disease, syphilis, subacute sclerosing panencephalitis, fungal meningoencephalitis, and Sjögren's syndrome; in these infectious conditions, most if not all immunoglobulin bands are directed against the respective pathogen.[10-13] Despite the presence of OCB in these CNS infections and inflammatory diseases, the presence of 10 or more bands is usually more frequently observed in MS.[14] Once present, OCB persist in the CSF of MS patients, pointing to a stable B-cell–mediated intrathecal immune response in MS. The sensitivity of OCB detection in IEF is higher than 85%, with a specificity of 92% and positive and negative predictive values of greater than 86.5% and 90%, respectively.[14]

OCB are detected by IEF and subsequent staining of the gels. A recent study combined IEF of oligoclonal IgG with alkaline phosphatase immunodetection and showed a higher sensitivity and specificity than MRI criteria.[15] Using this approach, it has been possible to reliably predict a second attack in patients with a clinically isolated demyelinating syndrome (CIS) and, consequently, to predict conversion to clinically definite multiple sclerosis (CDMS). Not only oligoclonal IgG, but also oligoclonal IgM may be detected by IEF.[16] The potential pathophysiologic importance of IgM is highlighted by the fact that IgM is the most potent activator of complement, which co-localizes with demyelinated areas in MS and NMO.[17,18] Early reports concerning oligoclonal IgM as a strong predictor of earlier conversion to CDMS and a more aggressive disease course have so far not been replicated in other studies.[19-24]

Anti-Myelin Antibodies

The pathologic role of autoantibodies in autoimmune disease is widely accepted. Among the potential autoantigens in MS, myelin basic protein (MBP) and myelin oligodendrocyte glycoprotein (MOG) are of particular interest because of their locations (in compact myelin and in the outer surface of the myelin sheath, respectively) and their pathogenicity in the experimental autoimmune encephalomyelitis (EAE) model. In a 2003 report, the presence of serum IgM autoantibodies specific for the extracellular domain of MOG and antibodies specific for MBP in CIS patients was highly predictive for conversion to CDMS.[25] Subsequent analysis of the prognostic value of anti-MOG and anti-MBP in eight different CIS cohorts produced controversial results, with correlations ranging from highly significant,[25-27] to significant in a subanalysis,[28,29] to not significant at all.[30-32] Because the same type of method (i.e., immunoblotting to recombinant MOG and human myelin–derived MBP) was used in all studies, the controversial results may primarily reflect differences in study populations (e.g., different genetic backgrounds) rather than methodologic problems.

It is a matter of ongoing debate whether pathogenic autoantibodies are reliably detected by binding to conformational or linear epitopes or glycosylated proteins.[33] Recently, high-sensitivity bioassays for the detection of autoantibodies that bind to the extracellular part of native MOG were reported.[34,35] To obtain MOG in its native form with all post-translational modifications, the full-length human MOG complementary DNA was expressed in a human glioblastoma cell line, and serum antibodies directed to the conformational epitopes of the extracellular domain of native MOG were detected by flow cytometry.[35] With the use of this approach, anti-MOG antibodies were found to be significantly elevated in the sera of MS patients compared with controls. These autoantibodies exerted cytotoxicity in vitro and enhanced demyelination as well as axonal damage after injection in susceptible rats.[35] It is not yet known whether the development of autoantibodies in MS patients reflects a response to myelin injury or is the cause for the insult. In the end, further studies are needed to elucidate whether these autoantibodies correlate with pathologic and clinical parameters.

In another study, a novel tetramer radioimmunoassay was presented, which was more sensitive than other methodologies for MOG autoantibody detection.[36] Autoantibodies from patients with acute disseminated encephalomyelitis (ADEM) selectively bound conformational MOG tetramers, whereas antibodies derived from adult-onset MS cases bound only rarely. Aberrant N-glycosylation was recently shown to be a fundamental determinant of autoantibody recognition in MS patients compared with controls.[37] A synthetic glycosylated peptide antigen called CSF114(Glc) was designed on the structural basis of myelin epitopes and proved to bind by enzyme-linked immunosorbent assay (ELISA) to specific IgM autoantibodies in the sera of MS patients, but not in healthy donors and other autoimmune conditions. The induction of anti-CSF114(Glc) antibodies correlated with clinical activity and brain lesions on MRI. So far, this novel immunoassay seems to represent a promising diagnostic and prognostic marker in a subgroup of MS patients.

Other promising candidate autoantibodies have been described, such as those against neurofascin,[38] which appear to be involved in axonal injury, but validation in independent studies is required.

Antibodies against Epstein-Barr Virus

Among the potential environmental triggers, recent data indicate that Epstein-Barr virus (EBV) may play an important role.[39] Despite the fact that the specificity spectrum of OCB is as yet poorly understood and a clear association of OCB with the pathogenesis of MS lacking, EBV appears to be one of the targets of OCB. An attempt to assess the specificity of OCB by screening protein expression arrays containing 37,000 tagged proteins led to the identification of two high-affinity epitopes derived from EBV proteins.[40] The frequency of the immunoreactivities toward these EBV proteins, BRRF2 and Epstein-Barr nuclear antigen-1 (EBNA1), was significantly higher in the serum and CSF of MS patients than in those of control donors. These findings point to a perturbed EBV-specific immune response in MS patients and corroborate the long-discussed association of EBV infection with the development of MS.

Further evidence for the importance of EBV stems from epidemiologic studies investigating EBNA1-specific antibodies. Analysis of blood samples collected before the onset of disease revealed that antibody titers to the EBNA complex and to EBNA1 were elevated in individuals who later developed MS, compared with those who remained healthy, and that elevated titers persisted after MS onset.[41-43] The risk of MS increased with higher antibody titers.[42] Teenagers and young adults experiencing infectious mononucleosis, an acute EBV-triggered febrile disease, are also to be at higher risk for development of MS some years later, compared with individuals who contracted EBV infection earlier in life.[44-46] The risk conferred by elevated EBNA1 antibody titers is independent from the major contributor of genetic risk in MS, the human leukocyte antigen (HLA)-DR15 allele.[47] Therefore, carriers of the risk allele HLA-DR15 who have elevated EBNA1 antibody titers may have an increased risk of MS.

Antibodies to EBV early antigens that indicate active viral replication may be associated with increased inflammatory activity, as assessed by gadolinium-enhanced MRI lesions, and with early MS.[48] Another study showed an association with clinical disease exacerbations in MS patients, but not with clinically stable disease.[49] It remains unclear how altered EBV-specific immunoglobulin responses are induced in MS patients.

The potential role of EBV in MS is supported not only by these observations regarding EBV-specific antibodies in MS, but also by the EBV-specific CD4- and CD8-positive T-cell response. The frequency, proliferative capacity, and antigen specificity of these cells were reported to be altered in MS patients compared with healthy individuals.[40,50,51] In addition, EBV persists and reactivates in the CNS of MS patients, but not in those with inflammatory neurologic diseases, and therefore might play an important role in MS immunopathology.[52] Taken together, these exciting studies point toward the possibility that a preceding state of altered EBV immunity and perturbed EBV infection predisposes for the development of autoimmunity. Still, EBV immunity–associated biomarkers and surrogate end points need to be defined more precisely in relation to the diagnosis of MS or prediction of the disease course.

Aquaporin-4 Antibodies

NMO is a severe inflammatory demyelinating disease that is characterized by immunopathology in the optic nerves and spinal cord.[53] It is hypothesized from serologic and clinical observations that antibody-mediated autoimmunity is prominent in a high proportion of patients with NMO.[18] Because immunomodulatory treatments of MS are not effective in NMO, treatment strategies differ considerably. The clinical significance of early accurate diagnosis and early aggressive intervention to prevent severe NMO relapses is high, because mortality is substantial and the risk of fast progression in disability is high in NMO compared with MS. Lennon and colleagues[53] identified serum IgG antibodies with high specificity for NMO by indirect immunofluorescence staining of mouse brain tissue. NMO-specific antibodies were detected in 73% of patients with definite NMO and in 46% of patients at high risk for NMO, but not in any single patient with classic MS. Showing a specificity of 91% in distinguishing NMO from MS, these NMO-IgG antibodies were considered to be a promising biomarker in patients with a first episode of myelitis.[54] Therefore, it was recently proposed to include NMO-IgG in the diagnostic criteria of NMO.[55] Subsequently, aquaporin-4 was identified as the target antigen of NMO-IgG.[56]

Aquaporin-4 is located in astrocytic foot processes at the blood–brain barrier and is the most abundant water channel in the brain, exhibiting an important role in brain water homeostasis. Although it is abundant in optic nerve and spinal cord, aquaporin-4 is found throughout the healthy brain and is completely lost in NMO lesions as opposed to MS lesions.[57,58] These findings have been corroborated by several studies on different patient populations using different assays.[59-62] For these reasons, NMO-IgG antibodies represent a novel disease-specific biomarker, the first discovered for any demyelinating disease affecting the human CNS, and they help distinguish NMO patients from those with classic MS and other inflammatory demyelinating variants of MS. NMO-IgG antibodies enable clinicians to reliably identify a subgroup of patients within the heterogeneous disease complex of MS before fulfillment of all traditional clinical diagnostic criteria and to direct them to early and specific treatments, such as plasmapheresis[63] or B-cell depletion by rituximab, a selective anti-CD20 (B-cell) monoclonal antibody.[64] However, it needs to be stressed that not all patients who fulfill clinical NMO criteria are NMO antibody positive.

CYTOKINES, CHEMOKINES, AND THEIR RECEPTORS

Cytokines are among the most intensively studied biomarkers in MS. Based on several reports in patients with MS and on numerous studies in the EAE model, pro-inflammatory cytokines that are characteristic for Th1 lineage, such as IFN-γ, tumor necrosis factor-α, and interleukin 12 (IL-12) are considered for the pathogenesis of MS. These cytokines were shown to be elevated in MS relapses, whereas anti-inflammatory cytokines such as the Th2 cytokines IL-4 and IL-10 and transforming growth factor-β, were associated with clinical remissions and a stable course of relapsing-remitting MS (RRMS).[65] The recently discovered Th17 lineage is characterized by the secretion of IL-17 and is one example for the notion that the cytokine network in MS is more complex than if reflected by the Th1/Th2 paradigm.[66] The production of IL-17 and IL-5 by MBP-induced $CD4^+$

T cells correlated with the number of active plaques on MRI scans in a recent report, indicating association with disease activity.[67] IL-12 and other related chemokines and their receptors have been considered as biomarkers for differentiation of progressive disease from relapsing-remitting disease course and as biomarkers of disease activity in progressive MS.[68-70]

Chemokines are chemotactic cytokines that are involved in the recruitment of immune cells within lymphoid organs and at sites of inflammation. The chemokine receptor CCR5 was described as correlating with symptomatic relapses.[71-73] In addition, CXCR3 expression in circulating T cells from MS patients was increased. Immunohistochemical analyses of autopsy brain sections containing active MS lesions have described CXCR3 expression on virtually all tissue-infiltrating T cells.[71,72] These CXCR3-positive perivascular cell infiltrates were uncommon in control brain specimens. It was suggested that the retention of $CXCR3^+$ T cells in patients with MS is a result of the presence of its ligand (IP-10) and that $CXCR3^+$ cells, in the absence of ligand, recirculate.[74] In active inflammatory MS lesions, $CCR1^+/CCR5^+$-expressing hematogenous monocytes were found in abundance in perivascular cell cuffs and at the demyelinating edges of evolving lesions, together with $CCR5^+$ microglia, but not in noninflamed brain sections.[75] Patients with MS show an enrichment of $CCR7^+$ memory T cells co-expressing CCR5, a candidate biomarker for Th1 cells, and CXCR3 in their CSF.[76,77] Chemokines and their receptors may become important in the study of disease heterogeneity and therefore need to be validated in larger cohorts, but they are unlikely candidates for surrogate end points in MS.

BIOMARKERS OF CELLULAR IMMUNE FUNCTION

Various changes related to T cells, B cells, natural killer (NK) cells, and other immune cells can be analyzed today in regard to a variety of parameters, such as phenotype, antigen specificity, frequency, proliferation capacity, activation status, susceptibility to apoptosis, special subpopulations, expression of specific surface molecules, cytokine production, and secretion, among others.

There are numerous interesting candidates among these parameters, but the assessment of most of them involves rather complex immunologic assays, which are difficult to perform, expensive, and often not standardized among different laboratories. In consequence, these analyses may be performed only in laboratories with expertise in this field and are not suited for routine use in clinical laboratories. Therefore, not only must observations on biomarkers for cellular immune function be validated in independent experiments by other groups, but it is essential to define the respective methods precisely and to standardize them (i.e., develop standard operating procedures).

The putative role of $CD4^+$ T cells in the autoimmune pathogenesis of MS is supported by many findings, which have been summarized in detail elsewhere.[1] Because the difficulties previously described with respect to validation and standardization apply to most of these studies and because of their sheer number, we will not list them here.

CSF mature B cells and plasma blasts were reported to correlate with acute brain inflammation measured by MRI and with inflammatory CSF parameters in CIS and RRMS, but not in chronic progressive MS.[78] Clonally expanded B cells, mainly of a memory phenotype, accumulate in chronic MS lesions and in the

CSF of MS patients.[79] A subset of B cells, called short-lived plasma blasts, were reported to be more frequent in the CSF in MS compared with other inflammatory and noninflammatory diseases, and the numbers of plasma blasts strongly correlated with intrathecal IgG synthesis and inflammatory parenchymal disease activity as shown by MRI.[80]

About 45% of patients with fulminant attacks of MS unresponsive to corticosteroids improve after therapeutic plasma exchange (TPE). TPE removes pathogenic humoral and plasma factors, indicating a therapeutic effect on B cell–mediated pathomechanisms in MS. Recently, lesion biopsies of 53% of a small cohort of patients with RRMS unresponsive to corticosteroids were classified as histopathologic pattern type II, according to the classification by Lucchinetti and colleagues.[17] The same patients experienced significant clinical improvement after TPE, but none of the patients with pattern I or pattern III had such improvement.[81] Because pattern type II is characterized by antibody/complement-associated demyelination, these findings clearly link TPE responsiveness in corticosteroid nonresponders to an MS subtype in which the pathophysiology is predominantly B cell driven. Patients with this subtype of disease could benefit from TPE or even rituximab treatment before application of corticosteroids. Whether the subgroup of MS patients with histopathologic pattern type II can be identified without brain biopsies (i.e., by alternative biomarkers using imaging or biochemical/immunologic constituents) remains to be shown.

A treatment study with daclizumab, a monoclonal antibody directed against CD25, demonstrated a profound inhibition of brain inflammatory activity.[82] The reduction of the inflammatory activity correlated highly with the absolute expansion of $CD56^{bright}$ NK cells, indicating an important immunoregulatory role for these cells in the MS pathogenesis.[83] The same population of NK cells was reduced in frequency in patients with untreated RRMS and in those with CIS, compared with healthy donors.[84] The same study revealed three distinct subpopulations of untreated RRMS patients by large-scale flow cytometry–based immunophenotyping (FACS). Further supporting the role of these cells, $CD56^{bright}$ NK cells were also reported to increase in frequency during the last trimester of pregnancy, a time of reduced MS relapses, in women with MS.[85] Similarly, an expansion of circulating $CD56^{bright}$ NK cells was noted in subjects with RRMS after treatment initiation with IFN-beta.[86] The expansion of $CX3CR1^{+}$ NK cells, however, correlated positively with disease activity in RRMS patients.[87]

MARKERS FOR HYPOXIC INJURY AND GLUTAMATE EXCITOTOXICITY

The biomarkers mentioned earlier focused on alterations of immune function and the autoimmune aspects of MS but provided little or no information about the effector mechanisms that lead to CNS tissue damage during MS. Because these mechanisms are ultimately responsible for the neurologic deficits of MS patients, it is particularly desirable to identify biomarkers reflecting these processes. According to the histopathologic classification by Lucchinetti and colleagues,[17] the demyelination pattern type III is characterized by an oligodendrocyte dystrophy that principally affects the most distant processes of these cells and leads to apoptosis of oligodendrocytes at later stages of lesion development. This pattern is associated with nuclear expression of hypoxia-inducible factor 1α (HIF-1α) and mimicks myelin destruction in acute white matter ischemia. So far, no MRI or clinical correlate to the histopathologic classification of demyelination has been identified, but, together with that classification system, HIF-1α clearly merits further exploration as a marker for pattern III MS.

Recently, a brain epitope (D-110) that is detectable by a monoclonal antibody against canine distemper virus and cross-reactive to an endogenous brain epitope was shown to be expressed at high levels in type III actively demyelinating MS lesions, but not, or to a much lesser extent, in other MS cases.[88] The presence of D-110 was significantly associated with expression of HIF-1α within the lesions. In addition, D-110 is liberated into the CSF, where it can be detected by ELISA in about 17% of patients. This proportion is similar to the reported incidence of cases with type III lesions found in histopathologic studies. Even though an elevated concentration of D-110 is not specific for type III lesions, being found also in acute lesions of white matter ischemia, D-110 may become a useful diagnostic tool to identify clinically a defined MS subtype. Further direct correlations between pathology and CSF values will be necessary to determine the reliability of this tool for diagnosis and subtyping of MS.

Because inflammation-induced hypoxia-like MS lesions occur in the absence of significant vascular pathology, these lesions have been suggested to result from a histotoxic hypoxia induced by mitochondrial damage.[89] Among the various molecules that are produced in effector cells in inflammatory lesions and mediate mitochondrial dysfunction, nitric oxide (NO) and reactive oxygen species are the most important ones implicated in axonal and myelin sheath vulnerability to hypoxia in MS pathogenesis.[90-92] Nevertheless, NO has also been linked to various beneficial and immunomodulatory effects in brain inflammation, such as inhibition of antigen presentation, T-cell proliferation, induction of apoptosis in T cells, and the downregulation of adhesion molecules.[92] Elevated levels of the NO metabolites nitrite and nitrate were found in CSF, serum, and urine in MS patients.[93-98] Intrathecal production of nitrite and nitrate was associated with clinical disease activity in the early phase of the disease as assessed by MRI parameters. Raised baseline levels of intrathecal NO metabolites were associated with clinical and MRI progression in MS patients over 3-year follow-up, suggesting that they could indicate a more aggressive disease course.[95] In another study, increased NO metabolites correlated with a presumed biomarker of axonal degeneration (neurofilaments) and clinical disability (Expanded Disability Status Scale [EDSS] score), suggesting that NO-mediated stress is related to the development of sustained disability in MS.[98] These results need to be replicated in larger cohorts with a high level of accuracy regarding the biochemical assessment of the metabolites, which is strongly dependent on the sampling procedure of the probes. An alternative way in which NO and other reactive oxygen species might affect the function of oligodendrocytes is by radical-mediated oxidation and breakdown of myelin components.[92] Cholesterol is the major component of the myelin sheath, and its breakdown product, 7-ketocholesterol, can activate and attract microglial cells in brain tissue, leading to neuronal damage. Indeed, higher levels of 7-ketocholesterol were detected in the CSF of patients with MS compared with control patients with other noninflammatory neurologic diseases.[99]

Oligodendrocytes also may be damaged by glutamate-mediated excitotoxicity mediated by the α-amino-3-hydroxy-5-methyl-4-isoxazolepropionic acid (AMPA)/kainate type of glutamate receptors, as was shown in the EAE model.[100]

Glutamate is released in excessive amounts by activated leukocytes and microglia and leads to increased calcium fluxes and excitotoxic death of oligodendrocytes and neurons on binding to AMPA/kainate receptors. Markers for glutamate production (e.g., glutaminase) are increased in macrophages and microglia in close proximity to dystrophic axons within active MS plaques.[100,101] A treatment with riluzole, a neuroprotective inhibitor of glutamate release from nerve terminals, reduced the rate of cervical cord atrophy and the development of T1-hypointense lesions.[102] However, due to small sample size, lack of a placebo group, short follow-up, and lack of statistical significance, these data must be interpreted cautiously. How biomarkers for glutamate excitotoxicity should be defined and how they can be assessed in the clinical setting remain to be determined.

Biomarkers Related to Disease Activity

BIOMARKERS RELATED TO MS-SPECIFIC ALTERATIONS OF THE IMMUNE SYSTEM

Soluble Proteins

Within sites of inflammation, a broad panel of receptors involved in immune response and regulation are upregulated on the surface of various cell types. This process involves exocytosis of inflammation-associated proteins and also shedding of soluble forms of cell surface receptors. In addition to their expression on the surface of most human cells, HLA class I antigens also occur naturally in the form of soluble HLA-A, -B, and -C (sHLA class I) antigens in body fluids. Increased concentrations of sHLA class I were observed in the CSF and serum of MS patients,[103] and both sHLA class I and sHLA class II are influenced reciprocally by immunomodulatory treatment.[104]

HLA-G is a nonclassic HLA class I molecule that differs from classic HLA class I by its limited polymorphism, its highly restricted tissue distribution, and its pattern of alternative splicing.[105] Expression of HLA-G can be induced in cases of cancer, transplantation, inflammatory disease, and viral infection, protecting target tissues from autoaggressive inflammation and exerting an immunotolerogenic function. Levels of soluble HLA-G (sHLA-G) are significantly increased in MS patients compared with patients with other neurologic diseases.[106] Recently, it was shown that a balance may exist between intrathecally produced sHLA class I and sHLA-G, which are inversely related to MRI and clinical disease activity.[107,108] It was suggested that these molecules serve opposing roles in the balance between inflammation (sHLA class I) and immunomodulation (sHLA-G). Consequently, sHLA molecules in sera and/or CSF of MS patients might be useful as biomarkers for monitoring of disease activity.

CD14 is expressed on mononuclear cells and, together with Toll-like receptor 4 (TLR4), represents a pattern recognition receptor of microbial products. In addition to mediating inflammation in the context of the innate host defense, CD14 was shown to be involved in the non-inflammatory phagocytosis of apoptotic cells by macrophages.[109,110] A soluble form of CD14 (sCD14) can be detected in serum or plasma, and elevated serum levels of sCD14 have been reported in both MS patients and those with other organ-specific autoimmune diseases.[111-118] The level of sCD14 correlates inversely with the clinical activity of the disease in MS patients. Corroborating this result, a decrease in sCD14 levels during relapse was observed in a longitudinal analysis.[118] The role of sCD14 in autoimmune disease is unknown, but the differences in sCD14 levels might reflect a differential activation and role of the innate immune system during inflammation in MS. Therapy with IFN-beta induced higher sCD14 serum levels in RRMS patients.[116,118] Further studies should validate these findings in different populations and correlate the biologic data with MRI imaging of brain inflammation.

Adhesion Molecules and Matrix Metalloproteases

Several adhesion molecules are involved in the transendothelial migration of leukocytes into the CNS, a central process in MS pathogenesis. Cytokines, which are secreted within an inflammatory focus in MS, induce the upregulation of adhesion molecules prior to disruption of the blood–brain barrier.[119] Adhesion molecules may also be released in a soluble form from activated endothelial cells, leukocytes, and platelets into serum and CSF.[120] Plasma levels of soluble adhesion molecules including soluble platelet endothelial cell adhesion molecule 1 (sPECAM-1), sP-selectin and sE-selectin were shown to be increased in RRMS compared with chronic progressive MS.[121] In addition, levels of sPECAM-1, sP-selectin and sE-selectin were increased during relapse, suggesting that they might be useful paraclinical markers of disease activity in MS with restriction to the clinical course of the disease.[122] Furthermore, increased levels of soluble intercellular adhesion molecule 1 (sICAM-1) were found in the serum of MS patients during a clinical relapse or with active MRI scans, and an association between high intrathecal sICAM-1 levels and IgG indices in RRMS patients was reported.[123] The increase of soluble vascular cell adhesion molecule-1 (sVCAM-1) was reported to be associated with a decrease in MRI lesions in MS patients treated with IFN-beta-1b.[124] In SPMS, early upregulation (1 to 6 months) of sVCAM-1 correlated inversely with less MRI activity in the 19- to 24-month treatment interval in the group treated with IFN-beta-1b.[125] Similar results were reported in RRMS patients treated with IFN-beta-1a.[126] However, downregulation of very late antigen 4 (VLA-4) showed higher sensitivity in predicting a favorable treatment response than did VCAM-1 upregulation, and VLA-4 was significantly upregulated during relapses.[126-129]

The matrix metalloproteases (MMPs) comprise a family of endopeptidases that degrade extracellular proteins; they are involved in the disintegration of the subendothelial basement membrane of the blood–brain barrier and subsequent CNS lesion formation in MS. Several family members (MMP-2, -3, -7, and -9) have been detected in autopsied brains of MS patients, and MMP-9 expression has been reported to be associated with acute lesions. Elevated messenger RNA and serum protein levels of MMP-9 were associated with disease activity as assessed by clinical and MRI parameters.[130,131] Using the ratio between serum protein levels of MMP-9 and its antagonistic tissue inhibitor of metalloproteinases 1 (TIMP-1), it was possible to predict the appearance of new active MRI lesions patients with SPMS.[131] Adhesion molecules, MMPs, and their inhibitors are clearly promising biomarkers in MS but require validation. However, because they predominantly reflect blood–brain barrier disruption when measured in blood, serum, or CSF samples, we find it unlikely that these molecules could become more useful than MRI-based markers of blood–brain barrier disruption.

Apoptosis-Related Molecules

Not only the formation of the repertoire of adaptive immune cells but also the regulation and termination of peripheral immune responses involves activation-induced cell death via apoptosis. There is evidence that a failure of apoptosis in potentially pathogenic T cells and B cells is involved in MS pathogenesis. An increased gene expression of anti-apoptotic mediators was demonstrated in a microarray analysis of blood cells from patients with RRMS (Blevins et al., in preparation). The pro-apoptotic factor and Bcl-2 family member Bcl-X_L (also called BCL2L1) was reported to be expressed at increased levels in peripheral blood cells of MS patients and to correlate directly with a resistance to activation-induced T-cell death.[132, 133] Consistent with these findings, the expression of Bcl-2 family members in blood cells from MS patients correlated with clinical features of disease activity, such as number of gadolinium-enhancing MRI lesions and clinical relapses.[133,134] Apart from Bcl-2–related proteins, the analysis of expression levels of the death-inducing ligand CD95 and the tumor necrosis factor–related apoptosis-inducing ligand (TRAIL), in either membrane-bound or soluble forms, has led to controversial results in different MS populations.[135-139]

In a longitudinal gene and protein expression analysis of patients under IFN-beta treatment, drug responders were distinguished from nonresponders by early and sustained induction of TRAIL.[139] Increased concentrations of soluble TRAIL in serum predicted treatment response to IFN-beta even before treatment was started. Therefore, TRAIL may be used as a prognostic marker of treatment response to IFN-beta in MS. However, the reported findings still await confirmation in a larger cohort of MS patients, and the significance of TRAIL in the pathogenesis of MS needs further clarification.

BIOMARKERS RELATED TO MS-SPECIFIC NEURODEGENERATIVE PROCESSES

Markers of Demyelination

Cholesterol is one of the main components of cell membranes; 24S-hydroxycholesterol is a metabolite that is synthesized exclusively in the brain and spinal cord and therefore is a marker for cell membrane homoeostasis within the CNS. Serum levels of 24S-hydroxycholesterol was reported to be increased in the CSF of patients with RRMS.[140] The increase was most pronounced in patients with gadolinium-enhancing lesions compared to patients without active scans. In contrast, serum 24S-hydroxycholesterol levels were reduced in the primary progressive clinical subtype.[141] Therefore, 24S-hydroxycholesterol may indicate the transition from a predominantly immune-mediated to a degenerative phase of the disease.

Markers of Axonal Damage and Regeneration and Astrocyte Activation

There has been increasing interest in the identification of biomarkers of axonal damage in MS, because such damage is now recognized as an important pathomechanism. Whereas markers of inflammation often correlate poorly with disability, markers of axonal degeneration are expected to provide helpful information on future disability of MS patients.

Neurofilaments, the major axonal cytoskeleton proteins, consist of three components that differ in molecular size: a light chain Nf-L, an intermediate chain Nf-M, and a heavy chain Nf-H.[142] Several studies have shown that the concentration of Nf-L is increased in the CSF of MS patients compared with healthy people or patients with other inflammatory or non-inflammatory neurologic disorders.[143] Increased CSF levels were most pronounced in RRMS and peaked in the third week after relapse, which suggests a delayed relation with disease activity.[144,145] However, the CSF concentrations of Nf-L correlate poorly with clinical disability measured by the EDSS. Apart from the protein itself, intrathecal anti-Nf-L autoantibodies were shown to occur more frequently in PPMS patients than in patients with RRMS or other neurologic disease or healthy controls.[146-148] The positive correlation of anti-Nf-L autoantibodies with MRI measures of brain atrophy suggests a correlation with disease progression.

Glial fibrillary acidic protein (GFAP), a monomeric intermediate filament protein, is a structural component of the cytoskeleton that is highly expressed in astrocytes. GFAP is considered to be the morphologic basis of astrogliosis, which is a prominent feature of MS.[149] Increased CSF levels of GFAP were reported in MS patients, although results were inconsistent.[145,149-152] Because it was also found intrathecally in patients with other neurologic diseases, GFAP represents a nonspecific marker of CNS tissue injury, although CSF levels of GFAP correlated with disability in MS patients.[153]

N-Acetylaspartate (NAA) is an amino acid that is almost exclusively expressed in neurons. NAA is important in osmoregulation: it functions as a water pump by transporting water molecules out of neurons against the water concentration gradient. Because of its neuronal specificity, NAA has been used as a marker of neuronal damage in pathology as well as magnetic resonance spectroscopy. Reduced neuronal levels of NAA, both in MS lesions and in the normal-appearing white matter, correlate inversely with the degree of disability.[143]

Nogo, a major component of CNS myelin, is a development-related molecule that inhibits axonal regeneration and sprouting of synaptic terminals. Three isoforms of Nogo exist (A, B, and C), generated by alternative splicing or differential promoter usage of a single gene. Intrathecal anti-Nogo-A autoantibodies are significantly more common in patients with RRMS compared with chronic progressive MS.[154] A study reporting an exclusive presence of soluble Nogo-A in the CSF of MS patients was later proved wrong.[155,156]

Even though they require further validation, the biomarker candidates for axonal damage are clearly promising to evolve into surrogate end points in MS.

Biomarkers for Treatment Responses

There is a strong need for baseline biomarkers and predictors of treatment responsiveness for a number of reasons. Early recognition of nonresponders to a treatment prevents the accumulation of disability and further relapses during ineffective therapy. The high costs of existing and future therapies encourage clinicians to direct the therapies to those who will most benefit from them. Furthermore, it is not conceivable to develop rational combination therapies without some readout for their effects on biologically relevant molecular pathways.

INTERFERON-BETA AND GLATIRAMER ACETATE

In the past, numerous molecules and immunologic functions were monitored during standard treatments of MS, particularly with IFN-beta and glatiramer acetate. Both drugs represent current first-line therapies for MS.[157] The mechanisms of action of IFN-beta are poorly understood, but it has been suggested that it blocks blood–brain barrier opening and skews the peripheral immune response from a pro-inflammatory, Th1-driven response to a more anti-inflammatory, Th2-driven response.[158] Nevertheless, the immunomodulatory effects of IFN-beta are far more complex, because treatment with IFN-beta affects the regulation of about 500 genes, including genes that encode pro-inflammatory mediators.[159] It has been shown by genome expression microarrays that IFN-beta nonresponder and responder phenotypes differ in their ex vivo gene expression profile.[160] Only a group of genes, rather than single genes, could reliably define the responder state. However, treatment response also depends on the underlying pathomechanisms of the disease, and this might be one reason why only a fraction of patients treated with these drugs have a good response.[161,162] With regard to the enormous treatment costs, individualization of patient management is needed urgently to improve the treatment of MS in the future.

Antibodies against IFN-beta can be induced on treatment, diminishing the bioavailability and treatment effect.[163,164] The bioactivity of interferon can be assessed by measuring interferon-stimulated genes. The most appropriate biomarker for IFN-beta is the myxovirus resistance protein-A (MxA), a guanosine triphosphatase with potent antiviral activity but no immunomodulatory effects.[165] There is no clear evidence that antibodies to glatiramer acetate inhibit clinical efficacy in vivo.[166] However, clinical response in glatiramer acetate–treated patients correlated not only to serum levels of IL-5 and IL-13 but also to an immunologic response profile that included a complex combination of assays monitoring cell-related parameters such as proliferation and secretion of IL-4 and IFN-γ.[167,168]

In summary, specific alterations in serum levels of sHLA class I, sHLA class II, VCAM-1, VLA-4, TRAIL, and MxA with IFN-beta therapy, or IL-5 and IL-13 with glatiramer acetate therapy, have been shown to be useful in a number of studies,[104,124-126,139,165,167] although none of these potential biomarkers has undergone rigorous validation in prospectively planned, confirmatory studies.

TREATMENT WITH MONOCLONAL ANTIBODIES

Daclizumab is a humanized monoclonal antibody directed against the IL-2 receptor α chain (CD25). It was considered as a means to limit T-cell expansion by blocking IL-2 signaling via its high-affinity receptor CD25, which is expressed especially on activated T cells. The drug is known to be well tolerated and was licensed in 1998 for the treatment of human T-cell lymphotropic virus 1–induced adult T-cell leukemia and for the prevention of renal allograft rejection. In a pilot trial in MS, daclizumab led to a 78% reduction in new contrast-enhancing lesions and significant improvement in several clinical outcome measures.[82] Surprisingly, the function of T cells appears to be affected only to a minor degree by daclizumab administration. In fact, only the expansion of CD56^{bright} NK cells, as measured by FACS staining, showed a strong inverse correlation with the treatment response and number of contrast-enhancing MRI lesions.[83] Therefore, expansion of the CD56^{bright} NK cells may be used as a biomarker of treatment response to daclizumab. Regarding bioavailability and function of the anti-CD25 treatment, blockade of Tac, the IL-2 binding epitope of CD25, can also be employed as a biomarker.

Rituximab is a monoclonal antibody that is directed against CD20, a molecule characteristically expressed on all B cells in the peripheral blood. It is a powerful immunosuppressant that eliminates mature circulating B cells with high efficiency for up to 9 months and has been approved for the treatment of CD20-positive B-cell non-Hodgkin's lymphoma and rheumatoid arthritis. Rituximab treatment reduced the number of new gadolinium-enhancing lesions and the number of relapses in a phase II trial.[169] The CD20^{+} B-cell count is useful as a marker of bioavailability, but a marker showing or even predicting response to rituximab treatment still remains to be defined.

Natalizumab is a humanized monoclonal antibody designed to bind VLA-4, an $\alpha_4\beta_1$ integrin expressed by all leukocytes except neutrophils.[170] Natalizumab is intended to prevent the extravasation of leukocytes into the target tissue by blocking the interaction of VLA-4 with its ligand VCAM-1 and the vessel wall. Unfortunately, two MS patients and one patient with Crohn's disease out of approximately 3000 individuals who had received the natalizumab during phase III trials, and 2 of 10,000 patients who were treated with rituximab for systemic lupus erythematosus (off-label use) developed progressive multifocal leukencephalopathy (PML) and later died.[171] PML is a demyelinating disorder of the CNS caused by infection with the human JC polyomavirus that leads to death in at least half of the cases.[172] To date, no reliable biomarker predictive of PML development has been described. These findings underscore the importance of immunomonitoring in patients receiving treatment with monoclonal antibodies. Table 6-1 summarizes biomarkers for treatment response.

Novel Technologies for the Identification of Novel Biomarkers

The increasing use of genomic information as well as large scale and high-throughput technologies is expected to fundamentally improve our understanding of the mechanisms that determine the onset and progression of complex diseases such as MS and offer unique chances to identify novel candidate biomarkers. Either as single markers or as sets of biomarkers, they should allow for identification of the "fingerprints" of MS subtypes and disease stages.

With methods such as genome-wide gene expression profiling, it is possible to measure or characterize families of cellular molecules (e.g., nucleic acids, proteins, intermediary metabolites) based on their ability to characterize all or most members of a family of molecules in a single, large-scale analysis. These methods are in summary termed "-omic" technologies—genomics, proteomics, glycomics, lipidomics, metabolomics, interactomics, and regulomics (Table 6-2). With these new tools, we can in principle obtain complete assessments of the functional activity of biochemical pathways, or of genetic differences among individuals, that were previously unattainable.

TABLE 6–1 Biological Markers Analyzed in Multiple Sclerosis

Biomarker	Sample	Method	Diagnosis	Prognosis	Disease Activity	Treatment Response/Effect	Validation
OCB IgG	CSF	IEF	+	+	–	–	*
OCB IgM	CSF	IEF	+	+	–	–	*
Anti-MOG Ab	Serum	Western-blot, ELISA, FACS, RBA	–	+	–	–	~
Aquaporin-4 Ab	Serum, CSF?	Immunofluorescence, FACS, RBA	+	+	–	–	*
CD20⁺ B cells	CSF	FACS	–	–	+	b.a. (rituximab)	n
CXC3	CSF	FACS	–	–	+	–	n
CD56^{bright} NK cells	Blood	FACS	–	–	+	t.r. (daclizumab, IFN-beta)	n
MxA	Blood	RT-PCR	–	–	–	b.a. (IFN-beta)	*
sHLA	Serum, CSF	ELISA	–	–	+	t.r. (IFN-beta)	~
sPECAM	Plasma	ELISA	–	–	+	–	*
sP-selectin, sE-selectin	Plasma, CSF	ELISA	–	–	+	–	n
sVCAM-1	Serum, CSF	ELISA	–	–	+	t.r. (IFN-beta)	*
VLA-4	Blood	FACS	–	–	+	t.r. (IFN-beta)	*
TRAIL	Serum	FACS, ELISA	–	–	–	p.m. (IFN-beta)	~
Nf-L Ab	Serum	ELISA	–	+	+	–	*
D-110	CSF	ELISA	+	–	–	–	n
Nitric oxide	CSF, serum, urine	Enzymatic reaction	–	+	+	–	~

+, the biomarker has been analyzed for respective outcome; –, the biomarker has not been analyzed for respective outcome; *, the respective outcome has been reanalyzed in at least one independent population; ~, the biomarker has been analyzed in at least one independent population with conflicting results; Ab, antibody; b.a., marker for bioavailability of a therapeutic; CSF, cerebrospinal fluid; CXC3, a chemokine; ELISA, enzyme-linked immunosorbent assay; FACS, flow cytometry–based immunophenotyping; IEF, isoelectric focusing; IFN-beta, interferon-beta; IgG, immunoglobulin G; IgM, immunoglobulin M; MOG, myelin oligodendrocyte glycoprotein; MxA, myxovirus resistance protein-A; n, the biomarker has not been validated in an independent population; NK, natural killer; OCB, oligoclonal bands; p.m., predictive marker of treatment response; RBA, radiobinding assay; RT-PCR, reverse transcriptase polymerase chain reaction; sHLA, soluble human leukocyte antigen; sPECAM, soluble platelet endothelial cell adhesion molecule; sVCAM-1, soluble vascular cell adhesion molecule 1; t.r., marker of treatment response; TRAIL, tumor necrosis factor–related apoptosis-inducing ligand; VLA-4, very late antigen 4.

TABLE 6-2 Novel Large-Scale Technologies for Detection of Biomarkers

Technique	Principle	Technique	Spectrum of Detection	State of Development
Genetics	SNP profiling	Oligonucleotide microarray	GW	+++
	CNV and CNP profiling by high-resolution sequencing	Oligonucleotide microarray	GW	++
		Pyrosequencing	GW	+
Epigenetics	High-resolution methylation profiling	Bisulfite sequencing	GW	+
Genomics	mRNA expression analysis	Oligonucleotide microarray	GW	+++
	Splice variant profiling	Oligonucleotide microarray	GW	+
Proteomics	Identification of proteins in complex mixtures	MALDI-MS, two-hybrid screening, immunoaffinity chromatography, mass spectrometry, protein binding microarray and antibody microarray, FACS profiling		+
	Protein–protein interaction profiling			
	Protein expression measurement			
Glycomics	Profiling of carbohydrates	Oligosaccharide and glycan arrays		–/+
Lipidomics	Profiling of lipids	Electrospray ionization, mass spectrometry, and liquid chromatography		–/+
Metabolomics	Small-molecule metabolite profiling	Mass spectrometry, NMR spectroscopy		++
Interactomics	Computational integration of interactions of all molecules	Systems biology and bioinformatic approaches		n
Regulomics	Computational integration of transcriptional and translational regulation of genes	Systems biology and bioinformatic approaches		n

CNP, copy number polymorphism; CNV, copy number variation; FACS, flow cytometry–based immunophenotyping; GW, genome-wide association screening is possible; MALDI-MS, matrix-assisted laser desorption/ionization mass spectrometry; mRNA, messenger RNA; n, necessitates the validation of each integrated approach as well as the development of suitable analysis strategies; NMR, nuclear magnetic resonance; SNP, single nucleotide polymorphism.

Genetic studies of complex diseases currently are witnessing major advances, which are based on platforms that enable researchers to study a large fraction of all single nucleotide polymorphisms, or SNPs (pronounced "snips"). SNPs are DNA sequence variations that occur when a single nucleotide in the genome sequence is altered. These polymorphisms make up about 90% of all human genetic variation and occur on average every 100 to 300 bases along the 3-billion-base human genome. SNPs are evolutionarily stable; they do not change much from generation to generation. This makes them useful for association studies relating genetic variation to disease. Because of their frequency and stability, SNPs are thought to be more informative than conventional methods in identifying risk-conferring genes in complex diseases such as MS. Commercial platforms with ever-increasing numbers of SNPs are commonly used and now comprise more than 500,000 SNPs covering 75% of the human genome. The first novel risk alleles for MS outside the MHC region, such as the interleukin-2 receptor alpha gene (*IL2RA*) and the interleukin-7 receptor alpha gene (*IL7RA*), were recently identified.[173] Showing odds ratios of 1.1 to 1.3, these risk alleles seem to confer only a moderate risk. However, it is expected that up to 20 novel low-risk alleles will be described in the near future, which together may confer a substantial risk for development of MS.

The HapMap project and the 1000 Genomes project represent international research efforts to establish a detailed catalog of human genetic variations. This information is crucial to develop novel more powerful SNP microarray platforms. In the end, rapid advancements in high-throughput sequencing, such as pyrosequencing, may allow researchers and consortia to analyze complete genomes of large populations and to increase the resolution of whole-genome association studies to highest fidelity. Compared with other SNP genotyping methods, sequencing is particularly suited to the identification of multiple SNPs in a small region (e.g., the highly polymorphic MHC region). Analysis of the genomic sequence is complicated by losses of large chunks of DNA sequence, varying from 10,000 to 5 million letters, that include genes. The contribution of allelic copy-number variation (CNV), including common copy-number polymorphisms (CNPs), to complex multifactorial diseases such as MS is unknown to date. The known role of CNVs in sporadic genomic disorders, combined with emerging information about inherited CNV, indicate the importance of systematically assessing CNVs and CNPs in complex diseases. This goal calls for high-resolution maps of common CNPs and techniques that accurately determine the allelic state of affected individuals. A related discipline, pharmacogenetics, encompasses the role of genes in an individual's response to drugs.

Genomics is a term that refers to the study of gene expression profiles generated from DNA oligonucleotide microarrays, which now cover all known genes. Gene expression patterns as a whole are already utilized in classification and predictive models to differentiate among tumors that appear to be common histologically and might be useful in the study of disease heterogeneity in MS. It has now become possible to assess systematically the splice variant profiles of all genes, but still these techniques require further refinement and validation. The ever-increasing description of new classes of noncoding RNA molecules that regulate the translation of gene transcripts (e.g., micro-RNA molecules) sets new dimensions to the regulome of the cell, which represents the complement of transcriptional and translational regulation of genes. In addition, novel insights into the dynamics of epigenetic regulation, which modulates the transcriptional activity of large chromosomal regions by methylation of DNA as well as by acetylation, methylation, and ubiquitination of histones, make the picture more complex, and epigenetic regulation patterns may also vary between healthy and diseased individuals.

Proteomic technologies attempt to separate, identify, and characterize a global set of proteins in an effort to provide information about protein abundance, location, and modification as well as protein–protein interactions. The proteome, unlike the fixed genome of the cell, possesses an even higher complexity and is in a constant state of flux. The benefit of protein analysis is its ability to take into account post-translational modifications, which can markedly alter the function and activity of a protein. Novel mass spectrometry–based technologies in particular, such as surface-enhanced laser desorption/ionization time-of-flight mass spectrometry (SELDI-ToF-MS), are available for the high-throughput analysis of complex protein samples and have shown promising results in the recent literature. Proteins unique to three major types of MS lesions (acute plaque, chronic active plaque, and chronic plaque) were identified by laser-capture microdissection and mass spectrometry techniques, illuminating potential therapeutic targets selective for specific pathologic stages of MS.[174] It is foreseeable that such proteomic analyses will be extended to CSF and blood screenings for biomarkers, but proteomic techniques still require advancement.

Metabolomics is a new discipline that intends to assay the full panel of small-molecule, nonprotein metabolites such as fatty acids, amino acids, and nucleosides present in a biologic sample. *Glycomics* and *lipidomics*, representing studies of the entirety of carbohydrates and lipid molecules in a sample, are expected to complete the picture of *interactomics*—the complement of interactions of all molecules in and outside the cell.

We strongly believe that technological and analytic advancements in the various imaging methods as well as the "-omic" methodologies and their integration and correlation with clinical profiles are crucial for the identification of novel biomarkers regardless of their relation to diagnosis, prognosis, or treatment response. Two technologies, genome-wide association studies based on SNP mapping (genetics) and genomics, have reached a level of commercial availability, high standardization, and good reliability. Other technologies, such as proteomics, are far from standardization. Still, all technologies heavily depend on the quality of electronic data banks, where information about the fine mapping of the human genome or of intracellular and extracellular signaling pathways is deposited. "Integrative functional informatics" will be needed for the interfacing and integration of different technologies. However, great emphasis must be placed on the need for development of rigorous standards and quality control procedures in sample acquisition, preparation, and storage; the preanalytic and analytic phases; and subsequent bioinformatics applied to analysis of the data. It is desirable to establish common standard operating procedures for all processes, including characterization and selection of patients to be studied, standardization of withdrawal and sampling of specimens, and biostatistical analysis of the results. Likewise, validation of the significance of any candidate biomarker in carefully designed, prospective, multicenter studies remains mandatory.

Concluding Remarks

In our summary of biomarkers in MS, the reader will note the discrepancy between the stressed urgency to develop and validate biomarkers on the one hand and the obvious lack of established biomarkers for any of the multitude of biologic processes that appear to be involved in MS on the other. This may at first glance be surprising, but, after considering the many reasons for this rather disappointing situation, one quickly realizes the main factors. The search for biomarkers often follows the latest trends of research, which offer quick rewards, rather than long-lasting efforts in the development of assay methodologies, confirmation and validation of findings, and correlation of clinical or imaging outcomes with a biologic marker. Furthermore, few centers, if any, follow patient cohorts that are of sufficient size and cover all clinical aspects of MS, and those that do often lack a strong laboratory with experience in immunology and/or neurobiology. Nevertheless, there is no doubt that a number of important questions in MS research and clinical care depend on the identification of suitable biomarkers. The development of combination therapies and the early identification of treatment responders and nonresponders are just two of the issues that need to be addressed. To conclude on a more optimistic note, it is only very recently that the tools have become available to address the complexities of a disease such as MS, and accepted biomarkers have already been identified in fields with much higher patient numbers and more robust clinical outcomes (e.g., cancer research). It is no question that similar paths will be followed in MS, and a number of U.S. and European initiatives[175] are currently underway in that direction. We expect, therefore, that the current situation will change in the next 10 years and that biomarkers will become an important aspect of research and treatment of MS.

REFERENCES

1. Sospedra M, Martin R: Immunology of multiple sclerosis. Ann Rev Immunol 2005;23:683-747.
2. Lepper ER, Nooter K, Verweij J, et al: Mechanisms of resistance to anticancer drugs: The role of the polymorphic ABC transporters ABCB1 and ABCG2. Pharmacogenomics 2005;6:115-138.
3. van Baarsen LG, Vosslamber S, Tijssen M, et al: Pharmacogenomics of interferon-beta therapy in multiple sclerosis: Baseline IFN signature determines pharmacological differences between patients. PLoS ONE 2008;3:e1927.
4. Bielekova B, Martin R: Development of biomarkers in multiple sclerosis. Brain 2004;127:1463-1478.
5. Biomarkers Definitions Working Group: Biomarkers and surrogate endpoints: Preferred definitions and conceptual framework. Clin Pharmacol Ther 2001;69:89-95.
6. Miller DH: Biomarkers and surrogate outcomes in neurodegenerative disease: Lessons from multiple sclerosis. NeuroRx 2004;1:284-294.
7. Bakshi R, Thompson AJ, Rocca MA, et al: MRI in multiple sclerosis: Current status and future prospects. Lancet Neurol 2008;7:615-625.
8. Polman CH, Reingold SC, Edan G, et al: Diagnostic criteria for multiple sclerosis: 2005 Revisions to the "McDonald Criteria." Ann Neurol 2005;58:840-846.
9. Kabat EA, Glusman M, Knaub V: Quantitative estimation of the albumin and gamma globulin in normal and pathologic cerebrospinal fluid by immunochemical methods. Am J Med 1948;4:653-659.
10. Wilske B, Schierz G, Preac-Mursic V, et al: Intrathecal production of specific antibodies against *Borrelia burgdorferi* in patients with lymphocytic meningoradiculitis (Bannwarth's syndrome). J Infect Dis 1986;153:304-314.

11. Porter KG, Sinnamon DG, Gillies RR: *Cryptococcus neoformans*-specific oligoclonal immunoglobulins in cerebrospinal fluid in cryptococcal meningitis. Lancet 1977;1:1262.
12. Vandvik B, Norrby E, Nordal HJ, Degre M: Oligoclonal measles virus-specific IgG antibodies isolated from cerebrospinal fluids, brain extracts, and sera from patients with subacute sclerosing panencephalitis and multiple sclerosis. Scand J Immunol 1976;5:979-992.
13. Vartdal F, Vandvik B, Michaelsen TE, et al: Neurosyphilis: Intrathecal synthesis of oligoclonal antibodies to *Treponema pallidum*. Ann Neurol 1982;11:35-40.
14. Bourahoui A, De Seze J, Guttierez R, et al: CSF isoelectrofocusing in a large cohort of MS and other neurological diseases. Eur J Neurol 2004;11:525-529.
15. Masjuan J, Alvarez-Cermeño JC, Garcia-Barragán N, et al: Clinically isolated syndromes: A new oligoclonal band test accurately predicts conversion to MS. Neurology 2006;66:576-578.
16. Sharief MK, Keir G, Thompson EJ: Intrathecal synthesis of IgM in neurological diseases: A comparison between detection of oligoclonal bands and quantitative estimation. J Neurol Sci 1990;96:131-142.
17. Lucchinetti C, Brück W, Parisi J, et al: Heterogeneity of multiple sclerosis lesions: Implications for the pathogenesis of demyelination. Ann Neurol 2000;47:707-717.
18. Lucchinetti CF, Mandler RN, McGavern D, et al: A role for humoral mechanisms in the pathogenesis of Devic's neuromyelitis optica. Brain 2002;125:1450-1461.
19. Villar LM, Sádaba MC, Roldán, et al: Intrathecal synthesis of oligoclonal IgM against myelin lipids predicts an aggressive disease course in MS. J Clin Invest 2005;115:187-194.
20. Perini P, Ranzato F, Calabrese M, et al: Intrathecal IgM production at clinical onset correlates with a more severe disease course in multiple sclerosis. J Neurol Neurosurg Psychiatry 2006;77:953-955.
21. Villar LM, Masjuan J, González-Porqué P, et al: Intrathecal IgM synthesis is a prognostic factor in multiple sclerosis. Ann Neurol 2003;53:222-226.
22. Schneider R, Euler B, Rauer S: Intrathecal IgM-synthesis does not correlate with the risk of relapse in patients with a primary demyelinating event. Eur J Neurol 2007;14:907-911.
23. Villar L, García-Barragán N, Espiño M, et al: Influence of oligoclonal IgM specificity in multiple sclerosis disease course. Mult Scler 2008;14:183-187.
24. Koch M, Heersema D, Mostert J, et al: Cerebrospinal fluid oligoclonal bands and progression of disability in multiple sclerosis. Eur J Neurol 2007;14:797-800.
25. Berger T, Rubner P, Schautzer F, et al: Antimyelin antibodies as a predictor of clinically definite multiple sclerosis after a first demyelinating event. N Engl J Med 2003;349:139-145.
26. Tomassini V, De Giglio L, Reindl M, et al: Anti-myelin antibodies predict the clinical outcome after a first episode suggestive of MS. Mult Scler 2007;13:1086-1094.
27. Greeve I, Sellner J, Lauterburg T, et al: Anti-myelin antibodies in clinically isolated syndrome indicate the risk of multiple sclerosis in a Swiss cohort. Acta Neurol Scand 2007;116: 207-210.
28. Kuhle J, Lindberg RL, Regeniter A, et al: Antimyelin antibodies in clinically isolated syndromes correlate with inflammation in MRI and CSF. J Neurol 2007;254:160-168.
29. Rauer S, Euler B, Reindl M, Berger T: Antimyelin antibodies and the risk of relapse in patients with a primary demyelinating event. J Neurol Neurosurg Psychiatry 2006;77:739-742.
30. Kuhle J, Pohl C, Mehling M, et al: Lack of association between antimyelin antibodies and progression to multiple sclerosis. N Engl J Med 2007;356:371-378.
31. Lim ET, Berger T, Reindl M, et al: Anti-myelin antibodies do not allow earlier diagnosis of multiple sclerosis. Mult Scler 2005;11:492-494.
32. Pelayo R, Tintoré M, Montalban X, et al: Antimyelin antibodies with no progression to multiple sclerosis. N Engl J Med 2007;356:426-428.
33. Reindl M, Khalil M, Berger T: Antibodies as biological markers for pathophysiological processes in MS. J Neuroimmunol 2006;180:50-62.
34. Lalive PH, Menge T, Delarasse C, et al: Antibodies to native myelin oligodendrocyte glycoprotein are serologic markers of early inflammation in multiple sclerosis. Proc Natl Acad Sci U S A 2006;103:2280-2285.
35. Zhou D, Srivastava R, Nessler S, et al: Identification of a pathogenic antibody response to native myelin oligodendrocyte glycoprotein in multiple sclerosis. Proc Natl Acad Sci U S A 2006;103:19057-19062.
36. O'Connor KC, McLaughlin KA, De Jager PL, et al: Self-antigen tetramers discriminate between myelin autoantibodies to native or denatured protein. Nat Med 2007;13:211-217.
37. Lolli F, Mazzanti B, Pazzagli M, et al: The glycopeptide CSF114(Glc) detects serum antibodies in multiple sclerosis. J Neuroimmunol 2005;167:131-137.

38. Mathey EK, Derfuss T, Storh MK, et al: Neurofascin as a novel target for autoantibody-mediated axonal injury. J Exp Med 2007;204:2363-2372.
39. Giovannoni G, Cutter GR, Lünemann J, et al: Infectious causes of multiple sclerosis. Lancet Neurol 2006;5:887-894.
40. Cepok S, Zhou D, Srivastava R, et al: Identification of Epstein-Barr virus proteins as putative targets of the immune response in multiple sclerosis. J Clin Invest 2005;115:1352-1360.
41. Sundström P, Juto P, Wadell G, et al: An altered immune response to Epstein-Barr virus in multiple sclerosis: A prospective study. Neurology 2004;62:2277-2282.
42. Levin LI, Munger KL, Rubertone MV, et al: Temporal relationship between elevation of epstein-barr virus antibody titers and initial onset of neurological symptoms in multiple sclerosis. JAMA 2005;293:2496-2500.
43. DeLorenze GN, Munger KL, Lennette ET, et al: Epstein-Barr virus and multiple sclerosis: Evidence of association from a prospective study with long-term follow-up. Arch Neurol 2006;63:839-844.
44. Thacker EL, Mirzaei F, Ascherio A: Infectious mononucleosis and risk for multiple sclerosis: A meta-analysis. Ann Neurol 2006;59:499-503.
45. Nielsen TR, Rostgaard K, Nielsen NM, et al: Multiple sclerosis after infectious mononucleosis. Arch Neurol 2007;64:72-75.
46. Hernan MA, Zhang SM, Lipworth L, et al: Multiple sclerosis and age at infection with common viruses. Epidemiology 2001;12:301-306.
47. De Jager PL, Simon KC, Munter KL, et al: Integrating risk factors: HLA-DRB1*1501 and Epstein-Barr virus in multiple sclerosis. Neurology 2008;70:1113-1118.
48. Buljevac D, van Doornum GJ, Flach HZ, et al: Epstein-Barr virus and disease activity in multiple sclerosis. J Neurol Neurosurg Psychiatry 2005;76:1377-1381.
49. Wandinger K, Jabs, Siekhaus A, et al: Association between clinical disease activity and Epstein-Barr virus reactivation in MS. Neurology 2000;55:178-184.
50. Lünemann JD, Edward N, Muraro PA, et al: Increased frequency and broadened specificity of latent EBV nuclear antigen-1-specific T cells in multiple sclerosis. Brain 2006;129:1493-1506.
51. Lünemann JD, Jelčić I, Roberts S, et al: EBNA1-specific T cells from patients with multiple sclerosis cross react with myelin antigens and co-produce IFN-gamma and IL-2. J Exp Med 2008;205:1763-1773.
52. Serafini B, Rosicarelli B, Franciotta D, et al: Dysregulated Epstein-Barr virus infection in the multiple sclerosis brain. J Exp Med 2007;204:2899-2912.
53. Lennon VA, Wingerchuk DM, Kryzer TJ, et al: A serum autoantibody marker of neuromyelitis optica: Distinction from multiple sclerosis. Lancet 2004;364:2106-2112.
54. Weinshenker BG, Wingerchuk DM, Vukusic S, et al: Neuromyelitis optica IgG predicts relapse after longitudinally extensive transverse myelitis. Ann Neurol 2006;59:566-569.
55. Wingerchuk DM, Lennon VA, Pittock SJ, et al: Revised diagnostic criteria for neuromyelitis optica. Neurology 2006;66:1485-1489.
56. Lennon VA, Kryzer TJ, Pittock SJ, et al: IgG marker of optic-spinal multiple sclerosis binds to the aquaporin-4 water channel. J Exp Med 2005;202:473-477.
57. Misu T, Fujihara K, Kakita A, et al: Loss of aquaporin 4 in lesions of neuromyelitis optica: Distinction from multiple sclerosis. Brain 2007;130:1224-1234.
58. Roemer SF, Parisi JE, Lennon VA, et al: Pattern-specific loss of aquaporin-4 immunoreactivity distinguishes neuromyelitis optica from multiple sclerosis. Brain 2007;130:1194-1205.
59. Jarius S, Franciotta D, Bergamaschi R, et al: NMO-IgG in the diagnosis of neuromyelitis optica. Neurology 2007;68:1076-1077.
60. Matsuoka T, Matsushita T, Kawano Y, et al: Heterogeneity of aquaporin-4 autoimmunity and spinal cord lesions in multiple sclerosis in Japanese. Brain 2007;130:1206-1223.
61. Paul F, Jarius S, Aktas O, et al: Antibody to aquaporin 4 in the diagnosis of neuromyelitis optica. PLoS Med 2007;4: e133.
62. Takahashi T, Fujihara K, Nakashima I, et al: Anti-aquaporin-4 antibody is involved in the pathogenesis of NMO: A study on antibody titre. Brain 2007;130:1235-1243.
63. Keegan M, Pineda AA, McClelland RL, et al: Plasma exchange for severe attacks of CNS demyelination: Predictors of response. Neurology 2002;58:143-146.
64. Cree BA, Lamb S, Morgan K, et al: An open label study of the effects of rituximab in neuromyelitis optica. Neurology 2005;64:1270-1272.
65. Link H: The cytokine storm in multiple sclerosis. Mult Scler 1998;4:12-15.
66. Kebir H, Kreymborg K, Ifergan I, et al: Human TH17 lymphocytes promote blood-brain barrier disruption and central nervous system inflammation. Nat Med 2007;13:1173-1175.

67. Hedegaard CJ, Krakauer M, Bendtzen K, et al: T helper cell type 1 (Th1), Th2 and Th17 responses to myelin basic protein and disease activity in multiple sclerosis. Immunology 2008;125: 161-169.
68. Balashov KE, Smith DR, Khoury SJ, et al: Increased interleukin 12 production in progressive multiple sclerosis: Induction by activated CD4+ T cells via CD40 ligand. Proc Natl Acad Sci U S A 1997;94:599-603.
69. Comabella M, Balashov K, Issazadeh S, et al: Elevated interleukin-12 in progressive multiple sclerosis correlates with disease activity and is normalized by pulse cyclophosphamide therapy. J Clin Invest 1998;102:671-678.
70. Filion LG, Matusevicius D, Graziani-Bowering GM, et al: Monocyte-derived IL12, CD86 (B7-2) and CD40L expression in relapsing and progressive multiple sclerosis. Clin Immunol 2003;106:127-138.
71. Sorensen TL, Tani M, Jensen J, et al: Expression of specific chemokines and chemokine receptors in the central nervous system of multiple sclerosis patients. J Clin Invest 1999;103:807-815.
72. Balashov KE, Rottman JB, Weiner HL, Hancock WW: CCR5(+) and CXCR3(+) T cells are increased in multiple sclerosis and their ligands MIP-1alpha and IP-10 are expressed in demyelinating brain lesions. Proc Natl Acad Sci U S A 1999;96:6873-6878.
73. Strunk T, Bubel S, Mascher B, et al: Increased numbers of CCR5+ interferon-gamma- and tumor necrosis factor-alpha-secreting T lymphocytes in multiple sclerosis patients. Ann Neurol 2000;47:269-273.
74. Sorensen TL, Trebst C, Kivisäkk P, et al: Multiple sclerosis: A study of CXCL10 and CXCR3 co-localization in the inflamed central nervous system. J Neuroimmunol 2002;127:59-68.
75. Trebst C, Sørensen TL, Kivisäkk P, et al: CCR1+/CCR5+ mononuclear phagocytes accumulate in the central nervous system of patients with multiple sclerosis. Am J Pathol 2001;159:1701-1710.
76. Trebst C, Ransohoff RM: Investigating chemokines and chemokine receptors in patients with multiple sclerosis: Opportunities and challenges. Arch Neurol 2001;58:1975-1980.
77. Sindern E, Patzold T, Ossege LM, et al: Expression of chemokine receptor CXCR3 on cerebrospinal fluid T-cells is related to active MRI lesion appearance in patients with relapsing-remitting multiple sclerosis. J Neuroimmunol 2002;131:186-190.
78. Kuenz B, Lutterotti A, Ehling R, et al: Cerebrospinal fluid B cells correlate with early brain inflammation in multiple sclerosis. PLoS ONE 2008;3:e2559.
79. Meinl E, Krumbholz M, Hohlfeld R: B lineage cells in the inflammatory central nervous system environment: Migration, maintenance, local antibody production, and therapeutic modulation. Ann Neurol 2006;59:880-892.
80. Cepok S, Rosche B, Grummel V, et al: Short-lived plasma blasts are the main B cell effector subset during the course of multiple sclerosis. Brain 2005;128:1667-1676.
81. Keegan M, König F, McClelland R, et al: Relation between humoral pathological changes in multiple sclerosis and response to therapeutic plasma exchange. Lancet 2005;366:579-582.
82. Bielekova B, Richert N, Howard T, et al: Humanized anti-CD25 (daclizumab) inhibits disease activity in multiple sclerosis patients failing to respond to interferon beta. Proc Natl Acad Sci U S A 2004;101:8705-8708.
83. Bielekova B, Catalfamo M, Reichert-Scrivner S, et al: Regulatory CD56(bright) natural killer cells mediate immunomodulatory effects of IL-2Ralpha-targeted therapy (daclizumab) in multiple sclerosis. Proc Natl Acad Sci U S A 2006;103:5941-5946.
84. De Jager PL, Rossin E, Pyne S, et al: Cytometric profiling in multiple sclerosis uncovers patient population structure and a reduction of CD8low cells. Brain 2008;131(Pt 7):1701-1711.
85. Airas L, Saraste M, Rinta S, et al: Immunoregulatory factors in multiple sclerosis patients during and after pregnancy: Relevance of natural killer cells. Clin Exp Immunol 2008;151:235-243.
86. Saraste M, Irjala H, Airas L: Expansion of CD56Bright natural killer cells in the peripheral blood of multiple sclerosis patients treated with interferon-beta. Neurol Sci 2007;28:121-126.
87. Infante-Duarte C, Weber A, Krätzschmar J, et al: Frequency of blood CX3CR1-positive natural killer cells correlates with disease activity in multiple sclerosis patients. FASEB J 2005;19:1902-1904.
88. Lassmann H, Reindl M, Rauschka H, et al: A new paraclinical CSF marker for hypoxia-like tissue damage in multiple sclerosis lesions. Brain 2003;126:1347-1357.
89. Aboul-Enein F, Lassmann H: Mitochondrial damage and histotoxic hypoxia: A pathway of tissue injury in inflammatory brain disease? Acta Neuropathol 2005;109:49-55.
90. Lu F, Selak M, O'Connor J, et al: Oxidative damage to mitochondrial DNA and activity of mitochondrial enzymes in chronic active lesions of multiple sclerosis. J Neurol Sci 2000;177:95-103.

91. Beltran B, Orsi A, Clementi E, Moncada S: Oxidative stress and S-nitrosylation of proteins in cells. Br J Pharmacol 2000;129:953-960.
92. Smith KJ, Lassmann H: The role of nitric oxide in multiple sclerosis. Lancet Neurol 2002;1:232-241.
93. Giovannoni G: Cerebrospinal fluid and serum nitric oxide metabolites in patients with multiple sclerosis. Mult Scler 1998;4:27-30.
94. Giovannoni G, Silver NC, O'Riordan J, et al: Increased urinary nitric oxide metabolites in patients with multiple sclerosis correlates with early and relapsing disease. Mult Scler 1999;5:335-341.
95. Rejdak K, Eikelenboom MJ, Petzold A, et al: CSF nitric oxide metabolites are associated with activity and progression of multiple sclerosis. Neurology 2004;63:1439-1445.
96. Yuceyar N, Taskiran D, Sagduyu A: Serum and cerebrospinal fluid nitrite and nitrate levels in relapsing-remitting and secondary progressive multiple sclerosis patients. Clin Neurol Neurosurg 2001;103:206-211.
97. Johnson AW, Land JM, Thompson EJ, et al: Evidence for increased nitric oxide production in multiple sclerosis. J Neurol Neurosurg Psychiatry 1995;58:107.
98. Rejdak K, Petzold A, Stelmasiak Z, Giovannoni G: Cerebrospinal fluid brain specific proteins in relation to nitric oxide metabolites during relapse of multiple sclerosis. Mult Scler 2008;14:59-66.
99. Diestel A, Aktas O, Hackel D, et al: Activation of microglial poly(ADP-ribose)-polymerase-1 by cholesterol breakdown products during neuroinflammation: A link between demyelination and neuronal damage. J Exp Med 2003;198:1729-1740.
100. Pitt D, Werner P, Raine CS: Glutamate excitotoxicity in a model of multiple sclerosis. Nat Med 2000;6:67-70.
101. Werner P, Pitt D, Raine CS: Multiple sclerosis: Altered glutamate homeostasis in lesions correlates with oligodendrocyte and axonal damage. Ann Neurol 2001;50:169-180.
102. Killestein J, Kalkers NF, Polman CH: Glutamate inhibition in MS: The neuroprotective properties of riluzole. J Neurol Sci 2005;233:113-115.
103. Filaci G, Contini P, Brenci S, et al: Soluble HLA class I and class II molecule levels in serum and cerebrospinal fluid of multiple sclerosis patients. Hum Immunol 1997;54:54-62.
104. Minagar A, Adamashvilli I, Jaffe SL, et al: Soluble HLA class I and class II molecules in relapsing-remitting multiple sclerosis: Acute response to interferon-beta1a treatment and their use as markers of disease activity. Ann N Y Acad Sci 2005;1051:111-120.
105. Carosella ED, Moreau P, Aractingi S, Rouas-Freiss N: HLA-G: A shield against inflammatory aggression. Trends Immunol 2001;22:553-555.
106. Wiendl H, Feger U, Mittelbronn M, et al: Expression of the immune-tolerogenic major histocompatibility molecule HLA-G in multiple sclerosis: Implications for CNS immunity. Brain 2005;128:2689-2704.
107. Fainardi E, Rizzo R, Melchiorri L, et al: Intrathecal synthesis of soluble HLA-G and HLA-I molecules are reciprocally associated to clinical and MRI activity in patients with multiple sclerosis. Mult Scler 2006;12:2-12.
108. Fainardi E, Rizzo R, Melchiorri L, et al: CSF levels of soluble HLA-G and Fas molecules are inversely associated to MRI evidence of disease activity in patients with relapsing remitting multiple sclerosis. Mult Scler 2008;14:446-454.
109. Devitt A, Moffatt OD, Raykundalia C, et al: Human CD14 mediates recognition and phagocytosis of apoptotic cells. Nature 1998;392:505-509.
110. Schlegel RA, Krahling S, Callahan MK, Williamson P: CD14 is a component of multiple recognition systems used by macrophages to phagocytose apoptotic lymphocytes. Cell Death Differ 1999;6:583-592.
111. Egerer K, Feist E, Rohr U, et al: Increased serum soluble CD14, ICAM-1 and E-selectin correlate with disease activity and prognosis in systemic lupus erythematosus. Lupus 2000;9:614-621.
112. Nockher WA, Wigand R, Schoeppe W, Scherberich JE: Elevated levels of soluble CD14 in serum of patients with systemic lupus erythematosus. Clin Exp Immunol 1994;96:15-19.
113. Takeshita S, Nakatani K, Tsujimoto H, et al: Increased levels of circulating soluble CD14 in Kawasaki disease. Clin Exp Immunol 2000;119:376-381.
114. Wuthrich B, Kagi MK, Joller-Jemelka H: Soluble CD14 but not interleukin-6 is a new marker for clinical activity in atopic dermatitis. Arch Dermatol Res 1992;284:339-342.
115. Yu S, Nakashima N, Xu BH, et al: Pathological significance of elevated soluble CD14 production in rheumatoid arthritis: In the presence of soluble CD14, lipopolysaccharides at low concentrations activate RA synovial fibroblasts. Rheumatol Int 1998;17:237-243.
116. Brettschneider J, Ecker D, Bitsch A, et al: The macrophage activity marker sCD14 is increased in patients with multiple sclerosis and upregulated by interferon beta-1b. J Neuroimmunol 2002;133:193-197.

117. Bas S, Gauthier BR, Spenato U, et al: CD14 is an acute-phase protein. J Immunol 2004;172: 4470-4479.
118. Lutterotti A, Kuenz B, Gredler V, et al: Increased serum levels of soluble CD14 indicate stable multiple sclerosis. J Neuroimmunol 2006;181:145-149.
119. Minagar A, Alexander JS: Blood-brain barrier disruption in multiple sclerosis. Mult Scler 2003;9:540-549.
120. Hartung HP, Reiners K, Archelos JJ, et al: Circulating adhesion molecules and tumor necrosis factor receptor in multiple sclerosis: Correlation with magnetic resonance imaging. Ann Neurol 1995;38:186-193.
121. Kuenz B, Lutterotti A, Khalil M, et al: Plasma levels of soluble adhesion molecules sPECAM-1, sP-selectin and sE-selectin are associated with relapsing-remitting disease course of multiple sclerosis. J Neuroimmunol 2005;167:143-149.
122. Minagar A, Jy W, Jimenez JJ, et al: Elevated plasma endothelial microparticles in multiple sclerosis. Neurology 2001;56:1319-1324.
123. Acar G, Idiman F, Kirkali G, et al: Intrathecal sICAM-1 production in multiple sclerosis: Correlation with triple dose Gd-DTPA MRI enhancement and IgG index. J Neurol 2005;252:146-150.
124. Calabresi PA, Tranquill LR, Dambrosia JM, et al: Increases in soluble VCAM-1 correlate with a decrease in MRI lesions in multiple sclerosis treated with interferon beta-1b. Ann Neurol 1997;41:669-674.
125. Rieckmann P, Kruse N, Nagelkerken L, et al: Soluble vascular cell adhesion molecule (VCAM) is associated with treatment effects of interferon beta-1b in patients with secondary progressive multiple sclerosis. J Neurol 2005;252:526-533.
126. Soilu-Hanninen M, Laaksonen M, Hanninen A, et al: Downregulation of VLA-4 on T cells as a marker of long term treatment response to interferon beta-1a in MS. J Neuroimmunol 2005;167:175-182.
127. Soilu-Hanninen M, Laaksonen M, Hanninen A: Hyaluronate receptor (CD44) and integrin alpha4 (CD49d) are up-regulated on T cells during MS relapses. J Neuroimmunol 2005;166:189-192.
128. Calabresi PA, Pelfrey CM, Tranquill LR, et al: VLA-4 expression on peripheral blood lymphocytes is downregulated after treatment of multiple sclerosis with interferon beta. Neurology 1997;49:1111-1116.
129. Muraro PA, Leist T, Bielekova B, McFarland HF: VLA-4/CD49d downregulated on primed T lymphocytes during interferon-beta therapy in multiple sclerosis. J Neuroimmunol 2000;111: 186-194.
130. Fainardi E, Castellazzi M, Bellini T, et al: Cerebrospinal fluid and serum levels and intrathecal production of active matrix metalloproteinase-9 (MMP-9) as markers of disease activity in patients with multiple sclerosis. Mult Scler 2006;12:294-301.
131. Waubant E, Goodkin D, Bostrom A, et al: IFNbeta lowers MMP-9/TIMP-1 ratio, which predicts new enhancing lesions in patients with SPMS. Neurology 2003;60:52-57.
132. Blevins G, Sung MH, Zhao Y, Campbell C, Bielekova B, McFarland HF, Martin R: Gene expression of heat shock proteins and molecules involved in apoptosis regulation differentiates multiple sclerosis patients from healthy controls. In preparation 2009.
133. Waiczies S, Weber A, Lünemann JD, et al: Elevated Bcl-X(L) levels correlate with T cell survival in multiple sclerosis. J Neuroimmunol 2002;126:213-220.
134. Sharief MK, Matthews H, Noori MA: Expression ratios of the Bcl-2 family proteins and disease activity in multiple sclerosis. J Neuroimmunol 2003;134:158-165.
135. Zipp F, Weller M, Calabresi PA, et al: Increased serum levels of soluble CD95 (APO-1/Fas) in relapsing-remitting multiple sclerosis. Ann Neurol 1998;43:116-120.
136. Gomes AC, Jönsson G, Mjörnheim S, et al: Upregulation of the apoptosis regulators cFLIP, CD95 and CD95 ligand in peripheral blood mononuclear cells in relapsing-remitting multiple sclerosis. J Neuroimmunol 2003;135:126-134.
137. Mahovic D, Petravic D, Petelin Z, et al: Level of sFas/APO 1 in serum and cerebrospinal fluid in multiple sclerosis. Clin Neurol Neurosurg 2004;106:230-232.
138. Huang WX, Huang MP, Gomes MA, Hillert J: Apoptosis mediators fasL and TRAIL are upregulated in peripheral blood mononuclear cells in MS. Neurology 2000;55:928-934.
139. Wandinger KP, Lünemann JD, Wengert O, et al: TNF-related apoptosis inducing ligand (TRAIL) as a potential response marker for interferon-beta treatment in multiple sclerosis. Lancet 2003;361:2036-2043.
140. Leoni V, Masterman T, Diczfalusy U, et al: Changes in human plasma levels of the brain specific oxysterol 24S-hydroxycholesterol during progression of multiple sclerosis. Neurosci Lett 2002;331:163-166.

141. Teunissen CE, Dijkstra CD, Polman CH, et al: Decreased levels of the brain specific 24S-hydroxycholesterol and cholesterol precursors in serum of multiple sclerosis patients. Neurosci Lett 2003;347:159-162.
142. Fuchs E, Cleveland DW: A structural scaffolding of intermediate filaments in health and disease. Science 1998;279:514-519.
143. Teunissen CE, Dijkstra C, Polman C: Biological markers in CSF and blood for axonal degeneration in multiple sclerosis. Lancet Neurol 2005;4:32-41.
144. Lycke JN, Karlsson JE, Andersen O, Rosengren LE: Neurofilament protein in cerebrospinal fluid: A potential marker of activity in multiple sclerosis. J Neurol Neurosurg Psychiatry 1998;64:402-404.
145. Malmestrom C, Haghighi S, Rosengren L, et al: Neurofilament light protein and glial fibrillary acidic protein as biological markers in MS. Neurology 2003;61:1720-1725.
146. Ehling R, Lutterotti A, Wanschitz J, et al: Increased frequencies of serum antibodies to neurofilament light in patients with primary chronic progressive multiple sclerosis. Mult Scler 2004;10:601-606.
147. Eikelenboom MJ, Petzold A, Lazeron RH, et al: Multiple sclerosis: Neurofilament light chain antibodies are correlated to cerebral atrophy. Neurology 2003;60:219-223.
148. Silber E, Semra YK, Gregson NA, Sharief MK: Patients with progressive multiple sclerosis have elevated antibodies to neurofilament subunit. Neurology 2002;58:1372-1381.
149. Petzold A, Eikelenboom MJ, Gveric D, et al: Markers for different glial cell responses in multiple sclerosis: Clinical and pathological correlations. Brain 2002;125:1462-1473.
150. Giovannoni G: Multiple sclerosis cerebrospinal fluid biomarkers. Dis Markers 2006;22:187-196.
151. Norgren N, Sundström P, Svenningsson A, et al: Neurofilament and glial fibrillary acidic protein in multiple sclerosis. Neurology 2004;63:1586-1590.
152. Rosengren LE, Lycke J, Andersen O: Glial fibrillary acidic protein in CSF of multiple sclerosis patients: Relation to neurological deficit. J Neurol Sci 1995;133:61-65.
153. Malmestrom C, Haghighi S, Rosengren L, et al: Neurofilament light protein and glial fibrillary acidic protein as biological markers in MS. Neurology 2003;61:1720-1725.
154. Reindl M, Khantane S, Ehling R, et al: Serum and cerebrospinal fluid antibodies to Nogo-A in patients with multiple sclerosis and acute neurological disorders. J Neuroimmunol 2003;145:139-147.
155. Jurewicz A, Matysiak M, Raine CS, Selmaj K: Soluble Nogo-A, an inhibitor of axonal regeneration, as a biomarker for multiple sclerosis. Neurology 2007;68:283-287.
156. Lindsey JW, Crawford MP, Hatfield LM: Soluble Nogo-A in CSF is not a useful biomarker for multiple sclerosis. Neurology 2008;71:35-37.
157. Noseworthy JH, Lucchinetti C, Rodriguez M, Weinshenker BG: Multiple sclerosis. N Engl J Med 2000;343:938-952.
158. Rudick RA, Ransohoff RM, Peppler R, et al: Interferon beta induces interleukin-10 expression: Relevance to multiple sclerosis. Ann Neurol 1996;40:618-627.
159. Wandinger KP, Stürzebecher CS, Bielekova B, et al: Complex immunomodulatory effects of interferon-beta in multiple sclerosis include the upregulation of T helper 1-associated marker genes. Ann Neurol 2001;50:349-357.
160. Sturzebecher S, Wandinger KP, Rosenwald A, et al: Expression profiling identifies responder and non-responder phenotypes to interferon-beta in multiple sclerosis. Brain 2003;126:1419-1429.
161. Stone LA, Frank JA, Albert PS, et al: Characterization of MRI response to treatment with interferon beta-1b: Contrast-enhancing MRI lesion frequency as a primary outcome measure. Neurology 1997;49:862-869.
162. Waubant E, Vukusic S, Gignoux L, et al: Clinical characteristics of responders to interferon therapy for relapsing MS. Neurology 2003;61:184-189.
163. Deisenhammer F, Reindl M, Harvey J, et al: Bioavailability of interferon beta 1b in MS patients with and without neutralizing antibodies. Neurology 1999;52:1239-1243.
164. Sorensen PS, Ross C, Clemmesen KM, et al: Clinical importance of neutralising antibodies against interferon beta in patients with relapsing-remitting multiple sclerosis. Lancet 2003;362:1184-1191.
165. Gilli F, Marnetto F, Caldano M, et al: Biological markers of interferon-beta therapy: Comparison among interferon-stimulated genes MxA, TRAIL and XAF-1. Mult Scler 2006;12:47-57.
166. Farina C, Weber MS, Meinl E, et al: Glatiramer acetate in multiple sclerosis: Update on potential mechanisms of action. Lancet Neurol 2005;4:567-575.
167. Wiesemann E, Klatt J, Wenzel C, et al: Correlation of serum IL-13 and IL-5 levels with clinical response to Glatiramer acetate in patients with multiple sclerosis. Clin Exp Immunol 2003;133:454-460.

168. Farina C, Wagenpfeil S, Hohlfeld R: Immunological assay for assessing the efficacy of glatiramer acetate (Copaxone) in multiple sclerosis: A pilot study. J Neurol 2002;249:1587-1592.
169. Hauser SL, Waubant E, Arnold DL, et al: B-cell depletion with rituximab in relapsing-remitting multiple sclerosis. N Engl J Med 2008;358:676-688.
170. Steinman L: Blocking adhesion molecules as therapy for multiple sclerosis: Natalizumab. Nat Rev 2005;4:510-518.
171. U.S. Food and Drug Administration: Information for Healthcare Professionals. FDA Alert: Rituximab (marketed as Rituxan). Dec. 2006. Available at http://www.fda.gov/CDER/Drug/InfoSheets/HCP/rituximab.pdf (accessed October 3, 2008).
172. Berger JR: Progressive multifocal leukoencephalopathy. Curr Neurol Neurosci Rep 2007;7:461-469.
173. International Multiple Sclerosis Genetics Consortium; Hafler DA, Compston A, Sawcer S, et al: Risk alleles for multiple sclerosis identified by a genomewide study. N Engl J Med 2007;357:851-862.
174. Han MH, Hwang SI, Roy DB, et al: Proteomic analysis of active multiple sclerosis lesions reveals therapeutic targets. Nature 2008;451:1076-1081.
175. Martin R, Bielekova B, Hohlfeld R, Utz U: Biomarkers in multiple sclerosis. Dis Markers 2006;22:183-185.

7 Cognitive and Psychiatric Disorders in Multiple Sclerosis

MARIA PIA AMATO • VALENTINA ZIPOLI

Whereas the attention of clinicians has tended to focus on the physical aspects of multiple sclerosis (MS), recognition and treatment of cognitive and psychiatric changes associated with the disease can be equally important in improving quality of life for the patient. Since the early 1980s, the systematic use of formal neuropsychological testing and the advent of magnetic resonance imaging (MRI) to assess possible clinicopathologic relationships have greatly contributed to improving understanding of the prevalence, clinical correlates, and underlying pathology of cognitive and psychiatric disorders in MS. More recently, the search for effective strategies for managing cognitive dysfunction (CD) has led to trials with pharmacologic agents and cognitive rehabilitation.

This chapter provides an overview of the current knowledge and implications for future research in the field.

Cognitive Dysfunction

PREVALENCE AND FUNCTIONAL IMPACT

In MS, CD typically consists of domain-specific deficits rather than global cognitive decline. It may be subtle, particularly in the early phases, and it is characterized by great interpatient variability. Overall, the estimated prevalence rates in the literature range from 43% to 65%, depending on the research setting (clinic-based or community-based studies) and the clinical characteristics of the study sample.[1] CD can have a dramatic impact on several aspects of quality of life, independently of the degree of physical disability, affecting the ability to maintain employment, daily living activities, and social life.[2-4] Cognitive impairment can also limit the capacity of the patient to benefit from inpatient rehabilitation.[5]

NEUROPSYCHOLOGICAL PROFILE

Because of the primary involvement of subcortical white matter, MS-related CD has traditionally been categorized as a "subcortical pattern," as opposed to the "cortical pattern" typical of cortical pathologies of the Alzheimer type. The concept of "subcortical dementia," however, is a controversial one. Moreover, taking into account the differences in neuropsychological profile in comparison with other neurologic diseases, as well as imaging findings that also document deep and cortical gray matter changes,[6] MS seems to be positioned between cortical and subcortical pathologies. The term *multiple disconnection syndrome* has been recently suggested to indicate that different cognitive domains can be interrupted in their afferent or efferent loop, producing a great variety of neuropsychological defects.[6]

Usually, in MS subjects, the intelligent quotient (IQ) is normal or shows only a moderate decline, primarily limited to performance IQ.[1] In general, impaired cognitive performance is more frequently observed on tests that assess complex attention and information-processing speed, verbal and visuospatial memory, and executive functions[1,7]; language, semantic memory, and attention span are rarely involved (Table 7-1). As for memory systems, within the long-term memory, explicit memory (memory for materials that the subject has been explicitly instructed to learn and repeat), and in particular episodic memory (e.g., memory of facts or conversations) are frequently affected. Semantic memory (e.g., memory of words or symbols) as well as implicit memory (learning and remembering that happens without conscious awareness) are usually preserved.[1,8] Short-term "working memory " (memory of materials that must be retained during thinking) is also commonly impaired. Both the processes of acquisition (encoding and storage) and retrieval of material are currently believed to be affected, although previous reports underlined prominent retrieval problems.[9]

Impaired attention and reduced information processing speed may represent a sensitive indicator of incipient CD.[1] The complex aspects of attention (e.g., selective, divided, and alternating attention) are most often impaired, whereas the simplest form of attention (attention span) is generally intact.[1] Moreover,

TABLE 7–1 Neuropsychological Profile

Cognitive Domain	% of Patients Impaired*
Episodic memory	22-31
Attention, concentration, processing speed	22-25
Verbal fluency	22
Executive functions	13-19
Visual perception	12-19
Language/semantic memory	8-10
Attention span	7-8

*Performance below the 5th percentile of normative values.

Modified from Rao SM, Leo GJ, Bernardin L, Unverzagt F: Cognitive dysfunction in multiple sclerosis: I. Frequency, patterns, and prediction. Neurology 1991;41:685-691.

MS patients may show a substantial decline in cognitive performance during tests that require sustained attention, a phenomenon known as "cognitive fatigue."[10,11] Deficits in executive functions involve abstract reasoning, problem solving, planning, monitoring, and cognitive estimation[12] and can affect performance on other cognitive and motor tasks and in daily living activities. Prevalence estimates of decline in visuospatial ability show great variability depending on the type of assessment.[1,13] Facial, visual form, and visuospatial perceptions are the most frequently impaired domains. Language deficits are observed in a minority of MS subjects[1] and may derive from damage to other cognitive faculties.[14,15] Slight problems in naming, reading, and verbal comprehension may be detected. Aphasic syndromes are rare. Verbal fluency impairment on both semantic and phonemic stimuli is common and depends on deficits in executive functions.

CLINICAL CORRELATES

On the whole, the available evidence suggests that CD in MS encompasses all disease stages and clinical phenotypes. There are, in general, modest correlations between the presence or degree of CD and disease duration, disability level as measured on the Expanded Disability Status Scale (EDSS),[16] and disease course.[1,17] The poor correlation with the EDSS is not surprising, because the scale is heavily weighted for motor abilities. However, in a large sample of patients with relapsing-remitting MS (RRMS) or secondary progressive MS (SPMS), a significant correlation of CD with the EDSS was found, particularly with the cerebral and cerebellar systems.[18]

CD has been consistently demonstrated in the early stages of the disease in patients with low disability levels[19] and even in patients with clinically isolated syndromes (CIS).[20,21] Achiron and Barak[20] found that 94% of patients with probable MS had an abnormal score on at least one of the tests administered. Glanz and associates[21] found that 49% of patients with CIS or with an MS diagnosis made within the last 3 years were impaired on one or more cognitive measures.

As for clinical phenotypes, there is consistent evidence in the literature that patients with RRMS show lesser degrees of CD compared with patients with chronic progressive disease.[22-24] Only a few studies have compared the frequency, severity, and pattern of CD in patients with primary progressive MS (PPMS) and SPMS, with inconsistent results.[25-28] Camp and colleagues[26] carried out the largest study published to date, including 63 patients with PPMS. The prevalence of CD was substantially higher than that previously reported in PPMS, reaching 29%. CD correlated moderately with the MRI lesion load in T2 and T1 studies and with cerebral volume. The authors suggested that, in PPMS, abnormalities in the normal-appearing white matter or cortical involvement may play a prominent role. In a comparative study,[28] patients with RRMS performed better than those with PPMS or SPMS, with the exception of the verbal fluency task. SPMS patients performed worse than PPMS patients on tests requiring higher-order working memory processes, with the exception of tests involving sustained attention and concentration. The authors suggested that the neuropsychological profile of deficits may be different in different disease phenotypes.

The cognitive functioning of 163 patients with so-called "benign MS" (EDSS score ≤ 3.0 at least 15 years from disease onset) was recently assessed.[29] In this study, CD was found in 45% of the patients, with a significant impact on work and social life despite complete preservation of motor abilities.

Approximately 5% of cases MS occur in children or adolescents.[30] Children may be especially vulnerable to cognitive impairment, because the neuropathologic changes of MS occur during the myelination process in the developing CNS. Moreover, disease-related difficulties occurring during key formative periods may have negative consequences on the individual and the family, as well as on school and other aspects of social functioning. Cognitive impairment in this age range was reported in two uncontrolled studies and revealed academic problems in a significant proportion of the cases.[31,32] A controlled, multicentric study in 63 childhood and juvenile cases[33] showed a 32% prevalence of cognitive impairment. Moreover, 26% of the patients had an IQ at the lower range and 9% were at the level classified as "mental insufficiency." The involvement of linguistic function was the most notable finding in pediatric and juvenile cases compared with adult cases.[31,33,34]

Specific attention has been given to the possible association of CD with fatigue and depression. Although the relationship between CD and fatigue is poorly understood, the two problems may often be associated. Positron emission tomography (PET) studies suggest that fatigue and CD may share a common physiopathologic substrate, due to involvement of common frontal-subcortical pathways.[35] Patients often report that fatigue lowers their cognitive performance, and on the other hand, CD may result in increased fatigue.[35] Self-reported depression seems to be only weakly related to overall cognitive function.[36] However, in more recent studies, depression correlated with deficits in information processing speed, working memory, and executive functions.[36] Finally, specific impairments of the frontal component of cognitive functions and of behavioral memory have been associated with a lower quality of life.[36]

NEUROIMAGING CORRELATES

Over the past decades, efforts toward detailed investigation of clinicopathologic correlations in MS have intensified, including both conventional MRI and new quantitative techniques with greater pathologic specificity. However, the relationship remains complex, and it seems to involve the contribution of various changes, including white matter lesions but also changes in brain tissue that appears to be normal on the conventional MRI, as well as involvement of both cortical and deep gray matter. In cross-sectional studies, CD shows mild to moderate relationships with brain lesion burden in T2- and T1-weighted sequences and with corpus callosum lesions.[37] Longitudinal assessments have confirmed an association with increasing T2 lesion burden, both total and in specific brain regions such as the frontoparietal areas.[37] Studies using magnetization transfer analysis have also highlighted the relevance of microscopic changes in the normal-appearing white matter.[37] Several studies have pointed to the importance of brain atrophy, including both generalized brain atrophy and central brain atrophy.[37] In their longitudinal study, Zivadinov and coworkers[38] documented that the best predictor of deteriorating cognitive performance over 2 years was progressing brain atrophy, independently of brain lesion loads. More recently, Ron and colleagues,[39] observed that the rate of global brain atrophy in the first year of their study accounted for significant variance in overall cognitive performance after 5 years; they suggested that early brain tissue loss and its rate of progression may predict cognitive impairment later in the disease course.

Recent evidence has also highlighted the role of gray matter pathology. In a cross-sectional survey involving patients with early-onset RRMS,[19] significant decreases in neocortical volumes were selectively found only in the subgroup who exhibited mild CD, compared with both cognitively preserved patients and a group of normal controls. Cortical atrophy showed a good relationship with performance on various cognitive tasks and with the total number of tests failed by the patients. On the contrary, there was no significant relationship between CD and whole brain atrophy or brain lesion loads. In the same cohort of subjects, reassessed after 2.5 years,[40] neocortical volume decrease was confirmed to be the only parameter discriminating between patients with a deteriorating cognitive performance and those with a stable or improving performance. Another study[41] found that white matter volume was the best predictor of processing speed and working memory performance, whereas gray matter volume predicted verbal memory performance, euphoria, and disinhibition. Significant relationships between cognitive tasks and atrophy of specific cortical regions[37] have also been found. Moreover, a recent study also pointed to the possible role of thalamic involvement.[42]

Research involving functional brain imaging has also provided valuable insight into the field. PET and single photon emission computed tomography (SPECT) studies have shown a relationship between CD and reduced cerebral blood flow and metabolism in specific brain areas.[37] To assess functional changes during neuropsychological performance, a series of functional MRI (fMRI) studies were conducted.[43] On the whole, in MS patients whose behavioral testing performance was comparable to that of healthy controls, cognitive and motor studies have found an increased number of activated regions and reduced laterality indices in the MS patients. This increased activation is not observed in patients with severe degrees of cognitive or motor dysfunction. The prevailing interpretation of these findings is that fMRI changes may reflect cortical reorganization resulting from neural plasticity. This adaptive mechanism may potentially allow MS patients to perform normally despite brain pathology. Impaired cognitive task performance might therefore reflect the failure of adequate compensatory strategies.[44]

NATURAL HISTORY

It is difficult to compare results from existing longitudinal studies, because they differ substantially in terms of clinical characteristics of the patients, neuropsychological measurements, and criteria for the definition of CD.[2,45-48] Kujala and colleagues,[48] in a 3-year follow-up study, found that the majority of subjects who were intact at baseline remained stable, but 77% of the patients who were impaired at baseline exhibited significant deterioration. This study showed that, although cognitive preservation may remain stable, incipient CD is widespread and progressive in nature and represents the major risk factor for further deterioration over the short term. In a long-term, controlled study,[47] the percentage of patients who exhibited mild or moderate deficits increased from 26% at baseline to 49% at the 4-year evaluation, and it reached the 56% by the end of the study, after 10 years. A higher EDSS score and a progressive course, as well increasing age, proved to be positively correlated with a worse cognitive outcome. This suggests that the severity of the disease course and the patient's cognitive outcome may tend to converge, at least in the long term. Camp and coworkers, in their 2-year study of PPMS,[49] observed a marked variability, with some patients deteriorating and others remaining stable or improving. Mean performance did not change significantly, but, in terms of individual changes, 37% of patients showed significant cognitive decline.

Taken as whole, available evidence suggests that cognitive outcome in MS patients may be quite heterogeneous. However, once CD is established, it does not remit to any significant extent, with the possible exception of transient cognitive changes reported during a relapse.[50] It may remain stable, but, during a sufficiently long follow-up period, it does tend to progress, albeit at different rates and within the context of great interpatient variability.

Assessment

In everyday clinical practice, a number of clinical "red flags" for CD should suggest the need for a specific neuropsychological evaluation These include complaints by the patient or a family member, frontal release signs at the objective examination, rapid disease progression, severe fatigue, treatment-resistant depression, and early employment retirement decisions that are not fully justified on the basis of the physical disability of the subject. MRI "red flags" are mainly large lesion load, extensive involvement of corpus callosum, and significant brain atrophy.[51]

Because it is impractical to refer all visited MS patients for comprehensive neuropsychological evaluation, clinicians should have at their disposal a brief and well-validated screening instrument to identify those subjects who need an extensive assessment. The Mini-Mental State Examination (MMSE)[52] has sensitivity levels ranging from 28% to 36% and specificity levels ranging from 89% to 100%. It is therefore insensitive for the detection of MS-related cognitive impairment, except for the most severe degrees of CD.[53] Other variants of the MMSE have similarly low sensitivity levels or have not been adequately validated.[53] Some authors have proposed the use of tests assessing complex attention and speed of information processing, such as the Paced Auditory Serial Addition Test (PASAT)[54] or the Symbol Digit Modality Test (SDMT),[55,56] although the use of these tests as screening instruments has not been thoroughly validated. Another proposed instrument is the Multiple Sclerosis Neuropsychological Screening Questionnaire (MSNQ), a 15-item questionnaire presented to patients or caregivers.[57,58] In validation studies, the MSNQ yielded 83% to 87% sensitivity and 84% to 97% specificity levels.[57,58] Patient self-reports were significantly influenced by depression, whereas caregiver reports seemed to be more reliable and were correlated with relevant clinical and MRI variables.[59]

A different approach is the development of brief batteries of neuropsychological tests that cover the functions most often compromised in MS. Among these, the Brief Repeatable Neuropsychological Battery (BRB)[60] is by far the most widely used for both clinical and research purposes. It has 68% sensitivity and 85% specificity, with an estimated administration time of 30 to 35 minutes. Two alternative versions are available for use in serial assessments, in order to minimize possible "practice effects" from repetition of the tests over time. Normative data have been published[61,62] and can enhance the applicability of the BRB in clinical practice when an appropriate control group is not available.

The use of comprehensive batteries is mandatory for specific issues, such as differential diagnosis, disability or employment issues, rehabilitation programs, and specific research purposes. In a recent consensus conference, the Minimal Assessment of Cognitive Function in Multiple Sclerosis (MACFIMS)[63] was developed. It includes a series of tests covering seven cognitive domains commonly impaired in MS, for which alternative versions are available, and it takes about 90 minutes to be completed. Its validation process is ongoing.

Finally, when assessing cognitive functioning in MS patients, it is necessary to take into account potential confounders of neuropsychological performance by providing concurrent measures of fatigue, depression, and degree of neurologic impairment and disability.

THERAPEUTIC APPROACHES

Tentative therapeutic approaches include both pharmacologic strategies and cognitive rehabilitation. To date, there is only preliminary evidence of efficacy provided by a few randomized, placebo-controlled, double-blind trials with disease-modifying drugs.[51] In a trial using interferon (IFN)-beta-1b, the high-dose group did significantly better than the low-dose and placebo groups on only one test of delayed visual recall. However, the study included only 30 patients, and there was no baseline neuropsychological assessment of the subjects in the pretreatment period. In a study of intramuscular IFN-beta-1a[64] including 276 patients, 166 completed the follow-up assessment at 2 years. Both the treated and the placebo group improved, probably due to practice effects. However, patients in the IFN-beta-1a group did significantly better than those in the placebo group on a series of tests evaluating memory and information processing speed. In a trial with glatiramer acetate including 251 subjects,[65] the cognitive performance of both the treated and the placebo group improved after 24 months, and there was no significant difference between the two groups. Participants in the open-label glatiramer acetate extension study were reassessed after approximately 10 years.[66] There was some decline in cognitive performance on specific tests, but mean scores on neuropsychological measures showed only minimal changes.

A number of small pilot trials have also tested symptomatic therapies for fatigue. Studies of amantadine, pemoline, 4-aminopyridine, and 3,4-aminopyridine provided mainly negative results,[51] as did a small trial with *Ginkgo biloba*.[67] Acetylcholinesterase inhibitors used to treat Alzheimer's disease have been tested in MS.[51,68] Krupp and associates[68] reported that 69 MS patients with initial CD were treated with donepezil (10 mg daily) or a placebo for 24 weeks. Sixty-five percent of the donepezil-treated patients showed significant improvement on a verbal learning and memory test, compared with 50% of those receiving placebo. Moreover, in the judgment of patients and clinicians, there was significantly greater memory improvement in the donepezil group. Other trials with acetylcholinesterase inhibitors and a variety of psychostimulant or symptomatic agents are ongoing.

Cognitive rehabilitation should be part of a comprehensive program involving the patient, family, and caregivers, taking into account neuropsychological performance, emotional disturbances, functioning in everyday activities, and family and social supports. To date, published studies on cognitive rehabilitation in MS have provided mainly inconsistent results.[51] Recent fMRI studies in MS patients[44] suggested the potential capacity for adaptation and compensation after cognitive training, hypothetically as a result of brain plasticity. MS patients with mild and severe cognitive impairment were compared before and after computerized training for attention; the authors found that both patient groups had activation in three additional areas involved in the attention network after training, including posterior cingulated cortex, precuneus, and dorsal frontal gyrus.

Further work is needed in this area to develop a comprehensive rehabilitative approach specifically tailored to the MS patients.

Psychiatric Disorders

The majority of the literature on psychiatric disorders is dedicated to depression, because it is the most frequent problem in MS patients.

DEPRESSION

Among MS outpatients, the prevalence of depression ranges from 18% to 54%; more representative, community-based studies have confirmed high prevalence figures ranging from 19% to 42%.[36] This is about three times higher than in the general population and exceeds the figures reported in patients with other chronic medical or neurologic illnesses.[36] However, a few methodologic issues suggest caution in interpreting these data. An important issue concerns the great variety of measures used to diagnose and quantify the severity of depression. Moreover, somatic symptoms of depression may overlap with disease-related symptoms such as fatigue, concentration difficulties, or sleep disturbances. In addition, limitations in activities of daily living may be caused both by depression and physical disability. Finally, depressive symptoms may be related to the direct effects of drugs (e.g., corticosteroids). Given this potential overlap, rating scales specific for the assessment of depression in patients with chronic medical illnesses have been developed, including the Chicago Multiscale Depression Inventory (CMDI)[69] and the Beck Fast Screen.[70]

There is consistent evidence that depression represents the single most important determinant of quality of life in MS patients, independent of the degree of neurologic disability.[36] Moreover, depressed patients show poor compliance to therapy with disease-modifying drugs, and treatment of depression may improve adherence to therapy.[71]

Depression in MS is also associated with the risk of suicide. In a Canadian cohort, the suicide rate in MS patients was 7.5 times higher than that observed in the general population,[72] and a Danish study reported that the number of suicides was twice as high as expected.[73] Major depression, severity of depressive symptoms, male gender, MS onset before 30 years of age, alcohol abuse, and living alone are the main risk factors for suicidal intent in MS patients.[73-75]

The pathogenesis of depression in MS is complex and multifactorial. Depression may be an expression of the distress caused by disease-related impairments and activity limitations and the uncertain prognosis.[36] An organic component may also play a role, related to involvement of relevant brain regions by the disease process. Neuroimaging studies have shown a variety of positive correlations between depression and lesions localized in the arcuate fasciculus, greater lesion load, frontal and parietal atrophy, and lesion load in the left medial inferior prefrontal region together with atrophy in the dominant anterior temporal lobe.[36] Furthermore, an association between depression and brainstem or basal limbic lesions has been reported.[36]

A common genetic susceptibility has also been investigated; however, to date, it has not been possible to identify any reliable genetic association between MS and depression.[36]

A possible role of IFN-beta therapy was suggested in some reports.[36] However, a review of available data[76] revealed that most studies discard an association between IFN-beta and depression or suicide. Overall, depression is not considered a contraindication to IFN-beta therapy, provided that close monitoring of the patient and adequate antidepressant treatment are offered.

In spite of the well-known high prevalence of depression in MS, a sizable proportion of depressed patients remain untreated.[36] In the pharmacologic treatment of depression, caution is needed due to possible worsening of MS symptoms such as constipation, urinary retention, spasticity, sleep disorders, and sexual disorders. Selective serotonin reuptake inhibitors (SSRIs) are probably preferred because of their better tolerability profile.[36]

OTHER PSYCHIATRIC DISTURBANCES

The prevalence of bipolar disorder in MS is 0.3%, significantly greater than the prevalence of in the general population (0.2%).[77] Research on its etiology is limited but has focused on genetic vulnerability, adverse reactions to steroid treatment, and MRI features.[77] To date, the reason for this association is not fully understood, and specific treatment guidelines are not available.

Euphoria is characterized by a persistently cheerful mood and overly optimistic state of mental and physical well-being despite significant neurologic disability. Lifetime prevalence estimates are approximately 25%.[78,79] Euphoria is usually considered a manifestation of advanced MS in patients with severe physical and cognitive disability, and it has been associated with extensive brain damage and atrophy.[41]

Pseudobulbar affect, also known as emotional lability, is characterized by frequent and inappropriate episodes of crying, laughing, or both.[77] It occurs in approximately 10% of MS patients, with varying degrees of severity.[77] The exact pathogenesis remains unknown, but recent evidence implicates the disruption of neural pathways emanating from the brainstem and cerebellum that normally control the expression of emotions.[77] Tricyclic antidepressants, SSRIs, and L-dopa are used to treat pseudobulbar affect. Positive results were obtained in a trial using dextromethorphan/quinidine.[80]

Finally, prevalence figures for psychosis in MS are conflicting, and a review concluded that the occurrence of psychotic disorders in MS is uncommon, probably not exceeding chance expectation.[81] MRI data, albeit scarce, suggest a possible pathogenetic role of temporal lobe involvement.[82,83]

REFERENCES

1. Rao SM, Leo GJ, Bernardin L, Unverzagt F: Cognitive dysfunction in multiple sclerosis: I. Frequency, patterns, and prediction. Neurology 1991;41:685-691.
2. Amato MP, Ponziani G, Pracucci G, et al: Cognitive impairment in early-onset multiple sclerosis: Pattern, predictors, and impact on everyday life in a 4-year follow-up. Arch Neurol 1995;52: 168-172.
3. Beatty WW, Paul RH, Wilbanks SL, et al: Identifying multiple sclerosis patients with mild or global cognitive impairment using the Screening Examination for Cognitive Impairment (SEFCI). Neurology 1995;45:718-723.
4. Rao SM, Leo GJ, Ellington L, et al: Cognitive dysfunction in multiple sclerosis: II. Impact on employment and social functioning. Neurology 1991;41:692-696.
5. Langdon DW, Thompson AJ: Multiple sclerosis: A preliminary study of selected variables affecting rehabilitation outcome. Mult Scler 1999;5:94-100.
6. Calabrese P, Penner IK: Cognitive dysfunctions in multiple sclerosis: A "multiple disconnection syndrome"? J Neurol 2007;254(Suppl 2):II18-II21.
7. Zakzanis KK: Distinct neurocognitive profiles in multiple sclerosis subtypes. Arch Clin Neuropsychol 2000;15:115-136.
8. Beatty WW, Monson N: Metamemory in multiple sclerosis. J Clin Exp Neuropsychol 1991;13: 309-327.
9. Lange G, Wang S, DeLuca J, Natelson BH: Neuroimaging in chronic fatigue syndrome. Am J Med 1998;105:50S-53S.
10. Krupp LB, Elkins LE: Fatigue and declines in cognitive functioning in multiple sclerosis. Neurology 2000;55:934-939.
11. Beatty WW, Goretti B, Siracusa G, et al: Changes in neuropsychological test performance over the workday in multiple sclerosis. Clin Neuropsychol 2003;17:551-560.
12. Arnett PA, Rao SM, Grafman J, et al: Executive functions in multiple sclerosis: An analysis of temporal ordering, semantic encoding, and planning abilities. Neuropsychology 1997;11:535-544.
13. Haase CG, Tinnefeld M, Lienemann M, et al: Depression and cognitive impairment in disability-free early multiple sclerosis. Behav Neurol 2003;14:39-45.
14. Kujala P, Portin R, Ruutiainen J: Language functions in incipient cognitive decline in multiple sclerosis. J Neurol Sci 1996;141:79-86.
15. Friend KB, Rabin BM, Groninger L, et al: Language functions in patients with multiple sclerosis. Clin Neuropsychol 1999;13:78-94.
16. Kurtzke JF: Neurologic impairment in multiple sclerosis and the disability status scale. Acta Neurol Scand 1970;46:493-512.
17. Ron MA, Callanan MM, Warrington EK: Cognitive abnormalities in multiple sclerosis: A psychometric and MRI study. Psychol Med 1991;21:59-68.
18. Lynch SG, Parmenter BA, Denney DR: The association between cognitive impairment and physical disability in multiple sclerosis. Mult Scler 2005;11:469-476.
19. Amato MP, Bartolozzi ML, Zipoli V, et al: Neocortical volume decrease in relapsing-remitting MS patients with mild cognitive impairment. Neurology 2004;63:89-93.
20. Achiron A, Barak Y: Cognitive impairment in probable multiple sclerosis. J Neurol Neurosurg Psychiatry 2003;74:443-446.
21. Glanz B, Holland C, Gauthier S, et al: Cognitive dysfunction in patients with clinically isolated syndromes or newly diagnosed multiple sclerosis. Mult Scler 2007;13:1004-1010.
22. Minden SL, Moes EJ, Orav J, et al: Memory impairment in multiple sclerosis. J Clin Exp Neuropsychol 1990;12:566-586.
23. Heaton RK, Nelson LM, Thompson DS, et al: Neuropsychological findings in relapsing-remitting and chronic-progressive multiple sclerosis. J Consult Clin Psychol 1985;53:103-110.
24. Filippi M, Alberoni M, Martinelli V, et al: Influence of clinical variables on neuropsychological performance in multiple sclerosis. Eur Neurol 1994;34:324-328.
25. Comi G, Filippi M, Martinelli V, et al: Brain MRI correlates of cognitive impairment in primary and secondary progressive multiple sclerosis. J Neurol Sci 1995;132:222-227.
26. Camp SJ, Stevenson VL, Thompson AJ, et al: Cognitive function in primary progressive and transitional progressive multiple sclerosis: A controlled study with MRI correlates. Brain 1999;122 (Pt 7):1341-1348.
27. Foong J, Rozewicz L, Chong WK, et al: A comparison of neuropsychological deficits in primary and secondary progressive multiple sclerosis. J Neurol 2000;247:97-101.

28. Huijbregts SC, Kalkers NF, de Sonneville LM, et al: Differences in cognitive impairment of relapsing remitting, secondary, and primary progressive MS. Neurology 2004;63:335-339.
29. Amato MP, Zipoli V, Goretti B, et al: Benign multiple sclerosis: Cognitive, psychological and social aspects in a clinical cohort. J Neurol 2006;253:1054-1059.
30. Duquette P, Murray TJ, Pleines J, et al: Multiple sclerosis in childhood: Clinical profile in 125 patients. J Pediatr 1987;111:359-363.
31. Banwell BL, Anderson PE: The cognitive burden of multiple sclerosis in children. Neurology 2005;64:891-894.
32. MacAllister WS, Belman AL, Milazzo M, et al: Cognitive functioning in children and adolescents with multiple sclerosis. Neurology 2005;64:1422-1425.
33. Amato M, Goretti B, Lori S, et al: An Italian multicentric study on cognitive functioning in childhood and juvenile multiple sclerosis. Neurology 2007;68. A241, P05100.
34. Banwell B, Ghezzi A, Bar-Or A, et al: Multiple sclerosis in children: Clinical diagnosis, therapeutic strategies, and future directions. Lancet Neurol 2007;6:887-902.
35. Bakshi R: Fatigue associated with multiple sclerosis: Diagnosis, impact and management. Mult Scler 2003;9:219-227.
36. Siegert RJ, Abernethy DA: Depression in multiple sclerosis: A review. J Neurol Neurosurg Psychiatry 2005;76:469-475.
37. Rovaris M, Comi G, Filippi M: MRI markers of destructive pathology in multiple sclerosis-related cognitive dysfunction. J Neurol Sci 2006;245:111-116.
38. Zivadinov R, Sepcic J, Nasuelli D, et al: A longitudinal study of brain atrophy and cognitive disturbances in the early phase of relapsing-remitting multiple sclerosis. J Neurol Neurosurg Psychiatry 2001;70:773-780.
39. Ron M, Summers MM, Fisniku L, et al: Cognitive impairment in relapsing-remitting multiple sclerosis can be predicted by imaging performed several years earlier. Mult Scler 2007;14:197-204.
40. Amato MP, Portaccio E, Goretti B, et al: Association of neocortical volume changes with cognitive deterioration in relapsing-remitting multiple sclerosis. Arch Neurol 2007;64:1157-1161.
41. Sanfilipo MP, Benedict RH, Weinstock-Guttman B, Bakshi R: Gray and white matter brain atrophy and neuropsychological impairment in multiple sclerosis. Neurology 2006;66:685-692.
42. Houtchens MK, Benedict RH, Killiany R, et al: Thalamic atrophy and cognition in multiple sclerosis. Neurology 2007;69:1213-1223.
43. Rocca MA, Filippi M: Functional MRI in multiple sclerosis. J Neuroimaging 2007;17(Suppl 1): 36S-41S.
44. Penner IK, Opwis K, Kappos L: Relation between functional brain imaging, cognitive impairment and cognitive rehabilitation in patients with multiple sclerosis. J Neurol 2007;254(Suppl 2):II53-II57.
45. Jennekens-Schinkel A, Laboyrie PM, Lanser JB, van der Velde EA: Cognition in patients with multiple sclerosis after four years. J Neurol Sci 1990;99:229-247.
46. Bernardin L, Rao S, Luchetta T: A prospective, long term longitudinal study of cognitive dysfunction in multiple sclerosis. J Clin Exp Neuropsychol 1993;15:17.
47. Amato MP, Ponziani G, Siracusa G, Sorbi S: Cognitive dysfunction in early-onset multiple sclerosis: A reappraisal after 10 years. Arch Neurol 2001;58:1602-1606.
48. Kujala P, Portin R, Ruutiainen J: The progress of cognitive decline in multiple sclerosis: A controlled 3-year follow-up. Brain 1997;120(Pt 2):289-297.
49. Camp SJ, Stevenson VL, Thompson AJ, et al: A longitudinal study of cognition in primary progressive multiple sclerosis. Brain 2005;128:2891-2898.
50. Foong J, Rozewicz L, Quaghebeur G, et al: Neuropsychological deficits in multiple sclerosis after acute relapse. J Neurol Neurosurg Psychiatry 1998;64:529-532.
51. Amato MP, Zipoli V: Clinical management of cognitive impairment in multiple sclerosis: A review of current evidence. Int MS J 2003;10:72-83.
52. Folstein MF, Folstein SE, McHugh PR: "Mini-mental state": A practical method for grading the cognitive state of patients for the clinician. J Psychiatr Res 1975;12:189-198.
53. Beatty WW, Goodkin DE: Screening for cognitive impairment in multiple sclerosis: An evaluation of the Mini-Mental State Examination. Arch Neurol 1990;47:297-301.
54. Rosti E, Hamalainen P, Koivisto K, Hokkanen L: PASAT in detecting cognitive impairment in relapsing-remitting MS. Appl Neuropsychol 2007;14:101-112.
55. Deloire MS, Bonnet MC, Salort E, et al: How to detect cognitive dysfunction at early stages of multiple sclerosis? Mult Scler 2006;12:445-452.
56. Parmenter BA, Weinstock-Guttman B, Garg N, et al: Screening for cognitive impairment in multiple sclerosis using the Symbol Digit Modalities Test. Mult Scler 2007;13:52-57.

57. Benedict RH, Cox D, Thompson LL, et al: Reliable screening for neuropsychological impairment in multiple sclerosis. Mult Scler 2004;10:675-678.
58. Benedict RH, Munschauer F, Linn R, et al: Screening for multiple sclerosis cognitive impairment using a self-administered 15-item questionnaire. Mult Scler 2003;9:95-101.
59. Benedict RH, Zivadinov R: Predicting neuropsychological abnormalities in multiple sclerosis. J Neurol Sci 2006;245:67-72.
60. Rao S: A Manual for the Brief Repeatable Battery of Neuropsychological Tests in Multiple Sclerosis. Milwaukee, Medical College of Wisconsin, 1990.
61. Amato MP, Portaccio E, Goretti B, et al: The Rao's Brief Repeatable Battery and Stroop Test: Normative values with age, education and gender corrections in an Italian population. Mult Scler 2006;12:787-793.
62. Boringa JB, Lazeron RH, Reuling IE, et al: The brief repeatable battery of neuropsychological tests: Normative values allow application in multiple sclerosis clinical practice. Mult Scler 2001;7: 263-267.
63. Benedict RH, Fischer JS, Archibald CJ, et al: Minimal neuropsychological assessment of MS patients: A consensus approach. Clin Neuropsychol 2002;16:381-397.
64. Fischer JS, Priore RL, Jacobs LD, et al: Neuropsychological effects of interferon beta-1a in relapsing multiple sclerosis. Multiple Sclerosis Collaborative Research Group. Ann Neurol 2000;48: 885-892.
65. Weinstein A, Schwid SR, Schiffer RB, et al: Neuropsychologic status in multiple sclerosis after treatment with glatiramer. Arch Neurol 1999;56:319-324.
66. Schwid SR, Goodman AD, Weinstein A, et al: Cognitive function in relapsing multiple sclerosis: Minimal changes in a 10-year clinical trial. J Neurol Sci 2007;255:57-63.
67. Lovera J, Bagert B, Smoot K, et al: Ginkgo biloba for the improvement of cognitive performance in multiple sclerosis: A randomized, placebo-controlled trial. Mult Scler 2007;13:376-385.
68. Krupp LB, Christodoulou C, Melville P, et al: Donepezil improved memory in multiple sclerosis in a randomized clinical trial. Neurology 2004;63:1579-1585.
69. Chang CH, Nyenhuis DL, Cella D, et al: Psychometric evaluation of the Chicago Multiscale Depression Inventory in multiple sclerosis patients. Mult Scler 2003;9:160-170.
70. Beck A, Steer R, Brown G: DI-Fast Screen for medical patients. San Antonio, Texas, The Psychological Corporation, 2000.
71. Mohr DC, Goodkin DE, Likosky W, et al: Treatment of depression improves adherence to interferon beta-1b therapy for multiple sclerosis. Arch Neurol 1997;54:531-533.
72. Sadovnick AD, Eisen K, Ebers GC, Paty DW: Cause of death in patients attending multiple sclerosis clinics. Neurology 1991;41:1193-1196.
73. Stenager EN, Stenager E, Koch-Henriksen N, et al: Suicide and multiple sclerosis: An epidemiological investigation. J Neurol Neurosurg Psychiatry 1992;55:542-545.
74. Feinstein A: An examination of suicidal intent in patients with multiple sclerosis. Neurology 2002;59:674-678.
75. Turner AP, Williams RM, Bowen JD, et al: Suicidal ideation in multiple sclerosis. Arch Phys Med Rehabil 2006;87:1073-1078.
76. Goeb JL, Even C, Nicolas G, et al: Psychiatric side effects of interferon-beta in multiple sclerosis. Eur Psychiatry 2006;21:186-193.
77. Chwastiak LA, Ehde DM: Psychiatric issues in multiple sclerosis. Psychiatr Clin North Am 2007;30:803-817.
78. Surridge D: An investigation into some psychiatric aspects of multiple sclerosis. Br J Psychiatry 1969;115:749-764.
79. Poser CM: Exacerbations, activity, and progression in multiple sclerosis. Arch Neurol 1980;37: 471-474.
80. Panitch HS, Thisted RA, Smith RA, et al: Randomized, controlled trial of dextromethorphan/ quinidine for pseudobulbar affect in multiple sclerosis. Ann Neurol 2006;59:780-787.
81. Feinstein A: The neuropsychiatry of multiple sclerosis. Can J Psychiatry 2004;49:157-163.
82. Feinstein A, du Boulay G, Ron MA: Psychotic illness in multiple sclerosis: A clinical and magnetic resonance imaging study. Br J Psychiatry 1992;161:680-685.
83. Reiss JP, Sam D, Sareen J: Psychosis in multiple sclerosis associated with left temporal lobe lesions on serial MRI scans. J Clin Neurosci 2006;13:282-284.

8 Gender Issues and Multiple Sclerosis

RHONDA VOSKUHL

For decades it has been known that females are more susceptible than males to MS. Sex hormones and/or sex-linked gene inheritance may be responsible for this enhanced susceptibility of females. In general, it has been documented that females have more robust immune responses than males.[1] However, an effect of gender on the immune response does not preclude additional effects on the target organ, the central nervous system (CNS), in multiple sclerosis (MS).[2,3] This chapter considers the gender bias in MS with respect to effects of sex hormones and sex chromosomes on both the immune system and the CNS.

Gender Differences in Multiple Sclerosis

During reproductive ages, there is a distinct female preponderance of autoimmune diseases including MS.[1] Sex hormones or sex chromosomes, or both, may be responsible for this enhanced susceptibility. In males, the onset of MS tends to be relatively later in life (thirties to forties), coinciding with the beginning of the decline in bioavailable testosterone (T).[4] Therefore, the female-to-male ratio is greater in patients presenting with MS before 20 years of age (3.2:1), compared with the MS population as a whole (2:1).[5] Interestingly, a recent Canadian study found a disproportionate increase in the incidence of MS among women.[6] This increased ratio, approaching 4:1, was theorized to possibly be of environmental origins. Alternatively, these data may merely reflect a propensity for neurologists to diagnose women with early MS. As time passes, neurologists have more sensitive tools for detecting early MS and a growing appreciation of the importance of early treatment in slowing disability accumulation. Notably, the relatively higher proportions of female patients with MS, as recently reported, remain consistent with the gender ratios that were previously known in other autoimmune diseases such as rheumatoid arthritis (RA) and systemic lupus erythematosus (SLE).

Although it is clear that there has been an increase in the incidence of MS among women compared with men, a different question is whether established disease progresses at a different rate in women and men. Clinical neurologists have had the impression that MS progresses more rapidly in men than in women. However, this observation may be confounded by the fact that their assessments have included primary progressive MS (PPMS). PPMS is distinct from relapsing-remitting MS (RRMS) and secondary progressive MS (SPMS) in that there is no gender bias in its incidence. It also differs with respect site of MS lesions, rate of progression, and response to anti-inflammatory treatments. PPMS primarily affects the spinal cord, is associated with relatively rapid progression of motor deficits, and is less responsive to anti-inflammatory treatments. Because the ratio of women to men is 1:1 in PPMS, there are relatively more men with PPMS, compared with RRMS and SPMS. This would make it appear that men have a more severe course of MS. However, many propose that, pathologically, PPMS is a different disease from RRMS and SPMS, and that it should be considered as such. Then the question becomes, do those men and women who have RRMS or SPMS progress at different rates? Most studies have not reported their outcome data according to gender. A National Multiple Sclerosis Society Task Force on Gender and MS suggested that placebo-treated MS patients in clinical trials should be assessed for effects of gender on their disease course.[1]

The data that currently exist suggest that early predictors of future disability in MS include gender, age at onset, and degree of recovery from first episode.[7,8] These parameters are not mutually exclusive. Men tend to have later age at onset and less recovery from relapses initially. Compared with men, women spend more years in an early relapsing-remitting phase before making the transition to the SPMS. Once the transition to a progressive course or given stage of disability was reached, however, there was no gender difference in the rate of further progression.[7] We propose that there may be an interaction between the aging CNS and the transition to SPMS. Women whose onset of MS occurred at age 20 to 30 years will spend approximately 15 years in the RRMS phase before approaching the transition at age 40 to 45; on the other hand, men who are 35 to 40 years of age at onset will spend much less time in the RRMS phase before beginning the transition to SPMS at age 40 to 45. The transition tends to occur at approximate the same age regardless of gender. Future neuropathologic studies should consider the role of the aging CNS in the development of SPMS. Future studies should also address why many relatively young men (ages 20 to 30 years) remain asymptomatic during their early years while women are already experiencing clinical relapses and remissions. Our group has postulated that relatively high levels of testosterone in young men may be playing a temporarily protective role in men who are otherwise genetically predisposed to ultimately developing MS.[9]

Given that the clinical picture of disease progression in women versus men is complex, neuroimaging studies were conducted in 413 MS subjects, comparing women and men with MS, in an effort to reveal some insights based on subclinical biomarkers of disease. Men had fewer contrast-enhancing lesions than women, but there was a higher likelihood for them to evolve into T1 "black holes"[10] (discussed in Chapter 5). Because enhancing lesions are considered a biomarker for relapses, these data were consistent with the observation that men are less likely to develop early RRMS. Further, because T1 black holes are thought to be destructive and potentially associated with permanent neurologic damage, they were also consistent with the suggestion that, when men develop MS, it tends to be more severe clinically.[4,7,11] However, a follow-up study of 35 women and 25 men with RRMS while confirming the finding of fewer enhancing lesions in men failed to corroborate an increased likelihood for lesions in men to evolve into T1 black holes, although this result was perhaps due to a smaller sample size.[12] Together, the data appear to confirm that men are less likely to develop clinical relapses and enhancing lesions on magnetic resonance imaging (MRI) at an early age, but it remains unclear whether the course of MS in men is more severe than that in age-matched women with MS.

Gender Differences in the Murine Model of Multiple Sclerosis

Although it is not perfect, experimental autoimmune encephalomyelitis (EAE) is the most widely used animal model for studying the pathogenesis of MS. EAE models vary according to the species and strain of the animal used and the method of EAE induction. Some models are monophasic, some are relapsing, and others are chronic progressive. Monophasic models (B10.PL strain) are best suited for studying mechanisms involved in downregulation of autoimmune responses, whereas relapsing models (SJL strain) are amenable to studying mechanisms involved in relapses. Chronic disability models (C57BL/6 strain) are suitable for studying mechanisms of inflammation-mediated neuronal degeneration.[13] It is of importance that genetic background appears to dictate in large measure what type of disease course will be induced.

Decades of work have described the immunology and the neuropathology of EAE. Immunologic studies have focused on myelin protein–specific immune responses, including those directed against myelin basic protein (MBP), proteolipid protein (PLP), and myelin oligodendrocyte protein (MOG). Much of what has been theorized in MS with respect to immune responses was based on initial findings in EAE, including the roles of Th1 cytokines, interleukin 17 (IL-17), chemokines, adhesion molecules, and costimulatory molecules. Regarding the neuropathology of EAE, past studies focused on detailed characterization of lesions with respect to inflammatory infiltrate composition, level of demyelination, level of oligodendrocyte loss, microglial activation, and astrocytic scar formation.[14-17] Less attention has focused on neurons, with only recent descriptions of a relationship between axonal loss and disability.[18] Our group and others have described CNS pathology "beyond the lesion" in normal-appearing white matter characterized by decreases in axon densities in white matter tracts of the dorsal spinal cord.[19-21] Another study described motor neuron dendritic abnormalities in gray matter of spinal cords of mice with EAE,[22] and our group showed that neuronal staining in spinal cord gray matter was abnormal even early during the course of EAE.[20] Regarding neuroimaging "beyond the lesion" in EAE, diffusion tensor imaging changes have been described in dorsal cord and optic nerve by others,[19,23] and cerebellar gray matter atrophy by our group.[24] Therefore, whereas EAE has been the prototypical Th1-mediated disease tool used by immunologists for decades, more recently it has also been characterized with respect to its neurodegenerative component by neuroscientists.

Because, like MS, EAE has both an inflammatory and a neurodegenerative component, one must begin to think of gender differences with respect to effects on both the immune system and the CNS. EAE in the SJL strain of mice has been characterized as having a gender bias that parallels that of MS, with males being less susceptible to disease than females.[25-29] In part, this difference may result from the protective effects of testosterone in male mice, as was suggested by studies demonstrating that removal of physiologic levels of testosterone from male mice via castration increased disease susceptibility.[30,31] Also, in animal models of other autoimmune diseases in which a similar gender dimorphism exists (nonobese diabetic mice, thyroiditis, and adjuvant arthritis), castration has been shown to increase disease prevalence or disease severity or both.[32-35] Further, testosterone levels have been shown to be decreased in male mice during EAE relapse.[36] Together, these data support the hypothesis that endogenous androgens may be protective at physiologic levels.

Notably however, while the SJL, the ASW and the NZW strains of mice have increased susceptibility to EAE in females compared with males, the B10.PL and PL/J strains have more susceptibility to disease in males,[37] and there is no gender bias in the C57BL/6 strain.[38,39] Effects of removal of androgens in EAE were previously shown to be dependent on genetic background,[39] and in MS some autosomal gene linkages to susceptibility have been identified in one gender but not the other.[40] Therefore, in the outbred human population, the genetic background of some, but not all, individuals may be permissive to effects of gender. Importantly, because overall there is a gender difference in many autoimmune diseases in humans, we hypothesize that relatively permissive genetic backgrounds are likely to be prevalent, not rare, in occurrence.

The Effects of Pregnancy in Clinical Multiple Sclerosis

Sex hormones and/or sex-linked gene inheritance may be responsible for the enhanced susceptibility of females to MS. Evidence consistent with a role for sex hormones as disease modifiers comes from well-documented effects of pregnancy on MS. The majority of MS patients have either RRMS or SPMS, and it is thought that these two phases represent a continuum of disease. The RRMS phase is primarily an early inflammatory phase, and the SPMS phase is a relatively later, neurodegenerative phase. Effects of intercurrent pregnancy have been better characterized in RRMS than in SPMS, probably because of the age of the patients in each group and their respective child-bearing capacities. Subsequent effects of prior pregnancies can be assessed in both RRMS and SPMS groups.

It has been appreciated for decades that symptoms of patients with autoimmune diseases are affected by pregnancy and the postpartum period. These effects have been best characterized in MS, rheumatoid arthritis (RA), and psoriasis. Patients experience clinical improvement during pregnancy, with a temporary "rebound" exacerbation after delivery.[1,41-47] In contrast, women with SLE may experience an exacerbation of symptoms with gestation.[48] The differential effect of pregnancy on these diseases is thought to reflect the difference in immunopathogenesis of SLE, compared with MS, RA, and psoriasis.

EFFECTS ON RELAPSES

What is the precise effect of pregnancy on MS? Through decades of observations that MS improved during late pregnancy, the early studies did not separate into RRMS and SPMS groups.[41,42,49] What was generally described was a period of relative "safety" with regard to relapses during pregnancy, followed by a period of increased relapses after delivery. These clinical observations were supported by a study of two patients who underwent serial cerebral MRIs during pregnancy and after delivery. In both women, there was a decrease in MRI disease activity (T2 lesion number) during the second half of pregnancy and a return of activity to prepregnancy levels during the first months after delivery.[50] Other studies found, in addition to this effect on disease activity in patients with established MS, that the risk of developing a first episode of MS was decreased in pregnancy compared with nonpregnant states.[47] The most definitive study of the effect of pregnancy on MS was published in 1998 by the Pregnancy in Multiple Sclerosis (PRIMS) Group.[43] Relapse rates were determined in 254 women with MS during 269 pregnancies and for up to 1 year after delivery. The rate of relapse was significantly reduced, from 0.7 per woman-year in the year before pregnancy to 0.2 during the third trimester; it then increased to 1.2 during the first 3 months after delivery before returning to the prepregnancy rate. No significant changes were observed between relapse rates in the first and second trimesters compared with the year before pregnancy. Together, these data clearly demonstrated that the later months of pregnancy are associated with a significant reduction in MS relapses, and there is a rebound increase in relapses after delivery.

In a 2-year follow-up report by the PRIMS group, clinical factors that predicted postpartum flares were examined. Neither breast feeding nor epidural anesthesia affected the likelihood of postpartum relapse. The best predictor of which subjects would relapse after delivery was their prepregnancy relapse rate: those with the most active disease before pregnancy were the most likely to relapse afterward.[51]

EFFECTS ON DISABILITY

Because late pregnancy is associated with a reduction in relapses and the postpartum period with a transient increase in relapses, what is the net effect of pregnancy on the accumulation of disability? In a short-term 2-year follow-up study, no net effect of a single pregnancy on disability accumulation was observed.[51] However, long-term follow-up studies suggested that disability accumulation may be reduced significantly in women who become pregnant after the onset of MS.[52] A study by Damek and Shuster indicated that a full-term pregnancy increased the time interval to reach a common disability end point (walking with the aid of a cane or crutch). In essence, pregnancy increased the time interval to a secondary progressive course.[45] Runmarker and Andersen compared the risk of transition from a relapsing-remitting to a secondary progressive course in women who were pregnant after MS onset with that in women who were not pregnant after MS onset. Importantly, the two groups were matched for neurologic deficit, disease duration, and age. There was a significantly decreased risk of a progressive course in the women who were pregnant after MS.[47] Although the longer time interval to reach a secondary progressive course might be predicted if there were a selection bias (i.e., women with less disability being more likely to get pregnant) the careful matching of the groups made this explanation unlikely. Therefore, the study indeed provided support for a net beneficial effect of pregnancy on the accumulation of disability in MS.

Whereas there is clearly a short-term effect of pregnancy on decreasing the relapse rate and possibly a long-term effect of pregnancy on increasing the time interval to reach a given level of disability, there appear to be no conclusive data supporting a long-term effect of pregnancy in healthy individuals in regard to their subsequent risk of developing MS. One study reported that women of parity 0-2 developed MS twice as often as women of parity 3 or more, implying a protective effect of multiple pregnancies, but the difference did not reach statistical significance.[53] Another found no association between parity and the subsequent risk of developing MS.[54] These data indicate that pregnancy in healthy women has no long-lasting effects with regard to reducing the risk of developing MS in the future. However, pregnancy in women with established MS is indeed associated with a temporary reduction in relapses during the pregnancy. The effect of pregnancy appears to be similar to what is observed when patients take the approved anti-inflammatory therapies for MS: relapses are reduced temporarily during treatment but return after they are discontinued.

Given that late pregnancy is a state of temporary immunomodulation lasting 4 to 5 months, one then returns to the question of whether multiple pregnancies would be expected to have permanent effects on disability. It is known that up to 5 years of continuous treatment with immunomodulatory treatments has only a modest impact on disability in MS, and therefore a temporary anti-inflammatory effect of the third trimester of pregnancy would not be expected to have an impact on long-term disability. However, a pregnancy-associated neuroprotective effect (as yet unidentified), combined with the temporary anti-inflammatory effect, could reconcile the finding of a beneficial effect of pregnancy on long-term disability.

EFFECTS ON THE IMMUNE SYSTEM

The mechanisms of action of approved injectable therapies for MS involve anti-inflammatory effects, and these treatments result primarily in a reduction in relapse rates. Therefore, it is logical to hypothesize that mechanisms underlying the protective effect of pregnancy on MS relapses involve anti-inflammatory effects. Indeed, pregnancy has been shown to have significant effects on the immune system.

Pregnancy is a challenge for the immune system. From the mother's standpoint, the fetus is an allograft, because it harbors antigens inherited from the father. It is evolutionarily advantageous for the mother to transiently suppress cytotoxic, cell-mediated, Th1-type immune responses involved in fetal rejection during pregnancy. However, not all immune responses should be suppressed, because humoral, Th2-type immunity is needed for passive transfer of antibodies to the fetus. Therefore, a shift in immune responses involving a downregulation of Th1 and an upregulation of Th2 is thought to be necessary for fetal survival.[55-58] Indeed, it has been shown in both mice and humans that failure to shift immune responses in this manner results in an increase in spontaneous abortion.[56,59,60] This shift from Th1 to Th2 responses occurs both locally at the maternal fetal interface[58,61,62] and systemically.[56,59,60,63-65] In two studies, MS subjects were observed longitudinally for immune responses during pregnancy and after delivery. Gilmore and colleagues demonstrated that ex vivo stimulated peripheral blood mononuclear cells (PBMCs) after delivery had increased production of interferon-γ (IFN-γ), compared to the third trimester, and that myelin protein–specific T-cell lines derived from subjects in the third trimester produced more IL-10.[66] Al-Shammri and associates found that ex vivo stimulated PBMCs in six of eight MS patients showed a distinct shift from a Th2 cytokine bias (IL-4 and IL-10) during pregnancy toward a Th1 cytokine bias (IFN-γ and tumor necrosis factor-α [TNF-α]) after delivery.[67] In light of these data, it becomes highly plausible that these alterations in the immune response (i.e., a relative shift to Th2 during pregnancy, with a rebound back to Th1 after delivery) could underlie both the improvement in putative Th1-mediated autoimmune diseases during pregnancy and the postpartum exacerbation.

EFFECTS ON THE CENTRAL NERVOUS SYSTEM

Pregnancy is a complex event characterized by changes in numerous factors that may affect the CNS, including increases in estriol, estradiol, progesterone, and prolactin.[68] Potential neuroprotective effects of estrogens are discussed later. Recently, it was shown that pregnant mice have an enhanced ability to remyelinate white matter lesions and that prolactin regulates oligodendrocyte precursor proliferation and mimics this regenerative effect of pregnancy.[69] This finding may be potentially exploited in pursuit of a therapeutic repair strategy to increase remyelination. However, when considering the effect of prolactin treatment in neuroimmunologic diseases such as MS, one must consider that prolactin has pro-inflammatory properties that could potentially exacerbate disease, as has been shown in the MS model, EAE.[70] Therefore, when considering any pregnancy factor, its effects on both the CNS and the immune system must be considered. Notably, breast feeding, which would be associated with a prolonged state of increased levels of prolactin, was found to have no effect, compared with no breast feeding, with respect to the postpartum relapse rate in MS.[51] This lack of a difference in relapse rate may suggest that the pro-inflammatory properties of increased prolactin during breast feeding are not clinically significant. On the other hand, relapse rate is a relatively insensitive, albeit important, outcome measure. Future studies should compare immune responses, enhancing lesions on MRI, and prolactin levels in women with MS who are or are not breast feeding their babies.

EFFECTS OF PREGNANCY: CONCLUSIONS FROM RESEARCH

In summary, what is striking about pregnancy is that it represents a state that is characterized by two important changes. First, there is a downregulation of cellular immune responses. This relative immunosuppression likely occurs to prevent fetal rejection as a semi-foreign graft. Second, pregnancy is characterized by the presence of potentially neuroprotective hormones such as estrogens, progesterone, and prolactin. It would seem evolutionarily advantageous to have such neuroprotective factors present as neuronal and oligodendrocyte lineage cells in the fetus progress through critical developmental windows.[71] Together, the combined anti-inflammatory and neuroprotective state of pregnancy, which is perhaps aimed at protecting the fetus, is precisely what is needed to protect the CNS from inflammatory attack in MS.

MEDICAL MANAGEMENT DURING PREGNANCY

Basic research and clinical observations as outlined here suggest that late pregnancy is beneficial in MS and that the postpartum period is characterized by vulnerability to increased relapses. Given these insights, what is the current best medical management of MS as it relates to pregnancy?

The first consideration regarding pregnancy is that women and men with MS do not suffer from infertility problems as part of the natural history of the disease process.[72] Despite theoretical possibilities of effects of MS on fertility due to abnormalities in the hypothalamic-pituitary-adrenal axis or the hypothalamic-pituitary-gonadal axis,[73] observations thus far indicate that women and men with MS are normal with respect to their ability to bear children.[72,74] However, some disease-modifying drugs used in MS can be associated with infertility.[143] Mitoxantrone and cyclophosphamide, for example, are known to affect fertility.[74] It remains unknown whether treatment with some of the more widely used disease-modifying drugs may be associated with altered fertility during intercurrent use. IFN-beta has been associated with menstrual irregularities, but whether this has any effect on fertility remains unknown. There are no reports of negative effects of glatiramer acetate (Copaxone) use on fertility. Further, one must keep in mind that women with MS can have infertility issues at a rate consistent with the normal age-matched population. In those women with MS who pursue in vitro fertilization

(IVF) treatments, the question is often posed as to whether infertility treatments may alter hormonal balance and thereby affect MS disease activity. To date, there are too few cases of IVF in MS to warrant firm conclusions. Anecdotal reports suggest that IVF may be associated with an exacerbation of relapse in MS.[75] The increased relapse rate occurred mainly in patients treated with gonadotrophin-releasing hormone (GnRH) agonists, but not in the patients treated with GnRH antagonists. A explanatory mechanism for this finding remains unknown, and larger studies are needed to determine whether certain forms of IVF indeed exacerbate MS. Currently, there are no large studies establishing that this is necessarily the case.

A second consideration entails the management of MS disease-modifying drugs in women who wish to become pregnant. Copaxone is pregnancy Category B, whereas the interferons (Rebif, Avonex, and Betaseron) are Category C. An increased potential for spontaneous abortion has been reported for the interferons.[76,77] Low birth weight of the fetus was observed in one study[76] but not in another.[77] Women with MS who plan to become pregnant should be informed of the potential hazards of interferon use with respect to their fetus. Copaxone treatment appears to be safer, because, to date, there has been no documentation of negative outcomes related to Copaxone treatment in pregnancy. Nevertheless, there are still insufficient data to assume that Copaxone treatment is safe during pregnancy. Therefore, the current recommendation is that women with MS who plan to become pregnant should discontinue use of disease-modifying drugs for one to two menstrual cycles before attempting conception, particularly if they are taking an interferon. The greatest risk for relapse is after a woman has discontinued use of disease-modifying treatments but before she is pregnant or in the early stages of pregnancy; it is the latter half of pregnancy that appears to provide some natural protection from MS relapses. Based on clinical trial designs, there is a wash-out period of approximately 3 months from when disease-modifying drugs are discontinued until the majority of their disease protection potential is lost. Therefore, women with MS who discontinue disease-modifying treatments and then cannot become pregnant for 6 months or longer are at risk for relapse.

During the postpartum period, there is an increased susceptibility for relapses, principally within 3 to 6 months after delivery.[43] To prevent relapses during this period, many women with MS choose to resume disease-modifying drugs within 2 weeks after delivery of their child. This is based on the idea that it will take up to 3 months for disease-modifying drugs to provide protection from relapses, depending on the particular disease-modifying therapy. For example, based on the temporal window of effects of various treatments on inflammation as assessed by enhancing lesions on MRI, high-dose interferons may act more rapidly (1 to 3 months) after initiation of treatment, compared with Copaxone (3 to 6 months). How aggressive one chooses to be in preventing postpartum relapses should principally be driven by insights into how frequently relapses occurred before pregnancy. Indeed, it is the prepregnancy relapse rate, not breast feeding, method of delivery, or anesthesia, that has been shown to be the best predictor of postpartum relapse.[51] In general, if relapses were relatively well controlled with a given disease-modifying treatment before pregnancy, then the treatment may be resumed based on this prior responsiveness. If relapses were poorly controlled with a given treatment before pregnancy, then one might consider switching to a more potent disease-modifying treatment afterward.

An additional consideration with respect to choice of post-partum treatment relates to depression. Postpartum depression is a well known phenomenon that occurs in many healthy women as well as in those with MS. The interferons, but not Copaxone, have been associated with depression. The physician should weigh the risk of developing postpartum depression in women with MS who take interferons after delivery. Small studies, which were not placebo controlled, suggested that treatment with intravenous immunoglobulin might prevent postpartum relapses,[78] but larger, well-controlled studies are needed before this is established as an efficacious treatment option.

The desire to breast feed confounds decisions concerning the resumption of disease-modifying therapies after delivery. It is not currently known whether disease-modifying treatments may pass through the mother's milk to the baby, so none of these treatments are generally recommended for use while breast feeding. Because there is no evidence that breast feeding in and of itself protects women with MS from relapse,[51] this postpartum period characterized by breast feeding and no use of disease-modifying therapy represents a particularly vulnerable period for relapse. The patient must weigh the overall benefits of breast feeding for mother and baby against the risk of relapse during this time. A highly supportive environment, put in place ahead of time, is advisable, not only to reduce fatigue in the mother but also to have assistance readily available in case the mother experiences a relapse.

The Effects of Ovarian Hormones in Multiple Sclerosis

ESTROGEN TREATMENT AMELIORATES THE MOUSE MODEL OF MULTIPLE SCLEROSIS

Gender differences in MS and the EAE model may be related to sex hormones, sex chromosomes, or both. With respect to sex hormones, female sex hormones or male sex hormones may play a role. Because pregnancy changes include alterations in female sex hormones, the changes in disease during pregnancy are consistent with a potential role of female sex hormones in disease.

It was shown more than a decade ago that EAE in guinea pigs, rats, and rabbits improved during pregnancy.[41] Further, it was shown that relapsing-remitting EAE in SJL mice improved during late pregnancy.[79,80] The EAE model was then used to determine whether an increase in levels of a certain hormone during pregnancy might be responsible for disease improvement. Because estrogens and progesterone increase progressively during pregnancy to the highest levels in the third trimester, these hormones were candidates for possibly mediating a protective effect. Two estrogens, estradiol and estriol, each increase progressively during pregnancy. Estradiol is otherwise present at much lower, fluctuating levels during the menstrual cycle in nonpregnant women and female mice. Estriol is made by the fetal placental unit and is not otherwise present in nonpregnant states. Over the last 10 years, it has been shown in numerous studies that estrogen treatment (both estriol and estradiol) can ameliorate both active and adoptive EAE in several strains of mice (SJL, C57BL/6, B10.PL, B10.RIII).[81-89] Estriol treatment has also been shown to be effective in reducing clinical signs in EAE when administered after disease onset.[88] Finally, both estradiol and estriol have been shown to be efficacious in both female and male mice with EAE.[90]

ESTROGEN TYPE AND DOSE IN THE MOUSE MODEL OF MULTIPLE SCLEROSIS

A clinical amelioration of EAE occurred when estriol was used at doses sufficient to induce serum levels that would be physiologic with pregnancy. On the other hand, estradiol had to be used at doses several-fold higher than pregnancy levels to induce the same degree of disease protection.[87] Therefore, although it is clear that high doses of estradiol are protective in EAE, it has not yet been clearly established whether low doses of estradiol are protective. Because of major differences in metabolic rates between humans and mice, it is difficult to determine the equivalent in a mouse of the low-dose estrogen contained in an oral contraceptive pill. One can only use available physiologic benchmarks, such as the dose needed to induce a level in blood equal to that in pregnant mice, or the dose needed to induce an estrus level in an ovariectomized mouse. Rigorous comparisons of blood levels in pregnant or estrus mice, assessed in parallel with levels in estradiol-treated mice, are needed. Because ovariectomy removes physiologic levels of estradiol as well as progesterone, data on the effect of ovariectomy on EAE is somewhat informative. Some reports have found that ovariectomy of female mice makes EAE worse,[84] and others have found that ovariectomy does not have a significant effect on disease.[80] Therefore, it remains controversial whether low levels of endogenous estradiol which fluctuate during the menstrual cycle have a significant influence on EAE.

EFFECTS ON THE IMMUNE SYSTEM IN THE MOUSE MODEL OF MULTIPLE SCLEROSIS

Protective mechanisms of estrogen treatment (both estriol and estradiol) in EAE clearly involve anti-inflammatory processes, with estrogen-treated mice having fewer inflammatory lesions in the CNS.[88] In adoptive EAE in SJL mice, an increase in IL-10, with no change in IFN-γ, was observed in ex vivo stimulated MBP-specific responses; this was accompanied by an increase in MBP-specific antibody of the IgG1 isotype but no change in that of the IgG2a isotype.[88] In active EAE in C57BL/6 mice, decreased levels of TNF-α, IFN-γ, and IL-6 were observed, with an increase in IL-5.[81,82,89,90] Estrogen treatment has also been shown to downregulate chemokines in the CNS of mice with EAE and may affect expression of matrix metalloprotease 9 (MMP-9), each of these changes leading to impaired recruitment of cells to the CNS.[84,86] In addition, estrogen treatment has been shown to impair the ability of dendritic cells to present antigen.[83,91] Finally, estrogen treatment has recently been shown to induce $CD4^{+}CD25^{+}$ regulatory T cells in EAE.[92,93] Therefore, estrogen treatment has been shown to be anti-inflammatory through a variety of mechanisms.

EFFECTS ON THE CENTRAL NERVOUS SYSTEM IN THE MOUSE MODEL OF MULTIPLE SCLEROSIS

An anti-inflammatory effect of estrogen treatment in EAE does not preclude an additional, more direct neuroprotective effect. Estrogens are lipophilic, readily traversing the blood–brain barrier, with the potential to be directly neuroprotective.[94-96] Numerous reviews have described estrogen's neuroprotective effects, both in vitro and in vivo,[95-97] in other model systems. Given the neuroprotective effect of estrogen treatment in other disease models, a possible neuroprotective effect of estrogen treatment in EAE was investigated. Estradiol treatment reduced clinical disease severity and was anti-inflammatory with respect to cytokine production in peripheral immune cells; it also decreased CNS white matter inflammation and demyelination. In addition, decreased neuronal staining, accompanied by increased immunolabeling of microglial/monocyte cells surrounding these abnormal neurons, was observed in gray matter of the spinal cords in placebo-treated EAE mice at the earliest stage of clinical disease, and treatment with estradiol significantly reduced this gray matter pathology. Therefore, estradiol treatment was not only anti-inflammatory but also neuroprotective in the prevention of both white and gray matter pathology in spinal cords of mice with EAE.[20]

ESTROGEN RECEPTORS THAT MEDIATE PROTECTION FROM THE MOUSE MODEL OF MULTIPLE SCLEROSIS

Determining which estrogen receptor mediates the protective effect of an estrogen treatment in disease is of central importance for the future development of selective estrogen receptor modifiers that aim to maximize efficacy and minimize toxicity. The actions of estrogen are mediated primarily by nuclear estrogen receptors, ERα and ERβ, although nongenomic membrane effects have also been described.[98] ERα and ERβ are expressed in both the immune system and the CNS.[99-102] Estrogen receptor knockout mice have been used to show that the protective effect of estrogen treatment (estradiol and estriol) in EAE was dependent on the presence of ERα but not ERβ.[85,89] A highly selective ERα ligand, propyl pyrazole triol (PPT),[103] was then used to determine whether stimulation of ERα in developmentally normal mice would be sufficient for the estrogen-mediated protection in EAE. Our group[20] and another[104] each found that treatment with this ERα-selective ligand was indeed sufficient for protection in EAE and was capable of mediating an anti-inflammatory effect on cytokine production. ERα ligand treatment also induced favorable changes in autoantigen-specific cytokine production in the peripheral immune system (i.e., decreased TNF-α, IFN-γ, and IL-6, with increased IL-5). It also protected from white and gray matter pathology in the CNS in a manner similar to that observed with estradiol treatment.

Subsequently, bone marrow chimers were used by Garidou and colleagues to show that the disease-ameliorating effects of estradiol treatment in EAE were not dependent on ERα signaling in blood-derived inflammatory cells.[105] This suggested that the functionally significant target for estrogen's actions in vivo during EAE are cells within the CNS. Given that treatment with either estradiol or the ERα ligand was anti-inflammatory and neuroprotective, the central question then became whether the neuroprotective properties of estrogen treatment in EAE were dependent on the anti-inflammatory properties. A recent study had suggested that an anti-inflammatory effect was necessary to observe estrogen-mediated neuroprotection in stroke.[106]

Differential neuroprotective and anti-inflammatory effects of ERα and ERβ ligand treatment revealed insights into this question. Our group contrasted the effects of treatment with an ERα versus an ERβ ligand in EAE.[21] Clinically, ERα ligand treatment abrogated disease at the onset and throughout the disease course. In contrast, ERβ ligand treatment had no effect at disease onset but promoted recovery during the chronic phase of the disease. ERα ligand treatment was anti-inflammatory in the systemic immune system, whereas ERβ ligand treatment was not. Also, ERα ligand treatment reduced CNS inflammation, but ERβ ligand treatment did not. Treatment with either the ERα or the ERβ ligand was neuroprotective, as evidenced by reduced demyelination and preservation of axon numbers in white matter as well as decreased neuronal abnormalities in gray matter. Therefore, by using the ERβ selective ligand, we dissociated the anti-inflammatory effect from the neuroprotective effect of estrogen treatment and showed that the neuroprotective effects of estrogen treatment were not necessarily dependent on anti-inflammatory properties.

ORAL CONTRACEPTIVE USE IN MULTIPLE SCLEROSIS

Levels of estrogens that are lower than those which occur during pregnancy, such as levels induced by oral contraceptives or hormone replacement therapy, may or may not be high enough to be protective in MS. Although some studies have attempted to simulate a situation of treatment with oral contraceptives in EAE mice and have shown an effect on disease,[81,86] the doses used in mice are not readily translatable to humans. In fact, the data in humans thus far has suggested that treatment with oral contraceptives is not likely to suppress MS. The incidence rate of MS onset in both former and current oral contraceptive users was not different from that in never-users.[107] It is not surprising that former use of oral contraceptives in healthy women would have no effect on subsequent risk of developing MS, because the effect of treatment on the immune system would not be expected to be permanent. However, the fact that incidence rates for MS in current oral contraceptive pill users were not decreased (compared with never-users) suggests that the estrogens in oral contraceptives are not of sufficient type or dose to ameliorate the immunopathogenesis of MS even temporarily during current use. This remains an unresolved issue, because controversial results have emerged with respect to the use of oral contraceptives and MS risk during current use.[54,108]

Studies of hormone replacement therapy and effects on disease activity in RA can provide further clues in regard to which doses of estrogens could potentially be protective in MS.[109] In a randomized, placebo-controlled trial of transdermal estradiol in 200 postmenopausal RA patients who also continued other antirheumatic medications, it was found that those who achieved a serum estradiol level greater than 100 pmol/L had significant improvements in articular index, pain scores, morning stiffness, and sedimentation rate, whereas those with lower estradiol levels did not demonstrate improvement.[110] There has been no consistent correlation between disease markers in MS or RA and hormone levels during the menstrual cycle. Based on these reports, it is likely that a sustained level of a sufficient dose of an estrogen is necessary to ameliorate disease activity in MS and RA.

A PILOT TRIAL OF ESTRIOL TREATMENT IN MULTIPLE SCLEROSIS

Because estriol is the major estrogen of pregnancy, and because an estriol dose that yielded a pregnancy level in mice was protective in EAE,[88] estriol was administered in a prospective pilot clinical trial to women with MS, in an attempt to recapitulate the protective effect of pregnancy on disease.[111] A crossover study was used whereby patients were monitored for 6 months before treatment to establish baseline disease activity; monitoring included cerebral MRI every month and neurologic examination every 3 months. The patients were then treated with oral estriol (8 mg/day) for 6 months, then observed for 6 more months in the post-treatment period. Six patients with RRMS and four with SPMS finished the 18-month study period. The RRMS subjects were then retreated with oral estriol and progesterone in a 4-month extension phase.

Estriol treatment resulted in serum estriol levels that approximated levels observed in untreated, healthy control women who were 6 months pregnant. When PBMCs were stimulated ex vivo, a favorable shift in cytokine profile (decreased TNF-α, increased IL-10 and IL-5) was observed during treatment, compared with baseline.[112] On serial MRIs, the RRMS patients demonstrated an 80% reduction in gadolinium-enhancing lesions within 3 months of treatment, compared with pretreatment,[111] and this improvement correlated with the favorable shift in cytokine profiles.[112] Importantly, gadolinium-enhancing disease activity gradually returned to baseline in the post-treatment period, and the favorable cytokine shift also returned to baseline. Further, during the 4-month extension phase of the study, both the decrease in brain-enhancing lesions and the favorable immune shift returned on retreatment with estriol in combination with progesterone in the RRMS group. These latter data have important translational implications, because progesterone treatment is needed in combination with estrogen treatment to prevent uterine endometrial hyperplasia when estriol is administered for 1 year or longer. These results indicate that treatment with progesterone in combination with estriol did not neutralize the beneficial effect of estriol treatment on these biomarkers of disease. A multicenter, double-blind, placebo-controlled trial of estriol treatment in RRMS is now ongoing.

SUMMARY OF ESTROGEN EFFECTS IN MULTIPLE SCLEROSIS

A protective effect of relatively high doses of estrogens (estradiol and estriol) within the late pregnancy range has been demonstrated in the MS model, but a role for lower, endogenous, fluctuating levels of estrogens during the menstrual cycle is controversial. Mechanisms underlying the protective effects of high-dose estrogens include both anti-inflammatory and neuroprotective properties. Anti-inflammatory properties of estrogen treatment in EAE are mediated primarily by ERα, not ERβ. However, there is a role for ERβ in neuroprotection. Whether treatment with supplemental estrogens may be protective in women with MS is currently being investigated through clinical trials.

The Effects of Testicular Hormones in Multiple Sclerosis

EFFECT OF ENDOGENOUS ANDROGENS IN THE MOUSE MODEL OF MULTIPLE SCLEROSIS

Gender differences in MS and the EAE model may be related to sex hormones, sex chromosomes, or both. This section discusses a possible role for male sex hormones. To begin to test the role of endogenous androgens in MS, the EAE model was used. Because EAE in the SJL strain of mice had previously been characterized to have a gender difference that paralleled that of MS, with males being less susceptible to disease than females,[28,29] the SJL strain was used. Protective effects of testosterone in male mice were shown by studies demonstrating that the removal of physiologic levels of testosterone from male mice via castration increased disease susceptibility.[30,39] Also, testosterone levels were shown to be decreased in male mice during EAE relapse.[36] Together, these data support the hypotheses that endogenous androgens are protective at physiologic levels in this MS model.

Because the MS population is genetically heterogeneous, it was then determined whether the protective effect of endogenous androgens was a phenomenon that was unique to the SJL strain. The C57BL/6 strain was used, because there is no gender bias in EAE in this strain.[37-39] Disease severity did not differ between castrated and sham-treated C57BL/6 male mice, and this lack of protective effect was not due to lower levels of endogenous androgens in the C57BL/6 strain compared with the SJL strain. Thus, equivalent levels of endogenous androgens were shown to be protective in males of one genetic background but not another.[39]

ANDROGEN TREATMENT IN THE MOUSE MODEL OF MULTIPLE SCLEROSIS

Treatment of EAE was done using either testosterone or 5-α-dihydrotestosterone (DHT), a form of testosterone that cannot be converted to estrogen. Both androgen treatments were shown to be protective in gonadally intact males of a strain in which endogenous androgens are protective (SJL), and they were also protective in a strain in which endogenous androgens are not protective (C57BL/6).[39] These data indicated that, even in genetic backgrounds that are not permissive to a protective effect of endogenous androgens, protection can still be provided by supplemental exogenous androgen treatment. This suggested that the mechanisms of disease protection may differ between endogenous physiologic androgens and supplemental supraphysiologic androgen treatment. These preclinical data laid the groundwork for clinical trials of testosterone treatment in the heterogeneous MS population.

MECHANISMS IN THE MOUSE MODEL OF MULTIPLE SCLEROSIS

Mechanisms underlying the protective effects of androgens have been previously investigated, and a number of studies have delineated immunologic changes in androgen-treated mice. One mechanism through which exogenous androgen treatment is protective in EAE involves effects on cytokine production.[113-116] Because testosterone can be converted to estrogen in vivo, and because estrogens have been shown to be neuroprotective in EAE (as discussed earlier), it is possible that testosterone treatment may be neuroprotective in EAE based on this conversion. However, this hypothesis has not been studied in MS or EAE.

TESTOSTERONE LEVELS IN MEN WITH MULTIPLE SCLEROSIS

MS disease onset in females typically occurs soon after puberty. In males, disease onset usually occurs later in life (age 30 to 40 years), coinciding with the age at which serum testosterone levels begin to decline in normal healthy men.[117-121] Interestingly, this phenomenon may be true of other autoimmune diseases as well.

The onset of RA in men also takes place later in life, with a reported fourfold increase in incidence rates in older men (age 35 to 74) compared with younger men (age 18 to 34). Further, the female-to-male ratio of RA is 4:1 between ages 35 and 44 and decreases to 1.1:1 by age 75.[122] Together, these observations suggested that relatively high levels of testosterone in young men after puberty may provide temporary protection from autoimmune disease onset in those men who are genetically predisposed to ultimately develop disease.

Additionally, it has been reported that 24% of male MS patients tested had significantly lower levels of testosterone than age-matched healthy men.[123] The reason for the decreased testosterone levels remains unclear. It may be due to gonadal failure or to effects on the hypothalamic-pituitary axis such as stress or hypothalamic lesions.[36] In men with MS and sexual dysfunction, low testosterone levels were shown to be associated with low levels of luteinizing hormone, thereby ruling out gonadal failure.[36] A decrease in free testosterone levels has also been reported in untreated men with new-onset RA,[124] making the possibility of hypothalamic lesions in the brain of men with MS less likely. An effect of the stress of chronic illness on the hypothalamic-pituitary axis may be the most likely explanation for the relatively lower levels of testosterone in men with chronic autoimmune diseases.

TESTOSTERONE TREATMENT IN MULTIPLE SCLEROSIS

Data from EAE studies suggested that supplemental, exogenous testosterone treatment might provide protection across genetic backgrounds in men of the heterogeneous MS population.[39] To investigate possible effects of testosterone treatment in MS, testosterone was administered via transdermal application (AndroGel) to men with RRMS in a small pilot trial (10 g of gel, containing 100 mg testosterone, per day).[9] A crossover design, using a within-arm comparison of 6 months pretreatment to 12 months treatment, was used to reduce the effect of disease heterogeneity given the small sample size, as previously described in MS.[125]

Ten subjects with RRMS completed the study. The average age was 46 years (range, 29 to 61 years). The median disease duration was 12.5 years (range, 0.5 to 25 years). The subjects were relatively mildly affected with MS, having a median Expanded Disability Status Scale (EDSS) score of 2.0 (range, 1.5 to 2.5). At baseline, all subjects had testosterone levels in the lower range of normal, with a mean concentration of 493 ng/dL (range, 321 to 732 ng/dL). During daily treatment with testosterone, serum testosterone levels rose 50% on average, to the higher range of normal. Lean body mass (muscle mass) increased significantly during treatment.

Scores from the Paced Auditory Serial Addition Task (PASAT) component of the Multiple Sclerosis Functional Composite (MSFC), a commonly used cognitive test for patients with MS, remained stable during the first 6 months of treatment (i.e., at months 3 and 6), trended upward after 9 months, and were significantly improved by month 12 of treatment. There was also a trend for improvement in spatial memory. These findings were consistent with previous reports of testosterone-mediated improvements in working and spatial memory in healthy, nonhypogonadal elderly men.[126,127] No significant changes were observed in classic MS disability measures of the EDSS, the nine-hole peg test, or the 25-foot timed walk. This was not surprising, because these measures generally require long-term observation (3 to 5 years) to detect changes.

The 10 subjects had low levels of enhancing lesion activity on brain MRI at baseline, and this low level was not significantly increased or decreased with treatment. The lack of a decrease in measures of inflammatory activity on MRI during treatment with testosterone may be related to the relatively low levels of inflammatory activity present at baseline. The exclusion of subjects undergoing disease-modifying treatments probably created a selection bias toward subjects with relatively milder clinical disease and less inflammatory activity on MRI. Therefore, in this subject group, it could be concluded only that testosterone treatment did not significantly increase inflammatory activity on otherwise relatively quiescent MRIs.

The most interesting finding of the study was the effect on brain atrophy. At study onset, the mean normalized whole brain volume was 0.82 (range, 0.78 to 0.84) and was negatively correlated with age ($P = .05$). During the first 9 months of the study, brain volumes decreased at an annualized rate of –0.81% ($P = .0001$). This was consistent with rates previously observed in MS patients.[128] During the subsequent 9 months of testosterone treatment, brain atrophy slowed to an annualized rate of –0.26%, representing a 67% reduction in the rate of brain volume loss compared with the pretreatment period. Interestingly, the timing of the cognitive improvements coincided with the slowing of brain atrophy on MRI. The protective effect of testosterone treatment on brain atrophy was observed in the absence of an appreciable anti-inflammatory effect, possibly suggesting direct neuroprotective effects. Larger, placebo-controlled trials of testosterone treatment in men with MS are warranted.

SUMMARY OF THE EFFECTS OF TESTICULAR HORMONES IN MULTIPLE SCLEROSIS

In the MS model EAE, endogenous androgens are protective in some strains but not others. However exogenous supplemental treatment with testosterone is protective across genetic backgrounds. An immunomodulatory role has been shown, but direct effects on the CNS have not been studied in the model. In humans with MS, we hypothesize that some, but not all, men may be of a genetic background that is permissive to a protective effect derived from the relatively high physiologic levels of testosterone that exist in young men. This effect may mask early presentation of the relapsing-remitting phase of the disease. As these men age, testosterone levels gradually decline, and clinical MS onset is observed. Later during the course of disease, it is possible that the stress of chronic disease may affect the hypothalamic-pituitary axis to suppress testosterone levels further, to within the low-normal range. Whether treatment with supplemental testosterone may offer some protection in men with MS is currently being investigated through clinical trials.

The Effects of Sex Chromosomes in Multiple Sclerosis

An alternative but not mutually exclusive explanation for sex hormone–induced differences in EAE and MS is a direct genetic effect. That is, specific gene products, which are not induced by gonadal hormones yet are expressed in a sexually dimorphic manner in either the immune system or the CNS, could induce gender-specific patterns of immune system or CNS development or function.

In male mammals, the Y-linked gene *Sry* is expressed in cells of the undifferentiated gonadal ridges, causing them to differentiate into Sertoli cells, which begins the differentiation of the testes.[129] Once the testes have formed, they secrete hormones distinct from those of the ovary, and these hormonal differences generate gender differences in many nongonadal tissues, including the external genitalia, immune system, and CNS. Indeed, the effects of these hormones account for the majority of gender differences in nongonadal tissues identified to date. However, there are other genetic differences between males and females that arise from the difference in sex chromosome complement and could also contribute to gender differences in phenotype.[130,131] There are other Y genes whose role in nongonadal tissues has been little studied, and there are also variations in X gene expression arising from differences in X chromosome complement. Because it has been much easier to study the effects of gonadal hormones than these possible direct effects of X and Y genes, the sexually differentiating effects of hormones are much better understood. This section focuses on whether direct actions of X or Y genes may also be important.

EFFECTS OF SEX CHROMOSOME COMPLEMENT ON IMMUNE RESPONSES

Because the study of gonadectomized female and male mice yields only limited information about putative effects of genes on sex chromosomes, our group employed a mouse strain that had been used by investigators studying sexually dimorphic development.[131-136] In these mice, the testis-determining gene *Sry* is "moved" from the Y chromosome to an autosome by successive deletion from the Y chromosome and insertion of a *Sry* transgene onto an autosome. Thus, the inheritance of genes causing testicular differentiation is separated from the Y chromosome; the Y chromosome can be present or absent in phenotypic male (testis-bearing) mice, and it can be present or absent in phenotypic female (ovary-bearing) mice. The Y chromosome that is deficient in the *Sry* gene is denoted Y⁻, and XY⁻*Sry* male mice carry the *Sry* transgene. When such a mouse is mated with an XX female, four progeny result: XX females, XY⁻ females, XX*Sry* males, and XY⁻*Sry* males. These four genotypes are informative with respect to discerning effects of genes normally located on sex chromosomes.

To determine the role of sex chromosome genes on autoantigen-specific immune responses, we backcrossed the outbred MF1Y⁻*Sry* mice onto the SJL strain. To address direct effects of sex chromosomes on immune responses, these responses were examined in SJL mice that differed in their complement of sex chromosomes while having the same gonadal type. This allowed determination of the effect of sex chromosomes on immune responses in the absence of confounding effects of exposure to different types of adult or developmental sex hormones. The effects of sex chromosome genotype on the immune response could be determined in the setting of a masculine endocrine environment by comparing XX*Sry* male mice with XY⁻*Sry* male mice. They could also be examined in a feminine endocrine environment by comparing XX female mice with XY⁻ female mice.

Using these informative experiments on mice that differed is sex chromosome complement while sharing a common gonadal type, autoantigen-specific immune responses were more robust with respect to the production of cytokines (IFN-γ, TNF-α, IL-10) in XY⁻ mice than in XX mice. An immunostimulatory effect of the XY⁻ chromosome complement was surprising, because wild-type males were known to have decreased immune responses compared with females, and testosterone was known to be inhibitory.[1,34,35,39,113-115,137,138] One would have predicted that the effects of the male sex chromosome complement would be synergistic with, not opposed to, the effects of the male hormone testosterone, and that the combined result would be a relatively low level of immune responsiveness in SJL males as compared with females.[1,28,114,139,140] Instead, the male sex chromosome complement was relatively stimulatory. This was the first experimental evidence of a compensatory "yin-yang" effect of sex chromosome complement and sex hormones on a biologic process.[141] Such an effect had previously been proposed only in a hypothetical fashion in brain development.[142]

The opposing actions of the male hormone and the male genome suggest the evolution of a compensatory relationship between the two, which would serve to decrease immune response differences between females and males in situations where extreme differences might be maladaptive. In the case of the autoantigen-specific immune response in the SJL mouse, testosterone has indeed overcompensated, in that intact, wild-type males have a less robust immune response than females. It is possible that these two forces may more precisely offset each other in other strains of mice, resulting in no net gender difference in response. This theory has broad implications for the study of the effects of sex hormones and sex chromosome complement even on biologic events that are not characterized by a sexual dimorphism. In essence, the two sexes may reach a common and equal biologic end point (phenotypic sexual equality) through opposing contributions of gender-specific (sexually unequal) hormonal or genetic signals. Whether a yin-yang (compensatory) effect or an additive (complementary) effect of sex hormones and sex chromosome complement exists in other organ systems remains to be determined. Evolutionary pressure may favor an antagonistic relationship in some organ systems and a synergistic relationship in others, depending on pressures on male and female animals.

SEX CHROMOSOME EFFECTS IN A MOUSE MODEL OF MULTIPLE SCLEROSIS

The finding that the XY^- sex chromosome complement, compared with the XX, resulted in relatively more robust autoantigen-specific cytokine responses supported the concept of direct effects of sex chromosomes on autoimmunity. However, because these cytokines can have both pro-inflammatory and anti-inflammatory roles in EAE, the role of sex chromosome complement in disease remained unknown. To directly assess this question, EAE was induced in mice with the informative sex chromosome complements.[143] SJL castrated male mice that were either XX*Sry* or XY^-Sry had active EAE induced with the PLP 139-151 peptide. The clinical disease course was significantly more severe in the XX*Sry* mice than in the XY^-Sry mice. This significant difference in disease severity also occurred in ovariectomized female XX versus XY^- mice. Further, in adoptive EAE, CNS pathology revealed higher levels of inflammation in mice that had received autoantigen-specific cells derived from XX mice, compared with those derived from XY^- mice. Together, these data showed that the XX sex chromosome complement, compared with XY^-, was associated with greater encephalitogenicity.

Because it had been shown previously that no gender bias exists in EAE in the C57BL/6 strain of mice,[37-39] we investigated whether an effect of sex chromosomes could be found in this strain.[143] C57BL/6 castrated male mice that were either XX*Sry* or XY⁻Sry had active EAE induced with the MOG 35-55 peptide. In contrast to results in the SJL mice, the clinical disease course was no different in XX*Sry* compared with XY⁻Sry mice. Likewise, there was no difference in disease course in ovariectomized female XX versus XY⁻ mice. Together, these data indicated the presence of a sex chromosome effect in a strain exhibiting gender difference in EAE (the SJL) but not in a strain characterized by no gender difference in EAE (the C57BL/6). This finding revealed an interaction between sex chromosome complement and genetic background. Significantly, the effects of sex hormones in EAE were also previously been shown to be dependent on genetic background,[39] and some autosomal gene linkages to susceptibility to MS in humans have been identified in one gender but not the other.[40] Therefore, in the outbred human population, the genetic background of some, but not all, individuals may be permissive to sex chromosome or sex hormone effects. Because there is a gender difference in many autoimmune diseases in humans, we hypothesize that relatively permissive genetic backgrounds are likely to be prevalent, not rare, in occurrence.

SUMMARY OF SEX CHROMOSOME COMPLEMENT EFFECTS

Data from studies of the informative *Sry* transgenic mice indicated that the XX sex chromosome complement was disease promoting, compared with the XY⁻ complement. It remains to be determined whether this effect results from (1) a gene or genes unique to the Y chromosome, (2) a higher dose of X genes that escape X-inactivation in XX mice, or (3) paternal imprinting of X genes that are present in XX but not XY⁻ mice.[131] Candidate autoimmune regulatory genes on the X chromosome include IL-13Rα (*IL13RA1*), CD40 ligand (*CD40LG*), forkhead box P3 (*FOXP3*), and toll-like receptor 7 (*TLR7*). Further studies mapping the gene on either X or Y are needed to discern the mechanisms that underlie direct sex chromosome effects in the MS model.

Conclusions

Gender differences in autoimmune diseases are prevalent across numerous human diseases, including MS, and in numerous animal models of these diseases, including EAE. Effects of sex hormones (estrogens and androgens) and sex chromosomes (XX and XY) have been shown in the immunopathogenesis of EAE. Further study is needed to determine the extent of these effects in the CNS.

Sex hormones and sex chromosomes can have synergistic or antagonistic effects, depending on the processes and the tissues being studied. Further, some hormone effects and sex chromosome complement effects are more readily observed on some autosomal genetic backgrounds than on others. The complexity of this system is not surprising given the prior precedent of numerous genetic contributions to complex polygenetic diseases, wherein some genes serving to enhance disease and others to suppress it.

Autoimmune diseases have classically been thought to result from interactions among environmental and genetic factors, with the latter generally referring to autosomal genetic background. This approach should be now be modified.

Autoimmune diseases should be considered to be caused by interactions among the environment, the autosomal genetic background, and gender-specific factors such as sex hormones and sex chromosomes.

REFERENCES

1. Whitacre CC, Reingold SC, O'Looney PA: A gender gap in autoimmunity. Science 1999; 283:1277.
2. Cerghet M, Skoff RP, Bessert D, et al: Proliferation and death of oligodendrocytes and myelin proteins are differentially regulated in male and female rodents. J Neurosci 2006;26:1439.
3. Spring S, Lerch JP, Henkelman RM: Sexual dimorphism revealed in the structure of the mouse brain using three-dimensional magnetic resonance imaging. Neuroimage 2007;35:1424.
4. Weinshenker BG: Natural history of multiple sclerosis. Ann Neurol 1994;36:S6.
5. Duquette P, Pleines J, Girard M, et al: The increased susceptibility of women to multiple sclerosis. Can J Neurol Sci 1992;19:466.
6. Orton SM, Herrera BM, Yee IM, et al: Sex ratio of multiple sclerosis in Canada: A longitudinal study. Lancet Neurol 2006;5:932.
7. Confavreux C, Vukusic S, Adeleine P: Early clinical predictors and progression of irreversible disability in multiple sclerosis: An amnesic process. Brain 2003;126:770.
8. Runmarker B, Andersson C, Odén A, Andersen O: Prediction of outcome in multiple sclerosis based on multivariate models. J Neurol 1994;241:597.
9. Sicotte NL, Giesser BS, Tandon V, et al: Testosterone treatment in multiple sclerosis: A pilot study. Arch Neurol 2007;64:683.
10. Pozzilli C, Tomassini V, Marinelli F, et al: "Gender gap" in multiple sclerosis: Magnetic resonance imaging evidence. Eur J Neurol 2003;10:95.
11. Hawkins SA, McDonnell GV: Benign multiple sclerosis? Clinical course, long term follow up, and assessment of prognostic factors. J Neurol Neurosurg Psychiatry 1999;67:148.
12. Tomassini V, Onesti E, Mainero C, et al: Sex hormones modulate brain damage in multiple sclerosis: MRI evidence. J Neurol Neurosurg Psychiatry 2005;76:272.
13. Voskuhl RR: Chronic relapsing experimental allergic encephalomyelitis in the SJL mouse: Relevant techniques. Methods 1996;10:435.
14. Mokhtarian F, McFarlin DE, Raine CS: Adoptive transfer of myelin basic protein-sensitized T cells produces chronic relapsing demyelinating disease in mice. Nature 1984;309:356.
15. Brown A, McFarlin DE, Raine CS: Chronologic neuropathology of relapsing experimental allergic encephalomyelitis in the mouse. Lab Invest 1982;46:171.
16. Raine CS, Cannella B, Hauser SL, Genain CP: Demyelination in primate autoimmune encephalomyelitis and acute multiple sclerosis lesions: A case for antigen-specific antibody mediation. Ann Neurol 1999;46:144.
17. Raine CS, Barnett LB, Brown A, et al: Neuropathology of experimental allergic encephalomyelitis in inbred strains of mice. Lab Invest 1980;43:150.
18. Wujek JR, Bjartmar C, Richer E, et al: Axon loss in the spinal cord determines permanent neurological disability in an animal model of multiple sclerosis. J Neuropathol Exp Neurol 2002;61:23.
19. Deboy CA, Zhang J, Dike S, et al: High resolution diffusion tensor imaging of axonal damage in focal inflammatory and demyelinating lesions in rat spinal cord. Brain 2007;130:2199.
20. Morales LB, Loo KK, Liu HB, et al: Treatment with an estrogen receptor alpha ligand is neuroprotective in experimental autoimmune encephalomyelitis. J Neurosci 2006;26:6823.
21. Tiwari-Woodruff S, Morales LB, Lee R, Voskuhl RR: Differential neuroprotective and antiinflammatory effects of estrogen receptor (ER)alpha and ERbeta ligand treatment. Proc Natl Acad Sci U S A 2007;104:14813.
22. Bannerman PG, Hahn A, Ramirez S, et al: Motor neuron pathology in experimental autoimmune encephalomyelitis: Studies in THY1-YFP transgenic mice. Brain 2005;128:1877.
23. Kim JH, Budde MD, Liang HF, et al: Detecting axon damage in spinal cord from a mouse model of multiple sclerosis. Neurobiol Dis 2006;21:626.
24. Mackenzie-Graham A, Tinsley MR, Shah KP: Cerebellar cortical atrophy in experimental autoimmune encephalomyelitis. Neuroimage 2006;32:1016.
25. Bebo BF Jr, Adlard K, Schuster JC, et al: Gender differences in protection from EAE induced by oral tolerance with a peptide analogue of MBP-Ac1-11. J Neurosci Res 1999;55:432.

26. Bebo BF Jr, Schuster JC, Vandenbark AA, Offner H: Gender differences in experimental autoimmune encephalomyelitis develop during the induction of the immune response to encephalitogenic peptides. J Neurosci Res 1998;52:420.
27. Bebo BF Jr, Vandenbark AA, Offner H: Male SJL mice do not relapse after induction of EAE with PLP 139-151. J Neurosci Res 1996;45:680.
28. Kim S, Voskuhl RR: Decreased IL-12 production underlies the decreased ability of male lymph node cells to induce experimental autoimmune encephalomyelitis. J Immunol 1999;162:5561.
29. Voskuhl RR, Pitchekian-Halabi H, MacKenzie-Graham A, et al: Gender differences in autoimmune demyelination in the mouse: Implications for multiple sclerosis. Ann Neurol 1996;39:724.
30. Bebo BF Jr, Zelinka-Vincent E, Adamus, et al: Gonadal hormones influence the immune response to PLP 139-151 and the clinical course of relapsing experimental autoimmune encephalomyelitis. J Neuroimmunol 1998;84:122.
31. Smith ME, Eller NL, McFarland HF, et al: Age dependence of clinical and pathological manifestations of autoimmune demyelination: Implications for multiple sclerosis. Am J Pathol 1999;155:1147.
32. Fitzpatrick F, Lepault F, Homo-Delarche F, et al: Influence of castration, alone or combined with thymectomy, on the development of diabetes in the nonobese diabetic mouse. Endocrinology 1991;129:1382.
33. Ahmed SA, Penhale WJ: The influence of testosterone on the development of autoimmune thyroiditis in thymectomized and irradiated rats. Clin Exp Immunol 1982;48:367.
34. Fox HS: Androgen treatment prevents diabetes in nonobese diabetic mice. J Exp Med 1992;175:1409.
35. Harbuz MS, Perveen-Gill Z, Lightman SL, Jessop DS: A protective role for testosterone in adjuvant-induced arthritis. Br J Rheumatol 1995;34:1117.
36. Foster SC, Daniels C, Bourdette DN, Bebo BF Jr: Dysregulation of the hypothalamic-pituitary-gonadal axis in experimental autoimmune encephalomyelitis and multiple sclerosis. J Neuroimmunol 2003;140:78.
37. Papenfuss TL, Rogers CJ, Gienapp I, et al: Sex differences in experimental autoimmune encephalomyelitis in multiple murine strains. J Neuroimmunol 2004;150:59.
38. Okuda Y, Okuda M, Bernard CC: Gender does not influence the susceptibility of C57BL/6 mice to develop chronic experimental autoimmune encephalomyelitis induced by myelin oligodendrocyte glycoprotein. Immunol Lett 2002;81:25.
39. Palaszynski KM, Loo KK, Ashouri JF, et al: Androgens are protective in experimental autoimmune encephalomyelitis: Implications for multiple sclerosis. J Neuroimmunol 2004;146:144.
40. Kantarci OH, Goris A, Hebrink DD, et al: IFNG polymorphisms are associated with gender differences in susceptibility to multiple sclerosis. Genes Immun 2005;6:153.
41. Abramsky O: Pregnancy and multiple sclerosis. Ann Neurol 1994;36(Suppl):S38.
42. Birk K, Ford C, Smeltzer S, et al: The clinical course of multiple sclerosis during pregnancy and the puerperium. Arch Neurol 1990;47:738.
43. Confavreux C, Hutchinson M, Hours MM, et al: Rate of pregnancy-related relapse in multiple sclerosis. Pregnancy in Multiple Sclerosis Group [see comments]. N Engl J Med 1998;339:285.
44. Da Silva JA, Spector TD: The role of pregnancy in the course and aetiology of rheumatoid arthritis. Clin Rheumatol 1992;11:189.
45. Damek DM, Shuster EA: Pregnancy and multiple sclerosis. Mayo Clinic Proc 1997;72:977.
46. Nelson JL, Hughes KA, Smith AG, et al: Remission of rheumatoid arthritis during pregnancy and maternal-fetal class II alloantigen disparity. Am J Reprod Immunol 1992;28:226.
47. Runmarker B, Andersen O: Pregnancy is associated with a lower risk of onset and a better prognosis in multiple sclerosis [see comments]. Brain 1995;118:253.
48. Jungers P, Dougados M, Pélissier C, et al: Lupus nephropathy and pregnancy: Report of 104 cases in 36 patients. Arch Intern Med 1982;142:771.
49. Birk K, Smeltzer SC, Rudick R: Pregnancy and multiple sclerosis. Semin Neurol 1988;8:205.
50. van Walderveen MA, Tas MW, Barkhof F, et al: Magnetic resonance evaluation of disease activity during pregnancy in multiple sclerosis. Neurology 1994;44:327.
51. Vukusic S, Hutchinson M, Hours M: The Pregnancy in Multiple Sclerosis Group: Pregnancy and multiple sclerosis (the PRIMS study): Clinical predictors of post-partum relapse. Brain 2004;127:1353.
52. Verdru P, Theys P, D'Hooghe MB, Carton H: Pregnancy and multiple sclerosis: The influence on long term disability. Clin Neurol Neurosurg 1994;96:38.
53. Villard-Mackintosh L, Vessey MP: Oral contraceptives and reproductive factors in multiple sclerosis incidence. Contraception 1993;47:161.

54. Hernan MA, Hohol MJ, Olek MJ, et al: Oral contraceptives and the incidence of multiple sclerosis. Neurology 2000;55:848.
55. Formby B: Immunologic response in pregnancy: Its role in endocrine disorders of pregnancy and influence on the course of maternal autoimmune diseases. Endocrinol Metab Clin North Am 1995;24:187.
56. Hill JA, Polgar K, Anderson DJ: T-helper 1-type immunity to trophoblast in women with recurrent spontaneous abortion [see comments]. JAMA 1995;273:1933.
57. Raghupathy R: Th1-type immunity is incompatible with successful pregnancy [see comments]. Immunology Today 1997;18:478.
58. Wegmann TG, Lin H, Guilbert L, Mosmann TR: Bidirectional cytokine interactions in the maternal-fetal relationship: Is successful pregnancy a TH2 phenomenon? [see comments]. Immunol Today 1993;14:353.
59. Krishnan L, Guilbert LJ, Wegmann TG, et al: T helper 1 response against Leishmania major in pregnant C57BL/6 mice increases implantation failure and fetal resorptions: Correlation with increased IFN-gamma and TNF and reduced IL-10 production by placental cells. J Immunol 1996;156:653.
60. Marzi M, Vigano A, Trabattoni D, et al: Characterization of type 1 and type 2 cytokine production profile in physiologic and pathologic human pregnancy. Clin Exp Immunol 1996;106:127.
61. Lin H, Mosmann TR, Guilbert L, et al: Synthesis of T helper 2-type cytokines at the maternal-fetal interface. J Immunol 1993;151:4562.
62. Sacks GP, Clover LM, Bainbridge DR, et al: Flow cytometric measurement of intracellular Th1 and Th2 cytokine production by human villous and extravillous cytotrophoblast. Placenta 2001;22:550.
63. Dudley DJ, Chen CL, Mitchell MD, et al: Adaptive immune responses during murine pregnancy: Pregnancy-induced regulation of lymphokine production by activated T lymphocytes. Am J Obstet Gynecol 1993;168:1155.
64. Elenkov IJ, Wilder RL, Bakalov VK, et al: IL-12, TNF-alpha, and hormonal changes during late pregnancy and early postpartum: Implications for autoimmune disease activity during these times. J Clin Endocrinol Metab 2001;86:4933.
65. Fabris N, Piantanelli L, Muzzioli M: Differential effect of pregnancy or gestagens on humoral and cell-mediated immunity. Clin Exper Immunol 1977;28:306.
66. Gilmore W, Arias M, Stroud N, et al: Preliminary studies of cytokine secretion patterns associated with pregnancy in MS patients. J Neurol Sci 2004;224:69.
67. Al-Shammri S, Rawoot P, Azizieh F, et al: Th1/Th2 cytokine patterns and clinical profiles during and after pregnancy in women with multiple sclerosis. J Neurol Sci 2004;222:21.
68. Voskuhl R: Sex hormomes and other pregnancy-related factors with therapeutic potential in multiple sclerosis. In Cohen D, Rudick R (eds): Multiple Sclerosis Therapeutics, vol 32. London, Martin Dunitz, 2003, p 535.
69. Gregg C, Shikar V, Larsen P, et al: White matter plasticity and enhanced remyelination in the maternal CNS. J Neurosci 2007;27:1812.
70. Riskind PN, Massacesi L, Doolittle TH, Hauser SL: The role of prolactin in autoimmune demyelination: Suppression of experimental allergic encephalomyelitis by bromocriptine. Ann Neurol 1991;29:542.
71. Craig A, Ling Luo N, Beardsley DJ, et al: Quantitative analysis of perinatal rodent oligodendrocyte lineage progression and its correlation with human. Exp Neurol 2003;181:231.
72. Giesser BS: Gender issues in multiple sclerosis. Neurologist 2002;8:351.
73. Grinsted L, Heltberg A, Hagen C, Djursing H: Serum sex hormone and gonadotropin concentrations in premenopausal women with multiple sclerosis. J Intern Med 1989;226:241.
74. Cavalla P, Rovei V, Masera S, et al: Fertility in patients with multiple sclerosis: Current knowledge and future perspectives. Neurol Sci 2006;27:231.
75. Laplaud DA, Lefrere F, Leray E, et al: [Increased risk of relapse in multiple sclerosis patients after ovarian stimulation for in vitro fertilization.] Gynecol Obstet Fertil 2007;35:1047.
76. Boskovic R, Wide R, Wolpin J, et al: The reproductive effects of beta interferon therapy in pregnancy: A longitudinal cohort. Neurology 2005;65:807.
77. Sandberg-Wollheim M, Frank D, Goodwin TM, et al: Pregnancy outcomes during treatment with interferon beta-1a in patients with multiple sclerosis. Neurology 2005;65:802.
78. Achiron A, Kishner I, Dolev M, et al: Effect of intravenous immunoglobulin treatment on pregnancy and postpartum-related relapses in multiple sclerosis. J Neurol 2004;251:1133.

79. Langer-Gould A, Garren H, Slansky A, et al: Late pregnancy suppresses relapses in experimental autoimmune encephalomyelitis: Evidence for a suppressive pregnancy-related serum factor. J Immunol 2002;169:1084.
80. Voskuhl RR, Palaszynski K: Sex hormones and experimental autoimmune encephalomyelitis: Implications for multiple sclerosis. Neuroscientist 2001;7:258.
81. Bebo BF Jr, Fyfe-Johnson A, Adlard K, et al: Low-dose estrogen therapy ameliorates experimental autoimmune encephalomyelitis in two different inbred mouse strains. J Immunol 2001;166:2080.
82. Ito A, Bebo BF Jr, Matejuk A, et al: Estrogen treatment down-regulates TNF-alpha production and reduces the severity of experimental autoimmune encephalomyelitis in cytokine knockout mice. J Immunol 2001;167:542.
83. Liu HY, Buenafe AC, Matejuk A, et al: Estrogen inhibition of EAE involves effects on dendritic cell function. J Neurosci Res 2002;70:238.
84. Matejuk A, Adlard K, Zamora A, et al: 17beta-Estradiol inhibits cytokine, chemokine, and chemokine receptor mRNA expression in the central nervous system of female mice with experimental autoimmune encephalomyelitis. J Neurosci Res 2001;65:529.
85. Polanczyk M, Zamora A, Subramanian S, et al: The protective effect of 17beta-estradiol on experimental autoimmune encephalomyelitis is mediated through estrogen receptor-alpha. Am J Pathol 2003;163:1599.
86. Subramanian S, Matejuk A, Zamora A, et al: Oral feeding with ethinyl estradiol suppresses and treats experimental autoimmune encephalomyelitis in SJL mice and inhibits the recruitment of inflammatory cells into the central nervous system. J Immunol 2003;170:1548.
87. Jansson L, Olsson T, Holmdahl R: Estrogen induces a potent suppression of experimental autoimmune encephalomyelitis and collagen-induced arthritis in mice. J Neuroimmunol 1994;53:203.
88. Kim S, Liva SM, Dalal MA, et al: Estriol ameliorates autoimmune demyelinating disease: Implications for multiple sclerosis. Neurology 1999;52:1230.
89. Liu HB, Loo KK, Palaszynski K, et al: Estrogen receptor alpha mediates estrogen's immune protection in autoimmune disease. J Immunol 2003;171:6936.
90. Palaszynski KM, Liu H, Loo KK, Voskuhl RR: Estriol treatment ameliorates disease in males with experimental autoimmune encephalomyelitis: Implications for multiple sclerosis. J Neuroimmunol 2004;149:84.
91. Zhang QH, Hu YZ, Cao J, et al: Estrogen influences the differentiation, maturation and function of dendritic cells in rats with experimental autoimmune encephalomyelitis. Acta Pharmacol Sin 2004;25:508.
92. Polanczyk MJ, Carson BD, Subramanian S, et al: Cutting edge: Estrogen drives expansion of the CD4+CD25+ regulatory T cell compartment. J Immunol 2004;173:2227.
93. Matejuk A, Bakke AC, Hopke C, et al: Estrogen treatment induces a novel population of regulatory cells, which suppresses experimental autoimmune encephalomyelitis. J Neurosci Res 2004;77:119.
94. Brinton RD: Cellular and molecular mechanisms of estrogen regulation of memory function and neuroprotection against Alzheimer's disease: Recent insights and remaining challenges. Learn Mem 2001;8:121.
95. Garcia-Segura LM, Azcoitia I, DonCarlos LL: Neuroprotection by estradiol. Prog Neurobiol 2001;63:29.
96. Wise PM, Dubal DB, Wilson ME, et al: Minireview: Neuroprotective effects of estrogen-new insights into mechanisms of action. Endocrinology 2001;142:969.
97. Sribnick EA, Wingrave JM, Matzelle DD, et al: Estrogen as a neuroprotective agent in the treatment of spinal cord injury. Ann N Y Acad Sci 2003;993:125.
98. Weiss DJ, Gurpide E: Non-genomic effects of estrogens and antiestrogens. J Steroid Biochem 1988;31:671.
99. Enmark E, Gustafsson JA: Oestrogen receptors: An overview. J Intern Med 1999;246:133.
100. Erlandsson MC, Ohlsson C, Gustafsson JA, Carlsten H: Role of oestrogen receptors alpha and beta in immune organ development and in oestrogen-mediated effects on thymus. Immunology 2001;103:17.
101. Igarashi H, Kouro T, Yokota T, et al: Age and stage dependency of estrogen receptor expression by lymphocyte precursors. Proc Natl Acad Sci U S A 2001;98:15131.
102. Kuiper GG, Shughrue PJ, Merchenthaler I, Gustafsson JA: The estrogen receptor beta subtype: A novel mediator of estrogen action in neuroendocrine systems. Front Neuroendocrinol 1998;19:253.

103. Harrington WR, Sheng S, Barnett DH, et al: Activities of estrogen receptor alpha- and beta-selective ligands at diverse estrogen responsive gene sites mediating transactivation or transrepression. Mol Cell Endocrinol 2003;206:13.
104. Elloso MM, Phiel K, Henderson RA, et al: Suppression of experimental autoimmune encephalomyelitis using estrogen receptor-selective ligands. J Endocrinol 2005;185:243.
105. Garidou L, Laffont S, Douin-Echinard V, et al: Estrogen receptor alpha signaling in inflammatory leukocytes is dispensable for 17beta-estradiol-mediated inhibition of experimental autoimmune encephalomyelitis. J Immunol 2004;173:2435.
106. Suzuki S, Brown CM, Dela Cruz CD, et al: Timing of estrogen therapy after ovariectomy dictates the efficacy of its neuroprotective and antiinflammatory actions. Proc Natl Acad Sci U S A 2007;104:6013.
107. Thorogood M, Hannaford PC: The influence of oral contraceptives on the risk of multiple sclerosis. Br J Obstet Gynaecol 1998;105:1296.
108. Alonso A, Jick SS, Olek MJ, et al: Recent use of oral contraceptives and the risk of multiple sclerosis. Arch Neurol 2005;62:1362.
109. Da Silva JA, Hall GM: The effects of gender and sex hormones on outcome in rheumatoid arthritis. Baillieres Clin Rheumatol 1992;6:196.
110. Hall GM, Daniels M, Huskisson EC, Spector TD: A randomised controlled trial of the effect of hormone replacement therapy on disease activity in postmenopausal rheumatoid arthritis. Ann Rheum Dis 1994;53:112.
111. Sicotte NL, Liva SM, Klutch R, et al: Treatment of multiple sclerosis with the pregnancy hormone estriol. Ann Neurol 2002;52:421.
112. Soldan SS, Retuerto AI, Sicotte NL, Voskuhl RR: Immune modulation in multiple sclerosis patients treated with the pregnancy hormone estriol. J Immunol 2003;171:6267.
113. Dalal M, Kim S, Voskuhl RR: Testosterone therapy ameliorates experimental autoimmune encephalomyelitis and induces a T helper 2 bias in the autoantigen-specific T lymphocyte response. J Immunol 1997;159:3.
114. Liva SM, Voskuhl RR: Testosterone acts directly on CD4+ T-lymphocytes to increase IL10 production. J Immunol 2001;167:2060.
115. Bebo BF Jr, Schuster JC, Vandenbark AA, Offner H: Androgens alter the cytokine profile and reduce encephalitogenicity of myelin-reactive T cells. J Immunol 1999;162:35.
116. Wilcoxen SC, Kirkman E, Dowdell KC, Stohlman SA: Gender-dependent IL-12 secretion by APC is regulated by IL-10. J Immunol 2000;164:6237.
117. Gray A, Berlin JA, McKinlay JB, Longcope C: An examination of research design effects on the association of testosterone and male aging: Results of a meta-analysis. J Clin Epidemiol 1991;44:671.
118. Morley JE, Kaiser FE, Perry HM 3rd, et al: Longitudinal changes in testosterone, luteinizing hormone, and follicle-stimulating hormone in healthy older men. Metabolism 1997;46:410.
119. Nankin HR, Calkins JH: Decreased bioavailable testosterone in aging normal and impotent men. J Clin Endocrinol Metab 1986;63:1418.
120. Tenover JS, Matsumoto AM, Plymate SR, Bremner WJ: The effects of aging in normal men on bioavailable testosterone and luteinizing hormone secretion: Response to clomiphene citrate. J Clin Endocrinol Metab 1987;65:1118.
121. Vermeulen A: Clinical review 24: Androgens in the aging male. J Clin Endocrinol Metab 1991;73:221.
122. Doran MF, Pond GR, Crowson CS, et al: Trends in incidence and mortality in rheumatoid arthritis in Rochester, Minnesota, over a forty-year period. Arthritis Rheum 2002;46:625.
123. Wei T, Lightman SL: The neuroendocrine axis in patients with multiple sclerosis. Brain 1997;120:1067.
124. Kanik KS, Chrousos GP, Schumacher HR, et al: Adrenocorticotropin, glucocorticoid, and androgen secretion in patients with new onset synovitis/rheumatoid arthritis: Relations with indices of inflammation. J Clin Endocrinol Metab 2000;85:1461.
125. Stone LA, Frank JA, Albert PS, et al: Characterization of MRI response to treatment with interferon beta-1b: Contrast-enhancing MRI lesion frequency as a primary outcome measure. Neurology 1997;49:862.
126. Janowsky JS, Chavez B, Orwoll E: Sex steroids modify working memory. J Cogn Neurosci 2000;12:407.
127. Cherrier MM, Asthana S, Plymate S, et al: Testosterone supplementation improves spatial and verbal memory in healthy older men. Neurology 2001;57:80.

128. Miller DH, Barkhof F, Frank JA, et al: Measurement of atrophy in multiple sclerosis: Pathological basis, methodological aspects and clinical relevance. Brain 2002;125:1676.
129. Capel B, Albrecht KH, Washburn LL, Eicher EM: Migration of mesonephric cells into the mammalian gonad depends on Sry. Mech Dev 1999;84:127.
130. Arnold AP: Sex chromosomes and brain gender. Nat Rev Neurosci 2004;5:701.
131. Arnold AP, Burgoyne PS: Are XX and XY brain cells intrinsically different? Trends Endocrinol Metab 2004;15:6.
132. Burgoyne PS, Lovell-Badge R, Rattigan A: Evidence that the testis determination pathway interacts with a non-dosage compensated, X-linked gene. Int J Dev Biol 2001;45:509.
133. Carruth LL, Reisert I, Arnold AP: Sex chromosome genes directly affect brain sexual differentiation. Nat Neurosci 2002;5:933.
134. De Vries GJ, Rissman EF, Simerly RB, et al: A model system for study of sex chromosome effects on sexually dimorphic neural and behavioral traits. J Neurosci 2002;22:9005.
135. Markham JA, Jurgens HA, Auger CJ, et al: Sex differences in mouse cortical thickness are independent of the complement of sex chromosomes. Neuroscience 2003;116:71.
136. Wagner CK, Xu J, Pfau JL, et al: Neonatal mice possessing an Sry transgene show a masculinized pattern of progesterone receptor expression in the brain independent of sex chromosome status. Endocrinology 2004;145:1046.
137. Ansar Ahmed S, Young PR, Penhale WJ: Beneficial effect of testosterone in the treatment of chronic autoimmune thyroiditis in rats. J Immunol 1986;136:143.
138. Sato EH, Ariga H, Sullivan DA: Impact of androgen therapy in Sjögren's syndrome: Hormonal influence on lymphocyte populations and Ia expression in lacrimal glands of MRL/Mp-lpr/lpr mice. Investig Ophthalmol Vis Sci 1992;33:2537.
139. Cua DJ, Coffman RL, Stohlman SA: Exposure to T helper 2 cytokines in vivo before encounter with antigen selects for T helper subsets via alterations in antigen-presenting cell function. J Immunol 1996;157:2830.
140. Cua DJ, Hinton DR, Stohlman SA: Self-antigen-induced Th2 responses in experimental allergic encephalomyelitis (EAE)-resistant mice: Th2-mediated suppression of autoimmune disease. J Immunol 1995;155:4052.
141. Palaszynski KM, Smith DL, Kamrava S, et al: A yin-yang effect between sex chromosome complement and sex hormones on the immune response. Endocrinology 2005;146:3280.
142. De Vries GJ: Minireview: Sex differences in adult and developing brains—Compensation, compensation, compensation. Endocrinology 2004;145:1063.
143. (a) Voskuhl R, Jackson Wu T: Do estroprogestinic homones protect against chemotherapy-induced amenorrhea in multiple sclerosis? Nat Clin Pract Neurol 2008.
(b) Smith-Bouvier DL, Divekar AA, Sasidhar M, Du S, Tiwari-Woodruff SK, King JK, Arnold AP, Singh RR, Voskuhl RR: A role for sex chromosome complement in the female bias in autoimmune disease. J Exp Med 2008;205:1099.

9 Pediatric Multiple Sclerosis

SUNITA VENKATESWARAN • BRENDA BANWELL

Pediatric-onset multiple sclerosis (MS), although rare, is being increasingly recognized worldwide. It is estimated that up to 10% of MS cases begin during childhood or adolescence.[1-8] Accurate and prompt diagnosis of MS in children is essential for the provision of MS-specific care and for the potential use of MS-targeted immunomodulatory therapies.

Historical Background

The first known case of MS may have been that of a teenager, St. Lidwina of Schiedam, during the 14th century, who developed a relapsing-remitting disease with visual loss and sensory changes that eventually led to severe disability.[9,10] Pediatric-onset MS was reported by Charcot's student, Pierre-Marie, in 1883, although careful review suggests that many of his patients may have actually been manifesting metabolic or infectious disorders.[11] The interest in pediatric MS did not truly emerge until the late 1950s, when Gall and colleagues described 40 MS patients whose disease began in childhood.[12] Limitations to the diagnosis of MS in children include the fact that the original MS criteria specifically excluded patients younger than 10 years of age.[13]

Many studies in pediatric MS have used 16 years as the upper age limit. Many have divided pediatric MS patients into those younger and older than 10 years of age, as a means of considering the impact of puberty on MS features. The youngest MS patients also represent a group of particular interest in studies of MS pathobiology; these patients have had a limited time for exposure to potential environmental triggers and may have a heightened genetic susceptibility to MS.

This chapter reviews the current understanding of the clinical features, natural history, pathobiology, differential diagnosis, investigations, and treatment of MS in children.

Epidemiology

Pediatric MS has been reported in many countries, although precise incidence and prevalence data are not yet available. Epidemiologic studies suggest that country of childhood residence may carry a significantly more important association with MS risk than country of birth. Children born in a region of low MS prevalence acquire the heightened MS risk of their adopted country, provided that they immigrate during childhood.[14-17] In a large multicultural Canadian city, the pediatric MS population was found to closely resemble the demographics of the local, largely recently diversified population. In contrast, the adult MS population cared for in the same city area was representative of the more restricted, largely northern European demographic of the region from 30 years earlier.[18] It is also possible that an earlier onset of MS could occur in individuals who immigrate from low- to high-risk MS regions, particularly if hypothesized protective factors against MS are less likely to be prevalent in regions of low MS risk.[18]

DEMOGRAPHIC FEATURES

Most children with MS experience their first attack between the ages of 9 and 13 years and onset of MS before age 6 years is rare.[19] Approximately 20% of childhood-onset MS occurs in children younger than 10 years.[21] The Italian Childhood Multiple Sclerosis study group and a recent review article on pediatric-onset MS examined the characteristics of children younger than 10 years of age who had a clear diagnosis of MS.[19-21] This will be outlined in the following sections.

The marked female preponderance seen in adult-onset MS is not a feature of MS in younger children (Fig. 9-1). In studies of very-early-onset MS, female-to-male ratios as low as 0.42 have been reported.[22] Female preponderance does emerge in adolescence. The female-to-male ratio in patients with MS onset between 13 and 17 years of age has been reported to be as high as 7.67,[7] although this is not a universal finding. The well-recognized reduction in MS relapse rates during pregnancy and an increased incidence of MS in postpubertal girls strongly implicates hormonal influences.

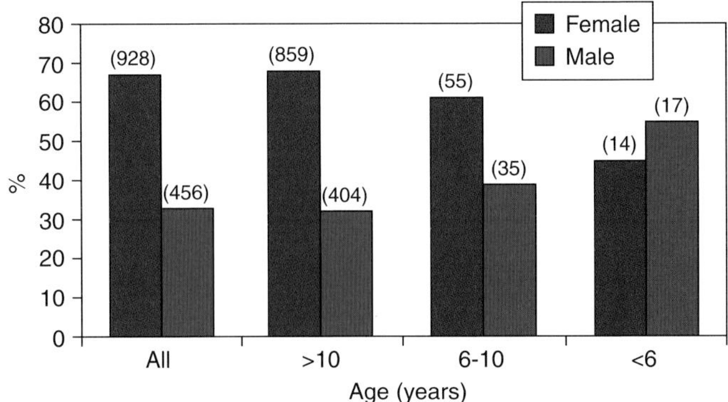

Figure 9–1 Relationships between age and gender in pediatric multiple sclerosis. Data were acquired from demographic information on 1384 children through a review of the literature and are summarized as the proportion of children of each gender subdivided by age group. (From Banwell B, Ghezzi A, Bar-Or A, et al: Multiple sclerosis in children: Clinical diagnosis, therapeutic strategies, and future directions. Lancet Neurol 2007;6:893, reproduced with permission by Lancet Neurology license #: 1890340083572.)

Clinical Characteristics

DIAGNOSTIC CRITERIA

The clinical diagnosis of MS in children requires evidence of recurrent, acquired demyelination, separated in location within the central nervous system (CNS) and disseminated over time.[23,24] Dissemination in space may be diagnosed either by findings on magnetic resonance imaging (MRI) according to the McDonald criteria[25] or by the combination of an abnormal cerebrospinal fluid (CSF) demonstrating an increased immunoglobulin G (IgG) index or oligoclonal bands (OCB) plus two lesions on MRI, one which must be in the brain. Dissemination in time may be determined by a new clinical event occurring 30 days after the onset of the first event or by visualization of a new T2 or gadolinium-enhancing lesion on MRI occurring 3 months after the onset of the initial attack.

The McDonald MRI criteria for dissemination in space may not be as sensitive to the diagnosis of MS in children as they are in adults.[26] In addition, even if new lesions are noted in subsequent imaging, many physicians wait for a second clinical event, especially in young children, before conveying a diagnosis of MS.

PRESENTING FEATURES

A polysymptomatic presentation seems more common in younger patients, whereas a monosymptomatic presentation is more common in adolescents and adults. Sensory symptoms and mild optic neuritis (ON) may be missed in younger children who cannot verbalize their symptoms. Younger children are more likely to have a first MS attack accompanied by polyfocal symptoms, encephalopathy, and ataxia, making the distinction from acute disseminated encephalomyelitis (ADEM) very difficult. In recognition of this issue, the recently proposed diagnostic criteria for pediatric MS specify that children with an initial demyelinating event meeting criteria for ADEM must experience two non-ADEM–like attacks before the diagnosis of MS can be conferred. If children who have an initial episode of ADEM at a young age eventually develop MS, they usually have their MS-defining attack at a younger age.[27,28] When clinical features were analyzed in 49 children with onset before 6 years of age, ataxia was found to be the most common presenting feature. [19] Seizures are also more commonly seen in these younger patients (22%). Presentation may also differ by the child's region of origin, with ADEM being more a more common presentation of MS in children from South America than in those from North America or Europe.[27]

Overall, the largest pediatric prospective study to date was that of a group of 296 children from France with a first episode of acquired central demyelination.[28] During the follow-up period of 2.9 ± 3 years, 168 children (56.7%) developed a second MS-defining episode. Most children presented with long-tract dysfunction consisting of sensory, motor, and sphincter abnormalities (76%), brainstem findings were present in 41%, ON in 22%, and transverse myelitis (TM) in 14%.

Clinical Presentations

OPTIC NEURITIS

Most physicians have a high index of suspicion for MS when adults present with ON, but ON is also a presentation of MS in 14% to 35% of pediatric cases.[2,3,5,7,28-32] Most studies on childhood ON have been retrospective,[32-35] but, together with a recent prospective study,[36] they have revealed important information. The majority of children recover well from the acute ON episode, with more than 85% returning to 20/40 vision or better.[34-36]

Bilateral ON appears to carry a higher risk for development of MS than unilateral ON.[32,36] The risk of MS after ON must be evaluated over many years, because some patients experience an MS-defining second event more than 10 years after ON.[33]

Lesions observed on MRI at the time of ON and the presence of other neurologic abnormalities on examination are associated with a markedly increased risk of future MS diagnosis.[36] Conversely, a normal brain MRI suggests a very low MS risk, at least in the short term. If the diagnosis of ADEM accompanies that of ON, the risk for MS also seems higher than in children with ADEM without optic nerve involvement.[28]

ACUTE DISSEMINATED ENCEPHALOMYELITIS

The term "ADEM" has been applied to a wide variety of clinical presentations, leading to considerable challenges in interpreting MS risk in this population. An international working group has proposed a standardized definition: "a first clinical event, with a presumed inflammatory or demyelinating cause, with acute or subacute onset that affects multifocal areas of the CNS. This presentation must be polysymptomatic and must be accompanied by encephalopathy (change in behavior or consciousness)."[23] The event may evolve over a 3-month period, during which fluctuations in clinical symptoms and MRI findings may be present. Typical MRI features include large, multifocal, hyperintense lesions with involvement of either supratentorial or infratentorial regions in addition to subcortical structures such as the thalami and basal ganglia. These types of lesions may also be found in the spinal cord.

The typical course of ADEM is monophasic. Recurrent ADEM is defined as a second demyelinating episode similar to the first episode of ADEM, occurring 3 or more months after onset of the initial event or 1 month after completion of steroid treatment. MRI does not reveal new areas of involvement. Multiphasic ADEM is defined as a second ADEM episode occurring 3 months after the onset of the initial episode, or 1 month after the cessation of steroid treatment, with a *new* polysymptomatic presentation and encephalopathy. In this subtype, imaging abnormalities occur in different locations compared to the initial episode. Importantly, silent new lesions do not emerge on MRI obtained between acute ADEM episodes.

ADEM is more commonly seen in children younger than 10 years of age, and the female-to-male ratio is almost 1:1.[37] Fever, headache, fatigue, and vomiting are often noted.[38] The CSF commonly demonstrates pleocytosis, elevated protein, and absence of oligoclonal bands (although OCBs may be detected in 5% to 10% of ADEM patients).

Hyperacute severe forms of ADEM include acute hemorrhagic leukoencephalitis (AHLE), acute hemorrhagic encephalomyelitis (AHEM), and acute necrotizing hemorrhagic leukoencephalitis (ANHLE).[37] Acute administration of high-dose intravenous corticosteroids and craniectomy can be life-saving.[39]

The majority of ADEM patients have monophasic disease and no or minimal sequelae.[40-42] Most patients had an Expanded Disability Status Scale (EDSS) score of less than 2.5 in follow-up in one series.[40] A prospective study of 132 children with ADEM in France revealed that 24 (18%) of the patients went on to experience relapses (diagnosed as MS), with none being diagnosed with relapsing or multiphasic ADEM.[28]

ACUTE TRANSVERSE MYELITIS

Acute TM (ATM) is an inflammatory disorder of the spinal cord that causes disturbances in sensory, motor, and autonomic function. It has a biomodal age distribution, affecting both children and adults.[43] Recently, the Transverse Myelitis Consortium developed criteria for diagnosis of idiopathic acute TM.[43] The diagnosis should include bilateral signs of sensory, motor, or autonomic dysfunction attributable to the spinal cord as a result of inflammation, with symptoms progressing over a period of 4 hours to 21 days and a definite sensory level. One must make sure to exclude spinal cord compression, a previous history of irradiation, connective tissue diseases (e.g., systemic lupus erythematosus), vascular causes (e.g., infarction, arteriovenous malformation), and infectious causes (e.g., Lyme disease, human immunodeficiency virus infection), because treatments differ for many of these diseases. Inflammation can be demonstrated by pleocytosis, elevated IgG index, or gadolinium enhancement.

ATM may accompany ADEM, a polysymptomatic CIS presentation, or ON, or it may be monolesional. ON and ATM may also occur as the presenting episode of neuromyelitis optica (NMO). Spinal cord symptoms have usually been seen in fewer than 10% of children during CIS[2,5,7,29,30] but in up to 30% in some European and South American case series.[6,42,44,45]

Children with a first episode of acute TM rarely go on to develop recurrent episodes or MS, but monophasic disease does not herald a good functional outcome. There has been only one large study of TM in children. In this retrospective study of 47 children with acute TM[46] using current diagnostic criteria, only 1 child developed MS. A bimodal peak was present even among the children, with almost 40% of cases occurring before the age of 3 years. The long-term sequelae were poor in these children. Forty percent of these children remained wheelchair dependent. Urinary dysfunction was present in almost 70%. Younger children fared worse in all activities of daily living. Good prognostic factors included a lower lesion level, fewer segments affected, normal white blood cell count in the CSF, older age at onset, and lack of T1-hypointense lesions during the acute phase.

NEUROMYELITIS OPTICA (DEVIC'S DISEASE)

The criteria for NMO requires the combination of TM and ON (either simultaneously or in succession) plus two of the following: (1) a longitudinally extensive spinal cord lesion (extending to more than 3 vertebral segments), (2) no brain lesions or lesions atypical for MS, and (3) NMO-IgG seropositivity.[47,48] NMO-IgG, the recently identified antibody to the water channel aquaporin-4,[49] has helped distinguish this entity from MS. In adults with NMO, this biomarker is 73% sensitive and 92% specific.[49,50] In children, the diagnosis may be suspected in anyone presenting with recurrent ON, with acute TM, especially if longitudinally extensive (LETM), or with LETM in the context of ADEM.

Children as young as 23 months have been diagnosed with NMO[51] and may make up 10% of NMO patients.[52] In contrast to acute TM, there is a female preponderance in both children and adults. In one small study of 9 children with NMO, all had monophasic disease, and all experienced near-complete resolution of motor and visual symptoms.[53] In the first study of the prevalence of NMO-IgG in children with acute CNS demyelinating disorders, 8 of 17 children with the diagnosis of NMO on clinical grounds and imaging features were positive for the NMO-IgG. [54] Most (78%) of these patients positive for the antibody had relapsing rather than monophasic NMO. These findings are similar to adult sensitivity rates for relapsing NMO (86%).[49] One patient with relapsing LETM and one patient with relapsing ON were also seropositive for the NMO-IgG. Again similar to adults,[49] only 1 child (12.5%) with monophasic NMO was seropositive for the antibody. None of the children diagnosed with relapsing-remitting MS (RRMS) and none with monophasic TM or ON were positive for the antibody.

MRI evidence of brain lesions may also occur in children with NMO, particularly lesions extending from the spinal cord into the brainstem, hypothalamus, and corpus callosum.[54] In adults with NMO, up to 10% of patients have brain lesions reminiscent of MS lesions.[52] MRI evidence of LETM, which is rare in both pediatric and adult MS populations, can nonetheless be detected in 14% of children with RRMS.[54] In adults, LETM is the most useful MRI feature in distinguishing NMO from MS.[47,56]

OTHER FEATURES OF MULTIPLE SCLEROSIS IN CHILDREN

The onset of MS in childhood or adolescence occurs during the key formative academic and social years. Since MS is not thought of as a disease of childhood, families may report feeling alone.[57] Multidisciplinary support for children and their families, including psychological and psychiatric services, plays an integral role in pediatric MS care.

Cognitive impairment is well recognized in adult-onset MS and also occurs in children.[58] Children with MS may be particularly vulnerable, perhaps due to MS-related disruption of related myelinogenesis and neural networking in areas responsible for cognition. In a small study of 10 children with MS, longer disease duration was associated with a greater degree of cognitive impairment ($P = .02$).[58] Similar findings were reported in a larger study of 37 children.[59] More than 30% of children were impaired on at least two cognitive measures, and 66% were impaired in at least one domain. Verbal fluency appears to remain intact in most of these children,[57,58] and this may serve to mask the degree of impairment in more complex cognitive tasks.[59,60]

Clinical Course of Multiple Sclerosis in Children

Most children have a complete recovery after their first episode,[2] and over 98% follow a relapsing remitting disease course.[4,7,27,30] Primary progressive MS is very rare in children. The time between the first and the second (typically, MS-defining) attack is 0.9 to 2.0 years, with longer intervals (median range: 4.6 to 6 years) in younger children.[4,21,61] Risk factors for an MS-defining second attack include female sex, age greater than 10 years, optic neuritis (especially with more than one lesion on MRI), and an MRI suggestive of MS at onset.[28]

The relapse rate is variable and, as in adults, is higher during the early stages of disease. The number of relapses per year ranges from 0.38 to 1.2 per year.[4,7,27,29,30,62] A higher number of relapses during the first 2 years appears to increase the risk of acquiring permanent disability.[4,5,7,30]

DISABILITY

The long-term prognosis of pediatric-onset MS is largely determined by the risk for development of secondary progressive disease (SPMS) and by the rate of accrual of physical and cognitive disabilities. To date, there exist very few outcome data from prospectively monitored pediatric MS cohorts.

As in adult MS, the EDSS score is widely used to measure physical disability, although this tool provides no information on cognitive performance and does not measure MS-related symptoms such as fatigue. Quality-of-life scales specific for pediatric MS would be of great value. Retrospective studies of pediatric MS outcome have used EDSS scores of 3 (moderate disability), 4 (deficits but ability to ambulate more than 500 m without assistance), 6 (requiring unilateral assistance to ambulate 500 m), or 7 (unable to ambulate despite bilateral assistance) as end points. EDSS scores of 6 or greater rarely occur during childhood years.

In one study, researchers formulated a model to predict EDSS scores based on age at onset of disease and disease duration.[5,63] This study included 43 children (2.9% of their MS population) and determined that EDSS scores of 4 and 6 would be reached after 25 and 40 years, respectively. A study by Simone and colleagues comparing adult- and pediatric-onset disease course found that an EDSS score of 4 occurred after a median disease duration of 20 years in cases with pediatric onset (10.5% of their population), compared with 10.8 years in their adult-onset patients.[5] In contrast, a score of 4 was predicted to occur in only 11 years by Kaplan-Meier analysis in a cohort of 296 CIS patients, particularly if children had residual deficits from their initial attack.[28] In another retrospective study, after 10 years of disease duration, fewer than 25% of pediatric-onset MS patients had an EDSS score between 3 and 6.5, and only 16% had a score greater than 7.[2] This same study showed that three quarters of children were still able to ambulate after 15 years. In a retrospective study of 28 pediatric-onset MS patients with a longer period of observation (28 years), the mean EDSS score was 5.8, with 70% of patients reaching an EDSS score of 6.0 after a mean of 18 years.[1] In one of the few prospective studies, 18 (33%) of 54 children had an EDSS greater than 4.0 after a mean follow-up period of 8 years.[30] In a prospective study of 197 children with MS, 1% developed an EDSS score of 4 after a mean of 5.5 years.[61]

Progression does not occur in a linear fashion and may happen as quickly in children once the stage of irreversible disability has been reached. This was demonstrated in a study of 113 children over an average of 20 years; the mean time to develop an EDSS score of 3.0 was 16 years (average age, 28 years), but further progression to a score of 6.0 occurred over the next 5 years.[7] A large, detailed, retrospective study demonstrated that the pediatric-onset MS group (n = 394) developed irreversible disability approximately 10 years later than did the adult-onset patients (n = 1775), and the rate of progression at the higher EDSS scores was similar. Younger-onset patients (<12 years) took longer to reach an EDSS score of 4.0 than did children who were older than 12 years of age at onset (median, 28.0 versus 19.1 years).[4]

The outcome of pediatric-onset MS in light of the increasing use of immunomodulatory therapies, the impact of MS on scholastic performance and vocational achievement, and the social and quality-of-life aspects of MS onset during childhood remain to be determined.

SECONDARY PROGRESSIVE MULTIPLE SCLEROSIS IN CHILDREN

The conversion to SPMS is a function of duration of disease and therefore occurs relatively rarely during the childhood and adolescent years. Approximately 4% to 5% of children develop SPMS after a median disease duration of 5 to 6 years.[27,61]

The 50% risk for patients with pediatric-onset MS to develop SPMS was determined to be 23 years by Kaplan-Meier analysis.[7] A large, retrospective study comparing adult-onset MS patients (n = 1775) and pediatric-onset MS patients (n = 394) found that conversion to SPMS occurred after a longer disease duration in the latter group (median, 28.1 versus 18.8 years), but at a much younger age (41 versus 52.1 years).[4]

Risk factors for progression to SPMS and for accrual of disability are outlined in Table 9-1.

Pathobiologic Studies in Children

GENETICS

Approximately 6% to 21% of children with MS have a first- or second-degree relative who also has the disease.[2,4,5,8,28] However, the true prevalence of familial MS in pediatric MS kindreds must consider the fact that parents and other relatives may themselves still be in the age range of MS onset at the time of diagnosis of the affected child. Longitudinal studies are required to accurately determine MS rates in families of pediatric MS patients.

TABLE 9–1 Factors Associated with an Increased Risk of Disability or Disability Progression in Children with Multiple Sclerosis

Risk Factor	Time to Development of Irreversible Disability*	Time to Develop Secondary Progression*
Short interval between episodes (<1 yr)	√[29, 61]	√[5]
Sequelae after first attack	√[28]	
Progressive course at onset	√[4, 28, 61]	
Secondary progressive course	√[5, 30]	
High number of relapses in first few years	√[4, 7, 29, 30]	√[5, 7]
Female gender	√[61]	
Suggestive MRI findings	√[61]	
Absence of encephalopathy	√[61]	
Sphincter involvement at onset	√[5]	
Brainstem involvement at onset		√[7]

MRI, magnetic resonance imaging.
*Numbers in parentheses refer to references cited in this chapter.

Children of one parent with MS have a 2.49% risk of developing MS, and children with both parents affected have a 30.5% risk.[64-66] However, the "children" in these studies were typically adults by the time they experience the first attack of MS.

The major histocompatibility complex (MHC), and in particular the human leukocyte antigen (HLA) *HLA-DRB1* locus has been linked with MS risk.[67-69] Aside from HLA-DRB1, other alleles within the HLA class II DR2 haplotype (DQA1*102, DQB1*602) have also been shown to have strong associations with MS, but these alleles tend to co-segregate in northern European populations with HLA-DRB1*1501.[70] Some studies have associated HLA-DR(15) with a younger age at onset of disease, although "younger" in this case refers to early adulthood.[71-73] Analysis of HLA class II DRB1 allele DR(15) in Russian children and adults with MS[74] did not find a relationship to age at onset.[75,76] It has been suggested that children with the DRB1*1501 allele are susceptible to MS with ON.[77,78]

Tumor necrosis factor-α polymorphisms studied in a group of 24 Turkish children with MS were comparable to those in healthy controls.[79] The myelin oligodendrocyte glycoprotein (MOG) gene, like MHC, has also been mapped to chromosome 6. Although polymorphisms within the MOG gene were detected, there was no association with predisposition for developing MS or with the course of disease in a group of 75 German children with MS.[80]

IMMUNOLOGIC INSIGHTS

The prevailing theory on MS pathogenesis implicates aberrant immunologic responses to environmental antigens in genetically susceptible individuals.[81] An advantage of studying children is the ability to analyze immune function closer to the biologic onset of disease.

Both the humoral and the cellular (adaptive) immune systems are implicated in MS, with a likely imbalance between Th1 (pro-inflammatory) and Th2 (anti-inflammatory) function as well as dysfunction of the newly recognized Th17 cells.[82]

In children, peripheral T-cell reactivity was examined in 63 children with CNS inflammatory demyelination (CIS and MS), compared with children with other CNS insults (trauma, epilepsy), type I diabetes, and healthy age-matched controls. T-cell reactivity was increased not only in children with CIS and MS but also in those children with other neurologic insults and diabetes.[83] Epitope-specific responses partially distinguished the more selective T-cell repertoire of the CIS/MS and neurologic patients from that of the children with diabetes. In addition, children with CNS and autoimmune diseases showed T-cell reactivity to specific cow milk protein antigens, which may implicate dietary exposures as putative environmental triggers. However, because the heightened T-cell reactivity to both self and environmental antigens was not specific to children with autoimmune disease, it is possible that such a response is a nonspecific immune response to tissue injury.

To date, the search for serologic biomarkers specific for MS has been largely unrewarding. In a subset of ADEM patients, but not in MS or CIS patients, autoantibodies were found to a certain conformation of MOG.[84] Whether these autoantibodies have a role in the pathogenesis of ADEM is still unknown.

Tau, an axonal microtubule protein, is a potentially useful biomarker in MS.[85] It reflects axonal injury and has been shown to be elevated in the CSF of adult MS patients. In the CSF of children with MS, tau levels were only slightly elevated compared with controls, and only in those children with more severe disease.[86] This may imply an early neurodegenerative aspect of the disease, but further studies are required.

HORMONAL FACTORS

In general, women have a 2.7 greater risk of developing autoimmune diseases.[87] Certain autoimmune diseases, such as systemic lupus erythematosus, have a 90% female predominance. Receptors for both androgens and estrogen are present on immune cells and may influence immunologic behavior. Females have more profound antibody-mediated humoral response than males and an increased production of autoantibodies[88-90]; testosterone and progesterone promote more of a Th2 response.[90] In girls, estrogen levels increase during puberty and fluctuate monthly; in boys, estrogen levels decrease after the growth spurt. Levels of prolactin and growth hormone also increase in females beginning at the time of puberty, and both of these hormones have a role to play in autoimmunity.[91,92] Insulin growth factor 1, a liver-derived hormone that is also present in higher concentrations in females from the onset of puberty, may play a role in neural tissue repair.[93] The role of sex hormones in MS pathobiology may be of particular interest in the pediatric MS population.

ENVIRONMENTAL FACTORS

Viral infection, and the subsequent requisite immunologic response, may play an important role in MS. Viral studies in pediatric MS patients are aided by the inherent temporal association between infectious exposures and disease onset. A retrospective Danish case-control study comparing childhood infection exposure in 455 cases of MS (onset after the age of 14) and 1801 age-matched controls, did not show a difference in frequency or timing of exposure to varicella, measles, mumps, rubella, pertussis, and scarlet fever between the two groups. [94] The same negative results were found when researchers looked for associations between certain common viral infections (cytomegalovirus, herpes simplex virus, parvovirus B19, and varicella) in children with MS compared with controls.[27] Recently, *Chlamydia pneumoniae* IgM antibodies were shown to be more prevalent in children with MS,[95] although similar results have not been found in adults.[96]

Epstein-Barr virus (EBV), a single-stranded DNA virus in the herpes family, has been associated with MS in both children and adults. Neurologic complications of primary infection with EBV include demyelination, such as TM. [97] Individuals with a history of infectious mononucleosis have been shown to have a fivefold increased risk of MS.[98]

Antibodies to EBV nuclear antigens (EBNA) are detected 3 to 6 weeks after the onset of symptoms. EBNA1 antibodies persist throughout life following infection while antibodies to EBV early antigen (EA) are detected transiently for approximately six months after exposure and again during periods of viral reactivation. IgM to VCA (viral capsid antigen) is present during acute disease but only for 2 to 3 months, whereas IgG persists for life. Adult studies have demonstrated that antibody titers to both VCA and EBNA are increased, possibly for as long as several years, before the onset of clinical disease.[99]

In children with clinically definite MS, serologic evidence of remote infection with EBV is significantly higher than in control patients.[100,101] None of a group of children with MS had experienced symptomatology consistent with infectious mononucleosis, and none had serologic evidence of a recent infection. Titers of antibodies were also significantly elevated in children with MS compared with controls.[27,101] A multinational study of 137 children with MS enrolled from South America, North America, and Europe confirmed the association of EBV and childhood MS and showed that this finding was present in multiple regions of the world.[27] The precise biologic importance of EBV infection in MS remains to be determined.

VACCINATIONS AND MULTIPLE SCLEROSIS

The role of vaccinations in triggering demyelinating events has also been of interest. Vaccination with the Semple rabies vaccine (derived from the CNS) was correlated with the development of ADEM.[102] Despite isolated case reports to the contrary, vaccination against tetanus, hepatitis B, or influenza has not been associated with MS or with MS relapse rate.[103] Similarly, a study of 356 children with CIS investigated whether exposure to hepatitis B or tetanus vaccines increased the risk of an MS-defining relapse. Children were monitored prospectively for a mean of 6 years and 61 of the 146 children who had relapses were exposed to either the hepatitis B vaccine (n = 33) or the tetanus vaccine (n = 28). The hazard ratios for developing a relapse within 3 years after being vaccinated were 0.78 (95% confidence interval, 0.32 to 1.89) and 0.99 (95% confidence interval, 0.58 to 1.67), respectively.[104]

VITAMIN D

Epidemiologic studies have linked MS with low vitamin D exposure.[105,106] For most individuals, the primary source of vitamin D is exposure to ultraviolet B radiation, which has strong geographic and seasonal variation.[107] Exposure to sunlight during childhood has been shown to decrease the risk of developing MS.[108,109] In monozygotic twins,[108] childhood sun exposure protected against the development of MS in late adolescence or adulthood, although this finding may have been influenced by recall bias. The risk of MS was also shown to be higher in individuals born in the spring, compared with those born in the fall,[110] raising the possibility of an important role for maternal vitamin D nutrition in fetal immunologic development. Detailed analyses of vitamin D in children with MS will be of considerable interest.

Investigations and Differential Diagnosis

Because pediatric-onset MS is one of several inflammatory CNS diseases of childhood, it is of great importance to have a high index of suspicion and a systematic approach when a child presents with presumed acquired CNS demyelination. As in adults, the clinical heterogeneity of presentations makes it difficult to immediately ensure that the clinical features are due to CNS demyelination. The features and time to maximal deficits of the presenting symptoms, as well as a detailed history of past events, help distinguish MS from entities such as genetic and metabolic diseases, vasculopathies, infectious diseases, and malignancies. Table 9-2 outlines an approach to the differential diagnosis to be considered in a child with possible acquired CNS demyelination.

Neuroimaging Features of Multiple Sclerosis in Children

Whereas the appearance of MS in older children and teenagers is fairly similar to that in adults, younger children tend to have ill-defined lesions that may not conform to the lesion distribution delineated in the McDonald MRI criteria for lesion dissemination in space.[111] Pediatric-specific MRI criteria are under development and will aid in establishing the diagnostic role for MRI in this population. The KIDMUS criteria consists of two criteria: discrete lesions and lesions perpendicular to the long axis of the corpus callosum.[112] This criteria had very high specificity but low sensitivity for relapse rate (MS-defining event). Of equal importance, identification of MRI features predictive of a monophasic demyelinating course, and thus a low risk of future MS diagnosis, would be of great value.

Treatment of Multiple Sclerosis in Children

Care of children with MS includes the use of medications for the treatment of acute relapses, for chronic immunomodulation, and for symptomatic relief of fatigue, spasticity, or pain. Rehabilitative services, including physiotherapy and occupational therapy, and neuropsychology are often required, and counseling and therapy for the psychological impact of MS are of enormous importance. Several resources are available for children and their families through the Multiple Sclerosis Societies in North America (available at http://www.mssociety.ca/en/help/YoungPersonsMS.htm and http://www.nationalmssociety.org, searching for "Pediatric MS Support Group"). In addition, we have designed a website discussing acute CNS demyelination for children and families (available at http://pedsdemyelination.ccb.sickkids.ca [accessed October 2008]).

TREATMENT OF ACUTE DEMYELINATION

Care of a child with an acute MS relapse depends on the clinical severity. Mild symptoms do not require pharmacologic intervention but do require discussion and should contribute to a detailed record of the child's MS disease course. Counseling of the child and family is much more in-depth in the situation of a first demyelinating event. With the advent of the Internet, many families are aware of the potential of MS even before the first neurology assessment, and a detailed discussion regarding MS risk is often a key aspect of care for the child with a first demyelinating event.

Children with acute demyelinating symptoms severe enough to interfere with function or to cause discomfort are treated with corticosteroids. Case series–level evidence and common clinical practice support the use of intravenous methylprednisolone, 20 to 30 mg/kg/day for 3 to 5 days.[113] If intravenous corticosteroid treatment leads to complete resolution of symptoms, then further treatment with oral prednisone is not required. Symptoms that markedly improve but have not resolved often benefit from a brief (14- to 28-day) course of oral prednisone. Prednisone, starting at a dose of 1 mg/kg/day and tapering by 5 mg every 2 to 3 days, is suggested.

Not all children respond to corticosteroids, and some children respond initially but have a recurrence of their symptoms as soon as the corticosteroid dose is lowered. Case report– and case series–level evidence exists for the use of intravenous immune globulin (IVIG) in such patients.[114-116] IVIG has also been shown to be benefit in adults with ADEM.[117-118] In our clinic, we use 2 g/kg IVIG divided over 2 days in children weighing less than 50 kg, or divided over 4 to 5 days in children who weigh more than 50 kg.[113]

IMMUNOMODULATORY THERAPY FOR RELAPSING-REMITTING DISEASE

The four immunomodulatory medications approved for treatment of RRMS in adults have also been used in the care of pediatric MS patients. There are no treatment trials of interferon (IFN)-beta (Rebif, Avonex, Betaseron) or glatiramer acetate (Copaxone) in children, but several retrospective reviews have documented a favorable side effect profile.[119-123] Importantly, younger pediatric MS patients appear to have a higher risk of elevation of liver enzymes after initiation of IFN therapy, and a gradual increase in dose is advised. Typically, children ultimately tolerate the same dosing as is prescribed for adults: IFN-beta-1b (Betaseron), 8 MIU by subcutaneous injection every second day; IFN-beta-1a (Rebif), 22 μg or 44 μg by subcutaneous injection three times weekly; IFN-beta-1a (Avonex), 30 μg via intramuscular injection once weekly; or glatiramer acetate (Copaxone), 20 mg daily by subcutaneous injection.

With a child and family centered education model, acceptance of injectable therapies is typically successful, even in the youngest patients. A teaching puppet is helpful to demonstrate injection technique, which is practiced by both parents and the child (even if the child will not be the one to administer the injection). Compliance is also enhanced by practicality. In our program, we specifically give "permission" for short medication "holidays" at such times as school trips or overnight camping excursions. Children welcome the short break, and the reduction in stress of not having to arrange injections, medication packing, and organization required to provide injectable therapies when away from parents is very much appreciated.

TABLE 9–2 Diagnoses and Investigations to Consider in a Child with Possible CNS Demyelination

Time to Maximal Deficit	Possible Conditions	Investigations to Consider*
<24 hr	Vascular causes	
	Stroke (arterial, venous)	Urgent imaging: CT, MRI, MRA, MRV
	Hemorrhage (traumatic, tumor-related)	Urgent imaging: include FLAIR, T2, T1 plus gadolinium, DWI
	Spinal disc herniation	MRI
	Spinal cord compression	MRI
	Infectious causes Meningitis/encephalitis	CBC, CSF
	Sickle cell crisis	Sickle cell screen
	Toxic causes	Toxin screen
	Seizure	Electroencephalogram
Few days to few months	Vascular Infarction Vasculitis	MRI (FLAIR, T2, T1 plus gadolinium, DWI) Possible angiogram Possible brain biopsy
	Malignancy	CSF cytology Brain biopsy
	Infectious HSV and other herpes family viruses HIV Mycoplasma Lyme disease HTLV-1 Neurosyphilis Neurocysticercosis	CBC: blood culture, viral serologies CSF: glucose, protein, WBC, bacterial C&S, viral PCR, cytology, parasitology
	Connective tissue disease Lupus Sarcoidosis Behçet's disease Antiphospholipid antibody syndrome	TSH, ESR, CRP, ANA, dsDNA, APLA, ACE, chest X-ray
	Macrophage activation syndrome	Ferritin, triglycerides
	Metabolic disease	Serum amino acids, urine organic acids, lactate, pyruvate

TABLE 9–2 Diagnoses and Investigations to Consider in a Child with Possible CNS Demyelination (Continued)

Time to Maximal Deficit	Possible Conditions	Investigations to Consider*
Progressive onset and course (± exacerbations)	Inherited leukodystrophies Adrenoleukodystrophy Metachromatic leukodystrophy Alexander's disease Krabbe's disease Vanishing white matter disease Mucopolysaccharidoses Peroxisomal disorders CADASIL Familial spastic paraparesis Pelizaeus-Merzbacher	EMG/NCS, VLCFA, arylsulfatase A, GFAP mutation analysis, galactocerebrosidase, eIFB2 mutation, urine MPS, NOTCH3 mutation, plasma cholestanol, PLP mutation
	Mitochondrial disease Leigh's disease MELAS LHON Pyruvate dehydrogenase deficiency	MRS, mitochondrial DNA mutation analysis, skin/muscle/nerve biopsy
	Metabolic disease Organic/amino acidopathies	See above
	Nutritional deficiencies	B_{12}, folate, MTHFR

ACE, angiotensin-converting enzyme; ANA, antinuclear antibodies; APLA, anti-phospholipid antibody; C&S, culture and sensitivity; CADASIL, cerebral autosomal dominant arteriopathy with subcortical infarcts and leukoencephalopathy; CBC, complete blood count; CNS, central nervous system; CRP, C-reactive protein; CSF, cerebrospinal fluid; CT, computed tomography; dsDNA, double-stranded DNA; DWI, diffusion-weighted imaging; eIFB2, eukaryotic initiation factor B2; EMG, electromyography; ESR, erythrocyte sedimentation rate; FLAIR, fluid-attenuated inversion recovery; GFAP, glial fibrillary acidic protein; HIV, human immunodeficiency virus; HSV, herpes simplex virus; HTLV-1, human T-cell lymphotropic virus 1; LHON, Leber's hereditary optic neuropathy; MELAS, mitochondrial encephalopathy lactic acidosis and stroke; MPS, mucopolysaccharides; MRA, magnetic resonance angiography; MRI, magnetic resonance imaging; MRS, magnetic resonance spectroscopy; MRV, magnetic resonance venography; MTHFR, methyltetrahydrofolate reductase; NCS, nerve conduction study; PCR, polymerase chain reaction; PLP, proteolipid protein; TSH, thyroid-stimulating hormone; VLCFA, very long chain fatty acids; WBC, white blood cell count.

*Supportive evidence for demyelination: electrophysiology (somatosensory evoked potential [SSEP], visual evoked potential [VEP], brainstem auditory evoked response [BAER]); CSF (oligoclonal bands, immunoglobulin index); serial MRI imaging.

IVIG has been studied in adult MS (reviewed in a meta-analysis[124]) and found to reduce the relapse rate, with a trend toward reduced disability. There are no data on the use of regularly scheduled IVIG in pediatric MS patients. However, IVIG has been administered monthly to children who have an exceptionally high relapse rate despite immunomodulatory therapy. IVIG has also been used in children who have received frequent or prolonged corticosteroid therapy and experience a relapse of symptoms when corticosteroid therapy is weaned. IVIG may permit elimination of corticosteroid dependence in these patients, with the obvious benefit of avoiding corticosteroid-related morbidity.

IMMUNOSUPPRESSIVE THERAPIES

Mitoxantrone has been approved for use in adults with aggressive RRMS (enhancing lesions on MRI and frequent MS relapses). Experience with the use of mitoxantrone in children with MS is extremely limited. Side effects reported in adults, including amenorrhea and a cumulative dose-dependent risk of cardiac toxicity, make mitoxantrone a less attractive therapeutic option in children.

Cyclophosphamide is an alkylating agent with potent immunosuppressive properties. The use of cyclophosphamide in MS is controversial, although many specialists use it for young adult patients with highly active MS disease. Anecdotal use of cyclophosphamide in children who have very high relapse rates (typically more than three relapses per year) or early evidence of relapse-related disability suggests a favorable impact on relapse rate and even an improvement in MS symptoms. A standardized protocol and multicenter studies are clearly required to evaluate the use of cyclophosphamide in these very ill pediatric MS patients. The risks of infertility and bladder carcinoma or other malignancies, as well as the short-term risks of alopecia, immune suppression, hemorrhagic cystitis, and nausea, clearly limit the use of this medication to only those children for whom other therapies are ineffective.

Natalizumab (Tysabri) has been approved for use in adults with severe MS. To date, there are no studies of the use of this medication in the pediatric population, and regulatory authorities have not approved its use in patients younger than 18 years of age.

TREATMENT OF SECONDARY PROGRESSIVE MULTIPLE SCLEROSIS

The management of SPMS remains largely symptomatic and supportive. Few children reach this stage of the MS disease process during their childhood.

SYMPTOMATIC MANAGEMENT

Fatigue is one of the most pervasive symptoms of MS in children, just as it is in adults. Management requires a careful history of daily activity. Carrying heavy backpacks to school, repeated trips up and down school stairs, and extensive homework assignments are a few examples of modifiable activities that can be reduced to allow a more meaningful expenditure of a child's energy. If lifestyle modification alone is insufficient, we have found medications such as modafinil (Provigil) or amantadine to be of benefit.[113]

The management of spasticity in children with severe MS is similar to that in children with other pediatric neurologic disorders. Localized injection of botulinum toxin[125] and oral medications such as tizanidine (reviewed by Weinstock-Guttman and Cohen[126]) and benzodiazepines may be effective.

Conclusion

MS onset in childhood and adolescence is now more readily diagnosed, although education of primary health care providers on the possibility of MS in children remains an area of high priority. Clinical care paradigms, therapeutic trials, and pediatric MS-specific outcome measures are urgently needed. Research into the inciting events in MS pathobiology and MRI features of the earliest aspects of inflammation and neurodegeneration are uniquely amenable to study in the youngest MS patient population. To address these important issues of education, clinical care, and research, the National Multiple Sclerosis Society in the United States, the Canadian Multiple Sclerosis Society, and other national MS organizations have partnered under the auspices of the Multiple Sclerosis International Federation to create the International Pediatric MS Study Group. The Study Group has an international collaborative mandate and will provide an invaluable means to advance understanding of MS in children.

REFERENCES

1. Deryck O, Ketelaer P, Dubois B: Clinical characteristics and long term prognosis in early onset multiple sclerosis. J Neurol 2006;253:720-723.
2. Duquette P, Murray TJ, Pleines J, et al: Multiple sclerosis in childhood: Clinical profile in 125 patients. J Pediatr 1987;111:359-363.
3. Ghezzi A, Deplano V, Faroni J, et al: Multiple sclerosis in childhood: Clinical features of 149 cases. Mult Scler 1997;3:43-46.
4. Renoux C, Vukusic S, Mikaeloff Y, et al: Natural history of multiple sclerosis with childhood onset. N Engl J Med 2007;356:2603-2613.
5. Simone IL, Carrara D, Tortorella C, et al: Course and prognosis in early-onset MS: Comparison with adult-onset forms. Neurology 2002;59:1922-1928.
6. Sindern E, Haas J, Stark E, Wurster U: Early onset MS under the age of 16: Clinical and paraclinical features. Acta Neurol Scand 1992;86:280-284.
7. Boiko A, Vorobeychik G, Paty D, et al: Early onset multiple sclerosis: A longitudinal study. Neurology 2002;59:1006-1010.
8. Cole GF, Stuart CA: A long perspective on childhood multiple sclerosis. Dev Med Child Neurol 1995;37:661-666.
9. Chabas D, Green AJ, Waubant E: Pediatric multiple sclerosis. NeuroRx 2006;3:264-275.
10. Medaer R: Does the history of multiple sclerosis go back as far as the 14th century? Acta Neurol Scand 1979;60:189-192.
11. Hanefeld F: Pediatric multiple sclerosis: A short history of a long story. Neurology 2007;68;(16 Suppl 2):S3-S6.
12. Gall JC Jr, Hayles AB, Siekert RG, Keith HM: Multiple sclerosis in children: A clinical study of 40 cases with onset in childhood. Pediatrics 1958;21:703-709.
13. Schumacher GA: Critique of experimental trials of therapy in multiple sclerosis. Neurology 1974;24:1010-1014.
14. Dean G, Elian M: Age at immigration to England of Asian and Caribbean immigrants and the risk of developing multiple sclerosis. J Neurol Neurosurg Psychiatry 1997;63:565-568.
15. Elian M, Dean G: Multiple sclerosis among the United Kingdom-born children of immigrants from the West Indies. J Neurol Neurosurg Psychiatry 1987;50:327-332.
16. Elian M, Nightingale S, Dean G: Multiple sclerosis among United Kingdom-born children of immigrants from the Indian subcontinent, Africa and the West Indies. J Neurol Neurosurg Psychiatry 1990;53:906-911.
17. Krupp L, Belman A, Cianciulli C, et al: Clinical, demographic and cognitive features of childhood onset multiple sclerosis. Mult Scler 2002;8(Suppl):S86.
18. Kennedy J, O'Connor P, Sadovnick AD, et al: Age at onset of multiple sclerosis may be influenced by place of residence during childhood rather than ancestry. Neuroepidemiology 2006;26:162-167.
19. Ruggieri M, Polizzi A, Pavone L, Grimaldi LM: Multiple sclerosis in children under 6 years of age. Neurology 1999;53:478-484.
20. Ruggieri M, Iannetti P, Polizzi A, et al: Multiple sclerosis in children under 10 years of age. Neurol Sci 2004;25(Suppl 4):S326-S335.
21. Banwell B, Ghezzi A, Bar-Or A, et al: Multiple sclerosis in children: Clinical diagnosis, therapeutic strategies, and future directions. Lancet Neurol 2007;6:887-902.

22. Haliloglu G, Anlar B, Aysun S, et al: Gender prevalence in childhood multiple sclerosis and myasthenia gravis. J Child Neurol 2002;17:390-392.
23. Krupp LB, Banwell B, Tenembaum S: Consensus definitions proposed for pediatric multiple sclerosis and related disorders. Neurology 2007;68(16 Suppl. 2):S7-S12.
24. Poser C, Paty D, Scheinberg L, et al: New diagnostic criteria for multiple sclerosis: Guidelines for research protocols. Ann Neurol 1983;13:227-231.
25. Polman C, Reingold S, Edan G, et al: Diagnostic criteria for multiple sclerosis: 2005 Revisions to the "McDonald Criteria." Ann Neurol 2005;58:840-846.
26. Hahn CD, Shroff MM, Blaser SI, Banwell BL: MRI criteria for multiple sclerosis: Evaluation in a pediatric cohort. Neurology 2004;62:806-808.
27. Banwell B, Krupp L, Kennedy J, et al: Clinical features and viral serologies in children with multiple sclerosis: A multinational observational study. Lancet Neurol 2007;6:773-781.
28. Mikaeloff Y, Suissa S, Vallée L, et al: First episode of acute CNS inflammatory demyelination in childhood: Prognostic factors for multiple sclerosis and disability. J Pediatr 2004;144:246-252.
29. Gusev E, Boiko A, Bikova O, et al: The natural history of early onset multiple sclerosis: Comparison of data from Moscow and Vancouver. Clin Neurol Neurosurg 2002;104:203-207.
30. Ghezzi A, Pozzilli C, Liguori M, et al: Prospective study of multiple sclerosis with early onset. Mult Scler 2002;8:115-118.
31. Pinhas-Hamiel O, Barak Y, Siev-Ner I, Achiron A: Juvenile multiple sclerosis: Clinical features and prognostic characteristics. J Pediatr 1998;132:735-737.
32. Riikonen R, Donner M, Erkkila H: Optic neuritis in children and its relationship to multiple sclerosis: A clinical study of 21 children. Dev Med Child Neurol 1988;30:349-359.
33. Lucchinetti CF, Kiers L, O'Duffy A, et al: Risk factors for developing multiple sclerosis after childhood optic neuritis. Neurology 1997;49:1413-1418.
34. Lana-Peixoto MA, Andrade GC: The clinical profile of childhood optic neuritis. Arq Neuropsiquiatr 2001;59(2-B):311-317.
35. Morales DS, Siakowski RM, Howard CW, Warman R: Optic neuritis in children. J Ophthalmic Nurs Technol 2000;19:270-274; quiz 5-6.
36. Wilejto M, Shroff M, Buncic JR, et al: The clinical features, MRI findings, and outcome of optic neuritis in children. Neurology 2006;67:258-262.
37. Tenembaum S, Chitnis T, Ness J, Hahn J: Acute disseminated encephalomyelitis. Neurology 2007;68(Suppl 2):S23-S36.
38. Brass SD, Caramanos Z, Santos C, et al: Multiple sclerosis vs acute disseminated encephalomyelitis in childhood. Pediatr Neurol 2003;29:227-231.
39. Payne ET, Rutka JT, Ho TK, et al: Treatment leading to dramatic recovery in acute hemorrhagic leukoencephalitis. J Child Neurol 2007;22:109-113.
40. Tenembaum S, Chamoles N, Fejerman N: Acute disseminated encephalomyelitis: A long-term follow-up study of 84 pediatric patients. Neurology 2002;59:1224-1231.
41. Murthy SN, Faden HS, Cohen ME, Bakshi R: Acute disseminated encephalomyelitis in children. Pediatrics 2002;110(2 Pt 1):e21.
42. Dale R, de Sousa C, Chong W, et al: Acute disseminated encephalomyelitis, multiphasic disseminated encephalomyelitis and multiple sclerosis in children. Brain 2000;123:2407-2422.
43. Transverse Myelitis Consortium Working Group: Proposed diagnostic criteria and nosology of acute transverse myelitis. Neurology 2002;59:499-505.
44. Boutin B, Esquivel E, Mayer M, et al: Multiple sclerosis in children: Report of clinical and paraclinical features of 19 cases. Neuropediatrics 1988;19:118-123.
45. Guilhoto LM, Osorio CA, Machado LR, et al: Pediatric multiple sclerosis report of 14 cases. Brain Dev 1995;17:9-12.
46. Pidcock F, Krishnan C, Crawford T, et al: Acute transverse myelitis in childhood: Center-based analysis of 47 cases. Neurology 2007;68:1447-1479.
47. Wingerchuk DM, Lennon VA, Pittock SJ, et al: Revised diagnostic criteria for neuromyelitis optica. Neurology 2006;66:1485-1489.
48. Wingerchuk DM, Hogancamp WF, O'Brien PC, Weinshenker BG: The clinical course of neuromyelitis optica (Devic's syndrome). Neurology 1999;53:1107-1114.
49. Lennon VA, Wingerchuk DM, Kryzer TJ, et al: A serum autoantibody marker of neuromyelitis optica: Distinction from multiple sclerosis. Lancet 2004;364:2106-2112.
50. Lennon VA, Kryzer TJ, Pittock SJ, et al: IgG marker of optic-spinal multiple sclerosis binds to the aquaporin-4 water channel. J Exp Med 2005;202:473-477.

51. Yuksel D, Senbil N, Yilmaz D, eYavuz Gurer YK: Devic's neuromyelitis optica in an infant case. J Child Neurol 2007;22:1143-1146.
52. Pittock SJ, Lennon VA, Krecke K, et al: Brain abnormalities in neuromyelitis optica. Arch Neurol 2006;63:390-396.
53. Jeffery AR, Buncic JR: Pediatric Devic's neuromyelitis optica. J Pediatr Ophthalmol Strabismus 1996;33:223-229.
54. Banwell B, Tenembaum S, Lennon VA, et al: Neuromyelitis optica-IgG in childhood inflammatory demyelinating CNS disorders. Neurology 2008;70:344-352.
55. Park KY, Ahn JY, Cho JH, et al: Neuromyelitis optica with brainstem lesion mistaken for brainstem glioma [case report]. J Neurosurg 2007;107(3 Suppl):251-254.
56. Wingerchuk DM, Weinshenker BG: Neuromyelitis optica: Clinical predictors of a relapsing course and survival. Neurology 2003;60:848-853.
57. MacAllister WS, Boyd JR, Holland NJ, et al: The psychosocial consequences of pediatric multiple sclerosis. Neurology 2007;68(16 Suppl 2):S66-S69.
58. Banwell BL, Anderson PE: The cognitive burden of multiple sclerosis in children. Neurology 2005;64:891-894.
59. MacAllister WS, Belman AL, Milazzo M, et al: Cognitive functioning in children and adolescents with multiple sclerosis. Neurology 2005;64:1422-1425.
60. MacAllister WS, Christodoulou C, Milazzo M, Krupp LB: Longitudinal neuropsychological assessment in pediatric multiple sclerosis. Dev Neuropsychol 2007;32:625-644.
61. Mikaeloff Y, Caridade G, Assi S, et al: Prognostic factors for early severity in a childhood multiple sclerosis cohort. Pediatrics 2006;118:1133-1139.
62. Deryck O, Ketelaer P, Dubois B: Clinical characteristics and long term prognosis in early onset multiple sclerosis. J Neurol 2006;253:720-723.
63. Trojano M, Liguori M, Bosco Zimatore G, et al: Age-related disability in multiple sclerosis. Ann Neurol 2002;51:475-480.
64. Ebers GC, Yee IM, Sadovnick AD, Duquette P: Conjugal multiple sclerosis: Population-based prevalence and recurrence risks in offspring. Canadian Collaborative Study Group. Ann Neurol 2000;48:927-931.
65. Sadovnick AD, Duquette P, Herrera B, et al: A timing-of-birth effect on multiple sclerosis clinical phenotype. Neurology 2007;69:60-62.
66. Robertson NP, O'Riordan JI, Chataway J, et al: Offspring recurrence rates and clinical characteristics of conjugal multiple sclerosis. Lancet 1997;349:1587-1590.
67. Olerup O, Hillert J: HLA class II-associated genetic susceptibility in multiple sclerosis: A critical evaluation. Tissue Antigens 1991;38:1-15.
68. Sotgiu S, Pugliatti M, Sanna A, et al: Multiple sclerosis complexity in selected populations: The challenge of Sardinia, insular Italy. Eur J Neurol 2002;9:329-341.
69. Oksenberg JR, Barcellos LF: Multiple sclerosis genetics: Leaving no stone unturned. Genes Immun 2005;6:375-387.
70. Dyment D, Ebers GC, Sadovnick AD: Genetics of multiple sclerosis. Lancet 2004;3:104-110.
71. Hensiek AE, Sawcer SJ, Feakes R, et al: HLA-DR 15 is associated with female sex and younger age at diagnosis in multiple sclerosis. J Neurol Neurosurg Psychiatry 2002;72:184-187.
72. Masterman T, Ligers A, Olsson T, et al: HLA-DR15 is associated with lower age at onset in multiple sclerosis. Ann Neurol 2000;48:211-219.
73. Weatherby SJ, Thomson W, Pepper L, et al: HLA-DRB1 and disease outcome in multiple sclerosis. J Neurol 2001;248:304-310.
74. Sudomoina MA, Boiko AN, Demina TL, et al: [Connection of multiple sclerosis in the Russian population with alleles of the major histocompatibility complex DRB1 gene.] Mol Biol (Mosk) 1998;32:291-296.
75. Boiko AN, Guseva ME, Guseva MR, et al: Clinico-immunogenetic characteristics of multiple sclerosis with optic neuritis in children. J Neurovirol 2000;6(Suppl 2):S152-S155.
76. Boiko AN, Gusev EI, Sudomoina MA, et al: Association and linkage of juvenile MS with HLA-DR2(15) in Russians. Neurology 2002;58:658-660.
77. Guseva MR, Boiko S, Sudomoina MA, et al: [Immunogenetics of optic neuritis in children with multiple sclerosis.]. Vestn Oftalmol 2002;118:15-19.
78. Ness JM, Chabas D, Sadovnick AD, et al: Clinical features of children and adolescents with multiple sclerosis. Neurology 2007;68(16 Suppl 2):S37-S45.
79. Anlar B, Alikasifoglu M, Kose G, et al: Tumor necrosis factor-alpha gene polymorphisms in children with multiple sclerosis. Neuropediatrics 2001;32:214-216.

80. Ohlenbusch A, Pohl D, Hanefeld F: Myelin oligodendrocyte gene polymorphisms and childhood multiple sclerosis. Pediatr Res 2002;52:175-179.
81. Bar-Or A: The immunology of multiple sclerosis. Semin Neurol 2008;28:29-45.
82. Bettelli E, Oukka M, Kuchroo VK: T(H)-17 cells in the circle of immunity and autoimmunity. Nat Immunol 2007;8:345-350.
83. Banwell B, Bar-Or A, Cheung R, et al: Abnormal T-cell reactivities in childhood inflammatory demyelinating disease and type 1 diabetes. Ann Neurol 2008;6:98-111.
84. O'Connor KC, McLaughlin KA, De Jager PL, et al: Self-antigen tetramers discriminate between myelin autoantibodies to native or denatured protein. Nat Med 2007;13:211-217.
85. Bielekova B, Martin R: Development of biomarkers in multiple sclerosis. Brain 2004;127(Pt 7):1463-1478.
86. Rostasy K, Withut E, Pohl D, et al: Tau, phospho-tau, and S-100B in the cerebrospinal fluid of children with multiple sclerosis. J Child Neurol 2005;20:822-825.
87. Jacobson DL, Gange SJ, Rose NR, Graham NM: Epidemiology and estimated population burden of selected autoimmune diseases in the United States. Clin Immunol Immunopathol 1997;84:223-243.
88. Shames RS: Gender differences in the development and function of the immune system. J Adolesc Health 2002;30(4 Suppl):59-70.
89. Whitacre CC: Sex differences in autoimmune disease. Nat Immunol 2001;2:777-780.
90. Whitacre CC, Reingold SC, O'Looney PA: A gender gap in autoimmunity. Science 1999;283:1277-1278.
91. Fink G: Oestrogen and progesterone interactions in the control of gonadotrophin and prolactin secretion. J Steroid Biochem 1988;30:169-178.
92. Ho KK, O'Sullivan AJ, Weissberger AJ, Kelly JJ: Sex steroid regulation of growth hormone secretion and action. Horm Res 1996;45:67-73.
93. Chesik D, Wilczak N, De Keyser J: The insulin-like growth factor system in multiple sclerosis. Int Rev Neurobiol 2007;79:203-226.
94. Bager P, Munk Nielsen N, Bihrmann K, et al: Childhood infections and risk of multiple sclerosis. Brain 2004;127:2491-2497.
95. Krone B, Pohl D, Rostasy K, et al: Common infectious agents in multiple sclerosis: A case control study in children. Mult Scler 2008;14:136-139.
96. Bagos PG, Nikolopoulos G, Ioannidis A: Chlamydia pneumoniae infection and the risk of multiple sclerosis: A meta-analysis. Mult Scler 2006;12:397-411.
97. Bray P, Luka J, Bray P, Culp K, Schlight J: Antibodies against Epstein-Barr nuclear antigen (EBNA) in multiple sclerosis CSF, and two pentapeptide sequence identities between EBNA and myelin basic protein. Neurology 1992;42:1708-1804.
98. Marrie RA, Wolfson C, Sturkenboom MC, et al: Multiple sclerosis and antecedent infections: A case-control study. Neurology 2000;54:2307-2310.
99. DeLorenze G, Munger KL, Lennette ET, et al: Epstein-Barr virus and multiple sclerosis: Evidence of association from a prospective study with long-term follow-up. Arch Neurol 2006;63:839-844.
100. Alotaibi S, Kennedy J, Tellier R, et al: Epstein-Barr virus in pediatric multiple sclerosis. JAMA 2004;291:1875-1879.
101. Pohl D, Krone B, Rostasy K, et al: High seroprevalence of Epstein-Barr virus in children with multiple sclerosis. Neurology 2006;67:2063-2065.
102. Javier RS, Kunishita T, Koike F, Tabira T: Semple rabies vaccine: Presence of myelin basic protein and proteolipid protein and its activity in experimental allergic encephalomyelitis. J Neurol Sci 1989;93:221-230.
103. Confavreux C, Suissa S, Saddier P, et al: Group ViMS: Vaccinations and the risk of relapse in multiple sclerosis. N Engl J Med 2001;344:319-326.
104. Mikaeloff Y, Caridade G, Assi S, et al: Hepatitis B vaccine and risk of relapse after a first childhood episode of CNS inflammatory demyelination. Brain 2007;130(Pt 4):1105-1110.
105. Munger K, Zhang S, O'Reilly E, et al: Vitamin D intake and the incidence of multiple sclerosis. Neurology 2004;62:60-65.
106. Munger KL, Levin LI, Hollis BW, et al: Serum 25-hydroxyvitamin D levels and risk of multiple sclerosis. JAMA 2006;296:2832-2838.
107. Holick M: The vitamin D epidemic and its health consequences. J Nutr 2005;135:2739S-2748S.
108. Islam T, Gaudermann W, Cozen W, Mack T: Childhood sun exposure influences risk of multiple sclerosis in monozygotic twins. Neurology 2007;69:381-388.

109. van der Mei I, Ponsonby A, Dwyer T, et al: Past exposure to sun, skin phenotype, and risk of multiple sclerosis: Case-control study. Br Med J 2003;327:316.
110. Soilu-Hänninen M, Airas L, Mononen I, et al: 25-Hydroxyvitamin D levels in serum at the onset of multiple sclerosis. Mult Scler 2005;11:266-271.
111. McDonald WI, Compston A, Edan G, et al: Recommended diagnostic criteria for multiple sclerosis: Guidelines from the International Panel on the diagnosis of multiple sclerosis. Ann Neurol 2001;50:121-127.
112. Mikaeloff Y, Adamsbaum C, Husson B, et al: MRI prognostic factors for relapse after acute CNS inflammatory demyelination in childhood. Brain 2004 Sep;127(Pt 9):1942-1947.
113. Banwell B: Treatment of children and adolescents with multiple sclerosis. Expert Rev Neurother 2005;5:391-401.
114. Hahn JS, Siegler DJ, Enzmann D: Intravenous gammaglobulin therapy in recurrent acute disseminated encephalomyelitis. Neurology 1996;46:1173–1174.
115. Nishikawa M, Ichiyama T, Hayashi T, et al: Intravenous immunoglobulin therapy in acute disseminated encephalomyelitis. Pediatr Neurol 1999;21:583-586.
116. Pradhan S, Gupta RP, Shashank S, Pandey N: Intravenous immunoglobulin therapy in acute disseminated encephalomyelitis. J Neurol Sci 1999;165:56-61.
117. Finsterer J, Grass R, Stollberger C, Mamoli B: Immunoglobulins in acute parainfectious, disseminated encephalo-myelitis. Clin Neuropharmacol 1998;21:258-261.
118. Sahlas DJ, Miller SP, Guerin M, et al: Treatment of acute disseminated encephalomyelitis with intravenous immunoglobulin. Neurology 2000;54:1370-1372.
119. Amato MP, Pracucci G, Ponziani G, et al: Long-term safety of azathioprine therapy in multiple sclerosis. Neurology 1993;43:831-833.
120. Beck RW, Cleary PA, Trobe JD, et al: The effect of corticosteroids for acute optic neuritis on the subsequent development of multiple sclerosis. The Optic Neuritis Study Group. N Engl J Med 1993;329:1764-1769.
121. Johnston JB, Silva C, Holden J, et al: Monocyte activation and differentiation augment human endogenous retrovirus expression: Implications for inflammatory brain diseases. Ann Neurol 2001;50:434-442.
122. Paty DW, Li DK: Interferon beta-1b is effective in relapsing-remitting multiple sclerosis: II. MRI analysis results of a multicenter, randomized, double-blind, placebo-controlled trial. UBC MS/MRI Study Group and the IFNB Multiple Sclerosis Study Group. Neurology 1993;43:662-667.
123. Trapp B, Ransohoff R, Rudick R: Neurodegeneration in multiple sclerosis: Relationship to neurological disability. Neuroscientist 1999;5:48-57.
124. Sorensen PS, Fazekas F, Lee M: Intravenous immunoglobulin G for the treatment of relapsing-remitting multiple sclerosis: A meta-analysis. Eur J Neurol 2002;9:557-563.
125. Hyman N, Barnes M, Bhakta B, et al: Botulinum toxin (Dysport) treatment of hip adductor spasticity in multiple sclerosis: A prospective, randomised, double blind, placebo controlled, dose ranging study. J Neurol Neurosurg Psychiatry 2000;68:707-712.
126. Weinstock-Guttman B, Cohen JA: Emerging therapies for multiple sclerosis. Neurologist 1996;2:342-345.

10 Clinically Isolated Syndromes

NUHAD E. ABOU ZEID • SEAN JOSEPH PITTOCK

A *clinically isolated syndrome* (CIS) is an isolated event that is suggestive of demyelination but does not fulfill the diagnostic criteria for a widespread demyelinating disease such as multiple sclerosis (MS). CIS most commonly manifests as an optic neuritis (ON), transverse melitis, or a brainstem syndrome. Because most MS patients present initially with a CIS, most practicing neurologists will deal with the challenges of managing these syndromes.

Understanding of CIS and early MS is rapidly evolving as more extensive pathologic studies and novel magnetic resonance imaging (MRI) techniques are developed. Recent clinical trials have established that the use of immunomodulatory treatments in patients with high-risk CIS could delay the development of MS, based on clinical and radiologic criteria. The application of these recent advances to everyday clinical practice is not straightforward. There are no robust prognostic factors that can be used to select those patients who are destined to progress to MS and to accrue disability. In view of this fact, some experts in the field have advocated initiating treatment with a disease-modifying agent (DMA) in a "treat all" approach, despite concerns regarding the magnitude of clinical benefit and the long-term efficacy in terms of disability and quality of life, not to mention the cost and parenteral mode of administration. All of these uncertainties make the management of CIS a very confusing topic to the practicing neurologist and create significant anxiety for the patients. In this chapter, we integrate evidence-based knowledge of the natural history of CIS with published clinical trial data and propose a practical guideline for the management of CIS.

Natural History of CIS

EPIDEMIOLOGY

The prevalence of MS is estimated to be 177 per 100,000 persons, and the incidence is about 7.5/100,000/year.[1] ON is the best studied CIS, with an estimated prevalence of 115/100,000 and an incidence of 5/100,000/year.[2,3] From natural history studies, it is estimated that 38% of patients with present with ON, 26% with a brainstem syndrome, 25% with a spinal cord syndrome, and 11% with multifocal symptoms.[4]

WHAT HAPPENS TO PATIENTS WITH CIS

Several retrospective and prospective studies have established an association between CIS and the future development of MS. The most recent prospective studies have estimated the long-term risk of MS after CIS to range between 45% and 75%.[2,9-20]

Various diagnostic criteria have been proposed to confirm the dissemination of demyelination and to establish a diagnosis of MS. Historically, the gold standard has been the occurrence of a second clinical event in a different anatomic location, confirming dissemination in time and in space. For a diagnosis of "clinically definite MS" by Poser's criteria, another clinical attack is required with objective clinical or paraclinical neurologic findings.[5] MRI criteria for the diagnosis of MS were proposed by Barkhof and colleagues in 1997 and modified by Tintoré and associates in 2000.[6,7] In 2001, an international panel proposed new MS diagnostic criteria by which MRI can be used to prove dissemination in time and in space, using the modified Barkhof/Tintoré criteria.[8]

Table 10-1 summarizes the results from the three most prominent recent CIS prospective natural history studies.[9,13-17] In the United Kingdom, a clinic-based cohort of CIS patients (*N* = 109) with ON, brainstem, spinal cord, or multifocal syndromes were monitored, and the prognostic value of baseline MRI abnormalities on development of CDMS and disability were investigated. The cumulative risk of CDMS was 43% at 5 years, 59% at 10 years, and 63% at 20 years. At 20 years, 61% of CDMS patients had an Expanded Disability Status Scale (EDSS) score greater than 3. Of patients who developed CDMS, 58% had relapsing-remitting disease (RRMS), whereas 42% had secondary progressive MS after 20 years.[12-15]

In a North American multicenter trial (*N* = 388) of steroids for the treatment of acute isolated ON (Optic Neuritis Treatment Trial), patients were monitored for the development of CDMS. The cumulative probability of developing CDMS was 13% at 2 years, 30% at 5 years, and 38% at 10 years. The risk of CDMS was greatest during the first 5 years, with 75% of CDMS patients converting within 5 years of their initial ON. Of those patients who had developed CDMS by 10 years, 35% had attained an EDSS score of 3 or greater.[9,17,21,22]

A study in Spain monitored patients who presented with CIS (*N* = 156) for a median of 7 years to investigate the rate of conversion to MS and the development of disability. The cumulative probability of developing MS was 42% by Poser's criteria and 51% by the McDonald criteria. The rate of conversion to CDMS was highest in the first 5 years after an episode of CIS, with 83% of patients who

TABLE 10–1 Long-Term Risk of Clinically Definite Multiple Sclerosis (CDMS) and Disability after an Episode of Clinically Isolated Syndromes (CIS)

Study	CIS	*N*	Risk of CDMS	Risk of CDMS Stratified by MRI	Risk of Disability in Patients with CDMS	Risk of Disability Stratified by Baseline MRI
UK study[12-15]	Mixed	109	43% at 5 yr 59% at 10 yr 63% at 20 yr	20 yr CDMS: 82% T2 lesions 21% No lesions	EDSS > 3 at 20 yr: 61%	EDSS > 3 at 20 yr: No T2 lesions, 26% 1-3 T2 lesions, 36% 4-9 T2 lesions, 50% ≥ 10 T2 lesions, 65%
ONTT[9,17,21,22]	ON	388	30% at 5 yr 38% at 10 yr	10 yr CDMS: 56% T2 lesions 22% No lesions	EDSS ≥ 3 at 10 yr: 35%	EDSS ≥ 3 at 10 yr (EDSS available only in CDMS patients): No T2 lesions, 10% ≥ 1 T2 lesions, 30%
Spanish study[16]	Mixed	156	42% at 7 yr	7 yr CDMS: 60% T2 lesions 8% No lesions	EDSS ≥ 3 at 8 yr: 40%	EDSS ≥ 3 at 8 yr: No T2 lesions, 5.8% 1-3 T2 lesions, 8.7% 4-9 T2 lesions, 11.1% ≥ 10 T2 lesions, 25.4%

CDMS, clinically definite multiple sclerosis; EDSS, Extended Disability Status Scale score; MRI, magnetic resonance imaging; ON, optic neuritis; ONTT, Optic Neuritis Treatment Trial.

eventually developed CDMS doing so within that period. At 8 years, 27% of CDMS patients had an EDSS score of 3 or more, compared with 6% of CIS patients.[16]

Clinical, Imaging, and Laboratory Predictors of Outcome in CIS

CLINICAL INDICATORS

Many studies have attempted to evaluate clinical predictors that could help determine long-term prognosis after an episode of CIS.[23-25] It has been reported in natural history studies that ON is associated with lower MS risk and better long-term outcome than other CIS presentations.[21,25,26] The United Kingdom prospective CIS cohort study reported that the type of CIS presentation did not affect the rate of conversion to MS or the development of disability,[12] but that study was underpowered. In a prospective study of 320 CIS patients in Spain, ON was found to have a lower rate of conversion to CDMS at 3 years, compared with the other CIS presentations (spinal cord, brainstem, and multifocal syndromes). However, the ON groups were more likely to have a normal MRI at baseline, which probably explains the lower rate of conversion to CDMS. When considering only patients with an abnormal baseline MRI of the head, no difference in rate of conversion to CDMS was found for ON compared with other CIS presentations, suggesting that MRI is the most important prognostic indicator.[27]

In a population-based cohort of 308 patients in Sweden, 220 patients with a clear CIS presentation were identified, and clinical predictors for development of MS by Poser's criteria and for long-term disability were analyzed. CIS patients who presented with weakness indicative of motor system involvement were twice as likely to develop MS, twice as likely to develop secondary progression, and three times as likely to reach an EDSS score of 7 at 25 years' follow-up than patients without motor involvement. In addition, patients who experienced incomplete remission were twice as likely to reach an EDSS score of 7 at 25 years than patients with complete recovery. Similar findings were reported in a natural history study of 1215 patients in France: patients with complete recovery from CIS were less likely to reach an EDSS score of 6 than those with incomplete recovery.[23] Both studies found that none of these clinical predictors had a significant impact on the rate of secondary progression in the long term.[23,25]

MAGNETIC RESONANCE IMAGING

Head MRI at baseline is the most important predictive tool for evaluating the risk of CDMS after an episode of CIS (see Table 10-1). The risk of MS 20 years after an episode of CIS is 82% if the initial brain MRI has T2 signal abnormality, but only 21% if the initial MRI is normal.[12] The presence of one versus multiple T2 lesions on the baseline brain MRI does not change the long-term risk of developing CDMS.[13,17] However, lesion number and burden on the baseline MRI does affect the time to a second clinical event leading to a diagnosis of MS, with higher lesion burden leading to a shorter duration between CIS and CDMS.[16]

Several long-term follow-up studies have shown a moderate correlation between baseline MRI measures of disease burden and the development of disability (see Table 10-1).[12,13,16,21] The development of disability at 5 years in the Spanish study, as defined by an EDSS score of 3 or greater, correlated with baseline brain MRI lesion burden—both with the number of baseline lesions (Spearman rho coefficient [ρ], 0.43) and with the number of Barkhof criteria fulfilled (ρ, 0.46). In addition, the accumulation of new T2 MRI lesions on follow-up was correlated with 5-year disability (ρ, 0.41).[16] In the United Kingdom study, the baseline T2 lesion volume was associated with the long-term (20-year) EDSS assessment (ρ, 0.48). MS patients who developed secondary progression had a higher rate of lesion accumulation than those who remained with RRMS, especially in the first 5 years after disease onset.[19]

The location of lesions on head MRI may also have prognostic implications. In a study of 42 patients with CIS who were monitored for a median of 8.7 years, using a proportional hazard regression analysis, the presence of two or more infratentorial lesions was a strong predictor of the time to reach an EDSS score of 3 (likelihood ratio, 11.3).[28]

LABORATORY STUDIES

In a prospective study of 415 CIS patients with baseline MRI and cerebrospinal fluid testing, Tintoré and coworkers[4] evaluated the value of oligoclonal band positivity in predicting the development of CDMS. Supernumerary oligoclonal bands were present in 61% of all CIS patients. Though MRI was the best predictor of CDMS risk after 4 years of follow-up, the presence of oligoclonal bands increased the risk of a second relapse independent of MRI, with an adjusted hazard ratio of 1.7. However, oligoclonal band positivity had no predictive value in terms of disability. In the subgroup of CIS patients with normal baseline head MRI, only 4% of patients lacking oligoclonal bands developed CDMS, compared with 23% of those with oligoclonal bands, suggesting that oligoclonal band assessment may have a role assessing MS risk in patients with normal baseline MRI.[4]

A recent prospective study of 73 patients presenting with acute partial transverse myelitis, with a mean follow-up of 46 months, found that not only oligoclonal band positivity but also an abnormal immunoglobulin G (IgG) index was associated with increased risk of conversion to MS by McDonald criteria, suggesting a role for IgG index evaluation.[29]

Antibodies to myelin basic protein (MBP) and myelin oligodendrocyte glycoprotein (MOG) have been proposed as serologic markers for MS, but the trials looking at correlation of these antibodies with the risk of MS have yielded conflicting results.[30,31] Recently, experimental biomarkers of axonal damage, such as tau, neurofilament, and Nogo A, have been under investigation in patients with CIS or MS. Elevated cerebrospinal fluid levels of these markers have been reported in patients with CIS and RRMS compared with controls, suggesting a potential future role in MS risk assessment if these results are corroborated by larger studies.[32,33] In summary, there are currently no data to support the routine use of any serologic testing in patients with CIS, except in neuromyelitis optica (NMO), as discussed later.

PATHOLOGY IN CIS

There is recent evidence that the pathology of early MS and CIS goes beyond the focal lesions, myelin, and the white matter. Trapp and colleagues demonstrated that axonal transection is present in MS, even in the early stages.[34] There have been several studies showing pathologic evidence of cortical MS plaques.[35] Novel MRI techniques have been used to demonstrate abnormalities in magnetization transfer histograms and magnetic resonance spectroscopic analysis of the so-called normal-appearing white and gray matter, even in early MS and CIS.[36,37] It is proposed that subclinical pathology accumulates in the early stages of MS until it reaches a threshold at which disability becomes clinically apparent.[38] Another important aspect of early MS and CIS that has become more obvious recently is cognitive dysfunction, which can occur even in CIS patients and can contribute to disruption of everyday functioning.[39,40]

CIS WITHIN THE NEUROMYELITIS OPTICA SPECTRUM

The NMO-IgG autoantibody is a validated clinical biomarker that distinguishes NMO and related relapsing CNS inflammatory demyelinating disorders from classic MS, which generally is less severe. NMO-IgG targets the astrocytic water channel aquaporin-4 (AQP4).[41,42] Clinical, radiologic, and immunopathologic data support a pathogenic role for this autoantibody. The severity of acute NMO is ameliorated by antibody-depleting therapies.[43,44] NMO attacks the optic nerves (ON) and the spinal cord (seen as a longitudinally extensive lesions on MRI) selectively and repeatedly. The advent of serologic testing for AQP4-IgG has revealed that NMO and its inaugural forms are not rare but are commonly misdiagnosed as MS, for which no specific biomarker is recognized.[45,46]

The initial event in NMO spectrum disorders is a CIS. Because patients with early NMO often have a negative head MRI, NMO-IgG serostatus may be helpful in therapeutic decision making, because seropositivity predicts early relapse (Fig. 10-1). NMO-IgG seropositivity is rare in patients with acute partial transverse myelitis, but it is found in approximately 40% of patients with longitudinally extensive transverse myelitis (LETM).[47] Detection of NMO-IgG in patients with CIS characterized by LETM predicts recurrence or development of ON (thus fulfilling criteria for NMO) within 1 year in 55% of cases.[48] Bilateral or relapsing ON may be a limited form of NMO, with an estimated 25% NMO-IgG seropositivity.[41,49] NMO-IgG seropositivity in these patients predicts poor visual outcome and future development of NMO.[49,50] NMO-IgG positivity is probably rare in isolated unilateral ON, and the role of NMO serology in this setting remains unclear, although seropositivity most likely suggests an NMO spectrum disorder and a higher likelihood of relapse.

Medical Management of CIS

TREATMENT OF THE ACUTE ATTACK

In clinical practice, the acute short-term management of an episode of CIS is similar to the management of an MS relapse. ON is the most studied CIS, and several trials have shown that treatment with steroids does not alter the long-term outcome but does reduce recovery time.[51,52] The American Academy of Neurology practice parameter for the treatment of acute ON concludes that there is no treatment that affects long-term visual outcome from acute ON, but very high-dose oral or intravenous methylprednisolone (0.5 to 1 g/day) or corticotropin (ACTH) may speed the recovery from an acute attack. Oral prednisone (1 mg/Kg/day) has no proven benefit in the acute treatment of ON.[53]

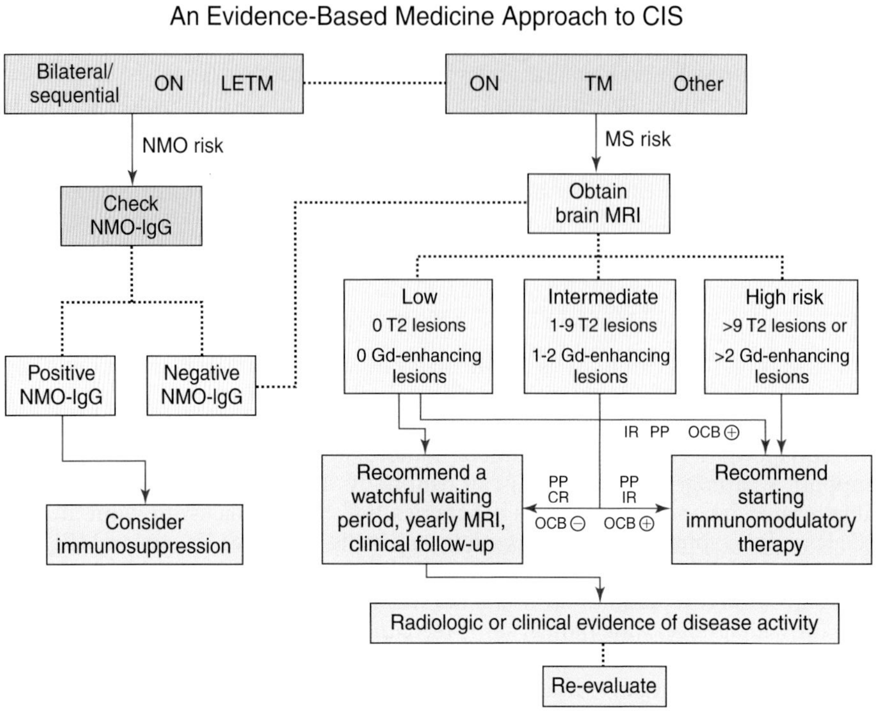

An Evidence-Based Medicine Approach to CIS

Bilateral/sequential ON LETM

ON TM Other

NMO risk

MS risk

Check NMO-IgG

Obtain brain MRI

Positive NMO-IgG

Negative NMO-IgG

Low 0 T2 lesions 0 Gd-enhancing lesions

Intermediate 1-9 T2 lesions 1-2 Gd-enhancing lesions

High risk >9 T2 lesions or >2 Gd-enhancing lesions

IR PP OCB ⊕

PP CR OCB ⊖

PP IR OCB ⊕

Consider immunosuppression

Recommend a watchful waiting period, yearly MRI, clinical follow-up

Recommend starting immunomodulatory therapy

Radiologic or clinical evidence of disease activity

Re-evaluate

Figure 10–1 An evidence-based suggested approach to the management of clinically isolated syndromes (CIS). Blue arrows reflect reasonable evidence, whereas red arrows reflect areas of controversy. CR, complete recovery; Gd, gadolinium; IgG, immunoglobulin G; IR, incomplete recovery; LETM, longitudinally extensive transverse myelitis; MRI, magnetic resonance imaging; MS, multiple sclerosis; NMO, neuromyelitis optica; OCB, oligoclonal bands; PP, patient preference; TM, transverse myelitis.

A randomized trial of 22 patients suggested that patients who have severe, steroid-unresponsive attacks of demyelination may benefit from therapeutic plasma exchange.[54] In a review of 59 patients with severe demyelination related to MS, NMO, or acute disseminated encephalomyelitis treated with plasma exchange, 44% of the patients had a good functional improvement.[43] A case series of plasma exchange in 10 patients with severe ON unresponsive to high-dose prednisone, improvement in visual acuity was demonstrated in 7 patients.[55] These studies suggest a role for plasma exchange in patients with severe CIS that is not responsive to corticosteroid treatment.

DISEASE-MODIFYING THERAPIES

Clinical observation was the paradigm for the long-term management of CIS until clinical trials addressed the possible use of immunomodulatory therapy in high-risk CIS patients. To date, there have been three randomized clinical trials: the Controlled High-Risk Subjects Avonex Multiple Sclerosis Prevention Study (CHAMPS), the Early Treatment of MS Study (ETOMS), and the Betaseron in Newly Emerging MS for Initial Treatment (BENEFIT) study. These investigations showed that use of DMAs in high-risk CIS groups can prolong the time to MS diagnosis (by Poser or McDonald's criteria) and modify the rate of development of new MRI lesions.[56-58] The characteristics of the trials and their main outcome results are summarized in Table 10-2.

Two of these trials had extension studies. The Controlled High-Risk Avonex Multiple Sclerosis Prevention Study in Ongoing Neurologic Surveillance (CHAMPIONS) was a 5-year, open-label extension study of CHAMPS.[59] At 3 years, the placebo patients who elected to go on treatment became the "delayed treatment" group, and the initial interferon treatment group became the "immediate treatment" group. These groups were compared at the 5-year time point for development of CDMS and MS-related disability. The risk of CDMS continued to be lower in the immediate treatment group, similar to the results in CHAMPS, but MRI outcomes and disability measures showed no difference between the two groups.[59] The major difficulty in interpreting the results of this study is that it was not prospectively planned and a significant proportion of the initial study cohort was lost to follow-up.

The second extension trial was the 5-year, prospectively planned extension of BENEFIT, which is ongoing. Disability was assessed in terms of EDSS progression, which was defined as an increase in EDSS of 1 point or more, sustained over repeat testing at 6 months. The 3-year prospectively planned analysis of this extension study showed that patients treated early had a 40% reduction in EDSS progression (24% versus 16%), compared with the delayed treatment group.[60] These results are promising but need to be interpreted with caution. The ultimate goal is meaningful clinical benefit as applied to patient care. The magnitude of clinical benefit at the 3-year point was small, with an absolute risk reduction of 8%. The median EDSS at baseline was 1.5, which is relatively low, and low EDSS scores have been shown to be less reproducible, with higher inter-rater variability compared with higher EDSS scores. Subgroup analysis showed that most of the benefit in terms of disability was in the higher-risk patients, those with multiple T2 lesions (>9) and gadolinium-enhancing lesions, whereas those with lower risk had minimal, if any, benefit.[61]

When applying the results of such trials to patient care, it is important to evaluate whether patients in daily clinical practice are clinically and radiologically similar to the selected high-risk patients who benefit from treatment in the trials. Table 10-2 summarizes the randomized CIS treatment trial results with an evidence-based approach.[56-60] The baseline median number of T2 lesions in the trial patients is significantly higher than in the natural history cohorts. The selection of patients with higher lesion burden for trials is also reflected in the higher rate of MS conversion in the trials at 2 to 3 years, compared with the rates in natural history CIS follow-up studies.[14,17,56-58,62]

THERAPEUTIC DECISION MAKING: EARLY TREATMENT OR WATCHFUL WAITING

With the advent of immunomodulatory therapy for MS and the recent trials showing potential benefit of early treatment initiation, there is significant controversy regarding the "who and when" to treat. In clinical practice, two approaches exist. One is early initiation of treatment in most CIS patients, and the other is to adoption of a "watchful waiting" approach in selected patients, to determine their natural course, with treatment those who are likely to be high risk[63,64] (see Fig. 10-1). The main arguments for these two approaches are summarized as follows.

TABLE 10–2 Summary of Randomized Treatment Trials for High-Risk CIS and Comparison to the UK Natural History Study of CIS

Study	Patient Population	MRI Inclusion Criteria	Treatment	Baseline MRI (Median No. of T2 Lesions)	Cumulative Probability of CDMS	ARR for CDMS	NNT to Prevent 1 CDMS	Days to conversion to CDMS
CHAMPS[56]	N = 383 Mean age: 33 yr Mixed CIS	≥2 T2 lesions	Avonex 30 μg/wk NA	Overall: 13	At 3 yr (P = .002): Placebo: 50% Interferon: 35%	15%	7	Not reported
ETOMS[57]	N = 308 Mean age: 29 yr Mixed CIS	≥4 T2 lesions *or* ≥3 lesions (infratentorial or enhancing)	Rebif 22 μg/wk NA	Placebo: 22 Interferon: 26	At 2 yr (P = .047) Placebo: 45% Interferon: 34%	11%	9	Placebo: 252 Interferon: 569 Delay: 317
BENEFIT[58]	N = 487 Mean age: 30 yr Mixed CIS	≥2 T2 lesions	Betaseron 250 μg/wk NA	Placebo: 17 Interferon: 18	At 2 yr (P < .0001) Placebo: 45% Interferon: 28%	17%	6	Placebo: 255 Interferon: 618 Delay: 363
UK natural history study[12-15]	N = 109 Mean age: 32 yr Mixed CIS	NA	NA	Overall: 2	43% at 5 yr	NA	NA	NA

BENEFIT, Betaseron in Newly Emerging MS for Initial Treatment; CDMS, clinically defined multiple sclerosis; CHAMPS, Controlled High-Risk Subjects Avonex Multiple Sclerosis Prevention Study; CIS, clinically isolated syndrome; ETOMS, Early Treatment of MS Study; MRI, magnetic resonance imaging; UK, United Kingdom. NA, not applicable; ARR, absolute risk reduction; the difference in the rates of adverse events between study and control populations (i.e., the difference in risk between the control group and the treated group: ARR = Control group risk – Treatment group risk; NNT, number needed to treat; the number of patients who must be exposed to an intervention before the clinical outcome of interest occurred. Equal to the inverse of the absolute risk reduction: NNT = 1/ARR.

Arguments for Treating Early

1. There is ample evidence from randomized trials that DMAs reduce the relative risk of CDMS in high-risk CIS patients by about one third and delay the development of CDMS by about 1 year after 2 to 3 years of treatment.
2. There are no reliable early clinical or paraclinical measures to accurately predict long-term outcome in individual patients with CIS or early RRMS; therefore, to maximize benefit, every patient should be treated early.
3. Early treatment could potentially limit the accumulation of early irreversible subclinical damage.
4. Long-term treatment with DMAs is relatively safe, with no significant serious or life-threatening side effects.
5. The long-term neuropsychiatric disability related to MS is underestimated, because most long-term natural history studies assess disability based on the EDSS, which is heavily weighted toward physical disability.[64,65]

Arguments for Watchful Waiting

1. DMAs have only a modest, short-term effect in high-risk CIS patients.
2. Some CIS patients never develop CDMS, and about 15% of those who do develop CDMS have a mild or benign MS disease course.[66,67]
3. Most high-risk CIS patients convert to CDMS early (within a few years); therefore, a brief early watchful waiting period might help select patients who are likely to develop CDMS and to have an active disease course, thus minimizing overtreatment of patients with mild disease burden who are less likely to benefit from treatment.
4. There is no robust evidence that long-term DMA treatment modifies the early accumulation of subclinical tissue damage or the long-term accumulation of physical or neuropsychiatric impairment.
5. Treatment is parenteral, is very expensive, and causes bothersome side effects.[63]

It is hard to predict how an individual patient with CIS will fare or who will benefit most from early initiation of treatment. The most reasonable approach is to explain the options for low-risk CIS patients and allow them to make an informed decision, whether to commit to DMAs or follow a watchful clinical and radiologic approach. On the other hand, high-risk patients, such as those with an aggressive initial episode and poor recovery, as well as patients with high disease burden or disease activity (enhancing lesions) on imaging, should be advised to commence immunomodulatory therapy (see Fig. 10-1). Helping patients make an informed decision may increase their compliance and satisfaction and decrease their uncertainty and anxiety

REFERENCES

1. Mayr WT, Pittock SJ, McClelland RL, et al: Incidence and prevalence of multiple sclerosis in Olmsted County, Minnesota, 1985-2000. Neurology 2003;61:1373-1377.
2. Rodriguez M, Siva A, Cross SA, et al: Optic neuritis: A population-based study in Olmsted County, Minnesota. Neurology 1995;45:244-250.
3. Transverse Myelitis Consortium Working Group: Proposed diagnostic criteria and nosology of acute transverse myelitis. Neurology 2002;59:499-505.

4. Tintoré M, Rovira A, Rio J, et al: Do oligoclonal bands add information to MRI in first attacks of multiple sclerosis? Neurology 2008;70(13 Pt 2):1079-1083.
5. Poser CM, Paty DW, Scheinberg L, et al: New diagnostic criteria for multiple sclerosis: Guidelines for research protocols. Ann Neurol 1983;13:227-231.
6. Barkhof F, Filippi M, Miller DH, et al: Comparison of MRI criteria at first presentation to predict conversion to clinically definite multiple sclerosis. Brain 1997;120(Pt 11):2059-2069.
7. Tintoré M, Rovira A, Martinez MJ, et al: Isolated demyelinating syndromes: Comparison of different MR imaging criteria to predict conversion to clinically definite multiple sclerosis. AJNR Am J Neuroradiol 2000;21:702-706.
8. McDonald WI, Compston A, Edan G, et al: Recommended diagnostic criteria for multiple sclerosis: Guidelines from the International Panel on the diagnosis of multiple sclerosis. Ann Neurol 2001;50:121-127.
9. The 5-year risk of MS after optic neuritis: Experience of the optic neuritis treatment trial. Optic Neuritis Study Group. Neurology 1997;49:1404-1413.
10. Ghezzi A, Torri V, Zaffaroni M: Isolated optic neuritis and its prognosis for multiple sclerosis: A clinical and paraclinical study with evoked potentials—CSF examination and brain MRI. Ital J Neurol Sci 1996;17:325-332.
11. Soderstrom M: The clinical and paraclinical profile of optic neuritis: A prospective study. Ital J Neurol Sci 1995;16:167-176.
12. Fisniku LK, Brex PA, Altmann DR, et al: Disability and T2 MRI lesions: A 20-year follow-up of patients with relapse onset of multiple sclerosis. Brain 2008;131:808-817.
13. Brex PA, Ciccarelli O, O'Riordan JI, et al: A longitudinal study of abnormalities on MRI and disability from multiple sclerosis. N Engl J Med 2002;346:158-164.
14. O'Riordan JI, Thompson AJ, Kingsley DP, et al: The prognostic value of brain MRI in clinically isolated syndromes of the CNS: A 10-year follow-up. Brain 1998;121(Pt 3):495-503.
15. Morrissey SP, Miller DH, Kendall BE, et al: The significance of brain magnetic resonance imaging abnormalities at presentation with clinically isolated syndromes suggestive of multiple sclerosis: A 5-year follow-up study. Brain 1993;116(Pt 1):135-146.
16. Tintoré M, Rovira A, Rio J, et al: Baseline MRI predicts future attacks and disability in clinically isolated syndromes. Neurology 2006;67:968-972.
17. Beck RW, Trobe JD, Moke PS, et al: High- and low-risk profiles for the development of multiple sclerosis within 10 years after optic neuritis: Experience of the optic neuritis treatment trial. Arch Ophthalmol 2003;121:944-949.
18. Hely MA, McManis PG, Doran TJ, et al: Acute optic neuritis: A prospective study of risk factors for multiple sclerosis. J Neurol Neurosurg Psychiatry 1986;49:1125-1130.
19. Francis G: The 5-year risk of MS after optic neuritis. Neurology 1998;51:1236; author reply1237-1238.
20. Sandberg-Wollheim M, Bynke H, Cronqvist S, et al: A long-term prospective study of optic neuritis: Evaluation of risk factors. Ann Neurol 1990;27:386-393.
21. Beck RW, Smith CH, Gal RL, et al: Neurologic impairment 10 years after optic neuritis. Arch Neurol 2004;61:1386-1389.
22. Beck RW, Cleary PA, Trobe JD, et al: The effect of corticosteroids for acute optic neuritis on the subsequent development of multiple sclerosis. The Optic Neuritis Study Group. N Engl J Med 1993;329:1764-1769.
23. Confavreux C, Vukusic S, Adeleine P: Early clinical predictors and progression of irreversible disability in multiple sclerosis: An amnesic process. Brain 2003;126:770-782.
24. Weinshenker BG, Rice GP, Noseworthy JH, et al: The natural history of multiple sclerosis: A geographically based study 4. Applications to planning and interpretation of clinical therapeutic trials. Brain 1991;114(Pt 2):1057-1067.
25. Eriksson M, Andersen O, Runmarker B: Long-term follow up of patients with clinically isolated syndromes, relapsing-remitting and secondary progressive multiple sclerosis. Mult Scler 2003;9:260-274.
26. Runmarker B, Andersen O: Prognostic factors in a multiple sclerosis incidence cohort with twenty-five years of follow-up. Brain 1993;116(Pt 1):117-134.
27. Tintoré M, Rovira A, Rio J, et al: Is optic neuritis more benign than other first attacks in multiple sclerosis? Ann Neurol 2005;57:210-215.
28. Minneboo A, Barkhof F, Polman CH, et al: Infratentorial lesions predict long-term disability in patients with initial findings suggestive of multiple sclerosis. Arch Neurol 2004;61:217-221.
29. Sellner J, Luthi N, Buhler R, et al: Acute partial transverse myelitis: Risk factors for conversion to multiple sclerosis. Eur J Neurol 2008;15:398-405.

30. Berger T, Rubner P, Schautzer F, et al: Antimyelin antibodies as a predictor of clinically definite multiple sclerosis after a first demyelinating event. N Engl J Med 2003;349:139-145.
31. Kuhle J, Pohl C, Mehling M, et al: Lack of association between antimyelin antibodies and progression to multiple sclerosis. N Engl J Med 2007;356:371-378.
32. Brettschneider J, Petzold A, Junker A, Tumani H: Axonal damage markers in the cerebrospinal fluid of patients with clinically isolated syndrome improve predicting conversion to definite multiple sclerosis. Mult Scler 2006;12:143-148.
33. Jurewicz A, Matysiak M, Raine CS, Selmaj K: Soluble Nogo-A, an inhibitor of axonal regeneration, as a biomarker for multiple sclerosis. Neurology 2007;68:283-287.
34. Trapp BD, Peterson J, Ransohoff RM, et al: Axonal transection in the lesions of multiple sclerosis. N Engl J Med 1998;338:278-285.
35. Pirko I, Lucchinetti CF, Sriram S, Bakshi R: Gray matter involvement in multiple sclerosis. Neurology 2007;68:634-642.
36. Traboulsee A, Dehmeshki J, Brex PA, et al: Normal-appearing brain tissue MTR histograms in clinically isolated syndromes suggestive of MS. Neurology 2002;59:126-128.
37. Brex PA, Gomez-Anson B, Parker GJ, et al: Proton MR spectroscopy in clinically isolated syndromes suggestive of multiple sclerosis. J Neurol Sci 1999;166:16-22.
38. Bjartmar C, Wujek JR, Trapp BD: Axonal loss in the pathology of MS: Consequences for understanding the progressive phase of the disease. J Neurol Sci 2003;206:165-171.
39. Amato MP, Zipoli V, Portaccio E: Multiple sclerosis-related cognitive changes: A review of cross-sectional and longitudinal studies. J Neurol Sci 2006;245:41-46.
40. Feuillet L, Reuter F, Audoin B, et al: Early cognitive impairment in patients with clinically isolated syndrome suggestive of multiple sclerosis. Mult Scler 2007;13:124-127.
41. Lennon VA, Wingerchuk DM, Kryzer TJ, et al: A serum autoantibody marker of neuromyelitis optica: Distinction from multiple sclerosis. Lancet 2004;364:2106-2112.
42. Lennon VA, Kryzer TJ, Pittock SJ, et al: IgG marker of optic-spinal multiple sclerosis binds to the aquaporin-4 water channel. J Exp Med 2005;202:473-477.
43. Keegan M, Pineda AA, McClelland RL, et al: Plasma exchange for severe attacks of CNS demyelination: Predictors of response. Neurology 2002;58:143-146.
44. Cree BA, Lamb S, Morgan K, et al: An open label study of the effects of rituximab in neuromyelitis optica. Neurology 2005;64:1270-1272.
45. Wingerchuk DM, Lennon VA, Pittock SJ, et al: Revised diagnostic criteria for neuromyelitis optica. Neurology 2006;66:1485-1489.
46. Wingerchuk DM, Weinshenker BG: Neuromyelitis optica. Curr Treat Options Neurol 2005;7:173-182.
47. Scott TF, Kassab SL, Pittock SJ: Neuromyelitis optica IgG status in acute partial transverse myelitis. Arch Neurol 2006;63:1398-1400.
48. Weinshenker BG, Wingerchuk DM, Vukusic S, et al: Neuromyelitis optica IgG predicts relapse after longitudinally extensive transverse myelitis. Ann Neurol 2006;59:566-569.
49. Matiello M, Lennon VA, Jacob A, et al: NMO-IgG predicts the outcome of recurrent optic neuritis. Neurology 2008;70:2197-2200.
50. Pirko I, Blauwet LK, Lesnick TG, Weinshenker BG: The natural history of recurrent optic neuritis. Arch Neurol 2004;61:1401-1405.
51. Vedula S, Brodney-Folse S, Gal R, Beck R: Corticosteroids for treating optic neuritis. Cochrane Database Syst Rev 2007: CD001430.
52. Beck RW, Gal RL, Bhatti MT, et al: Visual function more than 10 years after optic neuritis: Experience of the optic neuritis treatment trial. Am J Ophthalmol 2004;137:77-83.
53. Goodin DS: Corticosteroids and optic neuritis. Neurology 1993;43:632-633; author reply 633-634.
54. Weinshenker BG, O'Brien PC, Petterson TM, et al: A randomized trial of plasma exchange in acute central nervous system inflammatory demyelinating disease. Ann Neurol 1999;46:878-886.
55. Ruprecht K, Klinker E, Dintelmann T, et al: Plasma exchange for severe optic neuritis: Treatment of 10 patients. Neurology 2004;63:1081-1083.
56. Jacobs LD, Beck RW, Simon JH, et al: Intramuscular interferon beta-1a therapy initiated during a first demyelinating event in multiple sclerosis. CHAMPS Study Group. N Engl J Med 2000;343:898-904.
57. Comi G, Filippi M, Barkhof F, et al: Effect of early interferon treatment on conversion to definite multiple sclerosis: A randomised study. Lancet 2001;357:1576-1582.

58. Kappos L, Polman CH, Freedman MS, et al: Treatment with interferon beta-1b delays conversion to clinically definite and McDonald MS in patients with clinically isolated syndromes. Neurology 2006;67:1242-1249.
59. Kinkel RP, Kollman C, O'Connor P, et al: IM interferon beta-1a delays definite multiple sclerosis 5 years after a first demyelinating event. Neurology 2006;66:678-684.
60. Kappos L, Freedman MS, Polman CH, et al: Effect of early versus delayed interferon beta-1b treatment on disability after a first clinical event suggestive of multiple sclerosis: A 3-year follow-up analysis of the BENEFIT study. Lancet 2007;370:389-397.
61. Pittock SJ: Interferon beta in multiple sclerosis: How much BENEFIT? Lancet 2007;370: 363-364.
62. Beck RW, Arrington J, Murtagh FR, et al: Brain magnetic resonance imaging in acute optic neuritis. Experience of the Optic Neuritis Study Group. Arch Neurol 1993;50:841-846.
63. Pittock SJ, Weinshenker BG, Noseworthy JH, et al: Not every patient with multiple sclerosis should be treated at time of diagnosis. Arch Neurol 2006;63:611-614.
64. Frohman EM, Havrdova E, Lublin F, et al: Most patients with multiple sclerosis or a clinically isolated demyelinating syndrome should be treated at the time of diagnosis. Arch Neurol 2006;63:614-619.
65. Amato MP, Zipoli V, Goretti B, et al: Benign multiple sclerosis: Cognitive, psychological and social aspects in a clinical cohort. J Neurol 2006;253:1054-1059.
66. Pittock SJ, McClelland RL, Mayr WT, et al: Clinical implications of benign multiple sclerosis: A 20-year population-based follow-up study. Ann Neurol 2004;56:303-306.
67. Sayao AL, Devonshire V, Tremlett H: Longitudinal follow-up of "benign" multiple sclerosis at 20 years. Neurology 2007;68:496-500.

11 Acute Disseminated Encephalomyelitis

NATHAN P. YOUNG • BRIAN G. WEINSHENKER • CLAUDIA F. LUCCHINETTI

Acute disseminated encephalomyelitis (ADEM) is traditionally considered an uncommon monophasic, acute or subacute, multifocal, idiopathic inflammatory demyelinating disease (IIDD) that predominantly involves the white matter of the central nervous system (CNS). Fulminant presentations of ADEM, with early depressed level of conscious followed by death within days, are well described; pathologic descriptions highlight a unique pattern of perivenous demyelination that is not typical of the sharply demarcated plaques of demyelination in multiple sclerosis (MS). Most clinicians would not confuse such fulminant presentations of ADEM with typical presentations of MS. However, since the advent of modern critical care, effective short-term immunomodulatory treatments, and improved diagnostic testing, especially magnetic resonance imaging (MRI), patients with milder, nonfatal presentations of probable ADEM are more frequently encountered. These patients may present with symptoms, signs, and MRI abnormalities that are suggestive of MS, including optic neuritis (ON) and myelitis. In fact, most studies of clinically defined ADEM to date (in which most of the patients have survived with a favorable outcome) recognize considerable overlap of ADEM with presentations of patients eventually meeting criteria for MS. Now that long-term disease-modifying treatments for MS are available, there is an emphasis on early diagnosis and treatment of MS and its distinction from monophasic ADEM and other diseases that may mimic MS. Accurate diagnostic criteria that reliably distinguish monophasic ADEM from MS are needed, so that patients with monophasic ADEM are not unnecessarily exposed to the potential risks, side effects, and costs of current treatments for MS, especially the interferons. Although validated clinical criteria for ADEM are not yet established, recent clinical studies have advanced an understanding of ADEM for practicing clinicians and highlighted uncertainties that need further study.

In this chapter, we describe the recently proposed clinical and pathologic definitions of ADEM and discuss the clinical utility and limitations of individual criteria for ADEM. In addition, we outline a practical approach for evaluation and treatment of ADEM for clinicians and highlight uncertainties that require further study.

Definitions of Acute Disseminated Encephalomyelitis

CLINICAL DEFINITIONS

There are no accepted, prospective or pathologically verified, clinical diagnostic criteria for ADEM. Early retrospective studies suffered from broad inclusion criteria that most likely included patients with first presentations of MS[1-9] and neuromyelitis optica (NMO).[1,3,7,10] The first set of diagnostic criteria for ADEM in children (<10 years) were recently proposed by consensus of the International Pediatric MS Study Group (IPMSSG), a group of adult and pediatric neurologists and experts in genetics, epidemiology, neuropsychology, nursing, and immunology organized by The National Multiple Sclerosis Society (Table 11-1).[11,12] The ISPSSG criteria build on earlier, less rigorous criteria and clarify the terminology used to describe cases of possible ADEM that do have a monophasic clinical course (i.e., relapsing or recurrent). The IPMSSG criteria emphasize multifocal, polysymptomatic presentations, with encephalopathy as a key specific clinical feature that distinguishes ADEM from MS. Encephalopathy, broadly defined, is required for the diagnosis of ADEM in first and subsequent attacks of otherwise idiopathic CNS demyelination. The IPMSSG emphasizes the need for prospective validation and probable revision of the criteria over the next 10 to 20 years. Although these criteria are conservative by requiring encephalopathy, they should be used with caution in clinical practice, and they have not yet been reliably proven to distinguish between fulminant MS and other IIDDs.

Mikaeloff and associates used ADEM criteria similar to the IPMSSG criteria in a study of 132 pediatric patients presenting with first attacks of idiopathic CNS demyelination. The criteria predicted a monophasic course in 82% of patients over a mean follow-up of 5.5 ± 3.6 years. However, a substantial proportion of patients (18%) still went on to have a relapse at a different CNS site than the first attack and appeared to have a clinical course consistent with MS.[8] Relapsing patients tended to present with ON, a familial history of CNS demyelination, Barkhof MS criteria on MRI, and no neurologic sequelae after the first attack. Mikaeloff's group suggested a diagnosis of MS in patients with recurrence, but others have concluded that such cases provide evidence that ADEM can relapse or recur. This controversy is discussed in more detail later in this chapter.[3-5,7,13,14]

The IPMSSG criteria are largely based on earlier studies in pediatric patients and have not been tested in adults. In a retrospective study of 60 adults with fulminant first presentations of idiopathic demyelinating disease with multifocal MRI abnormalities mainly involving white matter, de Seze and colleagues analyzed patients with monophasic ADEM or relapsing MS at a mean follow-up of 37 months. They found that those patients who had monophasic ADEM at last follow-up tended to present with three major differences: (1) "atypical" clinical symptoms for MS (including consciousness alteration, hypersomnia, seizures, encephalopathy, aphasia, severe motor deficit, and bilateral ON); (2) absence of spinal fluid oligoclonal bands (OCB); and (3) gray matter involvement on MRI.[15] The authors determined that at least two of these three factors were present in most patients in the ADEM group (83%) and only one or none in the MS group (95%). These factors were proposed for further study as criteria for ADEM in adults. Although the IPMSSG criteria were not applied in this study, the similarities suggest that the IPMSSG criteria are worth further study in and may be applicable to adult patients. However, just as MS may present differently in children and adults, so may ADEM.

PATHOLOGIC DEFINITIONS

The pathologic hallmark of ADEM is perivenular inflammation with limited "sleeves of demyelination" (Fig. 11-1A).[16,17-20] In some cases, larger areas of demyelination occur secondary to coalescence of many perivenous demyelinating lesions (see Fig. 11-1B).[18-21] Although perivascular inflammation is also a feature of MS pathology, the patterns of demyelination in ADEM stand in contrast to the confluent sheets of macrophage infiltration admixed with reactive astrocytes in completely demyelinated regions that are typical of an MS plaque (see Fig. 11-1C).[22] Acute hemorrhagic leukoencephalitis (AHLE) is pathologically similar to ADEM but additionally exhibits petechial hemorrhage and venular necrosis.[16] A complete description of the pathology of ADEM and other IIDDs is beyond the scope of this text and is reviewed elsewhere.[16,17,19,22,23]

The pathologic differences between perivenous and confluent demyelination suggest that brain histopathology might be clinically useful as a diagnostic gold standard for distinguishing ADEM from MS or other IIDDs. However, the true utility of brain biopsy in distinguishing ADEM from MS or other IIDDs has not been examined. A large cohort of patients with biopsy-proven confluent demyelinating disease (excluding patients with perivenous demyelination) was found to be similar to a population-based MS cohort.[24] Perhaps confluent demyelination in such cases is predictive of future relapse or progression in a fashion typical of MS. Alternatively, it is also unknown whether a perivenous pattern of demyelination may predict a monophasic course typical of ADEM. So far, only rare case reports have clearly described the clinical and neuroimaging correlations in patients with perivenous demyelination since the last large clinicopathologic series published in 1975.[3,5,25-29] Importantly, all of these cases were monophasic, most were fatal,[5,25,27,28] and one patient presented with a focal brainstem syndrome.[26]

Clinical Characteristics of ADEM

Retrospective studies using various clinical criteria for ADEM have led to several clinical, laboratory, and imaging observations that are associated with a final diagnosis of ADEM versus MS (Table 11-2). The following sections discuss the utility and limitations of these observations for application in clinical practice. Although the power of these findings is limited by the lack of a diagnostic gold standard that distinguishes ADEM from MS to begin with, they may still be helpful to clinicians faced with this common diagnostic challenge.

TABLE 11–1 International Pediatric Multiple Sclerosis Study Group: Consensus Definitions

Monophasic Acute Disseminated Encephalomyelitis (ADEM)

A first clinical event with a presumed inflammatory or demyelinating cause, with acute or subacute onset that affects multifocal areas of the CNS. The clinical presentation must be polysymptomatic and must include encephalopathy, which is defined as one or more of the following:
1. Behavioral change (e.g., confusion, excessive irritability)
2. Alteration in consciousness (e.g., lethargy, coma)

Event should be followed by improvement (clinically, on MRI, or both), but there may be residual deficits

No history of a clinical episode with features of a prior demyelinating event

No other etiologies can explain the event

New or fluctuating symptoms, signs, or MRI findings occurring within 3 months of the inciting ADEM event are considered part of the acute event

Neuroimaging shows focal or multifocal lesion(s), predominantly involving white matter, without radiologic evidence of previous destructive white matter changes:
1. Brain MRI, with FLAIR or T2-weighted images, reveals large (>1-2 cm) lesions that are multifocal, hyperintense, and located in the supratentorial or infratentorial white matter regions; gray matter, especially basal ganglia and thalamus, is frequently involved
2. In rare cases, brain MRI shows a large single lesion (≥1-2 cm), predominantly affecting white matter
3. Spinal cord MRI may show confluent intramedullary lesion(s) with variable enhancement, in addition to abnormal brain MRI findings specified earlier

Recurrent ADEM

New event of ADEM with a recurrence of the initial symptoms and signs, occurring 3 or more months after the first ADEM event, without involvement of new clinical areas by history, examination, or neuroimaging

Event does not occur while on steroids, and it occurs at least 1 month after completing therapy

MRI shows no new lesions; original lesions may have enlarged

No better explanation exists

Multiphasic ADEM

ADEM followed by a new clinical event that also meets criteria for ADEM but involves new anatomic areas of the CNS as confirmed by history, neurologic examination, and neuroimaging

The subsequent event must occur at least 3 months after the onset of the initial ADEM event and at least 1 month after completion of steroid therapy

The subsequent event must have a polysymptomatic presentation including encephalopathy, with neurologic symptoms or signs that differ from those of the initial event (mental status changes may not differ from the initial event)

The brain MRI must show new areas of involvement but must also demonstrate complete or partial resolution of those lesions associated with the first ADEM event

CNS, central nervous system; FLAIR, fluid-attenuated inversion recovery; MRI, magnetic resonance imaging.

Reproduced from Krupp, LB, Banwell B, Tenembaum S: Consensus definitions proposed for pediatric multiple sclerosis and related disorders. Neurology 2007;68:S7-S12 with permission from Lippincott Williams & Wilkins; online at http://www.lww.com.)

Lucchinetti CF, Parisi J, Bruck W: The pathology of multiple sclerosis. Neurol Clin 2005;23:77-105, vi.

Marchioni E, Ravaglia S, Piccolo G, et al: Postinfectious inflammatory disorders: Subgroups based on prospective follow-up. Neurology 2005;65:1057-1065.

BACKGROUND: Acute disseminated encephalomyelitis (ADEM) refers to a monophasic acute multifocal inflammatory CNS disease. However, both relapsing and site-restricted variants, possibly associated with peripheral nervous system (PNS) involvement, are also observed, and a systematic classification is lacking. OBJECTIVE: To describe a cohort of postinfectious ADEM patients, to propose a classification based on clinical and instrumental features, and to identify subgroups of patients with different prognostic factors. METHODS: Inpatients of a neurologic and infectious disease clinic affected by postinfectious CNS syndrome consecutively admitted over 5 years were studied. RESULTS: Of 75 patients enrolled, 60 fulfilled criteria for ADEM after follow-up lasting from 24 months to 7 years. Based on lesion distribution, patients were classified as having encephalitis (20%), myelitis (23.3%), encephalomyelitis (13.3%), encephalomyeloradiculoneuritis (26.7%), and myeloradiculoneuritis (16.7%). Thirty patients (50%) had a favorable outcome. Fifteen patients (25%) showed a relapsing course. Poor outcome was related with older age at onset, female gender, elevated cerebrospinal fluid proteins, and spinal cord and PNS involvement. All but two patients received high-dose steroids as first-line treatment, with a positive response in 39 (67%). Ten of 19 nonresponders (53%) benefited from high-dose IV immunoglobulin; 9 of 10 had PNS involvement. The data were not controlled. CONCLUSIONS: A high prevalence of "atypical variants" was found in this series, with site-restricted damage or additional PNS involvement. Prognosis and response to steroids were generally good, except for some patient subgroups. In patients with PNS involvement and steroid failure, a favorable effect of IV immunoglobulin was observed.

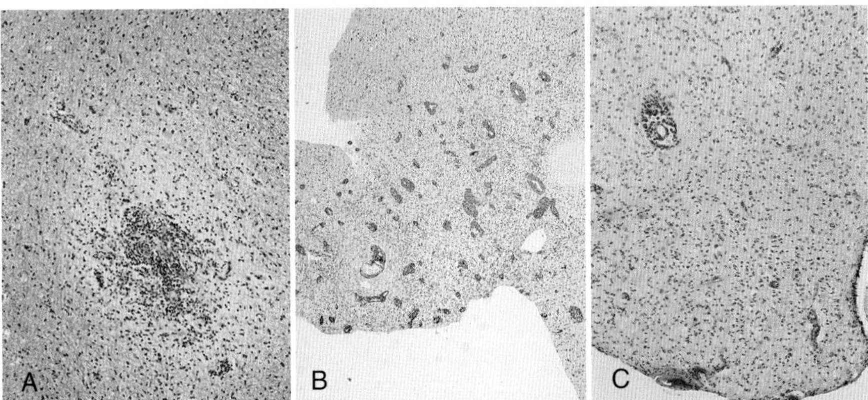

Figure 11–1 A, Luxol fast blue (LFB) stain for myelin (100×) demonstrates perivenous sleeves of demyelination. **B,** KiM1P immunohistochemical stain for macrophages (10×) highlights perivenous macrophages that co-localize with sleeves of demyelination (not shown). **C,** For comparison, LFB stain (20×) reveals a distinctly different, large, confluent demyelinating plaque typical of multiple sclerosis in which only fragments of LFB stain remain in a brain biopsy section.

ANTECEDENT INFECTION OR VACCINATION

Evidence of an infectious trigger for ADEM is supported by winter and spring seasonal peaks in presentation observed in some studies.[3,4] Infection may trigger the subsequent autoimmune attack on the CNS, possibly via "molecular

TABLE 11–2 Series of Clinically Defined Acute Disseminated Encephalomyelitis ($N > 40$)*

	Mikaeloff [20]	Tenembaum [1]	Dale [10]	Leake [6]	Anlar [11]	Schwarz [2]	Marchioni [12]	Lin [19]	de Seze [15]
Year	2006	2000	2000	2004	2003	2001	2005	2007	2007
Design	Prospective	Prospective	Retrospective	Retrospective	Retrospective	Retrospective	Prospective	Retrospective	Retrospective
Population	Pediatric	Pediatric	Pediatric	Pediatric	Pediatric	Adult	Adult	Any age	Adult
No. patients	132	84	48	42	46	40	60	42	35
Mean age in years (range)	6 (2.7-9.3)	(0.4-16)	(4-15)	6.5 (0.8-18)	8 (1-5)	(0.4-16)	51	32.8 (4-90)	36 (20-51)
Inclusion Criteria†									
Polysymptomatic	Y	Y	Y	N	N	N	N	N	N
Multifocal MRI abnormalities	Y	Y	N	N	Y	N	N	N	Y
White matter MRI abnormality	Y	Y	Y	Y	Y	Y	N	Y	Y
Encephalopathy	Y	Y	N	N	N	N	N	N	N
Post infection/ vaccination	N	N	N	N	N	N	Y	N	N
Monophasic	Y	N	N	N	N	Y	N	Y	N
Excluded isolated optic neuritis or transverse myelitis	Y	Y	Y	N	Y	Y	N	Y	Y
Presenting Symptoms (%)									
Post infection/ vaccination	64	74	69	33	45	46	100	59	74
Polysymptomatic	100	100	91	—	35	—	—	—	60
Encephalopathy	100	58	69	66	45	13	42	69	<74
Headache	—	27	58	41	33	—	—	—	—
Meningismus	—	36	31	5	24	15	27	—	—
Seizures	34	29	17	8	21	4	3	29	9
Optic neuritis (all)	6	23	23	—	15	4	—	7	11
Bilateral optic neuritis	—	18	23	—	11	4	12	—	6

TABLE 11–2 Series of Clinically Defined Acute Disseminated Encephalomyelitis ($N > 40$)* (Continued)

	Mikaeloff [20]	Tenembaum [1]	Dale [10]	Leake [6]	Anlar [11]	Schwarz [2]	Marchioni [12]	Lin [19]	de Seze [15]
Year	2006	2000	2000	2004	2003	2001	2005	2007	2007
Design	Prospective	Prospective	Retrospective	Retrospective	Retrospective	Retrospective	Prospective	Retrospective	Retrospective
Population	Pediatric	Pediatric	Pediatric	Pediatric	Pediatric	Adult	Adult	Any age	Adult
No. patients	132	84	48	42	46	40	60	42	35
Mean age in years (range)	6 (2.7-9.3)	(0.4-16)	(4-15)	6.5 (0.8-18)	8 (1-5)	(0.4-16)	51	32.8 (4-90)	36 (20-51)
Presenting Symptoms (%) (Continued)									
Cranial neuropathy	—	37	51	—	—	—	17	—	—
Pyramidal	85	85	71	50	65	66	82	76	51
Cerebellar	—	42	49	50	28	38	17	36	20
Myelopathy	—	—	23	—	—	15	78	—	—
Brainstem	52	—	—	—	—	—	—	64	23
Peripheral nerve	—	5	—	—	—	—	43	—	—
MRI Abnormalities (%)									
Juxtacortical	66	—	—	—	—	—	—	—	—
Subcortical	—	—	91	—	42	—	—	48	—
Periventricular	—	—	44	40	12	54	—	60	86
Cortical	19	—	12	—	—	8	61	43	31
Not-well-defined lesion	94	—	—	—	—	—	—	—	—
Large area	78	—	—	—	—	—	—	—	32
Thalamus or basal ganglia	63	—	69	60	—	—	23	62	60
Brainstem and/or cerebellar	68	—	87	73	87	88	—	77	46
Gadolinium enhancement	18	37	—	7	19	100	42	40	23
All lesions enhancing	—	80	—	—	0	71	—	—	—

Table continued on following page

TABLE 11–2 **Series of Clinically Defined Acute Disseminated Encephalomyelitis ($N > 40$)*** (Continued)

	Mikaeloff[20]	Tenembaum[1]	Dale[10]	Leake[6]	Anlar[11]	Schwarz[2]	Marchioni[12]	Lin[19]	de Seze[15]
Year	2006	2000	2000	2004	2003	2001	2005	2007	2007
Design	Prospective	Prospective	Retrospective	Retrospective	Retrospective	Retrospective	Prospective	Retrospective	Retrospective
Population	Pediatric	Pediatric	Pediatric	Pediatric	Pediatric	Adult	Adult	Any age	Adult
No. patients	132	84	48	42	46	40	60	42	35
Mean age in years (range)	6 (2.7-9.3)	(0.4-16)	(4-15)	6.5 (0.8-18)	8 (1-5)	(0.4-16)	51	32.8 (4-90)	36 (20-51)
Spinal Fluid Analysis (%)									
Pleocytosis	58	28	64	65	41	81	58	23	23
Oligoclonal bands	5	0	29	—	4	58	15 (all transient)	0	20
Clinical Course (%)									
Mean years of follow-up (range)	5.4 (2.1-8.7)	6.6	1.5 (0.2-3)	(1-5)	(0.25-10)	3.2 (0.7-11)	3 (2-7)	2.7 (0.2-10)	3.4 (1-8)
Monophasic	100	75	35	72	72	65	75	90	100
Relapses after initial diagnosis of ADEM	18	9	27	28	28	35	25	10	42
MS diagnosed in relapsing	Yes	No	Yes	No	Yes	Yes	No	Yes	Yes (32)
Recurrent or relapsing ADEM	No	Yes	No	Yes	Yes	No	Yes	No	Yes (10)
Mean years to relapse (range)	—	2.9 (0.1-8)	(0.15-2.5)	—	—	3.2 (0.67-11.4)	0.92	—	(mean, 0.7 relapses/yr)

—, not reported; ADEM, acute disseminated encephalomyelitis; CNS, central nervous syndrome; MRI, magnetic resonance imaging; MS, multiple sclerosis.

*All patients included presented with first acute or subacute idiopathic inflammatory demyelinating syndrome. Clinical, laboratory, and neuroimaging data are reported only for patients diagnosed with "ADEM" at last follow-up.

†All studies required first acute or subacute idiopathic CNS syndrome; other criteria are marked "Y" (required) or "N" (not required).

Modified from Young NP, Weinshenker BG, Lucchinetti CF: Acute disseminated encephalomyelitis: Current understanding and controversies. Semin Neurol 2008;28:84-94.

mimicry,"[30] a hypothesis supported by the pathologic similarities between ADEM and the experimental autoimmune encephalomyelitis (EAE) animal model of acute monophasic inflammatory demyelination.[16,17,22] Numerous infections, mostly viral, and other immunologic triggers such as vaccinations have been associated with ADEM and are listed elsewhere.[31-33] From a practical clinical standpoint, almost any infection or antigenic exposure might be associated with ADEM.

Although ADEM is often associated with recent vaccination or infection, the occurrence of these events has not been included in the definition of ADEM in most studies, nor in the new consensus clinical criteria.[1,4-6,9-11,14,34,35] Only four series required a clear antecedent history of infection or vaccination.[7,36-38] Omitting the presence of a preexisting infection or vaccination from the criteria for ADEM is supported by the significant proportion of likely ADEM patients who do not have such a history when evaluated prospectively,[8,14,34] retrospectively,[1,3,5,6,9,10] or pathologically.[16,18,19,25-28,39] A history of antecedent infection or vaccination may increase the likelihood of ADEM, but such a history also occurs with greater frequency among patients with first presentation of MS.[40,41] Therefore, a strict requirement of an antecedent infection or vaccination is neither specific nor sensitive for ADEM. Also, it may not be possible to obtain such a history in patients who tend to present with encephalopathy.

YOUNGER AGE AT PRESENTATION

ADEM is probably more frequent in children. with an estimated incidence of at least 0.4/100, 000/year.[5] The incidence of ADEM in adult patients has not been evaluated. Pediatric patients meeting the criteria of Mikaeloff and colleagues for ADEM presented at a mean age of 7.1 years, compared with a mean of 12.0 years for those presenting with MS.[34] Only about 5% of MS patients present before age 16, but MS patients have been reported to present as young as 1 year of age.[42] However, as the spectrum of pediatric MS has expanded, some evidence suggests that an "ADEM-like" presentation in pediatric MS may be under-recognized.[43] Although patients presenting with demyelinating disease before age 10 may be more likely to have ADEM than MS,[34,44] considerable overlap in age at presentation limits the utility of using age as a discriminating factor.[44] Few studies have attempted to characterize or define ADEM in adult patients,[6,7,9,15] perhaps because ADEM is rare in adults and possibly under-recognized.

POLYSYMPTOMATIC, MULTIFOCAL INITIAL PRESENTATION

Recent studies of ADEM have included only patients with polysymptomatic presentations, excluding those with monosymptomatic ON, transverse myelitis, brainstem encephalitis, or cerebellitis.[3,5,9,14,34,36] However, some have argued that many monosymptomatic patients have a monophasic course and therefore should be considered to have limited forms of ADEM.[1,7] In a retrospective study of 296 patients with a first attack of idiopathic demyelinating disease, Mikaeloff and associates required a polysymptomatic presentation with mental status change, multifocal MRI abnormalities, and a monophasic course over a mean of 2.9 years for the final diagnosis of ADEM.[34] A polysymptomatic presentation was not specific for ADEM and occurred in 67% of 168 patients with MS in the same series. ADEM is reported to be pathologically diffuse and multifocal.[16,17,20] A polysymptomatic presentation may be a marker of the diffuse underlying pathology of ADEM, but by itself it is probably nonspecific. In patients with a first presentation of an IIDD that is monosymptomatic, multifocal MRI abnormalities may be a surrogate marker of a multifocal process. However, complicating matters, patients who have monosymptomatic presentations but multifocal MRI abnormalities have a higher risk of a subsequent diagnosis of MS than those who do not.[45]

If the hallmark of ADEM pathology is perivenous demyelination, then brain biopsy of focal monosymptomatic lesions may help resolve the question of whether these cases should be included in the ADEM spectrum. Two well-documented cases of perivenous demyelination limited to the brainstem have been reported in the literature.[46,47] We are not aware of any reports of focal supratentorial lesions with well-documented perivenous pathology. On the contrary, most reported cases of focal supratentorial demyelination reveal confluent demyelination, which is pathologically more consistent with MS pathology, although some have argued these may be intermediate lesions along an ADEM-to-MS spectrum.[48] Much of the uncertainty in these cases arises from a lack of agreement on the clinical definitions of ADEM and emphasis on potential pathologic differences. The IPMSSG criteria are conservative in that ADEM could be diagnosed in patients with a single MRI lesion, but only if encephalopathy is also present (suggesting a more diffuse process than may be evident by MRI alone). Whether ADEM may present focally without encephalopathy is an important question that needs to be addressed, because such patients would likely be included within the spectrum of clinically isolated demyelinating syndromes.

SIGNS AND SYMPTOMS OF MENINGOENCEPHALITIS

Many patients with fatal ADEM have evidence of lymphocytic meningitis on histopathologic examination.[16,17] When compared with cases eventually diagnosed as MS, several clinical symptoms and signs of meningoencephalitis are consistently associated with ADEM, including encephalopathy, seizures, fever, headache, and meningeal signs.[3,9] However, these findings are not present in all patients with ADEM (see Table 11-2). Most would agree that a meningoencephalitic presentation is atypical of MS and should raise the clinical suspicion of ADEM. Meningoencephalitic symptoms may have merit in diagnostic criteria for ADEM, but the sensitivity may be low.

ENCEPHALOPATHY

Encephalopathy has been emphasized as a key distinguishing characteristic of ADEM in children.[8,11,12,34] This is best supported by fatal cases with pathologic confirmation of perivenous demyelination characteristic of ADEM in which early change in mental status and decline in level of consciousness was documented over days in all cases.[16,20] "Encephalopathy" as currently applied[8,11] is not precisely defined and may be confounded by postictal state or focal demyelinating lesions causing aphasia, frontal behavioral syndromes, or parietal-occipital visual spatial syndromes that may be confused with a diffuse encephalopathy. In cases of apparent ADEM with encephalopathy, the possibility of an unidentified infectious encephalitis remains in some cases, especially from retrospective series that did not apply a standardized broad infectious workup to each patient.[1,3,9,49] The specificity of encephalopathy probably depends on how precisely it is defined. A change in level of arousal or consciousness may be a more specific definition that more readily discriminates ADEM from even atypical presentations of MS.

BILATERAL OPTIC NEURITIS

Dale and coworkers found that 23% of 40 patients diagnosed with ADEM presented with bilateral ON. Conversely, in the same study, unilateral ON was present only among those patients who were eventually reclassified as having MS, none of whom had bilateral ON.[3] Though infrequently present, the occurrence of bilateral rather than unilateral ON was believed to potentially distinguish ADEM from MS; however, this robust difference was not reproduced in later studies using more restrictive diagnostic criteria (see Table 11-2).

Bilateral ON is uncommon in MS, but it is a well-recognized manifestation of NMO. Cases of NMO may contaminate some ADEM series.[1,3,7,13,14,36] Although early diagnostic criteria for NMO suggested that the brain MRI had to be relatively free of white matter lesions, recent publications provide evidence of a broader spectrum, including lesions consistent with ADEM and MS.[50] Patients with NMO have antibodies to the aquaporin-4 water channel, a recently identified novel biomarker that may be pathogenic.[51] NMO-IgG is positive in as many as 76% of cases of clinical NMO, but this is not an absolute criterion for diagnosis.[51-54] Early treatment of NMO may reduce the risk of severe disabling relapses.[52] NMO-IgG serologic testing became available only recently and has not been evaluated in the ADEM series published to date. Bilateral ON is likely to be less specific for ADEM than was originally suggested by Dale and colleagues,[3] and this exemplifies the potential confusion of ADEM with NMO, which is presumably a pathophysiologically different disease. Future studies of ADEM should include NMO-IgG testing in all clinically possible cases (ON or myelitis alone or in combination).

ASSOCIATED POLYRADICULONEUROPATHY

In a recent series,[7] adult patients presenting with a CNS syndrome after infection or vaccination were found to have peripheral nervous system (PNS) involvement that was usually demyelinating and subclinical. This finding was probably a result of the use of broad inclusion criteria (see Table 11-2) and the performance of extensive prospective neurophysiologic testing in all patients regardless of symptoms. ADEM was only rarely reported to be associated with PNS involvement before this study.[55-58] Further investigation is needed to determine whether PNS involvement is part of the ADEM spectrum.

MAGNETIC RESONANCE IMAGING CHARACTERISTICS

MRI neuroimaging is useful for the diagnosis of ADEM and the exclusion of other diagnoses. However, the consensus ADEM criteria emphasize clinical criteria and underplay the role of MRI in establishing a diagnosis. In clinically defined cases of ADEM, the MRI often demonstrates multifocal areas of increased T2-weighted signal abnormalities in the CNS white matter, frequently with additional gray

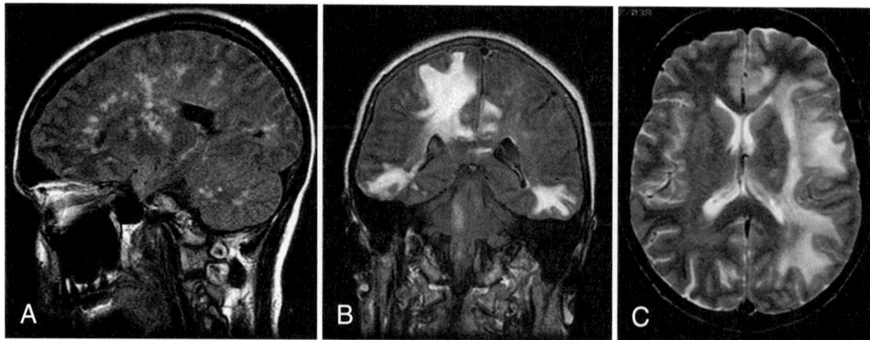

Figure 11–2 Sagittal fluid-attenuated inversion recovery (FLAIR) image (**A**), coronal FLAIR image (**B**), and axial T2-weighted magnetic resonance image from three different patients with acute disseminated encephalomyelitis (ADEM) evaluated at the Mayo Clinic with brain biopsy showing perivenous demyelination. These studies demonstrated multiple ill-defined, nonenhancing, periventricular lesions that also involved the deep gray matter and cerebellum (**A**); multiple bilateral, large, ill-defined, nonenhancing lesions involving white and gray matter and the brainstem (**B**); and a large, confluent hemispheric lesion (**C**) associated with faint punctuate foci of gadolinium enhancement (not shown).

matter involvement. Some authors have emphasized that ADEM lesions are indistinct or ill-defined and lack the sharply defined borders characteristic of MS lesions.[3,59] Examples of such MRI abnormalities from patients with ADEM evaluated at the Mayo Clinic with brain biopsy confirming perivenous demyelination are presented in Figure 11-2. Although ADEM lesions (of similar age) should all hypothetically enhance with gadolinium, this finding is rarely seen, and gadolinium enhancement may even be absent.[3,4,7,9,59-61]

Early MRI series identified overlap in lesion location and distribution between ADEM and MS but also highlighted features of ADEM that are unusual in MS, such as symmetric bilateral disease, relative sparing of the periventricular white matter, and cortical or deep gray matter involvement.[62] Absolute and relative periventricular sparing on MRI is typical of ADEM and was present in 78% patients with ADEM reported by Dale and colleagues; however, 22% of their ADEM patients had a periventricular lesion pattern indistinguishable from that seen in MS.[3]

Mikaeloff and coworkers prospectively found that corpus callosum long axis lesions (Dawson's fingers), together with the finding of only well-defined lesions, provided a completely specific predictor of relapse over a mean of 4.9 years and, accordingly, of MS.[59] However, only 21% of patients presenting with a first episode of demyelination had this combination of findings. This study highlights the difficulty of using the initial MRI to identify patients with increased risk of relapsing disease (MS) or those with a truly monophasic process. In contrast with other reports, lesions of the thalamus and basal ganglia were not significantly different between ADEM and MS patients in this study.[59]

Even when the MRI seems typical of either ADEM or MS, the findings remain relatively nonspecific, and a broad differential diagnosis of potential mimics of IIDD must be carefully considered.[63] MRI criteria may be most helpful in combination with clinical criteria that verify a multifocal demyelinating process or suggest an alternative pathology. Although the possibility of MRI-negative ADEM has been proposed,[3,36,37,64] it remains unclear whether an unidentified cause of encephalopathy other than ADEM may have been present in such cases. The recently published consensus criteria require an abnormal MRI and lesions larger than 1 to 2 cm for compatibility with ADEM. The current consensus criteria for ADEM suggest that a large focal lesion may rarely be compatible with ADEM,[11] even though some may regard this as a tumefactive presentation of MS. This question should be easily resolved by clear documentation of the pathology (perivenous or confluent demyelinating) in cases in which brain biopsy is performed to exclude neoplasm and correlation of the pattern of demyelination with clinical course.

ADVANCED NEUROIMAGING TECHNIQUES

Advanced neuroimaging techniques such as diffusion tensor imaging (DTI) and magnetic transfer imaging (MTI) may provide a better assessment of the underlying histopathology than an increase in T2-weighted signal on conventional MRI.[65,66] Quantitative MRI techniques have also suggested that progressive ventricular enlargement and gray matter atrophy are potential markers for MS in patients who present with clinically isolated syndromes.[67,68] Advanced neuroimaging techniques need to be studied further, ideally in patients who meet validated diagnostic criteria, to determine their utility in routine clinical practice.

SPINAL FLUID PLEOCYTOSIS WITHOUT OLIGOCLONAL BANDS

Before diagnosing ADEM, infection must be excluded by cerebrospinal fluid (CSF) analysis and culture. The CSF may be normal in ADEM, or a lymphocytic pleocytosis may be revealed (see Table 11-2); in contrast, patients with MS rarely have a pleocytosis exceeding 50 white blood cells per microliter. Detection of OCB may be helpful in predicting a subsequent diagnosis of MS, but the true utility is unknown, because as many as 58% of adult[9] and 29% of pediatric cases[3] of ADEM also exhibit OCB. Anecdotally, the OCB should resolve in ADEM but are more likely to persist in MS.[14,42] This was true in a series of 9 ADEM patients who initially had OCB that had resolved when analysis was repeated 6 days to 6 months later.[7] The presence of OCB on initial presentation is not specific for MS; however, if OCB persist, then a diagnosis of MS is more likely.[1] In a recent series, adult patients were more likely to have a monophasic course and a final diagnosis of ADEM if OCB were absent at presentation.[15]

RELAPSING AND RECURRENT ADEM

The monophasic clinical hallmark of ADEM is challenged by cases of recurrent "ADEM" reported mainly in isolated case reports without pathologic confirmation. A single case series reported presumed recurrent ADEM at the previously effected brain site, with accompanying pathology.[69] This series has been cited as evidence of the existence of recurrent ADEM. However, the description of pathology in this series was limited to "diffuse demyelination," and the one published photomicrograph was more typical of confluent demyelination, consistent with classic MS pathology. The diagnosis of recurrent ADEM was based on clinical presentation rather than characteristic perivenular ADEM pathology. The lack of pathologic evidence is a common limitation of many clinicopathologic reports of ADEM.

Even in the two large prospective studies of children with the most restrictive clinical criteria for ADEM, between 10% and 18% of patient subsequently had relapses.[8,14] In the cohort of Tenembaum and associates,[14] serial neuroimaging was performed at presentation, and follow-up examinations were performed over a mean of 6.6 years. This study identified 76 monophasic patients with a clinically and radiographically monophasic course. However, 10% of these 84 patients had one relapse at a previously unaffected site, with a mean interattack interval of 2.9 years (range, 2 months to 8 years), and subsequently remained relapse free for a mean of 8.2 years. After the relapse, these patients did not develop new subclinical lesions on yearly prospective repeat MRI scans. All were OCB negative. None of those with recurrences had biopsy verification of ADEM pathology. Based on these observations, the authors proposed a "biphasic" form of ADEM.[14] A similar group of relapsing patients were described in the Mikaeloff cohort[8] (18% of 132 patients); however, MS rather than "ADEM" was diagnosed in this circumstance.

The recent consensus criteria for ADEM attempt to clarify the terminology used to describe cases of possible ADEM that are not monophasic. A case is "recurrent" if a subsequent attack is stereotypical of the first attack and there is no evidence of involvement of a different part of the CNS clinically or by MRI. A case is "multiphasic" if there is evidence of new symptoms or involvement of a different part of the CNS than in the initial attack (see Table 11-1). Attacks occurring within 3 months after an initial attack or during a steroid taper are not considered to be new attacks based on the consensus clinical criteria. The terms "relapsing" and "biphasic" ADEM were discarded by the consensus group.[11] This clarification of terms is a step forward and will help guide prospective studies. Whether cases of clinically defined recurrent or relapsing ADEM represent a different pathogenetic process from monophasic ADEM or MS is a major question requiring further study.

We propose that ADEM be defined as a strictly monophasic disease until more definitive data prove otherwise. The duration of follow-up required to verify a monophasic course may be as long as 10 years, because the longest duration until first relapse was 8 years in a study using criteria similar to those of the IPMSSG.[3,8,14] The long-term prospective follow-up of patients diagnosed with ADEM by the IPMSSG will provide important natural history data on ADEM and its potential relationship with MS.

Practical Recommendations for Clinicians

EVALUATION AND MANAGEMENT

Although progress in defining ADEM has been made recently, reliable clinical diagnostic criteria are still not established, and clinicians are still faced with uncertainty about the true diagnosis and prognosis for relapse in patients who present with first attacks of CNS demyelination. Even the most restrictive criteria for ADEM do not reliably predict a monophasic course in patients presenting with first attacks of an IIDD. Recognition of the clinical and neuroimaging characteristics of encephalopathy; polysymptomatic presentation; MRI lesions that are large, ill-defined, multifocal, and involving deep gray matter and cortex; and CSF pleocytosis without OCB should support a diagnosis of ADEM. However, other mimickers of inflammatory demyelinating disease, as well as first presentations of MS, should be considered in addition to ADEM.[70] NMO should also be considered in patients with prominent myelitis or ON, in whom testing for NMO-IgG is indicated.

Once an CNS infectious process has been reasonably excluded, treatment with intravenous methylprednisolone (IVMP), 30 mg/kg/day in children and doses up to 1000 mg daily in adults for 3 to 5 days, is the most common approach based on anecdotal evidence from case reports and clinical series.[71] Intravenous immune globulin may be an effective alternative to corticosteroids.[72,73] If there is no response to IVMP, then plasma exchange once every other day for 7 days should be considered.[71] A brain biopsy is indicated if the diagnosis is uncertain and clinical or imaging features suggest an alternative diagnoses (e.g., neoplasm, vasculitis). Interpretation of brain biopsy specimens by an expert neuropathologist who can distinguish acute inflammatory demyelination from alternative processes and perivenous from confluent demyelination is essential.

Clinicians should avoid the potential pitfall of diagnosing ADEM simply because there are atypical clinical features of MS or NMO, assuming a probable benign monophasic course and delaying initiation of effective therapy to prevent recurrent attacks that may be disabling. ADEM is probably a monophasic illness that should not require long-term immunomodulatory treatment; therefore, it should be a diagnosis of exclusion. After a presenting attack, close follow-up with serial examination and MRI within the first 3 months is recommended, because new subclinical lesions may develop on MRI and suggest the diagnosis of MS. A yearly clinical follow-up, often with repeat neuroimaging looking for evidence of new subclinical lesions, is a possible surveillance strategy for patients with an unclear IIDD clinical phenotype in whom initiation of immunomodulatory therapy may eventually be indicated. The confidence in the diagnosis of ADEM should increase proportionally to the duration of follow-up without a subsequent attack.

SUMMARY

Multiple clinical factors should be considered in combination before arriving at a probable diagnosis of ADEM, including (1) presenting signs and symptoms; (2) conventional and advanced MRI abnormalities; (3) sufficient follow-up (perhaps as long as 10 years) confirming a monophasic course based on clinical and/or neuroimaging criteria; (4) lack of alternative diagnosis; and (5) brain histopathology if available. The IPMSSG has outlined a plan to prospectively study specific clinical diagnostic criteria in children.[11] Though these criteria will likely evolve with time, an agreement on terminology and suggestive clinical criteria is an important step forward. Because it is unclear whether ADEM presents differently in adults than in children (because the presentations of MS may be different), specific criteria should be applied with caution in adults. Although brain biopsy is uncommonly performed in most clinical practices, well-described clinicopathologic cases distinguishing between limited perivenous and confluent demyelination may help support pathology as a gold standard, verify cases, and refine future clinical diagnostic criteria for ADEM.

REFERENCES

1. Anlar B, et al: Acute disseminated encephalomyelitis in children: Outcome and prognosis. Neuropediatrics 2003;34:194-199.
2. Apak RA, et al: Acute disseminated encephalomyelitis in childhood: Report of 10 cases. J Child Neurol 1999;14:198-201.
3. Dale RC, et al: Acute disseminated encephalomyelitis, multiphasic disseminated encephalomyelitis and multiple sclerosis in children. Brain 2000;123(Pt 12):2407-2422.
4. Hynson JL, et al: Clinical and neuroradiologic features of acute disseminated encephalomyelitis in children. Neurology 2001;56:1308-1312.
5. Leake JA, et al: Acute disseminated encephalomyelitis in childhood: Epidemiologic, clinical and laboratory features. Pediatr Infect Dis J 2004;23:756-764.
6. Lin CH, et al: Acute disseminated encephalomyelitis: A follow-up study in Taiwan. J Neurol Neurosurg Psychiatry 2007;78:162-167.
7. Marchioni E, et al: Postinfectious inflammatory disorders: Subgroups based on prospective follow-up. Neurology 2005;65:1057-1065.
8. Mikaeloff Y, et al: Acute disseminated encephalomyelitis cohort study: Prognostic factors for relapse. Eur J Paediatr Neurol 2007;11:90-95.
9. Schwarz S, et al: Acute disseminated encephalomyelitis: A follow-up study of 40 adult patients. Neurology 2001;56:1313-1318.
10. Murthy SN, et al: Acute disseminated encephalomyelitis in children. Pediatrics 2002;110(2 Pt 1):e21.
11. Krupp LB, et al: Consensus definitions proposed for pediatric multiple sclerosis and related disorders. Neurology 2007;68;(16 Suppl. 2):S7-S12.
12. Tenembaum S, et al: Acute disseminated encephalomyelitis Neurology 2007;68(16 Suppl 2): S23-S36.
13. Murthy JM, et al: Clinical, electrophysiological and magnetic resonance imaging study of acute disseminated encephalomyelitis. J Assoc Physicians India 1999;47:280-283.
14. Tenembaum S, Chamoles N, Fejerman N: Acute disseminated encephalomyelitis: A long-term follow-up study of 84 pediatric patients. Neurology 2002;59:1224-1231.
15. de Seze J, et al: Acute fulminant demyelinating disease: A descriptive study of 60 patients. Arch Neurol 2007;64:1426-1432.
16. Hart MN, Earle KM: Haemorrhagic and perivenous encephalitis: A clinical-pathological review of 38 cases. J Neurol Neurosurg Psychiatry 1975;38:585-591.
17. Van Bogaert L: Post-infectious encephalomyelitis and multiple sclerosis: The significance of perivenous encephalomyelitis. J Neuropathol Exp Neurol 1950;9:219-249.
18. Oppenheimer DR: Demyelinating diseases. In Blackwood W, Corsellis JAN (eds): Greenfield's Neuropathology. London: Edward Arnold, 1976, pp 470-499.
19. Greenfield JG, Norman RM, Demyelinating diseases. In Blackwood W, et al ed: Greenfield's Neuropathology. London: Arnold, 1971.
20. Turnbull HM, McIntosh J: Encephalomyelitis following vaccination. Br J Exp Pahol 1926;7: 181-222.
21. Malamud N: Sequelae of postmeasles encephalomyelitis: A clinicopathologic study. Arch Neurol Psychiatry 1939;41:943-954.
22. Lucchinetti CF, Parisi J, Bruck W: The pathology of multiple sclerosis. Neurol Clin 2005;23:77-105, vi.
23. Greenfield JG: The pathology of measles encephalomyelitis. Brain 1929;52:171-195.
24. Pittock SJ, et al: Clinical course, pathological correlations, and outcome of biopsy proved inflammatory demyelinating disease. J Neurol Neurosurg Psychiatry 2005;76:1693-1697.
25. Shintaku M, Matsumoto R: Disseminated perivenous necrotizing encephalomyelitis in systemic lupus erythematosus: Report of an autopsy case. Acta Neuropathol (Berl) 1998;95:313-317.
26. Miller DH, et al: Acute disseminated encephalomyelitis presenting as a solitary brainstem mass. J Neurol Neurosurg Psychiatry 1993;56:920-922.
27. Hafler DA, Hedley-Whyte ET: Case records of the Massachusetts General Hospital: Weekly clinicopathological exercises. Case 37-1995: A 6-year-old boy with a rash, meningismus, and diplegia. N Engl J Med 1995;333:1485-1493.
28. Koch M, et al: A fatal demyelinating illness in a young woman 10 weeks post partum. Lancet Neurol 2005;4:129-134.
29. Silver B, et al: Fulminating encephalopathy with perivenular demyelination and vacuolar myelopathy as the initial presentation of human immunodeficiency virus infection. Arch Neurol 1997;54:647-650.

30. Fujinami RS, Zurbriggen A: Is Theiler's murine encephalomyelitis virus infection of mice an autoimmune disease? Apmis 1989;97:1-8.
31. Wingerchuk DM: Postinfectious encephalomyelitis. Curr Neurol Neurosci Rep 2003;3:256-264.
32. Mihai C, Jubelt B: Post-infectious encephalomyelitis. Curr Neurol Neurosci Rep 2005;5:440-445.
33. Menge T, et al: Acute disseminated encephalomyelitis: An update. Arch Neurol 2005;62:1673-1680.
34. Mikaeloff Y, et al: First episode of acute CNS inflammatory demyelination in childhood: Prognostic factors for multiple sclerosis and disability. J Pediatr 2004;144:246-252.
35. Mikaeloff Y, et al: Prognostic factors for early severity in a childhood multiple sclerosis cohort. Pediatrics 2006;118:1133-1139.
36. Hollinger P, et al: Acute disseminated encephalomyelitis in adults: A reappraisal of clinical, CSF, EEG, and MRI findings. J Neurol 2002;249:320-329.
37. Idrissova ZR, et al: Acute disseminated encephalomyelitis in children: Clinical features and HLA-DR linkage. Eur J Neurol 2003;10:537-546.
38. Hung KL, Liao HT, Tsai ML: The spectrum of postinfectious encephalomyelitis. Brain Dev 2001;23:42-45.
39. Prineas JW, McDonald WI, Franklin RJM: Demyelinating diseases. In Graham D, Lantos P (eds): Greenfield's Neuropathology. New York, Oxford University Press, 2002.
40. Marrie RA, et al: Multiple sclerosis and antecedent infections: A case-control study. Neurology 2000;54:2307-2310.
41. Sibley WA, Bamford CR, Clark K: Clinical viral infections and multiple sclerosis. Lancet 1985;1:1313-1315.
42. Banwell BL: Pediatric multiple sclerosis. Curr Neurol Neurosci Rep 2004;4:245-252.
43. Ruggieri M, et al: Multiple sclerosis in children under 10 years of age. Neurol Sci 2004;25 (Suppl 4):S326-S335.
44. Dale RC, Branson JA: Acute disseminated encephalomyelitis or multiple sclerosis: Can the initial presentation help in establishing a correct diagnosis? Arch Dis Child 2005;90:636-639.
45. Comi G, et al: Effect of early interferon treatment on conversion to definite multiple sclerosis: A randomised study. Lancet 2001;357:1576-1582.
46. Miller AA, Ramsden F: Acute necrotic myelitis and perivenous encephalomyelitis associated with hypertension and renal infection. J Clin Pathol 1967;20:821-825.
47. Hoffman HL, Norman RM: Acute necrotic myelopathy associated with perivenous encephalomyelitis. J Neurol Neurosurg Psychiatry 1964;27:116-124.
48. Kepes JJ: Large focal tumor-like demyelinating lesions of the brain: Intermediate entity between multiple sclerosis and acute disseminated encephalomyelitis? A study of 31 patients. Ann Neurol 1993;33:18-27.
49. Gupte G, et al: Acute disseminated encephalomyelitis: A review of 18 cases in childhood. J Paediatr Child Health 2003;39:336-342.
50. Pittock SJ, et al: Brain abnormalities in neuromyelitis optica. Arch Neurol 2006;63:390-396.
51. Lennon VA, et al: A serum autoantibody marker of neuromyelitis optica: Distinction from multiple sclerosis. Lancet 2004;364:2106-2112.
52. Wingerchuk DM: Diagnosis and treatment of neuromyelitis optica. Neurologist 2007;13:2-11.
53. Wingerchuk DM: Acute disseminated encephalomyelitis: Distinction from multiple sclerosis and treatment issues. Adv Neurol 2006;98:303-318.
54. Wingerchuk DM, et al: Revised diagnostic criteria for neuromyelitis optica. Neurology 2006;66:1485-1489.
55. Aimoto Y, et al: [A case of acute disseminated encephalomyelitis (ADEM) associated with demyelinating peripheral neuropathy]. No To Shinkei 1996;48:857-860.
56. Amit R, et al: Acute, severe, central and peripheral nervous system combined demyelination. Pediatr Neurol 1986;2:47-50.
57. Amit R, et al: Acute severe combined demyelination. Childs Nerv Syst 1992;8:354-356.
58. Kinoshita A, et al: [A case of acute disseminated encephalomyelitis with pathologically-proven acute demyelinating lesion in the peripheral nervous system]. Rinsho Shinkeigaku 1994;34:892-897.
59. Mikaeloff Y, et al: MRI prognostic factors for relapse after acute CNS inflammatory demyelination in childhood. Brain 2004;127(Pt 9):1942-1947.
60. Caldemeyer KS, et al: Gadolinium enhancement in acute disseminated encephalomyelitis. J Comput Assist Tomogr 1991;15:673-675.
61. Caldemeyer KS, et al: MRI in acute disseminated encephalomyelitis. Neuroradiology 1994;36:216-220.

62. Kesselring J, et al: Acute disseminated encephalomyelitis: MRI findings and the distinction from multiple sclerosis. Brain 1990;113(Pt 2):291-302.
63. Bastianello S, et al: Atypical multiple sclerosis: MRI findings and differential diagnosis. Neurol Sci 2004;25;(Suppl 4):S356-S360.
64. Murray BJ, Apetauerova D, Scammell TE: Severe acute disseminated encephalomyelitis with normal MRI at presentation. Neurology 2000;55:1237-1238.
65. Holtmannspotter M, et al: A diffusion tensor MRI study of basal ganglia from patients with ADEM. J Neurol Sci 2003;206:27-30.
66. Inglese M, et al: Magnetization transfer and diffusion tensor MR imaging of acute disseminated encephalomyelitis. AJNR Am J Neuroradiol 2002;23:267-272.
67. Dalton CM, et al: Progressive ventricular enlargement in patients with clinically isolated syndromes is associated with the early development of multiple sclerosis. J Neurol Neurosurg Psychiatry 2002;73:141-147.
68. Dalton CM, et al: Early development of multiple sclerosis is associated with progressive grey matter atrophy in patients presenting with clinically isolated syndromes. Brain 2004;127(Pt 5):1101-1107.
69. Cohen O, et al: Recurrence of acute disseminated encephalomyelitis at the previously affected brain site. Arch Neurol 2001;58:797-801.
70. Weinshenker BG, Lucchinetti CF: Acute leukoencephalopathies: Differential diagnosis and investigation. Neurologist 1998;4:148-166.
71. Keegan M, et al: Plasma exchange for severe attacks of CNS demyelination: Predictors of response. Neurology 2002;58:143-146.
72. Marchioni E, et al: Effectiveness of intravenous immunoglobulin treatment in adult patients with steroid-resistant monophasic or recurrent acute disseminated encephalomyelitis. J Neurol 2002;249:100-104.
73. Sahlas DJ, et al: Treatment of acute disseminated encephalomyelitis with intravenous immunoglobulin. Neurology 2000;54:1370-1372.

12 Transverse Myelitis: Pathogenesis, Diagnosis, and Management

CARRILIN C. TRECKER • DANA E. KOZUBAL • ADAM I. KAPLIN • DOUGLAS A. KERR

Transverse myelitis (TM) is a rare neuroinflammatory disease that causes neural injury to the spinal cord. Patients experience varying degrees of weakness, sensory alterations, and autonomic dysfunction. The first cases of acute TM were described in 1882 and were attributed to vascular lesions and other acute inflammations.[1] In England between 1922 and 1923, more than 200 postvaccinial cases were noted as complications of the smallpox and rabies vaccines.[2] Later reports revealed that TM was postinfectious in nature, and agents including measles, rubella, and mycoplasma were directly isolated from patient's spinal fluid. The term *acute transverse myelitis* was first used by an English neurologist in 1948 to describe a case of rapidly progressive paraparesis with a thoracic sensory level, occurring as a postinfectious complication of pneumonia.[3] Subsequently, the diagnostic criteria for acute transverse myelopathy has been debated and has evolved as more has been learned about this disease. In 2002, the Transverse Myelitis

Consortium Working Group delineated a diagnostic criterion (discussed later) for disease-associated TM and idiopathic TM along with a framework to differentiate TM from noninflammatory myelopathies.[4]

Clinical Features

TM usually manifests with weakness characterized by rapidly progressing paresis, beginning with the legs and potentially moving to the arms. Flaccidity may be noted initially, with pyramidal signs appearing gradually by the second week of the illness. In most cases, a sensory level is documented, most commonly in the midthoracic region in adults or in the cervical region in children.[5] Pain in the back, extremities, or abdomen is also common, and paresthesias are typical in adults.

Sexual dysfunction also results from sensory and autonomic involvement. Impaired sensation in both men and women is a consequence of genital anesthesia due to involvement of the pudendal nerve (S2 through S4) or ascending pathways from the pudendal nerve. Additional male sexual problems with parasympathetic (S2 through S4) and sympathetic (T10 through L2) dysfunction include erectile dysfunction, ejaculatory disorders, and difficulty reaching orgasm. Analogous female sexual problems include reduced lubrication and difficulty reaching orgasm. Increased urinary urgency, bowel or bladder incontinence, difficulty voiding or inability to void, and incomplete evacuation of bowel or constipation are other characteristic autonomic symptoms. Additionally, depression is often documented in TM patients and must be treated to prevent devastating consequences.

Natural History

In some cases, symptoms progress over hours; in other instances, the presentation is over days. Neurologic function tends to decline during the 4- to 21-day acute phase,[6] and 88% of cases reach their maximal deficit within 10 days after symptom onset.[4,7] At nadir, 50% of patients have lost all movement of their legs; 80% to 94% experience numbness, paresthesias or band-like dysesthesias; and almost all have some degree of bladder dysfunction.[8-13]

In 75% to 90% of cases, TM is monophasic, but a small percentage of patients experience recurrent (multiphasic) disease. After their initial attack, approximately one third of patients recover with little to no sequelae, one third are left with a moderate degree of permanent disability, and one third have virtually no recovery and are left severely functionally disabled. The rapid progression of clinical symptoms, the presence of back pain, and the presence of spinal shock, as well as paraclinical evidence such as absent central conduction on evoked potential testing and the presence of 14-3-3 protein in the cerebrospinal fluid (CSF) during the acute phase, are often indicators of a less complete recovery.

TM has a conservatively estimated incidence of between 1 and 8 new cases per 1 million population per year, or approximately 1400 new cases annually in United States .[8] Although this disease affects people of all ages, with a range of 6 months to 88 years, there are bimodal peaks between the ages of 10 to 19 years and 30 to 39 years.[8-11] In addition, our work at the Johns Hopkins Transverse

Myelitis Center (JHTMC) shows that 28% of cases occur in children (case series, manuscript in preparation). There is no sex or familial association with TM.[4]

Immunopathogenesis

The immunopathogenesis of TM is varied and multifaceted. For instance, lupus-associated TM is linked to central nervous system (CNS) vasculitis,[14-16] neurosarcoid is often associated with noncaseating granulomas within the spinal cord,[16,17] and multiple sclerosis (MS)-associated TM exhibits perivascular lymphocytic cuffing and mononuclear cell infiltration with variable complement and antibody deposition.[18] Other cases of TM may be connected with thrombotic infarction of the spinal cord.[19] Because the immunopathogenic and effector mechanisms of these diseases are varied and go beyond the scope of this review, the following discussion centers on non–disease-associated TM (i.e., idiopathic TM). Because TM is characterized by abnormal immune activation, an understanding of the mechanism by which an excessive immune response causes CNS injury is crucial to the development of diagnostic and treatment modalities.[20]

POSTVACCINATION TRANSVERSE MYELITIS

Although a causal relationship has not been established, TM has been reported to occur after influenza and booster hepatitis B vaccinations.[21,22] Thirty percent of children treated at an academic medical centers had received an immunization within 1 month of onset (JHTMC case series). On autopsy evaluation, lymphocytic infiltration of the spinal cord with axonal loss and demyelination was found among those with postvaccination TM, indicating that the vaccination may have excited an autoimmune process.[23] However, extensive research has demonstrated that vaccinations are safe, and the potential link to TM may only be coincidental or, at worst, an exceptionally rare complication.[20]

PARAINFECTIOUS TRANSVERSE MYELITIS

The term *parainfectious* suggests that the neurologic injury associated with TM may be related to (1) direct microbial infection and injury resulting from the infection, (2) direct microbial infection with immune-mediated damage against the agent, or (3) remote infection followed by a systemic response that induces neural injury. In 40% of pediatric TM cases, an illness characterized by nonspecific symptoms such as fever, nausea, and muscle pain preceded disease onset within 3 weeks (JHTMC case series). Between 30% and 60% of patients with TM demonstrated serologic evidence for acute infections, such as rubella, measles, infectious mononucleosis, influenza, enteroviruses, mycoplasma, or hepatitis A, B, or C.[24] In fewer cases, direct microbial infection of the CNS by herpesviruses—cytomegalovirus (CMV), varicella-zoster virus (VZV), herpes simplex virus 1 (HSV-1) and HSV-2, human herpesvirus 6 (HHV6), and Epstein-Barr virus (EBV)—or by human T-cell lymphotropic virus 1 (HTLV-1), human immunodeficiency virus 1 (HIV-1), *Borrelia burgdorferi* (Lyme neuroborreliosis), or *Treponema pallidum* (syphilis) has been linked with TM. Again, however, causality has not been established.

Molecular Mimicry

Two other mechanisms, molecular mimicry and superantigen-mediated disease, involve peripheral immune activation and may account for other cases of TM. Molecular mimicry was first noted in Guillain-Barré syndrome (GBS). Seventy-five percent of GBS cases are preceded by acute infection, 41% being with *Campylobacter jejuni*. Sialic acid, a characteristic component of human ganglioside found as a surface antigen within the lipopolysaccharide (LPS) outer coat on *C. jejuni*, is comparable to the ganglioside moieties within the cell walls of human neural tissue.[25-28] Antibodies against *C. jejuni* that cross-react with gangliosides have been identified in the serum of GBS patients[29-31] and have been implicated in the binding of peripheral nerves, which impairs neural transmission in experimental conditions that mimic GBS.[25,32-33] In TM cases of molecular mimicry, the development of autoantibodies is linked to an antecedent infection. After an *Enterobius vermicularis* (perianal pinworm) infection, one patient developed elevated titers of lupus anticoagulant immunoglobulin G (IgG), antisulfatide antibodies (1:6400), and anti-GM1 antibodies (1:600 IgG and 1:3200 IgM).[34] Because *E. vermicularis* has been shown to contain cardiolipin, ganglioside GM1, and sulfatides within its lipid composition, it was postulated that, in the proper genetic and hormonal background, the infection triggered the pathogenic antibodies that contributed to neural injury.[20]

Microbial Superantigen-Mediated Infection

Superantigens (SAGs) are microbial peptides that can activate the immune system and contribute to autoimmune disorders such as TM. Instead of binding to the highly variable peptide groove of the T-cell receptor as classic antigens do, SAGs interact with the more conserved Vβ region. Another unique feature of SAGs is that they can activate T lymphocytes in the absence of costimulatory molecules; one SAG can activate between 2% and 20% of circulating T lymphocytes, as opposed to 0.001% to 0.01% with conventional antigens.[35-37] The heightened lymphocyte response triggers autoimmunity by activating autoreactive T-cell clones.[20,38,39]

Humoral Derangements

The abnormal antibodies resulting from these processes can subsequently recruit other cellular components to the spinal cord. Studies have emphasized distinct autoantibodies in patients with neuromyelitis optica (NMO)[40-44] and recurrent TM, especially longitudinally extensive transverse myelitis (LETM).[45-47] The high prevalence of various autoantibodies in such patients suggests polyclonal derangement of the immune system. It may also be that some autoantibodies initiate direct and selective injury to neurons that contain antigens capable of cross-reacting with antibodies directed against infectious pathogens.[20]

Elevated levels of normal antibodies may also play a causative role in TM. Circulating antibodies can form immunocomplexes that deposit in focal areas of the spinal cord. This phenomenon was described in a patient with TM and high titers of hepatitis B surface antigen.[48] Immune complexes containing hepatitis B surface antigen were associated with disease activity during the acute phase but disappeared after treatment, correlating with functional recovery.[20]

PUTATIVE MECHANISMS OF IMMUNE-MEDIATED CENTRAL NERVOUS SYSTEM INJURY

Investigations of immune derangements have shown levels of spinal fluid interleukin 6 (IL-6) to be significantly increased in TM patients compared with normal and MS controls, and this represents a final common pathway of tissue injury in idiopathic TM.[20] IL-6 levels are positively correlated with disability in those with TM, whereas the same trend is not observed in MS patients. In addition, elevated IL-6 levels corresponded to increased nitric oxide metabolites, which also correlate with disability. It is hypothesized that the upregulation of IL-6 linked with immune activation parallels production of nitric oxide, which then predicts the tissue injury leading to clinical disability in TM.

Diagnosis and Classification of Transverse Myelitis

EVALUATION OF PATIENTS WITH ACUTE MYELOPATHY

A diagnostic approach for evaluating patients with acute myelopathies was proposed by the Transverse Myelitis Consortium Working Group in 2002.[6] This algorithm has been modified to more fully define the evaluation process of patients with inflammatory myelopathy (Fig. 12-1). The first priority is to rule out a compressive myelopathy. If a myelopathy is suspected based on history and physical examination, gadolinium-enhanced magnetic resonance imaging (MRI) of the spinal cord should be obtained as soon as possible. Disc herniations, epidural hematomas, vertebral body compression fractures, and spondylosis are among the most common causes of compressive myelopathy and may manifest without overt evidence or history of trauma. Identifying these disorders is critical, because immobilization to prevent further injury, neurosurgical consultation, and/or high-dose methylprednisolone may be warranted in certain cases. However, about one fifth of myelopathy patients treated at a UK neurosciences center had a normal MRI scan despite the presence of a spinal cord syndrome.[49] If TM is suspected despite a normal MRI, the physician is advised to re-examine the history, perform another physical examination, and evaluate the MRI with an experienced neuroradiologist.[50]

If no structural lesion is present, then the presence or absence of spinal cord inflammation should be assessed with a lumbar puncture. The best surrogate markers for inflammation are an inflammatory CSF (elevated white blood cell count and/or IgG index) and an inflammatory spinal MRI (gadolinium enhancement). It should be noted, however, that a significant percentage of individuals with a clinical pattern that otherwise resembles TM[51] do not meet these inflammatory features, and, therefore, the absence of inflammatory markers does not rule out TM. Noninflammatory myelopathies include those caused by arterial or venous ischemia, vascular malformations, radiation, fibrocartilaginous embolism, or nutritional/metabolic causes. Appropriate workups in these situations might include aortic ultrasonography, spinal angiography, or evaluation of prothrombotic risk factors.

For diagnosis of an inflammatory myelopathy, the primary indication is the development of bilateral signs and/or symptoms of sensory, motor, or autonomic dysfunction attributable to the spinal cord (Table 12-1). Additional diagnostic criteria are a clearly defined sensory level and evidence of inflammation, either on

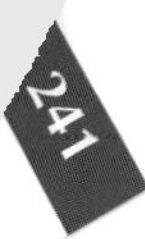

Workup of Suspected Acute Myelopathies

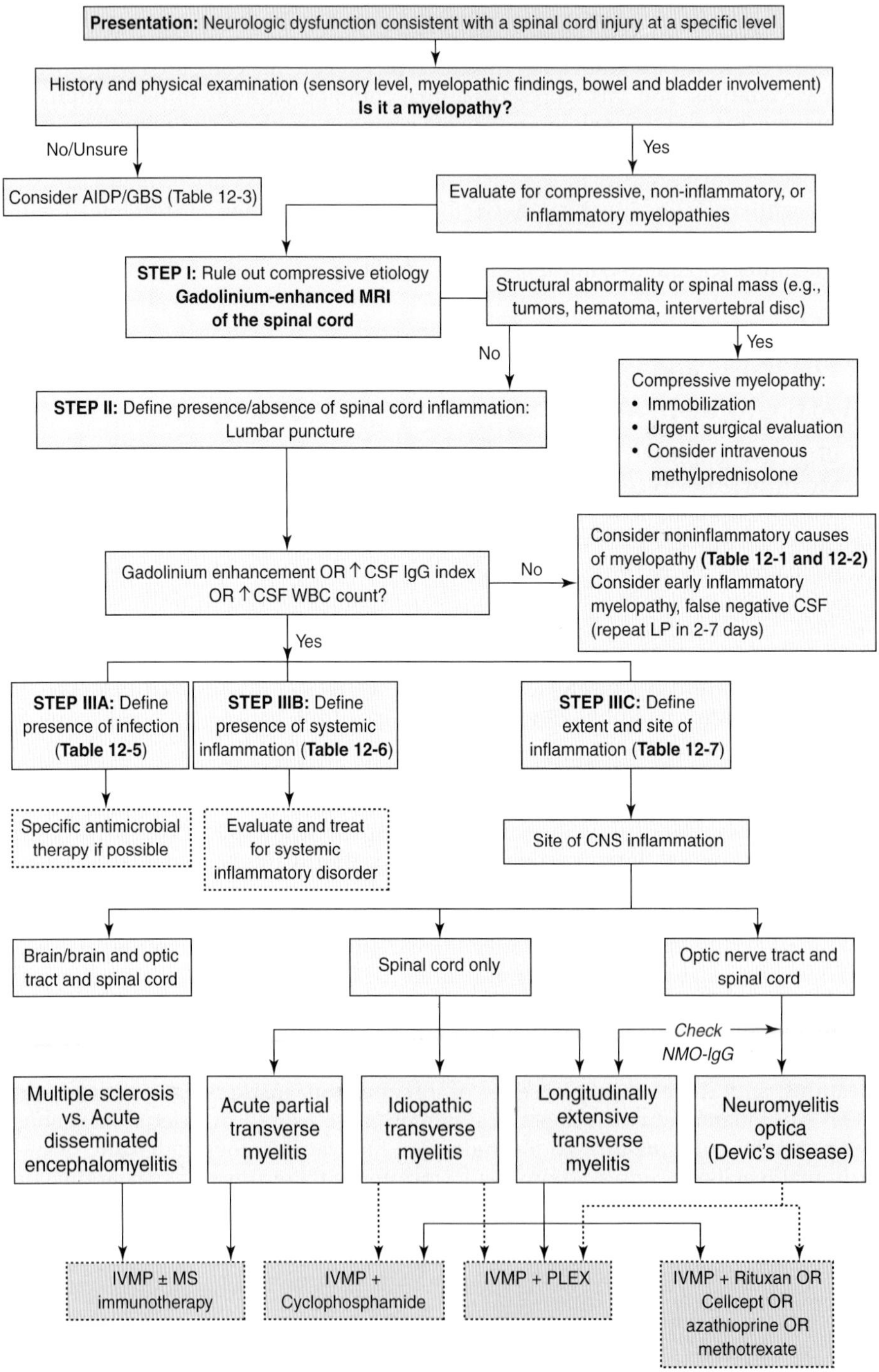

Presentation: Neurologic dysfunction consistent with a spinal cord injury at a specific level

↓

History and physical examination (sensory level, myelopathic findings, bowel and bladder involvement)
Is it a myelopathy?

- No/Unsure → Consider AIDP/GBS (Table 12-3)
- Yes → Evaluate for compressive, non-inflammatory, or inflammatory myelopathies

STEP I: Rule out compressive etiology
Gadolinium-enhanced MRI of the spinal cord

Structural abnormality or spinal mass (e.g., tumors, hematoma, intervertebral disc)

- Yes → Compressive myelopathy:
  - Immobilization
  - Urgent surgical evaluation
  - Consider intravenous methylprednisolone
- No → **STEP II:** Define presence/absence of spinal cord inflammation: Lumbar puncture

Gadolinium enhancement OR ↑ CSF IgG index OR ↑ CSF WBC count?

- No → Consider noninflammatory causes of myelopathy **(Table 12-1 and 12-2)**
  Consider early inflammatory myelopathy, false negative CSF (repeat LP in 2-7 days)
- Yes →
  - **STEP IIIA:** Define presence of infection (**Table 12-5**) → Specific antimicrobial therapy if possible
  - **STEP IIIB:** Define presence of systemic inflammation (**Table 12-6**) → Evaluate and treat for systemic inflammatory disorder
  - **STEP IIIC:** Define extent and site of inflammation (**Table 12-7**) → Site of CNS inflammation

Site of CNS inflammation:

- Brain/brain and optic tract and spinal cord → Multiple sclerosis vs. Acute disseminated encephalomyelitis → IVMP ± MS immunotherapy
- Spinal cord only →
  - Acute partial transverse myelitis → IVMP ± MS immunotherapy
  - Idiopathic transverse myelitis → IVMP + Cyclophosphamide; IVMP + PLEX
  - Longitudinally extensive transverse myelitis → IVMP + PLEX; IVMP + Cyclophosphamide; IVMP + Rituxan OR Cellcept OR azathioprine OR methotrexate
- Optic nerve tract and spinal cord → Neuromyelitis optica (Devic's disease) → IVMP + PLEX; IVMP + Rituxan OR Cellcept OR azathioprine OR methotrexate

Check NMO-IgG (Longitudinally extensive transverse myelitis ↔ Neuromyelitis optica)

Figure 12–1 Workup of suspected acute myelopathies. AIDP, acute idiopathic demyelinating polyneuropathy; CNS, central nervous system; CSF, cerebrospinal fluid; GBS, Guillain-Barré syndrome; IgG, immunoglobulin G; IVMP, intravenous methylprednisolone; LP, lumbar puncture; MRI, magnetic resonance imaging; MS, multiple sclerosis; NMO, neuromyelitis optica; PLEX, plasma exchange; WBC, white blood cells.

TABLE 12–1	Diagnostic Criteria for Transverse Myelitis
Sensory, motor, or autonomic dysfunction attributable to the spinal cord	
Bilateral signs and/or symptoms	
Clearly defined sensory level	
Inflammation defined by cerebrospinal fluid pleocytosis or elevated immunoglobulin G index or gadolinium enhancement	
Progression to nadir in 4 hours to 21 days	

MRI as gadolinium enhancement or on lumbar puncture as elevated white blood cell count or IgG index.

In the presence of an inflammatory process, one should determine whether there is an infectious cause (Table 12-2). Viral polymerase chain reaction assays should be performed to determine whether viral particles are present in the CNS; specifically, these should include assays for HSV-1 and HSV-2, VZV, CMV, EBV, and enterovirus. Detection of Lyme disease of the CNS typically is based on antibody detection methods (enzyme-linked immunosorbent assay with confirmatory Western blot), and the CSF/serum index is often helpful in determining whether neuroborreliosis is unequivocally present. Evidence of *Mycoplasma pneumoniae* infection may be determined by seroconversion, which is defined by a fourfold increase in titer or a single titer of 1:128 or less.

Patients with an inflammatory myelopathy should also be evaluated for the presence of a systemic inflammatory disease (e.g., Sjögren's syndrome, lupus, neurosarcoidosis) (Table 12-3). Sjögren's syndrome can manifest with acute TM or with a progressive myelopathy resembling MS, with clinical features such as unilateral sensory involvement, sphincter dysfunction, and optic neuropathy.[52] Invasive biopsy investigations or alpha-frodin antibodies are diagnostic markers for Sjögren's that often can differentiate this disease from primary progressive MS.[53] Acute TM is recognized in 2% of patients with lupus, either as the first presenting indicator of disease or as a sequela within 5 years after diagnosis.[54,55] An ischemic or vasculitic process is the supposed pathophysiology of TM in those with lupus.[50]

In the absence of a systemic inflammatory disease, the regional distribution of demyelination within the CNS should be defined, because several disorders (i.e., MS, NMO, and acute disseminated encephalomyelitis [ADEM]) may present with TM as the initial manifestation of a multiphasic disease (Table 12-4). NMO involves primarily, but not exclusively, the optic nerve and the spinal cord, and new criteria define NMO based on longitudinally extensive lesions regardless of

TABLE 12–2 Potential Workup for Infectious Disease-Associated Transverse Myelitis

Indicative Signs and Symptoms
Fever
Meningismus
Rash
Concurrent systemic infection
Immunocompromised state
Recurrent genital infection
Symptoms of zoster radiculopathy
Adenopathy
Residence in area endemic for parasitic infections
Lymphadenopathy
Potential Evaluation
CSF Studies
Gram's stain and bacterial culture
Polymerase chain reaction: HSV-1, HSV-2, HHV-6, VZV, CMV, EBV, enteroviruses, HIV
Viral culture
Acid-fast bacilli smear and tuberculosis culture
HSV, VZV, and HTLV-1 antibodies
Anti–*Borrelia burgdorferi* antibodies
VDRL
Serology
Antibodies to HSV, VZV, HTLV-1, *B. burgdorferi*
Hepatitis A, B, C and *Mycoplasma pneumoniae*
Parasites
Blood cultures
Chest radiology

CMV, cytomegalovirus; EBV, Epstein-Barr virus; HHV, human herpesvirus; HIV, human immunodeficiency virus; HSV, herpes simplex virus; HTLV, human T-cell lymphotropic virus 1; VDRL, Venereal Disease Research Laboratory test for syphilis; VZV, varicella-zoster virus.

optic nerve involvement.[56] A gadolinium-enhanced brain MRI and visual evoked potential (VEP) should be obtained to look for these entities. The absence of multifocal areas of demyelination would suggest a diagnosis of isolated TM and lead to appropriate treatment measures. In our case series at the JHTMC, approximately 64% of cases have been idiopathic, with recurrence rates of approximately 5%. In comparison, 36% of TM cases at our center have been disease-associated TM, with recurrence rates as high as 70%.[8,9,57]

SUBTYPES OF MYELITIS (LONGITUDINALLY EXTENSIVE AND PARTIAL MYELITIS)

Within the category of idiopathic TM, it may be of further value to differentiate groups of patients with acute partial TM, acute complete TM, and LETM, because these syndromes present distinct differential diagnoses and prognoses.

TABLE 12–3 Potential Workup for Systemic Inflammatory Disease in Patient with Transverse Myelitis

Indicative Signs and Symptoms
Rash
Oral or genital ulcers
Adenopathy
Livedo reticularis
Serositis
Photosensitivity
Inflammatory arthritis
Erythema nodosum
Xerostomia
Keratitis
Conjunctivitis
Contractures or thickening of skin
Anemia/leukopenia/thrombocytopenia
Raynaud's phenomenon
History of arterial and venous thrombosis
Potential Evaluation
Serum ACE/chest CT with intravenous contrast/gallium scan
Autoantibodies: ANA, ds-DNA, SS-A (Ro), SS-B (La), Sm (Smith), RNP
Complement levels
Urinalysis with microscopic analysis for hematuria
Lip/salivary gland biopsy
Chest CT with intravenous contrast
Shirmer's test
Chest radiograph
Anti-phospholipid antibodies, Russell viper venom time, partial thromboplastin time

ACE, Serum angiotensin-converting enzyme; NA, antinuclear antibodies; CT, computed tomography; ds-DNA, double-stranded DNA; SS, Sjögren's syndrome; RNP, ribonucleoprotein.

Acute partial TM refers to mild or grossly asymmetrical spinal cord dysfunction with an MRI lesion of less than 3 vertebral segments. *Acute complete TM* refers to those patients who have complete or near-complete clinical deficits below the lesion and an MRI lesion of less than 3 vertebral segments. Patients with *LETM* have a complete or incomplete clinical picture but an MRI lesion that is longer than or equal to 3 vertebral segments. The syndrome of severe "complete" acute TM has received attention in several studies, each involving dozens of patients.[8,58] By definition, cerebral MRI is considered to be negative in this population. These patients appear less likely to present with oligoclonal bands, are less likely to relapse with a second bout of TM, and have a very low transition rate to clinically definite MS (CDMS), probably <5%.

Patients with acute partial TM and normal cerebral MRI findings have a transition rate in the range of 10% to 33% for development of MS over a 5- to 10-year period.[59,60] For patients who present with acute partial TM and cerebral MRI showing lesions typical for MS, the transition rate to CDMS is known to be quite high, in the range of 80% to 90% within a few years.[61]

TABLE 12–4 Potential Workup for Multifocal Central Nervous System Inflammation

Indicative Signs and Symptoms
Previous demyelination event
Incomplete deficit clinically with MRI abnormality
<2 spinal segments and <50% of cord diameter (MS)
>3 spinal segments (NMO)
CSF oligoclonal bands
Optic pallor, red desaturation, visual field defect, afferent papillary defect
Presence of multiple autoantibodies (more common in NMO)
Potential Evaluation
Brain MRI (FLAIR with and without gadolinium)
Evoked potentials (VEP, BAER, SSEP)
Optical coherence tomography
NMO-IgG testing (Mayo Clinic)

BAER, brainstem auditory evoked response; CSF, cerebrospinal fluid; FLAIR, fluid-attenuated inversion recovery; IgG, immunoglobulin G; MRI, magnetic resonance imaging; MS, multiple sclerosis; NMO, neuromyelitis optica; SSEP, somatosensory evoked potential; VEP, visual evoked potential.

MONOPHASIC VERSUS RECURRENT DISEASE

Most patients (75% to 90%) experience monophasic disease. With appropriate and timely diagnosis and treatment, most symptoms improve within 3 months. However, in a subset of patients, who often manifest a history of systemic autoimmune disease, TM can be recurrent. Recurrence can often be predicted at the initial acute onset, based on multifocal lesions in the spinal cord, lesions in the brain, presence of anti-Rho antibody, underlying mixed connective tissue disease, presence of oligoclonal bands in the CSF, and/or NMO-IgG antibodies (Table 12-5).[62] Patients with very high levels of IL-6 have also been shown to be at risk for recurrence.[63]

DISCRIMINATION FROM MULTIPLE SCLEROSIS

TM can be the presenting feature of MS. Patients who are ultimately diagnosed with MS are more likely to have asymmetrical clinical findings, predominant sensory symptoms with relative sparing of motor systems, MR lesions extending over fewer than 2 spinal segments, abnormal brain MRI, and oligoclonal bands in the CSF.[57,61,64-66] A patient with monofocal CNS demyelination (TM or ON) whose brain MRI shows lesions consistent with demyelination has an 83% chance of meeting clinical criteria for MS over the subsequent decade, compared with an 11% chance in patients with a normal brain MRI.[67]

Management and Treatment of Transverse Myelitis

INTRAVENOUS STEROIDS

Intravenous steroid treatment is often instituted for patients with acute idiopathic TM. Corticosteroids have multiple mechanisms of action, including anti-inflammatory activity, immunosuppressive properties, and antiproliferative

TABLE 12–5 Distinguishing Features between Recurrent and Monophasic Transverse Myelitis

Tests	Monophasic	Recurrent
Spinal MRI	Single T2 lesion	Multiple distinct lesions or fusiform lesion extending over ≥3 spinal cord segments
Brain MRI	Normal	T2/FLAIR abnormalities
Blood serology	Normal	≥1 autoantibodies (ANA, dsDNA, APA, c-ANCA)
SS-A	Negative	Positive
NMO-IgG	Negative	Positive
CSF oligoclonal bands	Negative	Positive
Systemic disease	None	Connective tissue disorder
Optic nerve involvement	No	Likely

ANA, antinuclear antibodies; c-ANCA, cytoplasmic antineutrophilic cytoplasmic antibody; APA, antiphospholipid antibodies; CSF, cerebrospinal fluid; dsDNA, double-stranded DNA; FLAIR, fluid-attenuated inversion recovery; IgG, immunoglobulin G; MRI, magnetic resonance imaging; NMO, neuromyelitis optica; SS-A, Sjögren's syndrome A.

actions.[68,69] Although this approach has not been investigated in a randomized, double-blind, placebo-controlled study, it is supported by evidence from related disorders and clinical experience.[70-74] Additionally, there are several studies that support the administration of corticosteroids in patients with TM.[75-78] A study of five children with severe TM who received intravenous methylprednisolone (IVMP) at a dosage of 1 g/1.73 m^2/day (except one patient who received 0.5 g/1.73 m^2/day) for 3 or 5 consecutive days followed by oral prednisone for 14 days reported beneficial effects compared with the outcome in 10 historical controls.[77] The median time to walking was 23 days in the steroid-treated group versus 97 days in the control group; full recovery occurred in 80% versus 10%, and full motor recovery at 1 year was present in 100% versus 20%. No serious adverse effects from the steroid treatments occurred.[20]

Other investigations have suggested that intravenous steroid administration may not be effective in TM patients.[79-81] In the most significant of these studies, Kalita and Misra[79] compared 9 TM patients seen between 1995 and 1997 who received steroids with 12 patients seen between 1992 and 1994 who did not. The authors claimed that there was no statistically significant difference in outcomes between the groups; although it appears that the TM patients who received steroids were actually more likely to recover independent functionality, based on the Barthel Index (33% versus 67%). Therefore, the available evidence suggests that intravenous steroids are somewhat effective if given in the acute phase of TM. However, these studies did not rigorously define TM and therefore probably included patients with noninflammatory myelopathies.

At our center, the standard of care includes intravenous methylprednisolone (IVMP, 1000 mg) or dexamethasone (200 mg) for 3 to 5 days unless there are compelling reasons to avoid this therapy. The decision to offer continued steroids or to add a new treatment is often based on the clinical course and MRI appearance at the end of 5 days of steroids.

PLASMA EXCHANGE

Plasma exchange is often initiated if a patient has moderate to severe TM (i.e., inability to walk, markedly impaired autonomic function, and sensory loss in the lower extremities) and exhibits little clinical improvement after 5 to 7 days of intravenous steroids. Plasma exchange is believed to work in autoimmune CNS diseases through the removal of specific or nonspecific soluble factors that mediate, are responsible for, or contribute to inflammatory-mediated target organ damage. Plasma exchange has been shown to be effective in adults with TM and other inflammatory disorders of the CNS.[82-84] Predictors of good response to plasma exchange include early treatment (<20 days from symptom onset), male gender, and a clinically incomplete lesion (i.e., some motor function in the lower extremities, intact or brisk reflexes).[85] It is our experience that plasma exchange may significantly improve outcomes of patients with severe (although incomplete) TM and of patients who have not significantly improved on intravenous steroids.[20]

OTHER IMMUNOMODULATORY TREATMENTS

For patients with TM that continues to progress despite intravenous steroid therapy who seek treatment at Johns Hopkins, we consider pulse dose intravenous cyclophosphamide (800 to 1000 mg/m^2). Cyclophosphamide, a bifunctional alkylating agent, forms reactive metabolites that cross-link DNA. This results in apoptosis of rapidly dividing immune cells and is believed to underlie the immunosuppressive properties of this medication. In a recently published retrospective study, the efficacy of four treatment regimens was investigated, and subsets with better responses to specific therapies were identified.[86] The 122 patients who received the diagnosis of TM and were treated with 3 to 5 days of either (1) IVMP, (2) IVMP in combination with plasma exchange, (3) cyclophosphamide, or (4) both plasma exchange and cyclophosphamide were retrospectively assessed for recovery and outcomes. It was determined that plasma exchange provided an added benefit to steroids in patients who were not at American Spinal Injury Association (ASIA) disability level A and who did not have a history of autoimmune disease.[86] However, patients who were classified at a disability level of ASIA A at their nadir showed a significant benefit when given combination therapy with steroids, plasma exchange, and intravenous cyclophosphamide. It must be noted, however, that cyclophosphamide should be administered under the supervision of an experienced oncology team, and caregivers should monitor patients carefully for hemorrhagic cystitis and cytopenias.

CSF filtration is a new therapy, not yet available in the United States, in which spinal fluid is filtered for inflammatory factors (including cells, complement, cytokines, and antibodies) before being reinfused into the patient. In a randomized trial of CSF filtration versus plasma exchange for acute idiopathic demyelinating polyneuropathy (AIDP), CSF filtration was better tolerated and was at least as effective as plasma exchange.[87] Clinical trials for CSF filtration are currently being initiated. Chronic immunomodulatory therapy should be considered for the small subgroup of patients with recurrent TM. Although the ideal treatment regimen is not known, we consider a 2-year course of oral immunomodulatory treatment in patients with two or more distinct episodes of TM. We most commonly treat patients with azathioprine (150 to 200 mg/day), methotrexate (15 to 20 mg/wk), or mycophenolate (2 to 3 g/day), although oral cyclophosphamide (2 g/kg/day) may also be used in patients with systemic inflammatory disease. With any of these medicines, patients must be monitored for transaminitis or leukopenias.[20]

PROMISING NEUROPROTECTIVE THERAPIES

Substantial spinal cord axonal injury and loss occurs in TM and most likely correlates with permanent neurologic disability. In other demyelinating disorders, such as MS and the inherited demyelinating peripheral neuropathies, neurologic disability at a particular time point does not correlate with the number of demyelinating lesions but rather with the degree of axonal loss. The anti-inflammatory therapies previously mentioned would be expected to decrease the amount of inflammatory-mediated axonal damage occurring in acute TM, but a combination therapy that also includes a neuroprotective or "axonoprotective" agent would probably be more efficacious.[62]

Erythropoietin, neurotrophin-3, and the neuro-immunophilin ligands are promising agents with recently demonstrated axonoprotective properties.[62] A double-blind, randomized clinical trial investigating the efficacy of erythropoietin (in combination with intravenous steroids) in acute TM should be undertaken.

LONG-TERM MANAGEMENT

Many patients with TM will require rehabilitative care to improve their functional skills and prevent secondary complications of immobility. It is important to begin occupational and physical therapies early during the course of recovery, to prevent the inactivity-related problems of skin breakdown and soft tissue contractures that lead to a decreased range of motion. The principles of rehabilitation in the early and chronic phases after TM are summarized in Tables 12-6 and 12-7. During the early recovery period, family education is essential to develop a strategic plan for dealing with the challenges to independence that must be faced after return to the community. Assessment and fitting for splints designed to passively maintain an optimal position for limbs that cannot be actively moved is an important part of the management at this stage.[20]

The long-term management of TM requires attention to a number of issues. These are the residual effects of any spinal cord injury, including TM. In addition to chronic medical problems, there are the ongoing issues of ordering the appropriate equipment, reentry into school, re-socialization into the community, and coping with the psychological effects of this condition by the patients and their families.[20]

Patients with TM should be educated about the effect of TM on mood regulation and routinely screened for the development of symptoms consistent with clinical depression. Patient warning signs that should prompt a complete evaluation for depression include failure to progress with rehabilitation and self-care, worsening fixed low mood, pervasive decreased interest, and social and professional withdrawal. A preoccupation with death or suicidal thoughts constitutes a true psychiatric emergency and should lead to prompt evaluation and treatment.

TABLE 12–6 Chronic Management of Transverse Myelitis: Early Rehabilitation

General

Rehabilitation is critical
Strongly consider inpatient rehabilitation
Daily land-based and/or water-based therapy for 8-12 wk
Daily weight bearing for 45-90 min; standing frame if nonambulatory
Bone densitometry: vitamin D, calcium
Look for depression and treat if interfering with rehabilitation

Neuropsychiatric

Demoralization

Individual and group support*
Development of problem-focused coping skills; all members of medical care providers (e.g., neurologist, physiatrist, PT, OT, psychiatrist, psychologist, social worker) could contribute

Depression

Education about depression as a manifestation of brain involvement in conjunction with stressful circumstance
Warning about the lethality of depression (with suicide being one of the leading causes of death in TM)
Treatment of depression with antidepressants and talk therapy; SSRIs are common first-line agents, but consider a tricyclic antidepressant if there is the possibility of simultaneously treating depression, incontinence, and neuropathic pain with a single agent

Autonomic

Bladder Dysfunction

Assess ability to void spontaneously
Avoid Credé (bearing down to initiate urination), which may be dangerous
Check postvoid residual; if >80 mL, consider clean intermittent catheterization (goal: volumes < 400 mL)
Cystometrogram not required in acute phase
Anticholinergic therapy if significant urgency
Cranberry juice for urine acidification

Bowel Dysfunction

High-fiber diet
Increased fluid intake
Digital disimpaction
Bowel program: Colace, Senokot, Dulcolax, docusate PR, bisacodyl in a water base, MiraLax, enemas PRN

Motor

Weakness

Strengthening program for weaker muscles
Passive and active ROM
PT/OT consultation
Splinting or orthoses when necessary

Spasticity

ROM exercises
Aquatherapy

TABLE 12–6	Chronic Management of Transverse Myelitis: Early Rehabilitation (Continued)
Baclofen Tizanidine Diazepam Botulinum toxin Tiagabine	
Sensory	
Pain or Dysesthesias	
ROM exercises Gabapentin Carbamazepine Nortriptyline Tramadol Avoid narcotics if possible	

OT, occupational therapist; PRN, as needed; PT, physical therapist; ROM, range of motion; SSRIs, selective serotonin-reuptake inhibitors; TM, transverse myelitis.

*A useful resource is the Transverse Myelitis Association (TMA), which maintains a website at http://www.myelitis.org (accessed October 2008).

All patients should be educated about three main points related to depression.[20] First, patients should be educated that depression in TM is similar to the other neurologic symptoms they endure, which are mediated by the effects of the immune system on the brain. Depression is remarkably prevalent in TM, occurring in up to 25% of patients at any given time, and it is largely independent of the patient's degree of physical disability. Depression is not caused by personal weakness or the inability to "cope." Second, depression in TM can have devastating consequences; not only can it worsen physical disability (e.g., fatigue, pain, decreased concentration), but it can have lethal consequences. Suicide is the leading cause of death in TM, accounting for 60% of the deaths in the JHTMC patient population since its inception. Third, despite the severity of the clinical presentation of depression in many patients with TM, these patients generally show a very robust response to combined aggressive psychopharmacologic and psychotherapeutic interventions. With appropriate recognition and treatment of TM depression, complete symptom remission is standard.[20]

Spasticity is often a very difficult problem to manage. The goal is to maintain flexibility with a stretching routine, using exercises for active stretching and a bracing program with splints for a prolonged stretch. These splints are commonly used at the ankles, wrists, or elbows. Also recommended are appropriate strengthening programs for the weaker of the spastic muscles acting on a joint and an aerobic conditioning regimen. These interventions are supported by adjunctive measures that include antispasticity drugs (e.g., diazepam, baclofen, dantrolene, tizanidine), therapeutic botulinum toxin injections, and serial casting. The therapeutic goal is to improve the function of the patient in performing specific activities of daily living (e.g., feeding, dressing, bathing, hygiene, mobility) by improving the available joint range of motion, teaching effective compensatory strategies, and relieving pain.[62]

TABLE 12–7 Chronic Management of Transverse Myelitis: Late Rehabilitation

General

Avoid secondary complications
Examine for scoliosis in patients with high/severe lesions
Serial flexion/extension radiographs of back to follow angle
Skin hygiene to avoid breakdown
Treat fatigue: amantidine, methylphenidate, modafinil, coenzyme Q10
Bone densitometry: vitamin D, calcium, bisphosphonate therapy
Consider and treat depression

Neuropsychiatric

Demoralization

Biannual national TM symposiums organized through the JHTMC and TMA
Establish local TMA support group if none exists

Depression

Referral to psychiatrist if diagnosis is in doubt, initial trials of antidepressant treatment are unsuccessful, or there is concern about suicide potential
Ensure caregiver is receiving sufficient support to prevent burnout

Autonomic

Bladder Dysfunction

Urodynamics study for irritative or obstructive symptoms
Anticholinergic drug if detrusor hyperactivity: extended-release Ditropan or Detrol
Adrenergic blocker if sphincter dysfunction (e.g., Flomax)
Clean intermittent catheterization is safe for long-term use
Cranberry juice/vitamin C for urine acidification
Consider sacral nerve stimulation

Bowel Dysfunction

High-fiber diet
Increased fluid intake
Digital disimpaction
Bowel program: Colace, Senokot, Dulcolax, docusate PR, bisacodyl in a water base, MiraLax, enemas PRN

Sexual Dysfunction

Phosphodiesterase V inhibitors

Motor

Weakness

Strengthening program for weaker muscles
Passive and active ROM
Splinting or orthoses when necessary
Continued land-based and water-based therapy
Ambulation devices when appropriate
Daily weight bearing for 45-90 min; standing frame if nonambulatory
Orthopedics evaluation if joint imbalance is present

Spasticity

ROM exercises
Aquatherapy
Baclofen

TABLE 12–7 Chronic Management of Transverse Myelitis: Late Rehabilitation (Continued)

Tizanidine
Diazepam
Botulinum toxin
Tiagabine
Intrathecal baclofen trial
Sensory
Pain or Dysesthesias
ROM exercises
Gabapentin
Carbamazepine
Nortriptyline
Tramadol
Topical lidocaine (patch or cream)
Intrathecal baclofen or opioids

JHTMC, Johns Hopkins Transverse Myelitis Center; PRN, as needed; ROM, range of motion; TM, transverse myelitis; TMA, Transverse Myelitis Association.

Another major area of concern is effective management of bowel function. A high-fiber diet, adequate and timely fluid intake, and medications to regulate bowel evacuations are the basic components of success. Regular evaluations by medical specialists for adjustment of the bowel program are recommended to prevent potentially serious complications.[62]

Bladder function is almost always impaired, at least transiently, in patients with TM. Immediately after the onset of TM, as in the aftermath of traumatic spinal cord injury, there is frequently a period of transient loss or depression of neural activity below the involved spinal cord lesion. This phenomenon, often referred to as "spinal shock," lasts about 3 weeks, during which time there is an interruption of descending excitatory influence with resultant bladder flaccidity. After this period, bladder dysfunction can be classified into two syndromes, involving either upper motor neurons (UMN) or lower motor neurons (LMN).

UMN bladder dysfunction results from lesions above S1-S2. It is characterized by reflexive emptying with bladder filling if the injury is complete, or by urge incontinence if the neurologic involvement is incomplete. In addition, detrusor-sphincter dyssynergia results from impaired communication between the sacral and brainstem micturition centers. In the case of UMN dysfunction, anticholinergic medications, α-blockers, or electric stimulation is used to restore adequate bladder storage and drainage. LMN bladder dysfunction, with either direct involvement of S2-S4 or indirect involvement including the conus medullaris and cauda equina, results in detrusor areflexia and requires clean intermittent self-catheterization.[20]

TM-induced sexual dysfunction involves similar innervation and syndromes analogous to those observed in bladder dysfunction. Treatment of sexual dysfunction should take into account baseline function before the onset of TM. Of the utmost importance is adequate education and counseling about the known physical and neurologic changes that TM has on sexual functioning. Patients should be encouraged to discuss their concerns with their physicians as well as their partners. Because of the similarities in innervation between sexual and bladder function, patients with UMN-mediated sexual dysfunction should be encouraged to empty their bladders before sexual stimulation, to prevent inopportune incontinence. The mainstays of treatment of erectile dysfunction in men are inhibitors of cyclic guanosine monophosphate phosphodiesterase, type 5; these agents allow most men with TM to achieve adequate erections for success in intercourse through a combination of reflex and psychogenic mechanisms. Although they are less effective in women, these same types of medications have been shown capable of enhancing a woman's sexual functioning.[20]

The Future

Because little is known about the links between environmental triggers, individual predisposing factors, and TM, these areas will certainly be explored in future research. Current therapies for TM are largely nonspecific, but they are expected to become more targeted as more is learned about the disease's immunopathogenic events, such as the generation of autoantibodies and the presence of abnormally elevated cytokine levels in the spinal fluid. For example, evolving strategies will more effectively identify autoantibodies and the antigens to which they respond, making it possible to develop specific targets to block the effects of these autoantibodies.[88,89] Additionally, several strategies exist, and more are currently being developed, that specifically alter cytokine profiles or the effects of these cytokines within the nervous system. However, it is possible that when one pathway is blocked, secondary alterations in immune system function may occur, because tumor necrosis factor-α modulation has been shown to trigger demyelination in MS patients.[90] Hence, a "cocktail approach" aimed at halting multiple pro-inflammatory pathways may be ideal. Finally, for those patients who have already experienced extensive neurologic injury as a result of TM, neurorestorative treatments (perhaps involving stem cells) offer the best hope for meaningful functional recovery.[4]

REFERENCES

1. Bastian HC: Special diseases of the spinal cord. In: Quain R, ed. *A Dictionary of Medicine: Including General Pathology, General Therapeutics, Hygiene, and the Diseases Peculiar to Women and Children/By Various Writers*. London, England: Longmans, Green & Co; 1882;1:1479-1483.
2. Rivers TM: Viruses. JAMA 1929;92:1147-1152.
3. Suchett-Kaye AI: Acute transverse myelitis complicating pneumonia. Lancet 1948;255:417.
4. Krishnan C, Kaplin AI, Deshpande D: Transverse myelitis: Pathogenesis, diagnosis and treatment. Front Biosci 2004;9:1483-1499.
5. Pidcock F, Krishnan C, Crawford TO, et al: Acute transverse myelitis in childhood: Center-based analysis of 47 cases. Neurology 2007;68:1474-1480.
6. Transverse Myelitis Consortium Working Group: Proposed diagnostic criteria and nosology of acute transverse myelitis. Neurology 2002;59:499-505.
7. Knebusch M, Strassburg HM, Reiners K: Acute transverse myelitis in childhood: Nine cases and review of the literature. Dev Med Child Neurol 1998;40:631-639.
8. Berman M, Feldman S, Alter M, et al: Acute transverse myelitis: Incidence and etiologic considerations. Neurology 1981;31:966-971.
9. Jeffery DR, Mandler RN, Davis LE: Transverse myelitis: Retrospective analysis of 33 cases, with differentiation of cases associated with multiple sclerosis and parainfectious events. Arch Neurol 1993;50:532-535.

10. Christensen PB, Wermuth L, Hinge HH, et al: Clinical course and long-term prognosis of acute transverse myelopathy. Acta Neurol Scand 1990;81:431-435.
11. Altrocchi PH: Acute transverse myelopathy. Arch Neurol 1963;9:21-29.
12. Misra UK, Kalita J, Kumar S: A clinical, MRI and neurophysiological study of acute transverse myelitis. J Neurol Sci 1996;138:150-156.
13. Lipton HL, Teasdall RD: Acute transverse myelopathy in adults: A follow-up study. Arch Neurol 1973;28:252-257.
14. Piper PG: Disseminated lupus erythematosus with involvement of the spinal cord. JAMA 1953;153:215-217.
15. Adrianakos AA, Duffy J, Suzuki M, et al: Transverse myelitis in systemic lupus erythematosus: Report of three cases and review of the literature. Ann Intern Med 1975;83:616-624.
16. Nakano I, Mannen T, Mizutani T, et al: Peripheral white matter lesions of the spinal cord with changes in small arachnoid arteries in systemic lupus erythematosus. Clin Neuropathol 1989;8:102-108.
17. Ayala L, Barber DB, Lomba MR, et al: Intramedullary sarcoidosis presenting as incomplete paraplegia: Case report and literature review. J Spinal Cord Med 2000;23:96-99.
18. Garcia-Zozaya IA: Acute transverse myelitis in a 7-month-old boy. J Spinal Cord Med 2001;24: 114-118.
19. Sinkovics JG, Gyorkey F, Thoma GW: A rapidly fatal case of systemic lupus erythematosus: Structure resembling viral nucleoprotein strands in the kidney and activities of lymphocytes in culture. Tex Rep Biol Med 1969;27:887-908.
20. Kaplin AI, Krishnan C, Deshpande DM, et al: Diagnosis and management of acute myelopathies. Neurologist 2005;11:2-18.
21. Patja A, Paunio M, Kinnunen E, et al: Risk of Guillain-Barre syndrome after measles-mumps-rubella vaccination. J Pediatr 2001;138:250-254.
22. Schonberger LB, Bregman DJ, Sullivan-Bolyai JZ, et al: Guillain-Barre syndrome following vaccination in the National Influenza Immunization Program, United States, 1976-1977. Am J Epidemiol 1979;110:105-123.
23. Sindern E, Schroder JM, Krismann M, et al: Inflammatory polyradiculoneuropathy with spinal cord involvement and lethal [correction of letal] outcome after hepatitis B vaccination. J Neurol Sci 2001;186:81-85.
24. Kerr D: Transverse myelitis. In Johnson RT, Griffin JW, McArthur JC (eds): Current Therapy in Neurological Disease, 6th ed. St. Louis, Mosby, 2001.
25. Kusunoki S, Shiina M, Kanazawa I: Anti-Gal-C antibodies in GBS subsequent to mycoplasma infection: Evidence of molecular mimicry. Neurology 2001;57:736-738.
26. Jacobs BC, Endtz HP, Van der Meche FG, et al: Humoral immune response against *Campylobacter jejuni* lipopolysaccharides in Guillain-Barre and Miller Fisher syndrome. J Neuroimmunol 1997;79:62-68.
27. Lee WM, Westrick MA, Macher BA: High-performance liquid chromatography of long-chain neutral glycosphingolipids and gangliosides. Biochim Biophys Acta 1982;712:498-504.
28. Moran AP, Rietschel ET, Kosunen TU, et al: Chemical characterization of *Campylobacter jejuni* lipopolysaccharides containing *N*-acetylneuraminic acid and 2,3-diamino-2,3-dideoxy-D-glucose. J Bacteriol 1991;173:618-626.
29. Gregson NA, Rees JH, Hughes RA: Reactivity of serum IgG anti-GM1 ganglioside antibodies with the lipopolysaccharide fractions of *Campylobacter jejuni* isolates from patients with Guillain-Barre syndrome (GBS). J Neuroimmunol 1997;73:28-36.
30. Jacobs BC, Hazenberg MP, Van Doorn PA, et al: Cross-reactive antibodies against gangliosides and *Campylobacter jejuni* lipopolysaccharides in patients with Guillain-Barre or Miller Fisher syndrome. J Infect Dis 1997;175:729-733.
31. Hao Q, Saida T, Kuroki S, et al: Antibodies to gangliosides and galactocerebroside in patients with Guillain-Barre syndrome with preceding *Campylobacter jejuni* and other identified infections. J Neuroimmunol 1998;81:116-126.
32. Goodyear CS, O'Hanlon GM, Plomp JJ, et al: Monoclonal antibodies raised against Guillain-Barre syndrome-associated *Campylobacter jejuni* lipopolysaccharides react with neuronal gangliosides and paralyze muscle-nerve preparations. J Clin Invest 1999;104:697-708.
33. Plomp JJ, Molenaar PC, O'Hanlon GM, et al: Miller Fisher anti-GQ1b antibodies: Alpha-latrotoxin-like effects on motor end plates. Ann Neurol 1999;45:189-199.
34. O'Hanlon GM, Paterson GJ, Veitch J, et al: Mapping immunoreactive epitopes in the human peripheral nervous system using human monoclonal anti-GM1 ganglioside antibodies. Acta Neuropathol (Berl) 1998;95:605-616.

35. Drulovic J, Dujmovic I, Stojsavlevic N, et al: Transverse myelopathy in the antiphospholipid antibody syndrome: Pinworm infestation as a trigger? J Neurol Neurosurg Psychiatry 2000;68:249.
36. Brocke S, Gaur A, Piercy C, et al: Induction of relapsing paralysis in experimental autoimmune encephalomyelitis by bacterial superantigen. Nature 1993;365:642-644.
37. Racke MK, Quigley L, Cannella B, et al: Superantigen modulation of experimental allergic encephalomyelitis: Activation of anergy determines outcome. J Immunol 1994;152:2051-2059.
38. Brocke S, Hausmann S, Steinman L, et al: Microbial peptides and superantigens in the pathogenesis of autoimmune diseases of the central nervous system. Semin Immunol 1998;10:57-67.
39. Kotzin BL, Leung DY, Kappler J, et al: Superantigens and their potential role in human disease. Adv Immunol 1993;54:99-166.
40. Vanderlugt CL, Begolka WS, Neville KL, et al: The functional significance of epitope spreading and its regulation by co-stimulatory molecules. Immunol Rev 1998;164:63-72.
41. Fukazawa T, Hamada T, Kikuchi S, et al: Antineutrophil cytoplasmic antibodies and the optic-spinal form of multiple sclerosis in Japan. J Neurol Neurosurg Psychiatry 1996;39:203-204.
42. Leonardi A, Arata L, Farinelli M, et al: Cerebrospinal fluid and neuropathological study in Devic's syndrome: Evidence of intrathecal immune activation. J Neurol Sci 1987;82:281-290.
43. O'Riordan JI, Gallagher HL, Thompson AJ, et al: Clinical, CSF, and MRI findings in Devic's neuromyelitis optica. J Neurol Neurosurg Psychiatry 1996;60:382-387.
44. Reindl M, Linington C, Brehm U, et al: Antibodies against the myelin oligodendrocyte glycoprotein and the myelin basic protein in multiple sclerosis and other neurological diseases: A comparative study. Brain 1999;122(Pt 11):2047-2056.
45. Haase CG, Schmidt S: Detection of brain-specific autoantibodies to myelin oligodendrocyte glycoprotein, S100beta and myelin basic protein in patients with Devic's neuromyelitis optica. Neurosci Lett 2001;307:131-133.
46. Tippett DS, Fishman PS, Panitch HS: Relapsing transverse myelitis. Neurology 1991;41:703-706.
47. Pandit L, Rao S: Recurrent myelitis. J Neurol Neurosurg Psychiatry 1996;60:336-338.
48. Matsui M, Kakigi R, Watanabe S, et al: Recurrent demyelinating transverse myelitis in a high titer HBs-antigen carrier. J Neurol Sci 1996;139:235-237.
49. Moore AP, Blumhardt LD: A prospective survey of the causes of non-traumatic spastic paraparesis and tetraparesis in 585 patients. Spinal Cord 1997;35:361-367.
50. Wong SH, Boggild M, Enevoldson TP, et al: Myelopathy but normal MRI: Where next? Pract Neurol 2008;8:90-102.
51. Garcia-Merino A, Blasco MR: Recurrent transverse myelitis with unusual long-standing Gd-DTPA enhancement. J Neurol 2000;247:550-551.
52. Williams CS, Butler E, Roman GC: Treatment of myelopathy in Sjogren's syndrome with a combination of prednisone and cyclophosphamide. Arch Neurol 2001;58:815-819.
53. de Seze J, Dubucquoi S, Fauchais AL, et al: Alphafodrin autoantibodies in the differential diagnosis of MS and Sjogren syndrome. Neurology 2003;61:268-269.
54. Mok CC, Lau CS, Chan EYT, et al: Acute transverse myelopathy in systemic lupus erythematosus: Clinical presentation, treatment and outcome. J Rheumatol 1998;25:467-473.
55. Kovacs B, Lafferty TL, Brent LH, et al: Transverse myelopathy in systemic lupus erythematosus: An analysis of 14 cases and review of the literature. Ann Rheum Dis 2000;59:120-124.
56. de Seze J, Lanctin C, Lebrun C, et al: Idiopathic acute transverse myelitis: Application of the recent diagnostic criteria. Neurology 2005;65:1950-1953.
57. Wingerchuk DM, Lennon VA, Pittock SJ, et al: Revised diagnostic criteria for neuromyelitis optica. Neurology 2006;66:1485-1489.
58. de Seze J, Stojkovic T, Breteau G, et al: Acute myelopathies: Clinical, laboratory and outcome profiles in 79 cases. Brain 2001;124(Pt 8):1509-1521.
59. Bashir K, Whitaker JN: Importance of paraclinical and CSF studies in the diagnosis of MS in patients presenting with partial cervical transverse myelopathy and negative cranial MRI. Mult Scler 2000;6:312-316.
60. Scott TF, Kassab SL, Singh S: Acute partial transverse myelitis with normal cerebral magnetic resonance imaging: Transition rate to clinically definite multiple sclerosis. Mult Scler 2005;11:373-377.
61. Ford B, Tampieri D, Francis G: Long-term follow-up of acute partial transverse myelopathy. Neurology 1992;42:250-252.
62. Krishnan C, Kaplin AI, Pardo CA, et al: Demyelinating disorders: Update on transverse myelitis. Curr Neurol Neurosci Rep 2006;6:236-243.
63. Kaplin AI, Deshpande DM, Scott E, et al: IL-6 induces regionally selective spinal cord injury in patients with the neuroinflammatory disorder transverse myelitis. J Clin Invest 2005;115:2731-2741.

64. Miller DH, Ormerod IE, Rudge P, et al: The early risk of multiple sclerosis following isolated acute syndromes of the brainstem and spinal cord. Ann Neurol 1989;26:635-639.
65. Ungurean A, Palfi S, Dibo G, et al: Chronic recurrent transverse myelitis or multiple sclerosis. Funct Neurol 1996;11:209-214.
66. Bakshi R, Kinkel PR, Mechtler LL, et al: Magnetic resonance imaging findings in 22 cases of myelitis: Comparison between patients with and without multiple sclerosis. Eur J Neurol 1998;5:35-48.
67. O'Riordan JI, Losseff NA, Phatouros C, et al: Asymptomatic spinal cord lesions in clinically isolated optic nerve, brain stem, and spinal cord syndromes suggestive of demyelination. J Neurol Neurosurg Psychiatry 1998;64:353-357.
68. Miller JA, Munro DD: Topical corticosteroids: Clinical pharmacology and therapeutic use. Drugs 1980;19:119-134.
69. Hallam NF: The use and abuse of topical corticosteroids in dermatology. Scott Med J 1980;25:287-291.
70. Elovaara I, Lalla M, Spare E, et al: Methylprednisolone reduces adhesion molecules in blood and cerebrospinal fluid in patients with MS. Neurology 1998;51:1703-1708.
71. Sellebjerg F, Christiansen M, Jensen J, et al: Immunological effects of oral high-dose methylprednisolone in acute optic neuritis and multiple sclerosis. Eur J Neurol 2000;7:281-289.
72. Williams CS, Butler E, Roman GC: Treatment of myelopathy in Sjogren syndrome with a combination of prednisone and cyclophosphamide. Arch Neurol 2001;58:815-819.
73. Dumas JL, Valeyre D, Chapelon-Abric C, et al: Central nervous system sarcoidosis: Follow-up at MR imaging during steroid therapy. Radiology 2000;214:411-420.
74. Bracken MB, Shepard MJ, Collins WF, et al: A randomized, controlled trial of methylprednisolone or naloxone in the treatment of acute spinal-cord injury: Results of the Second National Acute Spinal Cord Injury Study. N Engl J Med 1990;322:1405-1411.
75. Defresne P, Meyer L, Tardieu M, et al: Efficacy of high dose steroid therapy in children with severe acute transverse myelitis. J Neurol Neurosurg Psychiatry 2001;71:272-274.
76. Lahat E, Pillar G, Ravid S, et al: Rapid recovery from transverse myelopathy in children treated with methylprednisolone. Pediatr Neurol 1998;19:279-282.
77. Sebire G, Hollenberg H, Meyer L, et al: High dose methylprednisolone in severe acute transverse myelopathy. Arch Dis Child 1997;76:167-168.
78. Kennedy PG, Weir AI: Rapid recovery of acute transverse myelitis treated with steroids. Postgrad Med J 1988;64:384-385.
79. Kalita J, Misra UK: Is methyl prednisolone useful in acute transverse myelitis? Spinal Cord 2001;39:471-476.
80. Knebusch M, Strassburg HM, Reiners K: Acute transverse myelitis in childhood: Nine cases and review of the literature. Dev Med Child Neurol 1998;40:631-639.
81. Dunne K, Hopkins IJ, Shield LK: Acute transverse myelopathy in childhood. Dev Med Child Neurol 1986;28:198-204.
82. Weinshenker BG: Plasma exchange for severe attacks of inflammatory demyelinating diseases of the central nervous system. J Clin Apheresis 2001;16:39-42.
83. Weinshenker BG: Therapeutic plasma exchange for acute inflammatory demyelinating syndromes of the central nervous system. J Clin Apheresis 1999;14:144-148.
84. Weinshenker BG, O'Brien PC, Petterson TM, et al: A randomized trial of plasma exchange in acute central nervous system inflammatory demyelinating disease. Ann Neurol 1999;46:878-886.
85. Keegan M, Pineda AA, McClelland RL, et al: Plasma exchange for severe attacks of CNS demyelination: Predictors of response. Neurology 2002;58:143-146.
86. Greenberg BM, Thomas KP, Krishnan C, et al: Idiopathic transverse myelits: Corticosteroids, plasma exchange or cyclophosphamide. Neurology 2007;68:1614.
87. Wollinsky KH, Hulser PJ, Brinkmeier H, et al: CSF filtration is an effective treatment of Guillain-Barre syndrome: A randomized clinical trial. Neurology 2001;57:774-780.
88. Robinson WH, Steinman L, Utz PJ: Protein arrays for autoantibody profiling and fine-specificity mapping. Proteomics 2003;3:2077-2084.
89. Robinson WH, Fontoura P, Lee BJ, et al: Protein microarrays guide tolerizing DNA vaccine treatment of autoimmune encephalomyelitis. Nat Biotechnol 2003;21:1033-1039.
90. Mohan N, Edwards ET, Cupps TR, et al: Demyelination occurring during anti-tumor necrosis factor alpha therapy for inflammatory arthritides. Arthritis Rheum 2001;44:2862-2869.

13 Neuromyelitis Optica

MARCELO MATIELLO • BRIAN G. WEINSHENKER

"How many a dispute could have been deflated into a single paragraph if the disputants had dared to define their terms."
Aristotle (384-322 BC)

Neuromyelitis optica (NMO)—also known as Devic's syndrome or Devic's disease—and the NMO spectrum disorders are severe idiopathic, inflammatory disorders of the central nervous system (CNS) with a remarkable predilection for the optic nerves and spinal cord. NMO was historically believed to be a monophasic syndrome characterized by bilateral optic neuritis (ON) and myelitis in rapid succession. Contemporary studies suggest that NMO most commonly manifests with unilateral ON or myelitis and usually follows a relapsing course, as does multiple sclerosis (MS); it thereby satisfies the defining characteristics of MS, a disease disseminated in time and space. Because MS has historically been the diagnosis applied to every patient with a relapsing inflammatory demyelinating disease satisfying the principle of "dissemination of lesions in time and space," the relapsing form of NMO was typically diagnosed as MS in the past. However, Asian investigators distinguished "optic-spinal multiple sclerosis" (OSMS) from classic MS, recognizing the distinction of NMO from prototypical MS before neurologists in Western countries. Recent studies on NMO natural history, neuroimaging, pathology, and immunology have confirmed that NMO is distinct from typical MS. Moreover, a specific and possibly pathogenic immunoglobulin G (IgG) antibody, known as NMO-IgG, was discovered in NMO patients. NMO-IgG targets the astrocytic water channel protein aquaporin-4 (AQP4). By contrast, no specific biomarker or antigenic target is recognized for MS. In a previous edition of this series, Wingerchuk and Weinshenker reviewed the clinical features, diagnostic criteria, and natural history of NMO and the pathologic characteristics that distinguish it from MS.[32] Here, we review these aspects briefly and then focus on recent developments: the NMO-IgG marker and how it has changed the clinical diagnosis of NMO, expanded the spectrum of disorders related to NMO, and is helping unravel the pathogenesis of this disorder.

History

Albutt provided the first known description of a patient with acute onset of optic symptoms after experiencing a spinal cord syndrome.[1] In 1894, reports by Devic and Gault summarized 16 patients with the concomitance of papillitis or retrobulbar neuritis and acute myelitis; subsequently, the disorder became eponymously known as Devic's disease.[2,3]

In 1927, Beck reviewed 70 patients whose dominant symptoms were paraplegia and blindness. He suggested that optic-spinal demyelinating disease may differ from other cases of MS: "Many of the cases reported as myelitis with ON may now be confidently diagnosed as disseminated sclerosis, but many cases remain in which a diffuse inflammatory myelitis was associated with a similar affection of the optic nerves, and the similarity of these cases to one another seems to establish them as belonging to a true disease entity."[4] He also identified a different distribution and size of pathologic lesions; some cases showed disseminated foci, whereas others had a continuous lesion involving a long segment of the cord. He wrote, "It is possible that these two types represent two distinct diseases with a common clinical picture."[4]

Stansbury described five patients whom he had examined personally and systematically reviewed other cases reported in the medical literature, 20 of which included autopsy findings. He concluded that NMO onset was typically between 30 and 50 years of age and was not limited to persons "of the white race." Severe and sometimes binocular vision loss was common, and respiratory paralysis was a common cause of early death.[5] Subsequent authors noted that NMO sometimes affected the brain,[6-8] although it was not until recently that brain involvement was accepted to be compatible with a diagnosis of NMO.

Okinaka[9] and Kuroiwa[10] and their colleagues characterized OSMS as an entity distinct from prototypical MS in Japan. These two types of MS were of comparable frequency in Japan in the 1960s. In retrospect, most of the OSMS cases reported at that time would probably be recognized as the relapsing form of NMO in Western countries today.

Clinical series[11,12] described characteristics of NMO, but the exact limits of the syndrome remained undefined, in particular the requirement for a short interval between index attacks of ON and myelitis and the requirement of bilateral rather than unilateral ON. Wingerchuk and associates[13] were the first to propose diagnostic criteria that rejected an arbitrary restriction of the interval between index episodes or a "monophasic course" (i.e., no relapses of ON or myelitis) as a requirement for the diagnosis. The proposed diagnostic criteria incorporated magnetic resonance imaging (MRI) findings that are now acknowledged as essential for distinguishing NMO from MS, the most important of which is the presence of a long spinal cord lesion (>3 vertebral segments) in the context of an attack of acute myelitis.[13]

The next major advance was the recognition of perivascular deposits of immunoglobulin and complement in immunopathologic studies; this suggested that

TABLE 13–1 Diagnostic Criteria for Neuromyelitis Optica

Optic neuritis
Acute myelitis
At least two of three supportive criteria:
- Contiguous spinal cord MRI lesions extending over ≥ 3 vertebral segments
- Brain MRI not meeting diagnostic criteria for multiple sclerosis
- NMO-IgG seropositive status

IgG, immunoglobulin G; MRI, magnetic resonance imaging; NMO, neuromyelitis optica.
From Wingerchuk DM, et al: Revised diagnostic criteria for neuromyelitis optica. Neurology 2006; 66:1485-1489.

the antigenic target in NMO most likely was concentrated in perivascular regions of the brain.[14] In parallel, Lennon and coworkers[15] recognized a specific antibody marker of NMO, which reacted with an antigen on the abluminal face of microvessels in the central nervous system. Her group subsequently identified the target antigen as the water channel, AQP4.[16] Those advances ushered in the modern era of understanding the pathogenesis of NMO.

The identification of NMO-IgG, the increased recognition of the high specificity of longitudinally extensive transverse myelitis (LETM) in distinguishing NMO, and the observation that brain lesions are compatible with a diagnosis of NMO led to revision of the diagnostic criteria in 2006 (Table 13-1).

Epidemiology

NMO usually manifests in adulthood, predominately in late middle age. A study of 71 patients diagnosed with NMO at the Mayo Clinic reported that the mean age of onset was 29 years (range, 1 to 54 years) for patients with a monophasic course and 39 years (range, 6 to 72 years) for patients with relapsing disease.[13] NMO has been reported in children as young as 23 months of age,[17] and NMO-IgG seropositivity is as frequent in children with NMO as in adults.[18] NMO may occur as late as the ninth decade.[19] The relapsing form of NMO is eight times more frequent in women than in men, although the monophasic form seems to occur with equal frequency in men and women.[13,20]

The incidence and prevalence of NMO are unknown in most Western countries. In Western nations, NMO has generally been considered a rare disorder, although it is almost certainly under-recognized and is frequently misdiagnosed as MS, (recurrent) transverse myelitis (TM), recurrent ON, lupus myelitis, or another "-connective tissue disease–associated" myelitis. The recognition of NMO has increased substantially since diagnostic criteria were articulated[13] and a specific biomarker was discovered.[15] Demyelinating disease in Asia has a strong predilection for the optic nerves and spinal cord. The prevalence of NMO in Asia is probably higher than in Europe or North America. The comparison is confounded by differences in diagnostic criteria used by Asian investigators, in particular the lack of requirement for a long spinal cord lesion at the time of an acute myelitis, which may result in misclassification (as OSMS) in Japan of some cases that would be regarded as prototypical MS in Western countries. Also, the presence of brain lesions is generally an exclusionary criterion in Japanese studies, contrary to the modified criteria proposed in Western countries.[20] Other factors complicate the diagnosis of MS. Confluent spinal cord lesions in chronic MS may conglomerate to yield to a long spinal cord lesion that is different from the homogeneous, usually well-delimited, long (>3 vertebral segments) spinal cord lesion that develops acutely in the context of an attack of NMO. Confluent small lesions in prototypical MS may be misinterpreted as satisfying the criterion for a myelitis-associated longitudinally extensive spinal cord lesion. The most recent Japanese nationwide survey of MS showed that about 20% of patients with demyelinating disorders had OSMS—a remarkable decrease from the series reported a half-decade earlier. This was largely due to an increase in the prevalence of prototypical MS rather than a decline in the optic-spinal form.[21] A similar proportion of "MS" that is truly NMO (25% of 32 patients) was reported in a hospital-based series from southern India.[22] Case series of patients with NMO phenotype (9 patients from Morocco and 8 from South Africa) suggested a relative higher frequency of NMO compared with MS in the African continent.[23,24] In Latin America, a population-based study of demyelinating diseases in French Afro-Caribbean countries from Martinique (West Indies)[25] showed that 17 (27%) of 62 patients had NMO. In Brazil,[26] a hospital-based series of 67 consecutive patients with demyelinating disease revealed that 28 (41.7%) had a predominantly optic-spinal form of MS. Prevalence studies are unavailable in Europe and North America. In North America, African Americans with demyelinating disease are more likely than Whites to have OSMS and TM.[27] Similarly, among the native populations, NMO seems to be the dominant form of inflammatory demyelinating disease.[28]

Clinical Presentation and Natural History

The cardinal features of ON and myelitis are essential for the diagnosis of NMO. They may occur simultaneously or, more commonly, separated from one another by months, years, or decades. Even though ON and myelitis also occur commonly in typical MS, they are, in general, more severe in NMO. For example, myelitis is commonly "complete" (symmetrical and with motor, sensory, and sphincter involvement) rather than "partial" (asymmetrical, either motor or sensory, with relatively little sphincter involvement).

A recent study comparing the clinical course of 96 NMO patients (median follow-up, 6.1 years) with MS natural history data demonstrated that neurologic disability in NMO is attack related and that a secondary progressive course is extremely rare.[29]

Spinal cord MRI scans also show distinctive findings: most patients have longitudinally extensive lesions extending over 3 or more vertebral segments. Brain MRI lesions are detected in approximately 60% of NMO patients. Although most brain lesions encountered in patients with NMO are nonspecific and asymptomatic, lesions in the brainstem and hypothalamus appear to be relatively characteristic and specific. Brain lesions have a predilection for regions known to have high levels of immunoreactivity for AQP4[30] (Fig. 13-1).

The specific serum biomarker for the disease (i.e., NMO-IgG; see later discussion) may help identify limited or inaugural presentations of NMO: idiopathic single or recurrent events of LETM (≥3 vertebral segment spinal cord lesion seen on MRI) and recurrent or simultaneous bilateral ON.[31] In prospective follow-up

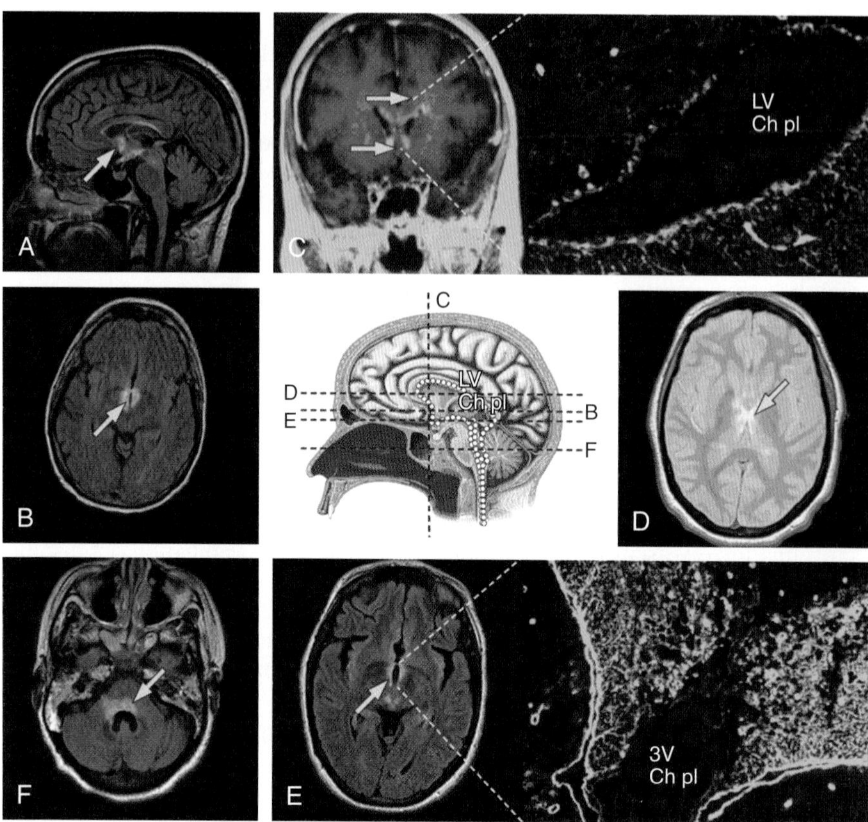

Figure 13–1 Brain lesions typical of neuromyelitis optica localize at the sites where aquaporin-4 expression is normally highest *(central diagram)*. **A** and **B,** Lesion around the third ventricle extending into the hypothalamus. **C,** Subependymal enhancement along the frontal horns and in the adjacent white matter. Linked immunofluorescence photomicrograph shows the binding pattern of the serum NMO-IgG from a patient with neuromyelitis optica in a mouse brain template (400×). Contiguous signal abnormality is shown throughout the periventricular tissues: diencephalon (**D**), third ventricle (**E**), and fourth ventricle (**F**). Immunofluorescence photomicrograph linked to image **E** shows the binding pattern of NMO-IgG from a patient with NMO in a mouse brain template (400×). (From Wingerchuk DM, Lennon VA, Lucchinetti CF, et al: The spectrum of neuromyelitis optica. Lancet Neurol 2007;6:805-815.)

of both ON and TM, seropositivity for the NMO-IgG marker is strongly predictive of the risk of relapse of myelitis and ON and the final disability outcome, as well as mortality. The spectrum of NMO should be widened to embrace patients who have isolated or recurrent ON or myelitis and who are seropositive for NMO-IgG. Clinical, imaging, and laboratory differences between NMO and MS were presented in the previous review that appeared in this series.[32]

The NMO-IgG Biomarker

NMO-IgG is a disease biomarker found in the serum of NMO patients. In 2004, Mayo Clinic investigators identified a characteristic immunostaining pattern in a few NMO patients studied using a protocol to detect paraneoplastic syndrome–associated autoantibodies. A larger and prospective study was then performed including sera of clinically defined NMO and OSMS patients, of individuals with high-risk syndromes (recurrent LETM and recurrent ON), and of controls consisting of MS patients and individuals with other neurologic or autoimmune disease. The sensitivity and specificity of the test were 73% (95% confidence interval, 60% to 86%) and 91% (79% to 100%), respectively, for NMO and 58% (30% to 86%) and 100% (66% to 100%) for OSMS.[15]

Several independent investigators have studied the performance characteristics of NMO-IgG using either the Neuroimmunology Laboratory at Mayo Clinic or one of a variety of different assays for AQP4 antibodies. The results of those studies are summarized in Table 13-2.[15,18,33-41]

Differences in performance characteristics could vary depending on criteria used to define cases, on the spectrum of controls used for comparison, and on the different immunoassays applied for NMO-IgG detection.

DIFFERENCES IN DEFINING NEUROMYELITIS OPTICA

The most commonly used gold standard for definition of NMO cases has been the diagnostic criteria published by Wingerchuk and colleagues in 1999.[13] However, there have been notable exceptions. Nakashima and co-authors[33] evaluated patients with an optic-spinal course, and those with brain lesions suggestive of MS were classified as having classic MS. It was subsequently appreciated in both the United States and Japan that brain lesions occur in NMO and often, although not always, differ from those seen in MS.[30] In another study of NMO-IgG in OSMS,[37] the seropositivity rate in the OSMS group was 27%, but patients with LETM with or without brain lesions had higher seropositivity rate (35%). In a different study, patients who were classified as having relapsing-remitting MS (RRMS) using the McDonald criteria were divided accordingly: LETM-MS, OSMS, and classic MS. Twenty-five (56%) of 45 patients with LETM had NMO-IgG antibodies; patients who did not have LETM, regardless of whether they had OSMS or classic MS, were seronegative, suggesting that patients with MS and LETM and are seropositive for NMO-IgG, regardless of whether they have brain lesions or not (i.e., OSMS or classic MS), may have NMO.[40]

Limited syndromes, such as isolated TM, differ in the frequency of seropositivity for NMO-IgG depending on characteristics of their myelitis. Only 1 of 22 cases with partial TM with MRI lesions extending over 2 or fewer spinal cord segments was seropositive.[34] The seropositivity rate in isolated LETM appears to be much lower in children: 1 relapsing LETM case was seropositive, but 9 single-event LETM cases were seronegative.[18]

SELECTION OF CONTROLS

Five studies[15,35,37,38,41] analyzed controls with a variety of inflammatory and noninflammatory diseases of the nervous system as well as those with other autoimmune disease and healthy controls. The most relevant controls are MS patients with ON and myelitis who, because of the detection of oligoclonal bands and either the presence or subsequent development of other brain lesions typical for MS, declare their true diagnosis as MS rather than NMO. Such controls were analyzed in seven studies. Lennon and colleagues studied 22 patients with what was initially suspected to be NMO that was subsequently classified as MS because the myelitis was

TABLE 13–2 Comparison of Studies That Independently Tested Patients with NMO and Controls for NMO-IgG

		Cases (positive for NMO-IgG)		*Controls (positive for NMO-IgG)*			*Methods*		*Diagnostic Properties*				
First Author and Year (Ref. No.)	**No. Tested**	**NMO/ OSMS**	**Inaugural/ Limited Forms of NMO**	**MS or Other IIDD**	**OND or AID**	**Healthy**	**Detection Assay**	**Gold Standard Comparison**	**Comparison**	**Sensitivity (%)**	**Specificity (%)**	**LR+**	**LR–**
Lennon, 2004 (15)	124	45 (33)	8 RON (2) 27Relapsing TM (14)	22 MS with ON or TM (2) 19 MS w/o ON or TM (0)	56 (0)	None	Indirect IF (mouse tissue)	Wingerchuk 1999	NMO vs MS NMO/limited forms vs MS	73 61	91 91	8.07 6.73	0.29 0.42
Nakashima, 2006 (33)	35	19 (12)	None	13 CMS (2) 3 Spinal cord MS (0)	None	None	Indirect IF (mouse tissue)	Wingerchuk 1999	NMO vs MS	63	85	4.11	0.44
Scott, 2006 (34)	32	4 (3)	None	6 MS (0) 22 TM w/o LETM (1)	None	None	Indirect IF (mouse tissue)	Wingerchuk 1999	NMO vs controls	75	95	16.5	0.26
Tanaka, 2007 (35)	91	26 (16)	None	6 OSMS w/o (0) LETM 21 MS (0)	28(0)	10 (0)	Indirect IF (AQP4 transfected cells)	Not mentioned	NMO vs MS	62	100	Inf.	0.38
Takahashi, 2007 (36)	148	22 (20)	13 (11)	53 MS (0) 10 CIS (0)	50 (0)	None	Indirect IF (AQP4 transfected cells)	Wingerchuk 2006	NMO vs MS NMO/limited forms vs MS	91 85	100 100	Inf. Inf.	0.09 0.15
Matsuoka, 2007 (37)	200	48 (13)	11 Brainstem-spinal MS (0) 4 TM (1)	54 MS (3)	52 (0)	35 (0)	Indirect IF (AQP4 transfected cells)	Kira 1996 (OSMS)	LETM with or without brain lesions vs CMS	35	94	10	0.47

TABLE 13–2 Comparison of Studies that Independently Tested Patients with NMO and Controls for NMO-IgG (Continued)

		Cases (positive for NMO-IgG)		*Controls (positive for NMO-IgG)*			*Methods*		*Diagnostic Properties*				
First Author and Year (Ref. No.)	**No. Tested**	**NMO/ OSMS**	**Inaugural/ Limited Forms of NMO**	**MS or Other IIDD**	**OND or AID**	**Healthy**	**Detection Assay**	**Gold Standard Comparison**	**Comparison**	**Sensitivity (%)**	**Specificity (%)**	**LR+**	**LR–**
Paul., 2007 (38)	334	37 (21)	6 LETM (6)	144 MS (4)	73 (1)	29 (0)	RIPA	Wingerchuk 1999	NMO vs MS NMO + LETM vs MS	57 63	98 98	12.49 13.81	0.45 0.39
Saiz, 2007 (39)	161	16 (10)	7 LETM (3) 7 RON (1)	115 MS (0) 4 TM w/o LETM (0)	None	None	Indirect im-muno-his-tochemistry (rat brain)	Wingerchuk 1999, 2006	NMO vs MS NMO/limited forms vs MS	63 45	100 100	Inf. Inf.	0.38 0.55
Tanaka, 2007 (40)	128	45 (25)	None	64 MS (0)	None	None	Indirect IF (AQP4 transfect-ed cells)	Cases were MS with LETM	MS with LETM vs MS w/o LETM	56	100	Inf.	0.44
Banwell, 2008 (18)	87	17 (8)	13 ON (1) 10 LETM (1)	41 MS (0) 3 TM w/o LETM (0) 3 ADEM (0)	None	None	Indirect IF (mouse tissue)	Wingerchuk 1999	NMO vs MS NMO/limited forms vs MS	47 24	100 100	Inf. Inf.	0.53 0.76
Marignier, 2008 (41)	135	26(14)	13 LETM (7) 21 ON (4)	52 MS (5) 8 TM w/o LETM (0)	43 (0)	None	Indirect IF (mouse tissue)	Wingerchuk 1999	NMO vs MS NMO/limited forms vs MS	54 45	90 95	5.6 4.64	0.51 0.61

ADEM, acute demyelinating encephalomyopathy; AID, autoimmune disease; AQP4, aquaporin-4; CIS, clinically isolated syndrome; CMS, classic multiple sclerosis; IF, immunofluorescence, IIDD, idiopathic inflammatory demyelinating disease; Inf., infinite number; LETM, longitudinally extensive transverse myelitis; LR+, positive likehood ratio; LR–, negative likehood ratio; MS, multiple sclerosis; NMO, neuromyelitis optica; ON, optic neuritis; OND, other neurologic disease; OSMS, optic-spinal multiple sclerosis; RIPA, radioimmunoprecipitation assay; RON, recurrent optic neuritis; w/o, without.

not longitudinally extensive and did not meet the Wingerchuk criteria.[15] Similarly, Tanaka and coworkers tested six patients with OSMS without LETM.[35] The studies by Scott[42] (n = 22), Marigner[41] (n = 8), Saiz[39] (n = 4), and Banwell[18] (n = 3) and their colleagues analyzed patients with acute TM shorter than 3 vertebral segments in length. Paul and associates studied 77 MS patients with at least one ON episode, 15 patients with TM without a large lesion, and 11 patients with isolated ON.[38]

IMMUNOASSAYS

Four different immunoassays have been described:

- Indirect immunofluorescence (IF) with a mouse CNS substrate as the AQP4 target
- Indirect IF with a substrate of cells stably transfected with a vector into which AQP4 complementary DNA was introduced
- Indirect immunohistochemistry assay with a rat CNS substrate as the AQP4 target
- Radioimmunoprecipitation assay using recombinant AQP4

The results of the sensitivity, specificity, and likelihood ratios were generally similar among the various assays. Two groups tested samples independently by comparing the new assay with the historical standard, the NMO-IgG by IF using rodent brain substrate. The results were contradictory, and no assay can be considered as the most sensitive based on these studies[36,37] (Table 13-3). Newer methods may ultimately prove to be more sensitive and, in the case of immunoprecipitation, more rapid and easier to quantitate. However, these new techniques must all be analyzed for specificity relative to the clinical gold standard.

NMO-IgG AND DISEASE OUTCOMES

The prognostic value of NMO-IgG was evaluated using both cross-sectional and longitudinal studies, although the data are limited. Other studies have evaluated whether seropositivity and titer predict relapse in patients presenting with possible limited or inaugural forms of NMO (isolated LETM or recurrent ON).

Takahashi and colleagues reported that antibody titers were higher in patients with permanent complete blindness compared with those with ON who experienced some degree of recovery. The length of spinal cord lesions also correlated with

TABLE 13–3 Comparison between Indirect Immunofluorescence Using Rodent Substrate (NMO-IgG) and Indirect Immunofluorescence with Aquaporin-4–Transfected Cells (New Assay)

First Author and Year (Ref. No.)	NMO-IgG Positive and New Assay Positive	NMO-IgG Negative and New Assay Positive	NMO-IgG Positive and New Assay Negative
Takahashi, 2007 (36)	15	6	0
Matsuoka, 2007 (37)	15	0	3

IgG, immunoglobulin G; NMO, neuromyelitis optica.

NMO-IgG titer. On serial studies of six patients, NMO-IgG antibody titers declined after high-dose intravenous methylprednisolone and remained low during relapse-free periods while the patient was receiving immunosuppressive therapy.[36]

Among patients with a single episode of LETM, 38% were seropositive for NMO-IgG. After 12 months' follow-up in 23 patients, none of 14 NMO-IgG seronegative experienced a relapse or developed ON, whereas 5 of 9 NMO-IgG seropositive developed a second neurologic event, including 4 (44%) with recurrent TM and 1 (11%) with ON (P = .004). The NMO-IgG titer was higher in the seropositive patients who had a relapse (median, 3840; range, 960 to 61,440), compared with the seropositive patients who did not relapse (median, 60; range, 60 to 120).[43]

Six (50%) of 12 NMO-IgG–seropositive patients with recurrent ON who did not satisfy criteria for MS or NMO experienced an attack of TM after a median follow-up of 8.4 years, compared with 1 (6.7%) of 15 seronegative patients. All 14 NMO-IgG–seropositive patients, compared with 11 (64.7%) of 17 seronegative patients, had at least one attack in which the visual acuity was worse than 20/200 in the affected eye (P = .05), and the final visual outcome at last follow-up (median, 8.4 years from the first ON episode) was also worse in the seropositive cases. Among the patients with recurrent ON who were seropositive, NMO-IgG titer was higher in those who developed myelitis than in those who did not. Specifically, 5 (71.4%) of 7 patients with an NMO-IgG titer greater than 1:480 developed myelitis, compared with only 1 (20%) of 5 patients who had a titer equal or less than 1:480 (P = .07).[44]

NMO-IgG IN CHILDREN

Banwell and colleagues analyzed clinical and neuroimaging data and assessed the NMO-IgG serologic status of 87 children with inflammatory demyelinating disease (RRMS, NMO, monophasic/recurrent ON, TM, or acute disseminated encephalomyelitis). Seven (78%) of nine children with relapsing NMO and one (12.5%) of eight with monophasic NMO were seropositive, similar to the seropositivity rates in adults with NMO. However, none of nine children with monophasic LETM was NMO-IgG seropositive, in contrast to observations in adults. Possibly, LETM in children is less frequently an NMO spectrum disorder than it is in adults.[18]

SUMMARY

Based on available evidence, NMO-IgG is highly specific for the diagnosis of NMO and related disorders and is useful in predicting the recurrence risk of myelitis and/or ON in patients with limited or inaugural presentations of NMO, such as myelitis associated with a LETM or recurrent ON. However, its correlation with disease activity and its utility as a surrogate measure of disease activity remain uncertain pending availability of more data.

Pathogenesis of Neuromyelitis Optica

TARGET ANTIGEN DISCOVERED

Immunopathologic studies provided the first major clues about the pathogenesis of NMO. The pathology of NMO was reviewed in a previous edition of this series.[32] Immunoglobulin is deposited in a characteristic perivascular rim or rosette pattern lining the outer rim of thickened microvessels co-localized with activated complement terminal components. Medium-sized spinal cord arteries are thickened and hyalinized.[14,45-47] In addition, histopathologic examination of brain lesions in an NMO patient revealed the typical abnormalities seen in spinal cord and optic nerves: extensive myelin loss, large number of macrophages, and perivascular prominent eosinophil infiltration (Fig. 13-2).[48]

The characteristic pattern of NMO-IgG immunostaining of the abluminal face of microvessels in the midbrain and cerebellum and also of the pia and subpial glia along the Virchow-Robin spaces in rodent brain was found to bear strong similarities to the distribution of human immunoglobulin and activated complement in NMO lesions (Fig. 13-3). This observation suggested that NMO-IgG might recognize an antigen similar or identical to that being recognized by pathogenic immunoglobulin

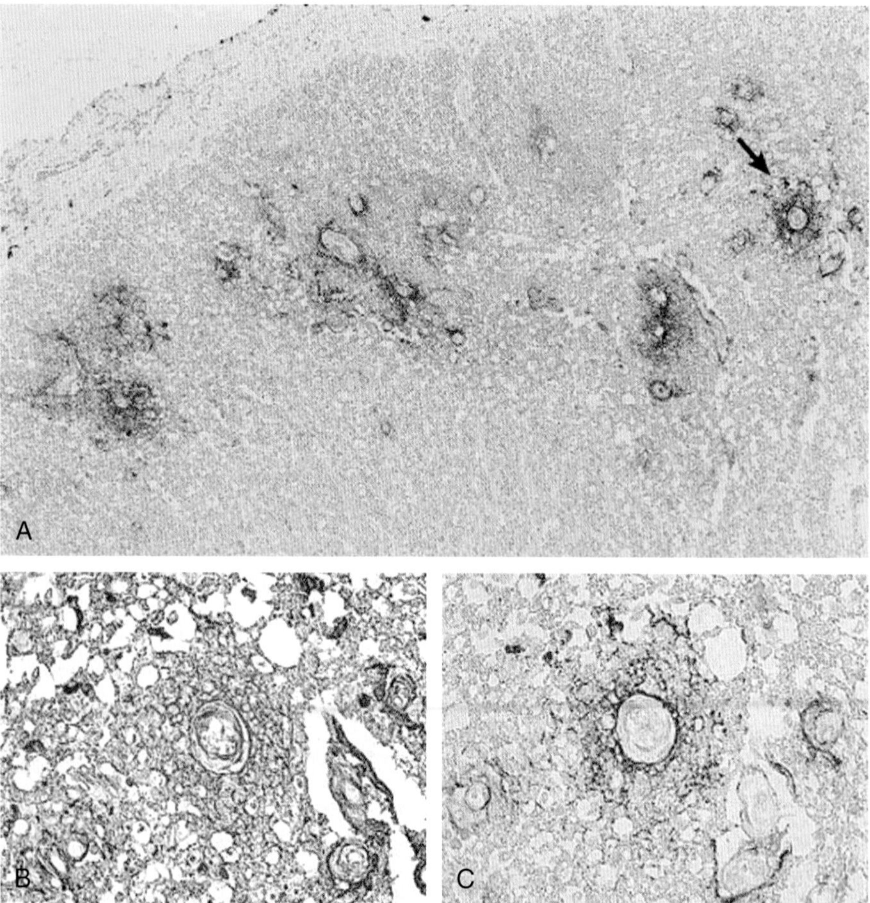

Figure 13–2 Immunopathology of neuromyelitis optica. **A,** Immunocytochemistry for C9neo antigen, complement activation products in a vasculocentric "rim and rosette" pattern (co-localization of immunoglobulin (**B,** immunocytochemistry for immunoglobulin G) and complement (**C,** immunocytochemistry for C9neo antigen) on sequential sections. (From Jacob A, Matiello M, Wingerchuk DM, et al: Neuromyelitis optica: Changing concepts. J Neuroimmunol 2007;187:126-138.)

in NMO. A series of definitive experiments established that AQP4 is the target of NMO-IgG; these studies included abolition of immunostaining in AQP4 knockout mice and immunoprecipitation of AQP4 to the exclusion of other proteins in the cell cytoskeleton complex that anchors AQP4 to the cell membrane.[16]

THE ROLE OF AQUAPORIN-4 IN THE PATHOGENESIS OF NEUROMYELITIS OPTICA

AQP4 is polarized by the dystrophin-dystroglycan complex to the membrane of astrocyte foot processes. It is a component of the blood–brain barrier with a major role in the regulation of the water transport to the cell (Fig. 13-4). AQP4-null mice are protected against cytotoxic edema, showing reduced blood–brain barrier water permeability and reduced rate of water flow into the brain parenchyma.[49] In a vasogenic edema model, brain edema is worsened by defective water elimination in AQP4-deficient animals.[50] AQP4 participates in the migration of reactive astrocytes to sites of injury, perhaps because transmembrane water fluxes are necessary for cell movement. In AQP4-null mice, glial scarring is impaired. AQP4 also influences neural excitability through slowed potassium reuptake resulting from impaired function of the inwardly rectified Kir4.1 channel in AQP4-deficient astroglia.[51]

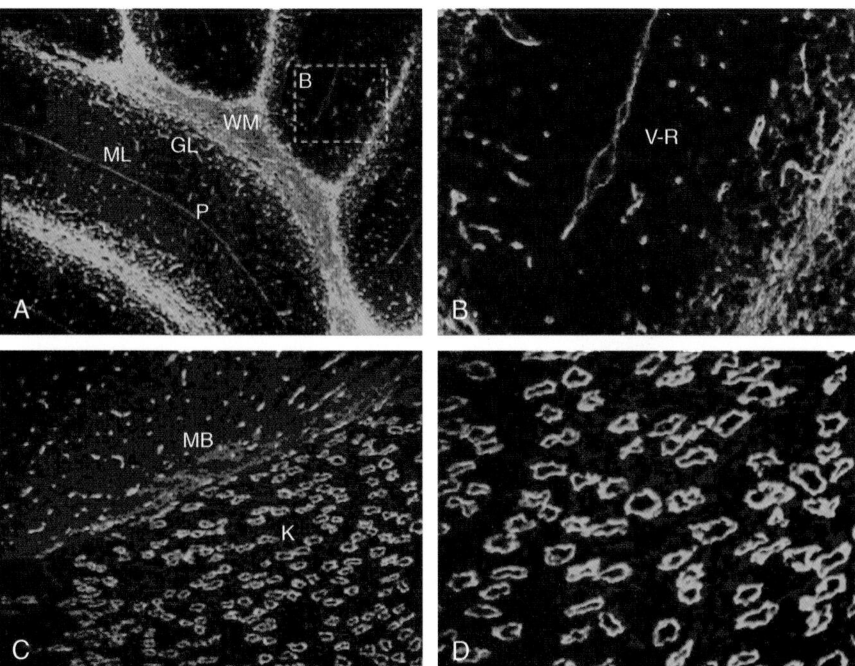

Figure 13–3 Immunofluorescence pattern of NMO-IgG binding to mouse central nervous system and kidney template. **A,** Cerebellar cortex, prominent staining of microvessels and pia (P) (100×). B; GL, granular layer; ML, molecular layer; WM, white matter. **B,** Detailed image from panel A showing the the outlined Virchow-Robin space (V-R) (400×). **C,** Midbrain (MB) and kidney (K) (200×). **D.** Kidney, collecting tubules of medulla (400×). (From Jacob A, Matiello M, Wingerchuk DM, et al: Neuromyelitis optica: Changing concepts. J Neuroimmunol 2007;187:126-138.)

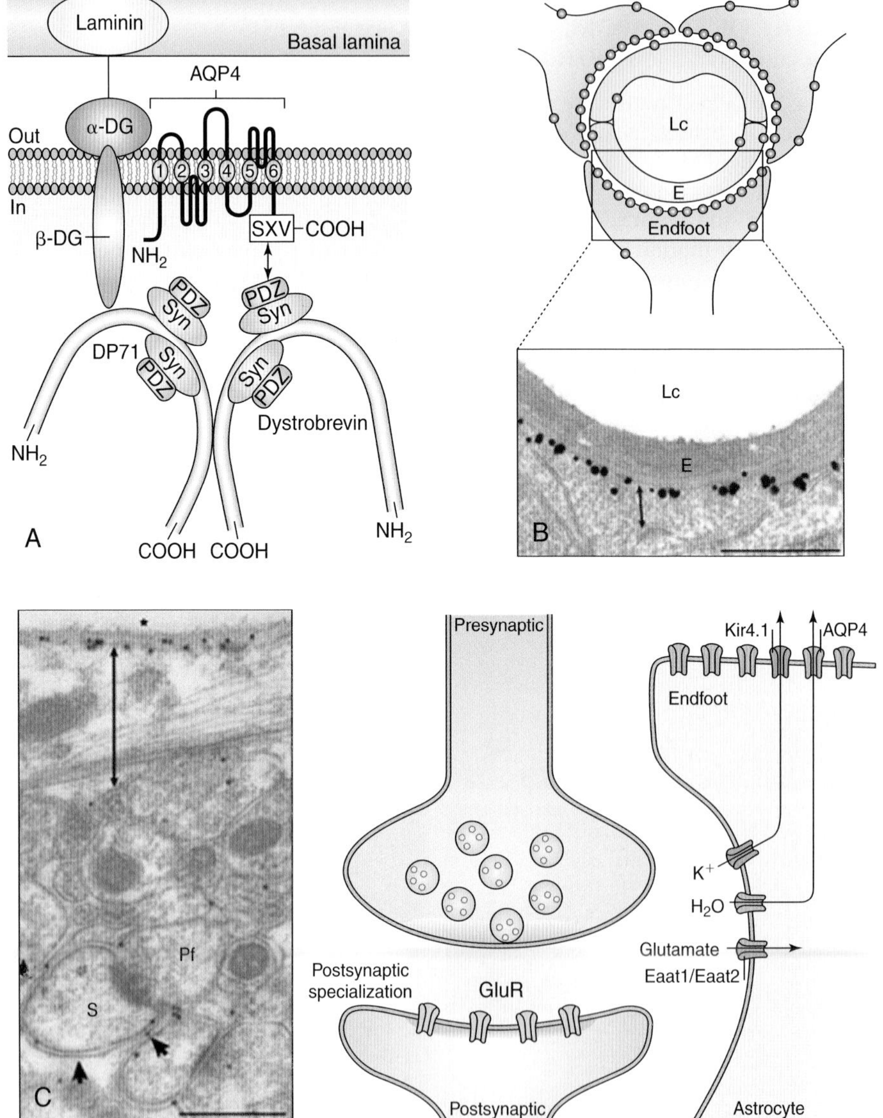

Figure 13–4 See legend on opposite page

In addition to the correspondence between the perivascular localization in astrocyte foot processes that abut cerebral microvessels and the infiltrate found in pathology specimens, other discoveries support the hypothesis that NMO-IgG is not merely an epiphenomenon useful for diagnosis but also pathogenic. Sites with high immunoreactivity for AQP4 in the brain (e.g., hypothalamus and periventricular regions) are those that are affected by the disease process as detected by MRI in NMO patients with NMO-IgG staining in mouse brain and with AQP4.[14,52,53] There is a striking loss of AQP4 in NMO lesions, regardless of the stage of demyelinating activity, the extent of tissue necrosis, or the site of CNS involvement. This was not the case in controls (MS, ischemic stroke, and normal brain).[54-56]

In a seminal study, Hinson and colleagues[57] demonstrated the selectivity and immunopathologic consequences of antibody binding to surface epitopes of cells expressing AQP4. Serum IgG from patients with NMO bound to the extracellular domains of AQP4 and led to a striking disappearance of AQP4 from the plasma membrane within minutes. Removal of the patients' serum in the absence of cycloheximide resulted in rapid reappearance of AQP4, indicating that reappearance was dependent on new synthesis of AQP4 protein. The AQP4-specific serum IgG was exclusively IgG1, the dominant complement-activating IgG subclass, in all NMO-IgG–positive patients tested. In the presence of NMO patient serum and human complement, AQP4-expressing cells were killed and C9neo, a marker of complement-mediated tissue injury, was deposited on the plasma membrane of cells, consistent with complement-mediated cytotoxicity as suggested by the immunopathologic studies on NMO autopsy material.[14,57]

The same study provided insights as to the possible mechanism whereby AQP4-mediated pathology might lead to demyelination. The immediate proximity of AQP4-specific immunoreactivity in astrocytic foot processes to the nodes of Ranvier was demonstrated by confocal microscopy with antibodies directed to AQP4 and to either sodium channel protein or the paranodal protein, Caspr. AQP4 co-localized with each of these proteins. Based on these observations, injury to the oligodendrocyte at paranodes where axons and paranodal myelin are in intimate contact with AQP4-containing astrocytic foot processes may result in axonal injury because of the alteration of the ionic microenvironment at the internode and secondary demyelination.[57]

Figure 13–4 Aquaporin-4 (AQP4) structure, localization, and function. **A,** Association of AQP4 and dystrophin-associated protein complex. **B,** Diagram of the expression pattern of AQP4 around brain microvessels and an electron micrograph showing strong AQP4 immunogold labeling in the perivascular membrane of an astrocytic endfoot. *, basal lamina; E, endothelium; Lc, capillary lumen. The *arrow* spans the two membranes of the endfoot, the top one abutting the endothelial cells of a capillary. Scale bar = 0.5 μm. **C,** Expression pattern of AQP4 in the superficial part of the cerebellar molecular layer. Gold particles labeling AQP4 occur in astrocytic lamellae *(arrowheads)*, parallel fibers (Pf) and Purkinje cell spines (S), and at higher density in endfoot membranes facing the pia and the subarachnoidal space *(asterisk)*. The double-headed *arrow* indicates a subpial endfoot. The accompanying drawing shows a simplified glutamatergic synapse and an astrocyte with molecules, rectifying K^+ channel (Kir4.1) and the glutamate transporters EAAt1 and EAAT2. Scale bar = 0.5 μm. GluR, glutamate receptors. (**A,** Reprinted from O'Riordan JI, Gallagher HL, Thompson AJ, et al: Clinical, CSF, and MRI findings in Devic's neuromyelitis optica. J Neurol Neurosurg Psychiatry 1996;60:382-387 with permission from the Society for Neuroscience. **B** and **C,** From Amiry-Moghaddam M, Ottersen OP: The molecular basis of water transport in the brain. Review. Nat Rev Neurosci 2003;4:991-1001. Nature Publishing Group © 2003.)

GENETIC SUSCEPTIBILITY TO NEUROMYELITIS OPTICA

Familial occurrence of NMO has been reported.[58-62] Genetic risk factors are suspected to increase NMO susceptibility. However, no study has demonstrated excess familial aggregation, and none has discovered a genetic association. The human leukocyte antigen HLA-DP*0501 has been reported to be over-represented in Japanese patients with OSMS[63]; however, the high frequency of this allele in the general Japanese population complicates the analysis of the supposed association. By contrast, in 24 British patients with NMO, only one had the DPB1*0501 allele, and no difference was found in the frequency of this allele between patients with NMO and healthy individuals.[64]

No mutation was found in the genes known to harbor the vast majority of mutations associated with Leber's hereditary optic neuropathy (LHON) in 32 NMO patients.[65]

Assuming that known single nucleotide polymorphism (SNPs) in the AQP4 gene could be in linkage disequilibrium with a causative mutation, seven SNPs were genotyped in 901 MS trio families, including 69 in which the affected offspring had clinical history of optic-spinal disease. No association was found. However, the results should not be considered definitive because of the small number of NMO patients included, the dependence of the conclusion on the assumption of linkage disequilibrium between a causative mutation and the SNPs tested, and the fact that the diagnosis of NMO was not clearly supported by serologic testing for NMO-IgG or other supporting clinical data.[66]

Treatment

No clinical trial has addressed treatment of NMO exacerbations or relapse prevention exclusively. Treatment recommendations have been based either on clinical trials that included patients with a broader spectrum of demyelinating disease or on small, open-label studies or case series. The use of high-dose methylprednisolone and oral prednisone to treat ON was substantiated by a randomized controlled trial that compared this treatment to oral prednisone alone or placebo: patients who received methylprednisolone recovered faster.[67] Therapeutic plasmapheresis is effective in treating CNS demyelinating episodes that do not respond do glucocorticoids. This recommendation is based on a randomized, controlled, crossover and double-blind trial that included patients with NMO ($n = 2$) and patients with acute TM ($n = 4$).

For long-term treatment, immunosuppressive therapy is recommended, rather than MS immunomodulatory therapies. Azathioprine 2.5 mg/kg/day target dose, low-dose oral corticosteroid (beginning at 60 mg/day, and decreasing to lowest possible maintenance dose), mycophenolate mofetil 2 g/day, mitoxantrone (12 mg/m^2 every three months, with maximum cumulative dose limited to 140 mg/m^2 primarily due to cardiotoxicity), and rituximab (1000 mg intravenously twice separated by 2 weeks; repeated every 6-9 months) have been claimed to be effective based on small, nonrandomized clinical series.[12,68-71] Interferon (IFN)-beta, commonly used for treatment of MS, is less effective or may be harmful for patients with NMO. Three of six patients with severe OSMS had a worse outcome after[72] In a retrospective study comparing the treatment results of NMO patients who received IFN-beta (n = 7) with those of patients treated with immunosuppressive drugs (n = 19), the IFN-beta group experienced significantly higher risk of a new relapse (hazard ratio, 27.92; P = .003).[73]

Treatment after a first attack of either LETM or ON for prophylaxis against further attacks of myelitis or ON should be considered for NMO-IgG–seropositive patients. This recommendation is based on two prognostic studies showing that that seropositive patients had a high risk of recurrence.[43,44]

Conclusion

Recent advances in NMO research have established that NMO is distinct from MS. NMO-IgG serologic testing has revolutionized the clinical diagnosis of NMO and facilitated early recognition of the condition, appreciation of a broader spectrum, and more specific diagnosis by distinguishing MS from NMO in patients with optic-spinal presentations of CNS demyelinating disease. Discovery of the target antigen, AQP4, promises to elucidate the pathogenesis of NMO, although animal models have not yet been established by active or passive immunization. Why patients develop the autoimmunity to AQP4 and why there is a predilection of the disease for the optic nerve and spinal cord are not yet understood and are the subjects of ongoing genetic and immunologic studies.

REFERENCES

1. Albutt TC: On the ophthalmoscopic signs of spinal disease. Lancet 1870;1:76-78.
2. Devic E: Myelite subaigue compliquee de neurite optique. Bull Med 1894:8.
3. Gault F: De la neuromyelite optique aigue [doctoral thesis]. Lyon, Lyon University, 1894.
4. Beck GM: A case of diffuse myelitis associated with optic neuritis. Brain 1927;50:687-703.
5. Stansbury FC: Neuromyelitis optica: Presentation of five cases, with pathologic study, and review of literature. Arch Ophthalmol 1949;42:465-501.
6. Dennis RH, Calkins LL: Optic neuroencephalomyelopathy (Devic's disease): Report of a case. Arch Ophthalmol 1949;42:768-775.
7. Van WG, Bethlem J: [A case of neuromyelitis optica with transverse lesions at the level of the brain stem.] Ned Tijdschr Geneeskd 1961;105:1786-1790.
8. Keefe RJ: Neuromyelitis optica with increased intracranial pressure. AMA Arch Ophthalmol 1957; 57:110-111.
9. Okinaka S, et al: Multiple sclerosis and allied diseases in Japan; Clinical characteristics. Neurology 1958;8:756-763.
10. Kuroiwa Y: Clinical features of demyelinating disease in Japan. Proc Aust Assoc Neurol 1968; 5:341-345.
11. O'Riordan JI, et al: Clinical, CSF, and MRI findings in Devic's neuromyelitis optica. J Neurol Neurosurg Psychiatry 1996;60:382-387.
12. Mandler RN, Ahmed W, Dencoff JE: Devic's neuromyelitis optica: A prospective study of seven patients treated with prednisone and azathioprine. Neurology 1998;51:1219-1220.
13. Wingerchuk DM, et al: The clinical course of neuromyelitis optica (Devic's syndrome). Neurology 1999;53:1107-1114.
14. Lucchinetti CF, et al: A role for humoral mechanisms in the pathogenesis of Devic's neuromyelitis optica. Brain 2002;125(Pt 7):1450-1461.
15. Lennon VA, et al: A serum autoantibody marker of neuromyelitis optica: Distinction from multiple sclerosis. Lancet 2004;364:2106-2112.
16. Lennon VA, et al: IgG marker of optic-spinal multiple sclerosis binds to the aquaporin-4 water channel. J Exp Med 2005;202:473-477.
17. Yuksel D, et al: Devic's neuromyelitis optica in an infant case. J Child Neurol 2007;22:1143-1146.

18. Banwell B, et al: Neuromyelitis optica-IgG in childhood inflammatory demyelinating CNS disorders. Neurology 2008;70:344-352.
19. Staugaitis SM, et al: Devic type multiple sclerosis in an 81 year old woman. J Neurol Neurosurg Psychiatry 1998;64:417-418.
20. Wingerchuk DM, et al: Revised diagnostic criteria for neuromyelitis optica. Neurology 2006; 66:1485-1489.
21. Kira J: [Epidemiology of multiple sclerosis in Japanese: With special reference to opticospinal multiple sclerosis.] Rinsho Shinkeigaku 2006;46:859-862.
22. Gourie-Devi D: Multiple sclerosis in south India. Presented at Asian Multiple Sclerosis Multiple Sclerosis Workshop. Japan, Kyushu University Press, 1982.
23. El Otmani H, et al: [Devic's neuromyelitis optica in Morocco: A study of 9 cases.] Rev Neurol (Paris) 2005;161(12 Pt 1):1191-1196.
24. Modi G, et al: Demyelinating disorder of the central nervous system occurring in black South Africans. J Neurol Neurosurg Psychiatry 2001;70:500-505.
25. Cabre P, et al: MS and neuromyelitis optica in Martinique (French West Indies). Neurology 2001; 56:507-514.
26. Lana-Peixoto MA, Lana-Peixoto MI: Is multiple sclerosis in Brazil and Asia alike? Arq Neuropsiquiatr 1992;50:419-425.
27. Cree BA, et al: Clinical characteristics of African Americans vs Caucasian Americans with multiple sclerosis. Neurology 2004;63:2039-2045.
28. Mirsattari SM, et al: Aboriginals with multiple sclerosis: HLA types and predominance of neuromyelitis optica. Neurology 2001;56:317-323.
29. Wingerchuk DM, et al: A secondary progressive clinical course is uncommon in neuromyelitis optica. Neurology 2007;68:603-605.
30. Pittock SJ, et al: Brain abnormalities in neuromyelitis optica. Arch Neurol 2006;63:390-396.
31. Wingerchuk DM, et al: The spectrum of neuromyelitis optica. Lancet Neurol 2007;6:805-815.
32. Wingerchuk D, Weinshenker B: Neuromyelitis optica. In McDonald I, Noseworthy J (eds): Multiple Sclerosis 2. Blue Books of Practical Neurology Series. Philadelphia, Butterworth Heinemann, 2003.
33. Nakashima I, et al: Clinical and MRI features of Japanese patients with multiple sclerosis positive for NMO-IgG. J Neurol Neurosurg Psychiatry 2006;77:1073-1075.
34. Scott TF, Kassab SL, Pittock SJ: Neuromyelitis optica IgG status in acute partial transverse myelitis. Arch Neurol 2006;63:1398-1400.
35. Tanaka K, et al: Anti-aquaporin 4 antibody in selected Japanese multiple sclerosis patients with long spinal cord lesions. Mult Scler 2007;13:850-855.
36. Takahashi T, et al: Anti-aquaporin-4 antibody is involved in the pathogenesis of NMO: A study on antibody titre. Brain 2007;130;(Pt 5):1235-1243.
37. Matsuoka T, et al: Heterogeneity of aquaporin-4 autoimmunity and spinal cord lesions in multiple sclerosis in Japanese. Brain 2007;130(Pt 5):1206-1223.
38. Paul F, et al: Antibody to aquaporin 4 in the diagnosis of neuromyelitis optica. PLoS Med 2007;4: e133.
39. Saiz A, et al: Revised diagnostic criteria for neuromyelitis optica (NMO): Application in a series of suspected patients. J Neurol 2007;254:1233-1237.
40. Tanaka M, et al: Anti-aquaporin 4 antibody in Japanese multiple sclerosis: The presence of optic spinal multiple sclerosis without long spinal cord lesions and anti-aquaporin 4 antibody. J Neurol Neurosurg Psychiatry 2007;78:990-992.
41. Marignier R, et al: NMO-IgG and Devic's neuromyelitis optica: A French experience. Mult Scler 2008;14:440-445.
42. Scott TF: Nosology of idiopathic transverse myelitis syndromes. Acta Neurol Scand 2007; 115:371-376.
43. Weinshenker BG, et al: Neuromyelitis optica IgG predicts relapse after longitudinally extensive transverse myelitis. Ann Neurol 2006;59:566-569.
44. Matiello M, et al: NMO-IgG predicts the outcome of recurrent optic neuritis. Presented at ECTRIMS 2007: Multiple Sclerosis. Prague, Czech Republic, 2007.
45. Mandler RN, et al: Devic's neuromyelitis optica: A clinicopathological study of 8 patients. Ann Neurol 1993;34:162-168.
46. Ortiz de Zarate JC, et al: Neuromyelitis optica versus subacute necrotic myelitis: II. Anatomical study of two cases. J Neurol Neurosurg Psychiatry 1968;31:641-645.
47. Lefkowitz D, Angelo JN: Neuromyelitis optica with unusual vascular changes. Arch Neurol 1984; 41:1103-1105.

48. Hengstman GJ, et al: Neuromyelitis optica with clinical and histopathological involvement of the brain. Mult Scler 2007;13:679-682.
49. Manley GT, et al: Aquaporin-4 deletion in mice reduces brain edema after acute water intoxication and ischemic stroke. Nat Med 2000;6:159-163.
50. Papadopoulos MC, et al: Aquaporin-4 facilitates reabsorption of excess fluid in vasogenic brain edema. FASEB J 2004;18:1291-1293.
51. Nagelhus EA, et al: Immunogold evidence suggests that coupling of K+ siphoning and water transport in rat retinal Muller cells is mediated by a coenrichment of Kir4.1 and AQP4 in specific membrane domains. Glia 1999;26:47-54.
52. Pittock SJ, et al: Neuromyelitis optica brain lesions localized at sites of high aquaporin 4 expression. Arch Neurol 2006;63:964-968.
53. Wingerchuk DM: Neuromyelitis optica: New findings on pathogenesis. Int Rev Neurobiol 2007; 79:665-688.
54. Roemer SF, et al: Pattern-specific loss of aquaporin-4 immunoreactivity distinguishes neuromyelitis optica from multiple sclerosis. Brain 2007;130;(Pt 5):1194-1205.
55. Sinclair C, et al: Absence of aquaporin-4 expression in lesions of neuromyelitis optica but increased expression in multiple sclerosis lesions and normal-appearing white matter. Acta Neuropathol 2007;113:187-194.
56. Misu T, et al: Loss of aquaporin 4 in lesions of neuromyelitis optica: Distinction from multiple sclerosis. Brain 2007;130;(Pt 5):1224-1234.
57. Hinson SR, et al: Pathogenic potential of IgG binding to water channel extracellular domain in neuromyelitis optica. Neurology 2007;69:2221-2231.
58. McAlpine D: Familial neuromyelitis optica: Its occurrence in identical twins. Brain 1938;61:430-438.
59. Ch'ien LT, et al: Neuromyelitis optica (Devic's syndrome) in two sisters. Clin Electroencephalogr 1982;13:36-39.
60. Yamakawa K, et al: Familial neuromyelitis optica (Devic's syndrome) with late onset in Japan. Neurology 2000;55:318-320.
61. Keegan M, et al: Plasma exchange for severe attacks of CNS demyelination: Predictors of response. Neurology 2002;58:143-146.
62. Braley T, Mikol DD: Neuromyelitis optica in a mother and daughter. Arch Neurol 2007;64:1189-1192.
63. Yamasaki K, et al: HLA-DPB1*0501-associated opticospinal multiple sclerosis: Clinical, neuroimaging and immunogenetic studies. Brain 1999;122(Pt 9):1689-1696.
64. Jacob A, et al: HLA DPB1*0501 allele is not associated in neuromyelitis optica. Presented at ECTRIMS 2007: Multiple Sclerosis. Prague, Czech Republic, 2007.
65. Hudson G, et al: Does mitochondrial DNA predispose to neuromyelitis optica (Devic's disease)? Brain 2007;131(Pt 4):e93.
66. Ban M, et al: Polymorphisms in the neuromyelitis optica auto-antigen AQP4 and susceptibility to multiple sclerosis. J Neurol 2007;254:398-399.
67. Beck RW, et al: A randomized, controlled trial of corticosteroids in the treatment of acute optic neuritis. The Optic Neuritis Study Group. N Engl J Med 1992;326:581-588.
68. Watanabe S, et al: Low-dose corticosteroids reduce relapses in neuromyelitis optica: A retrospective analysis. Mult Scler 2007;13:968-974.
69. Weinstock-Guttman B, et al: Study of mitoxantrone for the treatment of recurrent neuromyelitis optica (Devic disease). Arch Neurol 2006;63:957-963.
70. Falcini F, et al: Sustained improvement of a girl affected with Devic's disease over 2 years of mycophenolate mofetil treatment. Rheumatology (Oxf) 2006;45:913-915.
71. Cree BA, et al: An open label study of the effects of rituximab in neuromyelitis optica. Neurology 2005;64:1270-1272.
72. Warabi Y, Matsumoto Y, Hayashi H: Interferon beta-1b exacerbates multiple sclerosis with severe optic nerve and spinal cord demyelination. J Neurol Sci 2007;252:57-61.
73. Papeix C, et al: Immunosuppressive therapy is more effective than interferon in neuromyelitis optica. Mult Scler 2007;13:256-259.

14 Attack Therapies in Multiple Sclerosis

RALF GOLD • RALF A. LINKER • ALEXANDRA SCHRÖDER

New symptoms that persist for more than 24 hours are considered to be relapses of multiple sclerosis (MS) if other causes are excluded. In particular, in MS patients with significant disability (mostly with Expanded Disability Status Scale [EDSS] scores > 4), infections may lead to deterioration via cytokine release and fever and must be excluded. These "pseudoexacerbations" first require adequate antibiotic therapy, before further decisions are made. There is broad consensus that relapses with motor, brainstem, or cranial nerve symptoms should be treated, whereas pure sensory symptoms may receive only follow-up and symptomatic therapy if they do not progress.

Traditionally disabling relapses of MS are treated with glucocorticosteroids (GS). In the 1980s, high-dose intravenous pulse therapy was introduced,[1] although the available evidence for its efficacy is limited. Data from the optic neuritis trial support at least a short-term effect on remission of symptoms.[10] In clinical practice, only a proportion of patients respond well to GS, with repeated administration at higher dosages (2000 mg/day) as recommended by guidelines.[2] This is not surprising in view of the heterogeneity of disease mechanisms in MS. A large series of diagnostic brain biopsies from acute inflammatory lesions has increased knowledge of molecular effector pathways: Lassmann, Lucchinetti, and Brück defined the most prevailing T cell/macrophage inflammation pattern (pattern I), in contrast to local deposition of antibodies and complement (pattern II), which speaks for B-cell mechanisms.[3] Clearly, the value of GS in pattern II is limited. At best, these drugs may downregulate associated cellular cytotoxicity and lead to death of activated B cells,[4] yet in the short term they will not modulate tissue destruction or conduction blockade by local antibody deposition. The following sections briefly summarize the available evidence for GS and plasma exchange (PE) as attack therapies in MS.

Glucocorticosteroid Therapy for Acute Multiple Sclerosis Relapses

The GS are the most potent immunosuppressive and anti-inflammatory drugs available, even in modern molecular medicine. In 1938, natural steroid hormones were first extracted and purified from the suprarenal (adrenal) gland. Soon after the discovery of natural GS, synthesis of steroid hormones was achieved in 1947, opening immediate access to steroid therapy for human autoimmune disorders.[5] In the 1950s, further progress was made in the development of new and more potent GS derivatives. Nevertheless, treatment with corticotropin (ACTH) of hypophyseal origin, which was based on the "indirect" release of endogenous GS and mineralocorticosteroid hormones, was still widely used until 1970. It is estimated that ACTH may equal the release of a maximum of 80 mg endogenous GS. ACTH has now been abandoned for virtually all neuroimmunologic diseases.

Over the 6 decades that have passed since their discovery, a variety of *genomic* effector mechanisms of steroid hormones that are mediated by the cytosolic steroid receptor have been described. Also, the relative potency of GS effects has been ascertained for the various derivatives. Recent evidence supports a direct effect of GS on cellular membranes that occurs at higher hormone concentrations; this is termed a *nongenomic* effect. These mechanisms can easily be delineated in vitro.[6] In vivo, nongenomic steroid effects may interfere with bioenergetic processes, including signaling pathways. Both mechanisms may act in concert and lead to a qualitatively distinct mode of steroid action resulting in cellular apoptosis. In the animal model for MS, experimental autoimmune encephalossmyelitis (EAE), a clear dose-response curve has been shown for induction of T-cell apoptosis and, consequently, termination of inflammation. Interestingly, methylprednisolone doses up to 50 mg/kg were most efficient.[7] T-cell apoptosis was also shown to be augmented in peripheral blood lymphocytes from MS patients treated with GS for acute deterioration.[8]

The efficacy of high-dose treatment with intravenous GS was first examined by Dowling and colleagues in 1980,[9] followed by a number of uncontrolled studies. All of these described a rapid clinical improvement but lacked appropriate controls. The first study of class I evidence was published by Milligan and associates.[1] In this randomized, placebo-controlled trial, 50 patients received either 500 mg IV methylprednisolone for 5 days or placebo. Patients with acute relapses and with deterioration of progressive MS were included. In relapsing MS, IV GS was associated with significantly faster remission. Patients with chronic progressive disease had benefit in motor function only during the first 4 weeks.

Beck and colleagues[10] conducted a study of class I evidence in optic neuritis. The patients received either 1000 mg methylprednisolone for 3 days, followed by oral tapering at 1 mg/kg body weight for 11 days, or 1 mg/kg oral prednisone for 14 days, or a placebo. High-dose IV GS pulses were associated with more rapid improvement of vision. Statistical significance for this parameter disappeared after 6 months, although positive effects on visual field, contrast, and color vision were still maintained in the high-dose GS group. This modern study design may be viewed as the first clinically isolated syndrome (CIS) study in MS. The three groups were later followed up for relapses in the further disease course, to fulfill classic diagnostic criteria for MS.[11] It came as a surprise that GS pulses diminished subsequent relapses: 14.7% of oral GS recipients, but only 7.5% of high-dose GS patients, fulfilled criteria for MS within 2 years. It was speculation that low-dose oral GS may impair suppressor mechanisms, but a good explanation is still not available. Because no other long-term immunotherapy was established at the time of this study, further follow-ups by the Beck group rather reflect the natural variability of MS and will not be discussed here.

It was always a question whether intravenous administration is necessary or whether oral GS at a comparable dosage could be substituted. Sellebjerg and coworkers[12] conducted a randomized study wherein 25 patients with an attack of MS lasting less than 4 weeks received placebo treatment, and 26 patients received oral methylprednisolone (500 mg once a day for 5 days plus a 10-day tapering period). The patients were scored according to the Scripps Neurological Rating Scale (NRS) and the Kurtzke Expanded Disability Status Scale. After 1, 3, and 8 weeks, 4%, 24%, and 32% in the placebo group and 31%, 54%, and 65% in the methylprednisolone group, respectively, had improved 1 point on the EDSS (all $P < .05$). The efficacy of oral high-dose GS was further supported in a group of 60 patients with optic neuritis,[13] yet significant effects of GS disappeared after 3 weeks. Of note, an oral dosage of 500 mg GS is in most countries equivalent to 10 tablets of 50 mg each, which the patients have to take at breakfast.

These clinical data were further supported by magnetic resonance imaging (MRI) tomography, by which suppression of gadolinium-enhancement could be observed after GS therapy. Oliveri and colleagues[14] addressed the dose-response relationship by means of MRI. Their double-blind, randomized study compared 2000 mg versus 500 mg GS per day, followed by MRI tomography at 7, 15, 30, and 60 days and serial clinical examinations. The higher dose of intravenous methylprednisolone was significantly more effective than the lower dose in reducing the number of MRI contrast-enhanced lesions at 30 and 60 days, mainly by decreasing the rate of new lesion formation. MRI may also provide additional advice as to whether oral tapering should be performed. Miller and coworkers[15] observed rapid re-enhancement of lesions despite maintained clinical efficacy without tapering of GS.

OPEN QUESTIONS IN GLUCOCORTICOSTEROID THERAPY

In view of expired patents, the interest in systematic modern studies with GS is limited. Most neurologists use methylprednisolone for pulse therapy, but no data exist as to whether this is superior to prednisone or dexamethasone (at equivalent genomic dosage). Also, there is no general consensus as to which kind of steroid derivative should be given, whether for 3 days or 5, and with or without oral tapering. In view of the lack of evidence, it may help that, in virtually all modern MS studies, 1000 mg methylprednisolone given intravenously for 3 days is recommended. We also consider the patient's history of GS treatment response in determining whether to use oral tapering. With regard to dose-response, experimental data only suggest use of higher GS dosages in severe inflammation. At least short-term tolerability is good, as has been demonstrated in spinal cord injury with 30 mg/kg body weight of GS.[16] The tolerability of short-term, high-dose GS is very good in a routine clinical or outpatient setting; some patients may complain about sleeplessness, increased sweating, or accelerated pulse. β-Blockers or short-acting hypnotic drugs typically lead to immediate relief. In older patients, blood glucose levels should be monitored carefully. Only some transient and mild declines in memory function have been observed.[17] Finally, targeting of GS to the site of inflammation may be greatly facilitated by the use of liposomal encapsulation.[18]

Plasma Exchange Therapy for Acute Deterioration in Relapsing and Secondary Progressive Multiple Sclerosis

The term *plasmapheresis* was coined in 1914 to describe removal of potentially pathogenic plasma factors from the blood of patients. Nowadays, it can be performed more selectively, either by PE or by immunoadsorption, wherein pathogenic antibodies bind to a specific matrix. PE is a nonselective immune therapy; for example, 150 g of plasma proteins must be removed to eliminate about 1 g of pathogenic autoantibodies. The effects of PE mainly comprise the elimination of humoral factors such as immunoglobulins, complement, or cytokines. The subsequent modulation of cellular immune responses seems likely but is less well characterized.

PE entered into neurology in the 1980s, after its efficacy for treatment of myasthenic crisis[19] and Guillain-Barré syndrome[20] was shown. Before then, passive transfer studies from human to mouse had proven the pathogenic nature of these autoantibodies.[21] PE typically requires central venous access, which can lead to severe complication such as thrombosis, septic infections, or pneumothorax. Nowadays, PE is easily accessible, and medication costs are mainly restricted to protein replacement with albumin or fresh-frozen plasma (used mostly in the 1980s).

HISTORY AND MODERN APPROACH OF PLASMA EXCHANGE IN MULTIPLE SCLEROSIS

Already in the 1980s, plasmapheresis was used for treatment of severe MS.[22] However, this three-armed trial focused on progressive forms of MS, and only cyclophosphamide and ACTH had some efficacy in slowing disease progression.

The approach experienced a revival when modern molecular histopathology led to a new classification of MS lesions. The international cooperating group of investigators around Lassmann, Lucchinetti, and Brück coined a four-pattern classification of the inflammatory MS lesion.[3] The most prevalent pattern, type II, reflected deposition of antibodies and complement, thus opening the minds of investigators for therapeutic approaches aimed at humoral factors. In clinical practice, persistence of severe symptoms after steroid pulse therapy (e.g., visual acuity < 0.3, disabling paresis, ataxia) should alert the physician to discuss PE with the patient.

A randomized, sham-controlled, double-masked PE study by Brian Weinshenker and colleagues[23] focused on patients with acute, severe neurologic deficits caused by MS or other inflammatory demyelinating diseases of the central nervous system who had had a failed response to high-dose GS. PE without concomitant immunosuppressive treatment was performed in 22 patients who had recently acquired severe neurologic deficits resulting from attacks of inflammatory demyelinating disease. Patients who did not achieve moderate or greater improvement after the first treatment phase crossed over to the opposite treatment. Moderate or greater improvement in neurologic disability occurred during 8 (42.1%) of 19 courses of active treatment, compared with 1 (5.9%) of 17 courses of sham treatment. Improvement occurred early in the course of treatment and was sustained on follow-up. However, four of the patients who responded to the active treatment experienced new attacks of demyelinating disease during 6 months of follow-up.

In this first trial, the patients who were included had a mean of 6 weeks since onset of symptoms, but the inclusion criteria allowed an interval of up to 3 months. A subsequent analysis of 59 patients by the same group of investigators[24] showed that the most powerful predictor of response to PE was early initiation of treatment—less than 6 weeks after onset of symptoms. Male gender and preserved tendon reflexes were further predictors, with the latter perhaps indicating that the damage to the nervous system was limited.

In the controlled study by Weinshenker's group, patients with optic neuritis, a frequent symptom of early MS, were under-represented. This issue was addressed in a prospective case series of 10 consecutive patients treated with PE for acute, severe optic neuritis largely unresponsive to previous high-dose IV GS.[25] PE was associated with improvement of visual acuity in 7 of 10 patients. On follow-up, three of these patients continued to improve, two remained stable, and two had worsened visual acuity, underscoring the need for adequate long-term therapy in these patients. The series included six patients with a first clinical attack, now designated as CIS. Of note, treatment success was best when residual visual acuity was greater than 0.05. One may speculate that, with fulminant affliction of the optic nerve, swelling in the optic channel may lead to irreversible secondary ischemia.

The ultimate proof for the underlying pathogenetic concept was given when a retrospective study correlated response to PE with results of diagnostic brain biopsy. Here, a hitherto undescribed "black and white" picture of treatment success was reported[26]: Of 19 patients, only those 10 with a pattern II lesion type exhibited moderate or substantial neurologic improvement, whereas patients with other lesion types did not respond to PE. The tight correlation between PE response and histopathology underscores the concept that efficacy of PE may result from the elimination of humoral factors, leading only to conduction block at first but to irreversible tissue damage after longer periods; in other cases, the serum may contain anti-myelin antibodies that lead to demyelination.[27] Amelioration typically occurred after a mean of three PE sessions. The need for sufficient long-term therapy was underscored in the follow-up period of this study. Later, an uncontrolled series of 16 patients with severe optic neuritis and also motor impairment or severe ataxia was reported. Emphasis was put on a maximum time interval of 6 weeks between onset of symptoms and start of PE; a significant effect of PE was again observed in about 70% of patients.[28]

During early phases of secondary progressive MS, relapses may still occur. Although these patients start from a much higher EDSS level, the relapses may result in loss of the ability to walk at least short distances at home. For these reasons, the decision for PE may be made on an individual basis in these patients. Successful PE, as described by Zettl[29] and Linker[30] and their associates, leads to clearly improved quality of life. This is the only scenario in which PE should be considered in progressive MS.

A prototype of MS in which humoral disease mechanisms prevail is neuromyelitis optica (Devic's disease). This notion was supported by the recent identification of antibodies to aquaporin-4, which are expressed on astrocytic processes,[31] although the pathologic mechanism is incompletely understood. PE was also effective in neuromyelitis optica.[32]

OPEN QUESTIONS IN PLASMA EXCHANGE THERAPY

The high percentage of pattern II lesions in acute MS contrasts with the rare cases of steroid nonresponders for whom PE is needed. A possible explanation may be that aggressive T cells exist in pattern II lesions and are eliminated by steroids, leading to improvement. Furthermore T cells and B cells are in immunologic interaction, and this may also influence responsiveness to steroids.

It is important to be aware that, in any case of PE-treated MS, a modification of the preceding immunotherapy should be sought, or, in the case of CIS, initiation of immunotherapy is recommended. Of course, no standard follow-up is available. In view of the humoral mechanisms that obviously dominate in these patients, one may consider anti–B cell therapies such as anti-CD20,[33] which is typically an off-label use. Mitoxantrone also has anti-B cell activity[34] and may be easier to prescribe, despite substantial toxicity. In our experience, we prefer high-dose interferon(IFN)-beta as follow-up after PE. Only one patient that suffered a relapse under this regimen, a 27-year-old woman who had made a full recovery after four PE cycles, which she received because of severe optic neuritis of the left eye. Subsequent to the PE treatment, we started an immunomodulatory therapy with interferon-beta-1b. Three weeks later, the patient again suffered from recurrent, severe loss of visual acuity (<0.1) in the left eye associated with retrobulbar pain. The visual evoked response showed no response in the left eye. She then received another four cycles of PE, and visual acuity normalized to 1.0 after three treatment sessions. Thereafter, three mitoxantrone infusions were given before IFN-beta was started again. She has now been stable for 18 months. Some physicians consider potent immunosuppressants such as mitoxantrone or cyclophosphamide immediately after a severe attack; we typically recommend PE first and then modify long-term treatment.

In view of the substantial overlap in efficacy of PE and intravenous immunoglobulins (IVIG) in neurologic diseases,[35] one may also consider treatment with IVIG instead of PE. IVIG has been used for several aspects of MS, with limited success. So far only a small study addressed the benefit from IVIG in steroid-refractory optic neuritis.[36] Elaborate formal studies are urgently needed.

Conclusion

The gold standard treatment for relapses of MS is still high-dose GS therapy. Despite the lack of sufficient evidence-based trials, intravenous administration of 500 to 1000 mg GS over 3 to 5 days is widely recommended. Based on experimental data and limited clinical evidence, higher doses (20 to 30 mg/kg body weight) may lead to faster remission by apoptotic clearance of the inflammatory lesion.

However, some patients with severe MS relapses do not respond sufficiently to corticosteroids. In such cases, knowledge of the value of PE in steroid-resistant MS relapses has greatly expanded. The molecular basis of therapeutic efficacy has been defined by local deposition of antibodies and complement, which is accessible to PE through the damaged blood–brain barrier. From a double-blind, randomized study and a number of prospective open trials, a beneficial effect has been described in up to 70% of the patients. The median time point of improvement is after the third plasmapheresis session, and early initiation of PE therapy (within 1 month after the beginning of relapse) is associated with better outcome.

REFERENCES

1. Milligan NM, Newcombe R, Compston DAS: A double-blind trial of high dose methylprednisolone in patients with multiple sclerosis: 1. Clinical effects. J Neurol Neurosurg Psychiatry 1987;50: 511-516.
2. Bassetti C, Beer K, Beer S, et al: Escalating immunotherapy of multiple sclerosis: New aspects and practical application. J Neurol 2004;251:1329-1339.
3. Lassmann H, Brück W, Lucchinetti C: Heterogeneity of multiple sclerosis pathogenesis: Implications for diagnosis and therapy. Trends Mol Med 2001;7:115-121.
4. Gold R, Buttgereit F, Toyka KV: Mechanism of action of glucocorticosteroid hormones: Possible implications for therapy of neuroimmunological disorders. J Neuroimmunol 2001;117:1-8.
5. Hench PS, Kendall EC, Slocumb CH, Polley HF: The effect of a hormone of the adrenal cortex (17-hydroxy-11-dehydrocorticosterone, compound E) and of pituitary adrenocorticotropic hormone on rheumatoid arthritis. Proc Staff Meet Mayo Clin 1949;24:181-197.
6. Song IH, Buttgereit F: Non-genomic glucocorticoid effects to provide the basis for new drug developments. Mol Cell Endocrinol 2006;246:142-146.
7. Schmidt J, Gold R, Schönrock L, et al: T-cell apoptosis in situ in experimental autoimmune encephalomyelitis following methylprednisolone pulse therapy. Brain 2000;123:1431-1441.
8. Leussink VI, Jung S, Merschdorf U, et al: High-dose methylprednisolone therapy in multiple sclerosis induces apoptosis in peripheral blood leukocytes. Arch Neurol 2001;58:91-97.
9. Dowling PC, Bosch VV, Cook SD: Possible beneficial effect of high-dose intravenous steroid therapy in acute demyelinating disease and transverse myelitis. Neurology 1980;30:33-36.
10. Beck RW, Cleary PA, Anderson MMJ, et al: A randomized, controlled trial of corticosteroids in the treatment of acute optic neuritis. The Optic Neuritis Study Group [see comments]. N Engl J Med 1992;326:581-588.
11. Beck RW, Cleary PA, Trobe JD, et al: The effect of corticosteroids for acute optic neuritis on the subsequent development of multiple sclerosis. N Engl J Med 1993;329:1764-1769.
12. Sellebjerg F, Frederiksen JL, Nielsen PM, Olesen J: Double-blind, randomized, placebo-controlled study of oral, high-dose methylprednisolone in attacks of MS. Neurology 1998;51:529-534.
13. Sellebjerg F, Nielsen HS, Frederiksen JJ, Olesen J: A randomized, controlled trial of oral high-dose methylprednisolone in acute optic neuritis. Neurology 1999;52:1479-1484.
14. Oliveri RL, Valentino P, Russo C, et al: Randomized trial comparing two different high doses of methylprednisolone in MS: A clinical and MRI study. Neurology 1998;50:1833-1836.
15. Miller DH, Thompson AJ, Morrissey SP, et al: High dose steroids in acute relapses of multiple sclerosis: MRI evidence for a possible mechanism of therapeutic effect. J Neurol Neurosurg Psychiatry 1992;55:450-453.
16. Bracken MB, Shepard MJ, Collins WF, et al: A randomized, controlled trial of methylprednisolone or naloxone in the treatment of acute spinal-cord injury: Results of the Second National Acute Spinal Cord Injury Study [see comments]. N Engl J Med 1990;322:1405-1411.
17. Uttner I, Muller S, Zinser C, et al: Reversible impaired memory induced by pulsed methylprednisolone in patients with MS. Neurology 2005;64:1971-1973.
18. Schmidt J, Metselaar JM, Wauben MH, et al: Drug targeting by long-circulating liposomal glucocorticosteroids increases therapeutic efficacy in a model of multiple sclerosis. Brain 2003;126: 1895-1904.
19. Newsom-Davis J, Pinching AJ, Vincent A, Wilson SG: Function of circulating antibody to acetylcholine receptor in myasthenia gravis: Investigation by plasma exchange. Neurology 1978;28:266-272.
20. Plasmapheresis and acute Guillain-Barré syndrome: The Guillain-Barré syndrome Study Group. Neurology 1985;35:1096-1104.
21. Toyka KV, Drachman DB, Pestronk A, Kao I: Myasthenia gravis: Passive transfer from man to mouse. Science 1975;190:397-399.
22. Hauser SL, Dawson DM, Lehrich JR, et al: Intensive immunosuppression in progressive multiple sclerosis: A randomized, three-arm study of high-dose intravenous cyclophosphamide, plasma exchange, and ACTH. N Engl J Med 1983;308:173-180.

23. Weinshenker BG, O'Brien PC, Petterson TM, et al: A randomized trial of plasma exchange in acute central nervous system inflammatory demyelinating disease. Ann Neurol 1999;46:878-886.
24. Keegan M, Pineda AA, McClelland RL, et al: Plasma exchange for severe attacks of CNS demyelination: Predictors of response. Neurology 2002;58:143-146.
25. Ruprecht K, Klinker E, Dintelmann T, et al: Plasma exchange for severe optic neuritis: Treatment of 10 patients. Neurology 2004;63:1081-1083.
26. Keegan M, Konig F, McClelland R, et al: Relation between humoral pathological changes in multiple sclerosis and response to therapeutic plasma exchange. Lancet 2005;366:579-582.
27. Zhou D, Srivastava R, Nessler S, et al: Identification of a pathogenic antibody response to native myelin oligodendrocyte glycoprotein in multiple sclerosis. Proc Natl Acad Sci U S A 2006;103:19057-19062.
28. Schilling S, Linker R, Konig F, et al: Plasma exchange therapy for steroid-unresponsive multiple sclerosis relapses: Clinical experience with 16 patients. Nervenarzt 2006;77:430.
29. Zettl UK, Hartung HP, Pahnke A, et al: Lesion pathology predicts response to plasma exchange in secondary progressive MS. Neurology 2006;67:1515-1516.
30. Linker RA, Chan A, Sommer M, et al: Plasma exchange therapy for steroid-refractory superimposed relapses in secondary progressive multiple sclerosis. J Neurol 2007;254:1288-1289.
31. Lennon VA, Wingerchuk DM, Kryzer TJ, et al: A serum autoantibody marker of neuromyelitis optica: Distinction from multiple sclerosis. Lancet 2004;364:2106-2112.
32. Watanabe S, Nakashima I, Misu T, et al: Therapeutic efficacy of plasma exchange in NMO-IgG-positive patients with neuromyelitis optica. Mult Scler 2007;13:128-132.
33. Stuve O, Cepok S, Elias B, et al: Clinical stabilization and effective B-lymphocyte depletion in the cerebrospinal fluid and peripheral blood of a patient with fulminant relapsing-remitting multiple sclerosis. Arch Neurol 2005;62:1620-1623.
34. Chan A, Weilbach FX, Toyka KV, Gold R: Mitoxantrone induces cell death in peripheral blood leucocytes of multiple sclerosis patients. Clin Exp Immunol 2005;139:152-158.
35. Gold R, Stangel M, Dalakas MC: Drug Insight: The use of intravenous immunoglobulin in neurology—Therapeutic considerations and practical issues. Nat Clin Pract Neurol 2007;3:36-44.
36. Tselis A, Perumal J, Caon C, et al: Treatment of corticosteroid refractory optic neuritis in multiple sclerosis patients with intravenous immunoglobulin. Eur J Neurol 2008;15:1163-1167.

15 Current Disease-Modifying Therapeutic Strategies in Multiple Sclerosis

ANU JACOB • DEAN M. WINGERCHUK

Six disease-modifying treatments (DMTs) are currently approved for multiple sclerosis (MS) in the United States, and many more are in various stages of development. This chapter aims to summarize and integrate the evidence supporting the use of these agents, as well as other available but unapproved treatments, by outlining contemporary treatment strategies. This review focuses on early-course treatment decisions for established MS; the clinically isolated syndromes (CIS), management of aggressive MS, and future approaches are detailed elsewhere in this text.

General Therapeutic Strategies for Multiple Sclerosis

MS is a potentially disabling, lifelong disease with a wide spectrum of clinical manifestations and tremendous interindividual variability of disease course.[1] Despite advances in neuroimaging and other technologies that facilitate earlier and more accurate MS diagnosis, the clinical course remains relatively unpredictable from the standpoint of the individual patient, especially in its early relapsing-remitting (RR) stage. Even when the disease converts to a secondary progressive (SP) phenotype—the milestone that is most strongly predictive of future neurologic impairment—the rate of progression varies widely among patients. Clinical trial methodology has steadily improved over the past 3 decades, resulting in confirmation of short-term efficacy for several therapies including interferon-beta (IFNB), glatiramer acetate (GA), mitoxantrone, and natalizumab. However, the limitations of these therapies, and of controlled trials themselves, have added new dimensions of uncertainty. For example, all current therapies have been shown to reduce the relapse rate, but by varying degrees. Some reduce accrual of neurologic disability as measured by the Expanded Disability Status Scale (EDSS). None has been convincingly demonstrated to delay or prevent the occurrence of SP disease in the long term. Furthermore, the duration of benefit is unknown, with controlled trials lasting 2 to 4 years and all subsequent data subject to the biases of uncontrolled observational studies. This constellation of uncertainties is unsettling for individuals affected with MS, who are typically otherwise healthy young adults entering the most productive occupational and personal portions of their lives, and also for their physicians, who may have difficulty making sense of the data. Knowledge of the current evidence base can assist the clinician in both counseling these patients and in choosing therapies that are backed by experimental evidence or, at least, grounded in solid hypotheses about disease mechanisms.

Because the early, more "inflammatory" phase of RRMS is probably also the most treatable with current DMTs, initiation of early therapy for prevention of future disability is a popular current mantra.[2] Nevertheless, it should be recognized that many patients are diagnosed with evidence that they have had MS for several years. The decision to initiate DMT in a treatment-naïve patient with established MS therefore requires integration of several factors. These include the suspected or confirmed duration of disease (based on historical or imaging evidence), disease course (RR versus progressive), characteristics of clinical relapses (symptom type, frequency, severity, and sequelae), perceived rate of progression, presence of medical comorbidities, regional/national differences in prescribing practices, and patient desires and preferences. Although there is much interest in stratification for risk of future disability or response to specific therapies, our current ability to predict such outcomes with useful precision is extremely limited and requires new developments in the fields of biomarkers and pharmacogenomics. Until those technologies are available, clinical and patient preference factors will continue to direct therapeutic decisions.

The standard current treatment paradigm employs DMT monotherapy for patients with established RRMS or SPMS. Increasingly, MS investigators are seeking to determine whether alternative early treatment strategies, such as combination therapy or more aggressive induction therapy followed by maintenance treatments, can provide better clinical outcomes with acceptable risk (Table 15-1). For those patients who are taking and tolerating a DMT, the on-treatment clinical course usually dictates the next series of questions, including "Should I change therapy?" and "To which therapy should I switch?" Uncommonly, in the case of a patient with a lengthy remission, the question arises, "Can I safely stop therapy?" The remaining sections of this chapter deal with these issues, beginning with a review of available agents, followed by strategies for management of relapsing and progressive forms of MS.

TABLE 15–1 General Therapeutic Strategies for Multiple Sclerosis

Disease Course

Relapsing
- Typical
- "Benign"
- Aggressive

Secondary progressive
- With relapses
- Without relapses

Primary progressive

Therapeutic Approach

Monotherapy
- Sequential monotherapy using an "escalation" approach

Combination therapy
- At initiation
- After treatment failure

Induction therapy followed by maintenance therapy

TABLE 15–2 Currently Available Disease-Modifying Therapies

Drug (Trade Name, Manufacturer)	Dose	Indications
IFN-beta-1a (Avonex, Biogen IDEC)	30 μg IM weekly	USA and EU: RRMS and CIS
IFN-beta-1a (Rebif, Serono)	22 or 44 μg SC three times weekly	USA and EU: RRMS
IFN-beta-1b (Betaseron/ Betaferon, Bayer)	250 μg SC, alternate days	USA and EU: RRMS and SPMS with relapses
Glatiramer acetate (Copaxone, Teva)	20 mg SC daily	USA and EU: RRMS
Mitoxantrone (Novantrone, Serono)	12 mg/m^2 BSA IV every 3 mo (maximum, 140 mg/m^2)	USA: Worsening RRMS and SPMS EU: Active RRMS and SPMS
Natalizumab (Tysabri, Biogen IDEC/Elan)	300 mg IV monthly	USA and EU: relapsing forms of MS

BSA, body surface area; CIS, clinically isolated syndrome; EU, European Union; IFN, interferon: IV, intravenously; RRMS, relapsing-remitting multiple sclerosis; SPMS, secondary progressive multiple sclerosis; USA, United States.

Overview of Currently Approved Therapies

This section summarizes each of the therapies approved for relapsing forms of MS. Table 15-2 summarizes features of the available DMTs, and Tables 15-3 and 15-4 describe the pivotal trial data and clinically relevant interpretation of relapses and disability using the number needed-to-treat (NNT).

TABLE 15–3 **Summary of Efficacy Data for Approved Therapies for Relapsing-Remitting Multiple Sclerosis**

Outcome	Trial	NNT* vs Placebo
Placebo-Controlled Trials		
Prevent one relapse per year	Pivotal Betaseron	2.3 (8 MIU)
	PRISMS (Rebif)	2.7 (22 μg), 2.4 (44 μg)
Prevent one relapse over 2 yr	Pivotal Copaxone	2.7
Preserve one patient relapse-free for 1 yr	PRISMS (Rebif)	6.7 (22 μg), 4.3 (44 μg)
	Natalizumab monotherapy	4.8
Preserve one patient relapse-free for 2 yr	Pivotal Betaseron	5.6 (8 MIU)
	PRISMS (Rebif)	9.1 (22 μg), 6.3 (44 μg)
	Natalizumab monotherapy	3.8
Prevent one moderate/severe attack per year	Pivotal Betaseron	4.5
Prevent one moderate/severe attack over 2 yr	PRISMS (Rebif)	3.6 (22 μg), 2.7 (44 μg)
Prevent 1 EDSS point progression for 2 yr	Pivotal Avonex	7.7
	PRISMS (Rebif)	12 (22 μg), 9 (44 μg)
	Natalizumab monotherapy	8.5
Comparison Trials		
Preserve one patient relapse-free for 2 yr on Betaseron	INCOMIN (Betaseron vs Avonex)	7
Preserve one patient relapse-free for 24 wk on Rebif	EVIDENCE (Rebif vs Avonex)	9
Preserve one patient relapse-free for 48 wk on Rebif	EVIDENCE (Rebif vs Avonex)	10

EDSS, Expanded Disability Status Scale; EVIDENCE, Evidence of Interferon Dose-Response: European North American Comparative Efficacy; INCOMIN, Independent Comparison of Interferon; MIU, million international units; PRISMS, Prevention of Relapses and Disability by Interferon-beta-1a Subcutaneously in Multiple Sclerosis.

*The number needed to treat (NNT) is the most clinically useful measure of therapeutic efficacy. It is calculated by taking the reciprocal of the absolute risk reduction (expressed as a decimal). For example, if a treatment reduces the absolute risk of an event by 5% compared with placebo, NNT = 1/0.05 = 20. This value is best interpreted as "one needs to treat 20 patients with the intervention to prevent one undesirable outcome over and above the effects of placebo or the comparator agent."

Reprinted with permission from Wingerchuk DM: Current evidence and therapeutic strategies for multiple sclerosis. [Erratum in: Semin Neurol 2008;28:389.] Semin Neurol 2008;28:56-68.

INTERFERON-BETA PREPARATIONS

Three IFNB preparations are approved for relapsing MS: IFNbeta-1a (Avonex, which is administered intramuscularly weekly, and Rebif, which is administered subcutaneously three times a week) and IFN-beta-1b (Betaseron, administered subcutaneously on alternate days). The beneficial mechanisms of IFNB for MS are not clear but may include cytokine modulation, inhibition of T-cell costimulation or activation, and inhibition of antigen presentation, among others. Pivotal trials demonstrated that each of the IFNB drugs reduced the relapse rate by

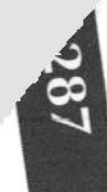

TABLE 15–4 Number Needed to Treat (NNT) for Secondary Progressive Multiple Sclerosis (SPMS)

Study	NNT
European IFN-beta-1b SPMS study[21]	
To prevent EDSS progression	9.2 over 3 yr
IMPACT study[22]	
To prevent progression on MSFC	Unable to determine from publication
To prevent progression on EDSS	Not applicable*
North American Study Group trial[23]	Not applicable*
SPECTRIMS study[24]	Not applicable*
MIMS study[27]	
To prevent worsening of 1.0 EDSS point from baseline EDSS	6.0 over 2 yr
To maintain one patient free of relapses	4.8 over 2 yr

EDSS, Expanded Disability Status Scale; IFN, interferon; IMPACT, International Multiple Sclerosis Secondary Progressive Avonex Controlled Trial; MIMS, Mitoxantrone in Multiple Sclerosis; MSFC, Multiple Sclerosis Functional Composite measure; SPECTRIMS, Secondary Progressive Efficacy Clinical Trial of Recombinant Interferon-beta-1a in Multiple Sclerosis.

*Primary outcome was negative.

approximately one third over a 2- to 4-year period.[3-9] Available evidence supports a modest benefit against accumulation of neurologic impairment. Studies comparing one IFNB to another suggest that more frequent administration (three times weekly versus once weekly) may be associated with more favorable clinical and MRI outcomes. There is some evidence for a dose-response effect among the IFNB preparations, specifically from the Independent Comparison of Interferon (INCOMIN) and Evidence of Interferon Dose-Response: European North American Comparative Efficacy (EVIDENCE) studies, but these trials were of very short duration and relied almost completely on MRI results and unblinded clinical measures.[10,11] Newer data, discussed in more detail later, suggest that differences between the drugs are modest and may be related to dose frequency rather than total drug dose per unit time. Extension studies were interpreted as showing that early treatment with IFNB was associated with better outcome than delayed treatment up to 4 years later.[7]

Adverse effects include injection site reactions, flu-like symptoms, hematologic and hepatic function abnormalities, depression, menstrual disorders, and neutralizing antibody (N Ab) formation.

GLATIRAMER ACETATE

Glatiramer acetate(GA) is a random polymer of four amino acids that are found in myelin basic protein. Its mechanism of action is unclear but may primarily involve regulatory Th2 cells. The standard dose of GA (20 mg/day SC) reduces the relapse rate by approximately one third.[12] Individual controlled trials and a subsequent meta-analysis[13] did not demonstrate an effect on disability progression as measured by EDSS, although another meta-analysis using individual patient data (n = 540) showed a 28% reduction in annualized relapse rate and lower risk of disability accumulation (risk ratio, 0.6; 95% confidence interval, 0.4 to 0.9).[14] A dose comparison study of 20 mg versus 40 mg daily showed trends favoring the higher dose.[15] GA has less impact than the IFNB drugs on MRI measures of inflammatory MS activity such as gadolinium-enhancing lesions and accumulation of T2 lesions. Observational extension studies conducted after the close of the pivotal GA trial confirmed an excellent safety profile, but the purported long-term benefits on relapse rates and neurologic status could not be validated owing to the lack of an intact control group.[16-18]

NATALIZUMAB

Natalizumab (Tysabri, administered IV every 4 weeks) is a humanized monoclonal antibody that binds to the $\alpha_4\beta_1$ and $\alpha_4\beta_7$ integrins on the surface of all leukocytes except neutrophils.[19] This interaction prevents binding of leukocytes to the vascular endothelium, which is considered a key step in the process of cellular migration across the blood–brain barrier and subsequent initiation of inflammatory MS lesions. In the 2-year, maximum 128-week, placebo-controlled AFFIRM trial (the Natalizumab Safety and Efficacy in Relapsing Remitting Multiple Sclerosis study) of 942 patients with relapsing MS, natalizumab reduced the relapse rate by 68% and progression of sustained disability by 42%.[20] MRI data were congruent, showing strong effects on enhancing lesion number and new lesion development as well as reduced brain atrophy during the second year of the study.[21] The Safety and Efficacy of Natalizumab in Combination with Interferon Beta-1a in Patients with Relapsing Remitting Multiple Sclerosis (SENTINEL) study showed that the combination of natalizumab with IFNB-1a (Avonex) was more effective than Avonex alone for relapse reduction (53% at 120 weeks of total study duration).[22]

Natalizumab was approved by the U.S. Food and Drug Administration in November 2004, but it was withdrawn by its manufacturers 3 months later after the development of progressive multifocal leukoencephalopathy (PML) in two patients with MS (both of whom were also taking Avonex) and another with Crohn's disease; only one MS patient survived.[23-26] A comprehensive review that included 91% of 3417 patients exposed to natalizumab in trials estimated the risk of PML to be 1:1000 in patients exposed for an average of 17.9 monthly doses.[27] Natalizumab became available again in 2006 but only under a restricted prescribing and distribution program called TOUCH (Tysabri Outreach: Unified Commitment to Health), which provides safety surveillance for all treated patients. Guidelines for patient selection and monitoring have been published, including the recommendation of a washout period for other immunomodulatory and immunosuppressive therapies.[28] Natalizumab is otherwise well tolerated. Hypersensitivity reactions occur in 1% to 4% of patients within the first 2 hours of the infusion, in which case it should be stopped and the reaction treated symptomatically with fluids, corticosteroids, antihistamines, or acetaminophen if necessary. About 6% of patients develop antibodies against the drug, increasing the risk of infusion reaction and reducing the drug's efficacy; this result requires discontinuation of therapy. Natalizumab may increase the risk for infection, and it is recommended for monotherapy only. Hepatic enzyme monitoring is now recommended because of elevations noted as early as 6 days after therapy initiation.

MITOXANTRONE

Mitoxantrone, an anthracenedione that exerts its immunosuppressive effect through antimitotic effects on T and B cells, is approved in the United States for its effects on reducing disease activity and slowing progression of worsening in relapsing, SP, or progressive relapsing MS.[29] It is reserved for patients with more active or treatment-refractory RRMS or SPMS.[30] Its advantages include rapid onset of action and infrequent administration schedule. It is administered intravenously at a dose of 12 mg/m^2 once per quarter for a total of eight doses.

Adverse effects include temporary discoloration of urine and sclerae, mild alopecia, amenorrhea, and teratogenicity. Mitoxantrone is associated with cumulative dose-dependent cardiotoxicity at a rate as high as 6% in patients receiving up to 140 mg/m^2, but cardiotoxicity may occur with smaller cumulative doses, and therapy is usually stopped at 96 mg/m^2.[31-33] Evaluation of cardiac ejection fraction is required before each dose, and the drug should be discontinued if the ejection fraction falls below 50% or by more than 10% on serial studies. Additional risks include bone marrow suppression (usually maximal at about 2 weeks after infusion, recovering by about day 24), amenorrhea, oligospermia, and an association with malignancy. Acute leukemia is of primary concern; its incidence after mitoxantrone therapy was 0.21% in one study but may be greater.[34]

Treatment Strategies: Relapsing-Remitting Disease

TREATMENT-NAÏVE PATIENTS

For purposes of clinical decision-making, one might consider DMT-naïve RRMS patients as belonging to one of three categories based on disease course: typical, benign, or aggressive. Attack frequency is not necessarily the most important feature to consider in treatment decisions, but it does play a significant role. Patients with a "typical" course experience a clinical relapse every 12 to 16 months, on average, in the first few years of the disease. However, we frequently encounter patients who unequivocally have RRMS but who have experienced remissions lasting 10 years or longer without therapy and who maintain a near-normal or normal neurologic examination. Such patients are very likely to maintain their clinical status over the next 10 years and would seem to have the greatest likelihood of populating the "benign" subgroup of MS patients. Finally, a small minority of RRMS patients demonstrate an unusually aggressive early course with more severe and frequent relapses, placing them in the "aggressive" disease category. From a treatment perspective, the ability to place an individual patient into one of these three categories can provide useful initial direction.

Typical Active RRMS

Most RRMS patients fall into the "typical" category. For definition purposes, the Association of British Neurologists suggests that two clinically significant relapses in the last 2 years, one disabling relapse in the last year, or an active MRI scan containing new or gadolinium-enhancing lesions that have developed during the last year should be considered signs of active disease.[35] Such patients are generally representative of those who were recruited into the placebo-controlled clinical trials that led to approval of IFNB drugs and GA. Based on trial data, one can expect this patient group to experience one third fewer relapses when receiving an IFNB preparation or GA, compared with placebo, over a period of 2 to 4 years.

Which Disease-Modifying Treatment Has Greatest Short-Term Efficacy?

When selecting DMT monotherapy, evidence from randomized, head-to-head trials that evaluate either different dosages of the same drug or different drugs would be optimal, because inferences from comparisons of individual placebo-controlled studies may not be valid. Based on brief head-to-head trials and between-study comparisons, it has been argued that there is likely a dose-response relationship for the IFNB drugs, with high-frequency injections (and, therefore, higher weekly dosage) having somewhat greater efficacy, as measured by MRI and, to a lesser degree, clinical relapse measures.[6,10,36,37] There are, however, some opposing results; for example, weekly administration of 60 µg of Avonex was no more effective than 30 µg.[38] In another trial, weekly low-dose (22 µg SC) IFNB 1a (Rebif) appeared as effective as alternate-day IFNB 1b (Betaferon).[39] However, newer, randomized, head-to-head trials have demonstrated that the differences between these agents may be modest. Moreover, these studies suggested that higher dose frequency, rather than dose amount, may be the important factor that differentiates the IFNB preparations.

Table 15-5 shows data from some of the large and high-profile recent studies. The REbif vs GA in Relapsing MS Disease (REGARD) study compared Rebif (44 µg SC given three times weekly) against GA (20 mg SC given daily) in 756 patients; no difference was observed in time to first relapse or in relapse rate over 2 years.[40] Although Rebif had a greater effect on gadolinium-enhancing MRI lesions, there was no difference in new and enlarging T2 lesions. Drug tolerability was similar in the two study arms, with drug discontinuation rates being 6% for Rebif and 5% for GA. The Betaferon/Betaseron Efficacy Yielding Outcomes of a New Dose (BEYOND) study was a head-to-head comparison of Betaseron at standard dose (250 µg SC every other day) versus double dose (500 µg) versus GA (20 mg SC daily) in 2241 patients over 2 years.[41] There was no difference between the groups with respect to relapse rate (the primary end point); however, this study, like the REGARD study, was compromised by much lower than expected event rates. Despite being underpowered, these head-to-head studies suggest that the efficacies of IFNB and GA at standard doses may be rather similar, at least in the short-term, and that any differences between IFNB preparations may have to do with dose frequency rather than dose amount. The CombiRx study, which is comparing IFNB-1a plus GA versus IFNB-1a plus placebo versus GA plus placebo in a randomized, double-blind, 3-year, three-arm parallel group design, is expected to be completed in 2012.[42] It will involve approximately 1000 patients and should provide the best direct comparative data regarding these agents.

The larger head-to-head studies are either not yet published or not completed. In the meantime, some have tried to compare DMTs over short periods using observational methods. One approach is the use of post–controlled trial extension studies,[7,17,43] but the rigor of having a blinded comparator group and full evaluation of dropouts, among other problems, limits the inferences that may be drawn from this approach.[44]

TABLE 15–5 Recent Large, Head-to-Head Comparison Trials of Disease-Modifying Treatments in Multiple Sclerosis

Study	Interventions	Study Design	Outcomes and Comments
BEYOND (Betaferon/ Betaseron Efficacy Yielding Outcomes of a New Dose) Sponsor: Bayer	Betaferon 250 μg vs 500 μg vs GA for up to 3.5 yr	Randomized multicenter trial, *n* = 2244 treatment-naïve RRMS patients	Primary outcome (relapse rate) was negative; similar rates in all three arms; low relapse rate in all study arms
REGARD (REbif vs GA in Relapsing MS Disease) Sponsor: Serono	Rebif vs GA at standard doses for 96 wk	Randomized trial, *n* = 764 RRMS patients meeting 2001 McDonald criteria	No difference in primary end point of time to first relapse, but very insensitive due to low overall event rate
CombiRx Sponsors: NIH-NINDS, Biogen Idec, Teva Pharmaceuticals	Avonex plus placebo vs GA plus placebo vs Avonex/GA combination for 3 yr	Randomized, double-blind trial for RRMS, *n* = 1000	Primary outcome is relapse rate; EDSS progression is one secondary outcome; study completion in 2012

EDSS, Expanded Disability Status Scale; GA, glatiramer acetate; MS, multiple sclerosis; NIH, National Institutes of Health; NINDS, National Institute of Neurological Disorders and Stroke; RRMS, relapsing-remitting multiple sclerosis.

Other investigators have compared agents using open-label, prospective, observational studies without randomization. One example was an open-label study comparing the effects of all three IFNBs and GA versus no therapy on the relapse rate in 156 patients with RRMS.[45] At 18 months, only 78% of the subjects remained on their original therapy. The authors found that GA and IFNB-1b significantly reduced mean annualized relapse number, whereas IFNB-1a did not. Again, few valid conclusions may be drawn from these studies because of their typically small sample size, short duration, and nonrandomized and unblinded design.

Larger efforts have included a recent study reporting on the use of a large database to analyze the effectiveness of a DMT program in delaying disability progression in a population-based cohort of 590 relapse onset MS patients in Nova Scotia.[46] DMT effectiveness was examined by comparing individuals' estimated annual changes in EDSS in the years preceding and following treatment. Estimates of EDSS increase avoided per treatment year were significant for the group that remained as RRMS (−0.103), the group that converted to SPMS (−0.065), and the combined group (−0.162), with relative effect size estimates of 112%, 21%, and 105%. The authors concluded that DMTs had a significant impact on disability progression, a finding that was actually more prominent than in the pivotal controlled trials. A thoughtful editorial by Trojano[47] encouraged the investigators and suggested efforts to find better methodologies that may help maximize the validity of observational studies, which are much cheaper and more generalizable than controlled trials. Some believe that very large and long-duration observational studies could detect important clinical benefits and overcome some of the biases inherent in this design (see later discussion on whether DMTs alter the long-term course of MS).

Tolerability of first-line DMTs is also a major factor in determining choice of initial therapy and subsequent adherence. Patient preference plays a major role here. Some patients who abhor injections of any type will favor weekly IFNB, whereas those who are swayed more by the needle bore and adverse effects may be more likely to select GA because of its well-tolerated injections and absence of flu-like symptoms or requirements for blood monitoring.

In summary, the choice of first-line DMT for typical early RRMS requires a careful and balanced discussion of the advantages and drawbacks of each drug. Patients with more active disease, as measured by relapse frequency, relapse recovery, and accumulated neurologic impairment, might be steered toward selection of a high-frequency subcutaneous IFNB preparation because of the evidence supporting a greater effect on inflammatory disease measures as well as confirmed effects on disability. On the other hand, those with milder disease activity may gain benefit from once-weekly IFNB or GA with an acceptable adverse effect profile that allows them to maintain treatment adherence.

"Benign" Multiple Sclerosis

Up to 20% of MS patients do very well for decades and fall into the category of "benign" MS, for which there is no consensus definition and no strong predictive factors.[48,49] At times, the diagnosis of MS is made after a patient has experienced a first inter-attack interval of a decade or more. Other patients carry a diagnosis of MS but maintain a prolonged clinical remission without therapy. Although recent data indicate that patients with long-standing MS and minimal impairment have up to an 90% likelihood of maintaining their "benign" clinical status over the subsequent 10 years, some will still experience late deterioration. It is very unlikely that current DMTs are cost-effective in this scenario, and even more so because they have not been shown to delay the onset of SP disease. We typically recommend observation without DMT for this subgroup if we are confident in the validity of the diagnosis, duration of disease, and documentation of lasting clinical remission with normal or near-normal neurologic findings. The unlikely emergence of new clinical relapse activity would prompt re-evaluation of this strategy for an individual patient.

Very Active Relapsing-Remitting Multiple Sclerosis

A small subgroup of relapsing MS patients display a highly inflammatory early course signaled by moderately severe relapses, short interattack intervals, incomplete clinical recovery, and numerous gadolinium-enhancing lesions on brain MRI. It is rather easy to justify more aggressive initial therapy in such patients. Approved drug options include natalizumab, which is otherwise typically a second-line agent, or mitoxantrone. The therapeutic strategy depends on the subsequent clinical response. The purpose of mitoxantrone is to induce a lasting remission, with the recognition that transition to a viable long-term drug will be required before the threshold for cumulative dose-related cardiotoxicity is reached. Some clinicians employ a more rapid induction approach, with monthly doses of mitoxantrone for 3 months, followed by a standard DMT such as GA.[50] A similar approach may be taken with unapproved therapies such as cyclophosphamide. Alternatively, one may consider beginning with natalizumab monotherapy and continuing it indefinitely if the clinical response is favorable. Such strategies have not been subjected to rigorous trials, and this patient subgroup is also the most likely to experience regression to the mean level of disease activity, limiting the validity of short-term observational studies that seem to show benefit for these therapies. However, as discussed later, the principle of "induction" therapy is gaining interest for treatment of early established RRMS, regardless of the level of disease activity, with the hope of influencing mechanisms that lead to later development of progressive disease.

TREATED PATIENTS WITH CHANGING DISEASE STATUS

Declaring Treatment Failure

When clinical or MRI "breakthrough" MS activity occurs in a treated patient, a verdict about the viability of continuing the current therapy is required, especially with the knowledge that all therapies are only partially effective and some disease activity is expected at some time for most treated patients. Although there is no consensus definition of "treatment failure," most would agree that clinical status (relapses, progression) should carry greater weight than MRI for decision-making, and the occurrence of more than one moderate or two minor definite relapses on any therapy should prompt consideration of an alternative approach. In some cases, the need to change therapy is obvious to all parties, but in many instances, the emergent activity is mild and consists of a typical relapse with good recovery or with asymptomatic new brain MRI lesions detected on serial imaging. There are no validated methods to define a therapeutic nonresponder or treatment failure, but evaluation of clinical activity (relapses and worsening of neurologic examination findings) and MRI activity have been proposed.[51-53] The OPTimization of Interferon dose for MS (OPTIMS) study showed that one active scan, revealing a new T2 or gadolinium-enhancing lesion during the first 6 months of IFNB treatment, was associated with a positive predictive value of 59% for development of clinical activity (occurrence of relapses or of EDSS 1.0 score confirmed progression) during further follow-up.[54] Disability progression may be the most important predictor; during the first 2 years of IFNB therapy, confirmed worsening by 1 or more EDSS points was associated with high risk of reaching EDSS 6 at year 6.[53] Until better models and predictive biomarkers are available, systematic clinical follow-up that evaluates the number, severity, and recovery of relapses; examination changes; MRI activity; and neutralizing antibody (NAb) status (if applicable) must all be utilized to determine whether the post-treatment course is acceptable or DMT change is required.

Assessing Adherence to Therapy

The proportion of patients remaining on treatment (adherence) is most likely associated with overall efficacy. Nonadherence rates vary from 15% to 40% in patients treated with DMTs; the main contributing factors are perceived lack of drug efficacy (30% to 50% of those discontinuing) and adverse effects (22% to 70% of dropouts).[54-59] Direct questioning of patients about their adherence to their DMT dosage schedule and reasons for nonadherence could result in recommendations that would reduce adverse effects and better control disease activity.

Switching Therapies

The decision-making process for changing therapy is not well informed by controlled trials. One approach is to consider the evidence for individual placebo-controlled trials and incorporate a "step-up" approach. For example, one might consider switching to three times weekly IFNB-1a in a patient who exhibits significant breakthrough activity on weekly IFNB-1a. Some might consider a switch from GA to an IFNB because the latter therapy is supported by more controlled trials with similar relapse rate reduction data, a confirmed effect on disability progression, and more impact on MRI measures. Although they are intuitive and are commonly used in the absence of better data, such between-trial comparisons have uncertain validity because of differences among study protocols and participants. Furthermore, the placebo-controlled studies do not actually address the clinical question of how to manage breakthrough activity on therapy.

Currently, numerous controlled trials are underway for patients who have active disease despite the use of a DMT, in part because most patients are already using a DMT, and testing of new drugs in treatment-naïve patients is becoming a greater challenge. An earlier example was the AFFIRM study of natalizumab, in which relapsing MS patients who experienced disease activity while using weekly IFNB-1a (Avonex) were randomized to add either placebo or natalizumab.[22] The results favored the combination IFNB-plus-natalizumab arm; the study lacked a natalizumab-plus-placebo arm for optimal comparison. Similar designs are now being used to study drugs such as adjunctive oral cladribine in patients taking three-times-weekly IFNB-1a (Rebif). Although these study designs are useful, they also have limitations because they do not address situations of clear treatment failure, in which keeping a patient on his or her current regimen is not a viable option.

Some patients develop NAbs against IFNB; when they are persistent and at high titer, these are associated with a reduction in the radiographic and clinical effectiveness of IFNB treatment, including the benefits on EDSS progression.[60-65] Reanalysis of the Prevention of Relapses and Disability by Interferon-1a Subcutaneously in Multiple Sclerosis (PRISMS) placebo-controlled Rebif RRMS trial demonstrated that the rate of confirmed 1-point EDSS progression over 4 years was significant only for the NAb-positive group.[64] The European Interferon Beta-1a IM Dose Comparison Study (Avonex given at 30 μg or 60 μg IM weekly) showed a greater mean EDSS increase for NAb-positive patients than for those who were NAb negative.[65]

Weekly intramuscular IFNB-1a is less immunogenic than the current subcutaneous IFNB-1a and IFNB-1b preparations given multiple times per week, but low titer NAbs are transient in many patients, even with continued treatment.[62,66] NAbs usually develop within 24 months after therapy initiation. Although the American Academy of Neurology did not make recommendations for integration of NAbs into clinical decision making in their practice guideline,[67] other groups have put forth stronger recommendations.[68] It seems reasonable to assess NAb status in patients who have disease activity on IFNB therapy, especially because cross-reactivity of NAbs for different IFNB preparations means that Nab-positive patients who require a change in DMT should use a non-IFNB therapy. Neutralizing antibodies may persist for years after IFNB discontinuation.[69] There are no proven strategies for prevention or elimination of NAbs.

Based on dose-response data and controlled trial evidence for effects on relapses, EDSS, and MRI activity, one might consider switching patients taking GA to an IFNB and switching patients taking a low-dose weekly IFNB to a more frequently dosed IFNB preparation (i.e., from Avonex to either Betaseron or Rebif) if NAbs are absent. Some data suggest that switching from high-dose to low-dose IFNB may be detrimental.[37] Treatment failure for patients who are taking a high-dose IFNB or who have persistent, high-titer NAbs should prompt consideration of strategies beyond first-line therapies. There are several potential approaches[70]:

1. *Escalation* from one monotherapy to a more potent single drug (e.g., natalizumab, mitoxantrone,[71] cyclophosphamide[72]), with the choice depending on the presence of relative contraindications.
2. *Combination therapy*, which usually entails continuing a first-line therapy such as IFNB or GA and adding a second agent; this is attractive when two agents with different mechanisms of action are used.[73] The Avonex Combination Trial (ACT) evaluated the combination of methotrexate and Avonex; it showed only trends for benefit of the combination compared with monotherapy.[74] A variety of available general immunosuppressants, including azathioprine, mycophenolate, and cyclophosphamide, have been used in combination with other therapies for patients with active disease.[75-77] Several trials are in progress, including CombiRx (GA plus Avonex), ERAZMUS (Avonex plus Azathioprine), ASPIRE (azathioprine plus Avonex), and ASSERT (GA plus prednisone).[73,74]
3. *Induction therapy*, a term used to describe initiation of a potent immunosuppressant followed by maintenance therapy with a less toxic drug. Induction therapy with mitoxantrone followed by nonstandard maintenance treatment with mitoxantrone, azathioprine, GA, or methylprednisone was associated with good clinical outcomes up to 5 years later.[78] Mitoxantrone induction followed by overlapping and maintenance GA showed similar results for 18 months.[50]

The gradually increasing number of approved therapies, together with the recognition that these agents affect relapses but not later progressive mechanisms, is increasing the attractiveness of combination and induction therapy approaches and many more studies will emerge in coming years.

DO DISEASE-MODIFYING TREATMENTS ALTER THE LONG-TERM COURSE OF MULTIPLE SCLEROSIS?

Does the reduction in clinical relapses and MRI activity seen in the initial years of treatment translate into prevention of disability and progression of disease? Controlled clinical trials, especially randomized ones, are by nature rather short and cannot be expected to answer this question. Several pivotal trials have been followed by observational extension studies in attempts to gather more information about efficacy and safety. However, the patients followed up are more likely to be "responders" to therapy (or to have experienced a milder course regardless of treatment allocation), whereas dropouts are more likely to be "nonresponders." This fact biases interpretations of the data.

Some believe that several of the limitations of observational studies might be overcome if the magnitude of the benefit of an intervention was very clinically significant. For example, if a drug could prevent a significant proportion of treated patients from requiring a cane or wheelchair at a future time point, perhaps a large enough, long enough observation of a completely ascertained cohort could demonstrate such benefits.

There have been a few large-scale studies of several years' duration. A Danish registry study of 2393 patients treated between 1996 and 2003 showed that 1252 patients (52.3%) were still receiving their initial therapy; the remainder had either discontinued therapy or switched to a different drug.[79] A major predictor of sustained 1-point EDSS progression was use of the 44 μg subcutaneous IFNB-1a preparation using IFNB-1b as reference, perhaps due to patient selection. In another study, Ebers and colleagues identified 328 (88.2%) of 372 patients treated in the pivotal Betaseron clinical trial 16 years later; 293 were alive, and 35 were deceased.[80] Patients were categorized as having "always,", "never," or "ever" been exposed to IFNB-1b. Data from 260 patients showed that 30% were currently taking IFNB-1b, with a median length of exposure of almost 10 years. Wheelchair use was required by 44.2% of the "never" and 29.4% of the "always" groups, and time to EDSS score 6 was 6 years longer for the latter group. Adverse effects were uncommon. Although still subject to biases, this study has some advantages over other observational studies, including the effort to evaluate all patients (rather than only those who continued treatment). Another recent 5-year study of 175 IFNB-treated patients showed that the proportion of patients with fixed disability was significantly less than in a cohort of matched historical control subjects; disability progression was related to failure of IFNB to completely suppress relapses and to higher initial EDSS.[81]

In sum, these studies illustrate somewhat different observational approaches (extension studies, registry studies, historical control studies) that collectively, if the magnitude and direction of effect of treatment were consistent, could support long-term treatment benefits for current DMTs.

Strategies for Secondary Progressive Multiple Sclerosis

EVIDENCE FOR APPROVED THERAPIES

Controlled trials of IFNB for SPMS have shown mixed results (see Table 15-2). Two studies demonstrated that subcutaneous IFNB-1b (Betaferon; European SPMS study) and weekly intramuscular IFNB-1a (Avonex; International Multiple Sclerosis Secondary Progressive Avonex Controlled Trial [IMPACT]) at 60 μg (twice the dose approved for RRMS) both slowed progression rates over 2 to 3 years.[82,83] The primary outcome measure in the European study was the EDSS, whereas IMPACT used the MS Functional Composite (MSFC) measure. Although the MSFC has been shown to be reproducible, has good inter-rater and intrarater reliability, and predicts later change in the EDSS score, some point to the fact that the only component of the MFSC that showed a significant treatment benefit was the nine-hole peg test, a measure of upper extremity function.

Cognitive testing showed a nonsignificant trend, and timed ambulation did not show a treatment effect.

In contrast, in two other large, controlled trials of IFNB-1a and IFNB-1b at doses effective for RRMS failed to slow disability progression but did improve several secondary clinical outcomes (relapse rate and severity) and MRI measures (disease activity and total burden of disease).[84-86]

Mitoxantrone showed benefit in a placebo-controlled trial of relapsing or SPMS with "recent rapid worsening," but the sample size was relatively small, the dropout rate was high, and patients were not stratified according to disease course. Most patients had recently experienced active inflammatory disease (74% had experienced a relapse during the 2 years before enrollment), and treatment benefit was dose-related, favoring 12 mg/m^2 over 5 mg/m^2 dosage regimens.[29,30]

There are no study data that demonstrate a role for GA in the treatment of SPMS. Natalizumab has not been evaluated in progressive forms of MS, and, at present, the drug is not recommended for use in such cases because of concern that symptoms of treatment-related PML may not be easily detectable in the context of progressive disease. A randomized, placebo-controlled trial of intravenous immune globulin (1 g/kg/month) to reduce the rate of progression in SPMS was negative.[87]

DECISION MAKING IN SECONDARY PROGRESSIVE MULTIPLE SCLEROSIS

Current data suggest that the rate of disability progression in SPMS may be slowed by IFNB therapy if the course is accompanied by evidence of superimposed relapses. In contrast, older SPMS patients, those who have been in the SP phase for many years, and those who have not had superimposed relapses in the last 2 years and do not have continued inflammatory disease activity on MRI seem to receive no benefit from IFNB therapy.[88,89] Patients who are progressing rapidly, especially if there are superimposed relapses or MRI evidence of active inflammatory disease, may stabilize with mitoxantrone therapy. There are no current roles for GA, natalizumab, or intravenous immune globulin in the treatment of SPMS. Some patients may respond to pulse IV methylprednisolone therapy[90] or methotrexate,[91] but the utility of these approaches has not been established.

Strategies for Primary Progressive Multiple Sclerosis

There are no approved therapies for primary progressive MS (PPMS). The PROMiSe study showed no benefit of GA compared with placebo, and the study was terminated for futility.[92] Although the overall study results were negative, a post hoc subgroup analysis suggested that male patients might derive some benefit from GA; however, this finding may be explained by the relatively poorer performance of the male placebo control group. Other therapeutic trials have failed, very likely reflecting the relatively minor influence of inflammatory mechanisms in PPMS.[93-96] Some patients with PPMS will develop relapses at some point during the disease course ("progressive relapsing" disease) and, like SPMS patients, might be expected to derive some benefit from DMTs for relapse prevention. However, there are no studies that directly address this question.

Strategies for Very Stable Patients: Stopping Therapy

Some patients express a desire to completely discontinue use of DMTs. This may occur in the setting of very advanced disease in which further treatments are considered futile. It is almost impossible in individual patients to conclude that treatment is providing no benefit. However, the Association of British Neurologists guidance (2007) suggests that nonrelapsing SPMS with loss of ability to ambulate (EDSS 7 or greater) be used as a guideline for stopping all DMT .[35] In situations that do not seem futile, such as relapsing disease in an ambulatory patient, the reasons for stopping must be clearly understood. Very often, changes in technique or treatment of other disease symptoms (depression, sleep disorders, spasticity, bladder symptoms, pain) may improve quality of life and change the patient's perspective about continued DMT use.

Less commonly, a subgroup of relapsing MS patients appear to have completely quiescent disease during many years of therapy. Such patients naturally wonder whether they may sustain their remission off therapy. This scenario should again prompt a careful evaluation of motivating factors such as "treatment fatigue" or adverse effects. However, if a patient has had clinical and radiographic evidence of complete remission for several years, it is reasonable to entertain his or her request to stop therapy, with the caveat that an agreement should be reached concerning surveillance for re-emergent disease activity, ideally by clinical and imaging methods, so that treatment may be restarted if indicated. Such a decision can be more difficult to reach than starting therapy, and decision making is aided by a good physician-patient relationship, because there are no firm data to guide stopping therapy after long-term remission.

Conclusions

Therapeutic options continue to expand for patients with MS. Those with early RRMS are still best served by initiating treatment with an IFNB or GA. Treatment intolerance or declaration of treatment failure should lead to switching therapy. Some evidence suggests greater efficacy for more frequently administered IFNB preparations compared with the once-weekly dosage form; in the absence of persistent, high-titer NAbs, switching to a more frequent IFNB seems logical. If treatment failure occurs in an NAb-positive patient, then non-IFNs such as natalizumab or mitoxantrone should be used. SPMS that worsens relatively rapidly or has superimposed clinical relapses is likely to be slowed by IFNB and may respond to mitoxantrone. There are still no proven therapies for PPMS. Future therapeutic approaches will incorporate combination or induction therapies earlier in the disease course; although logical, these approaches require rigorous evaluation in randomized clinical trials. This general approach is similar to that outlined by an international consensus group.[97] If feasible, every MS patient should be encouraged to consider participation in a clinical trial, especially those patients who have breakthrough disease despite therapy, rapidly worsening MS, or progressive forms of the disease. The emergence of new oral therapies and powerful parenteral drugs, especially monoclonal antibodies, guarantees that the future of MS therapy will become more complex, but also hopefully more effective for individual patients.

REFERENCES

1. Noseworthy JH, Lucchinetti CF, Rodriguez M, Weinshenker BG: Multiple sclerosis. N Engl J Med 2000;343:938-952.
2. Frohman EM, Havrdova E, Lublin F, et al: Most patients with multiple sclerosis or a clinically isolated demyelinating syndrome should be treated at the time of diagnosis. Arch Neurol 2006;63:614-619.
3. The IFNB Multiple Sclerosis Study Group: Interferon beta-1b is effective in relapsing remitting multiple sclerosis: I. Clinical results of a multicenter, randomized, double-blind, placebo-controlled trial. The IFNB Multiple Sclerosis Study Group. Neurology 1993;43:655-661.
4. The IFNB Multiple Sclerosis Study Group and the University of British Columbia MS/MRI Analysis Group. Interferon beta-1b in the treatment of MS: Final outcome of the randomized controlled trial. Neurology 1995;45:1277-1285.
5. Jacobs LD, Cookfair DL, Rudick RA, et al: Intramuscular interferon beta-1a for disease progression in relapsing multiple sclerosis. Ann Neurol 1996;39:285-294.
6. PRISMS (Prevention of Relapses and Disability by Interferon-1a Subcutaneously in Multiple Sclerosis) Study Group: Randomized double-blind placebo-controlled study of interferon beta-1a in relapsing/remitting multiple sclerosis. Lancet 1998;352:1498-1504.
7. PRISMS Study Group, and the University of British Columbia MS/MRI Analysis Group: PRISMS-4: Long-term efficacy of interferon-β-1a in relapsing MS. Neurology 2001;56:1628-1636.
8. Goodin DS, Frohman EM, Garmany GP, et al: Disease modifying therapies in multiple sclerosis. Report of the Therapeutic and Technology Assessment Subcommittee of the American Academy of Neurology and the MS Council for Clinical Practice Guidelines. Neurology 2002;58:169-178.
9. Fillippini G, Munari L, Incorvaia B, et al: Interferons in relapsing remitting multiple sclerosis: A systematic review. Lancet 2003;361:545-552.
10. Durelli L, Verdun E, Barbero P, et al: Every-other-day interferon beta-1b versus once-weekly interferon beta-1a for multiple sclerosis: Results of a 2-year prospective randomised multicentre study (INCOMIN). Lancet 2002;359:1453-1460.
11. Panitch H, Goodin DS, Francis G, et al: Randomized, comparative study of interferon beta-1a treatment regimens in MS: The EVIDENCE Trial. Neurology 2002;59:1496-1506.
12. Johnson KP, Brooks BR, Cohen JA, et al: Copolymer 1 reduces relapse rate and improves disability in relapsing-remitting multiple sclerosis: Results of a phase III multicenter, double-blind placebo-controlled trial. Neurology 1995;45:1268-1276.
13. Boneschi FM, Rovaris M, Johnson KP, et al: Effects of glatiramer acetate on relapse rate and accumulated disability in multiple sclerosis: Meta-analysis of three double-blind, randomized, placebo-controlled clinical trials. Mult Scler 2003;9:349-355.
14. Munari L, Lovati R, Boiko A: Therapy with glatiramer acetate for multiple sclerosis. Cochrane Database Syst. Rev 2003;(4). CD004678.
15. Cohen J, Rovaris M, Goodman AD, et al: Randomised, double-blind, parallel-group, dose-comparison study of glatiramer acetate in relapsing-remitting multiple sclerosis. Neurology 2007;68:939-944.
16. Johnson KP, Brooks BR, Cohen JA, et al: Extended use of glatiramer acetate (Copaxone) is well tolerated and maintains its clinical effect on multiple sclerosis relapse rate and degree of disability. Neurology 1998;50:701-708.
17. Ford CC, Johnson KP, Lisak RP, et al: A prospective open-label study of glatiramer acetate: Over a decade of continuous use in multiple sclerosis patients. Mult Scler 2006;12:309-320.
18. Debouverie M, Moreau T, Lebrun C, et al: A longitudinal observational study of a cohort of patients with relapsing-remitting multiple sclerosis treated with glatiramer acetate. Eur J Neurol 2007;14:1266-1274.
19. Rice GP, Hartung HP, Calabresi PA: Anti-alpha4 integrin therapy for multiple sclerosis: Mechanisms and rationale. Neurology 2005;64:1336-1342.
20. Polman CH, O'Connor PW, Havrdova E, et al: A randomized, placebo-controlled trial of natalizumab for relapsing multiple sclerosis. N Engl J Med 2006;354:899-910.
21. Miller DH, Soon D, Fernando KT, et al: MRI outcomes in a placebo-controlled trial of natalizumab in relapsing MS. Neurology 2007;68:1390-1401.
22. Rudick RA, Stuart WH, Calabresi PA, et al: A randomized, placebo-controlled trial of natalizumab plus interferon beta-1a for relapsing multiple sclerosis. N Engl J Med 2006;354:911-923.
23. Kleinschmidt-DeMasters BK, Tyler KL: Progressive multifocal leukoencephalopathy complicating treatment with natalizumab and interferon beta-1a for multiple sclerosis. N Engl J Med 2005;353:369-374.

24. Van Assche G, Van Ranst M, Sciot R, et al: Progressive multifocal leukoencephalopathy after natalizumab therapy for Crohn's disease. N Engl J Med 2005;353:362-368.
25. Langer-Gould A, Atlas SW, Green AJ, et al: Progressive multifocal leukoencephalopathy in a patient treated with natalizumab. N Engl J Med 2005;353:375-381.
26. Berger JR, Koralnik IJ: Progressive multifocal leukoencephalopathy and natalizumab: Unforeseen consequences. N Engl J Med 2005;353:414-416.
27. Yousry TA, Major EO, Ryschkewitsch C, et al: Evaluation of patients treated with natalizumab for progressive multifocal leukoencephalopathy. N Engl J Med 2006;354:924-933.
28. Kappos L, Bates D, Hartung H-P, et al: Natalizumab treatment for multiple sclerosis: Recommendations for patient selection and monitoring. Lancet Neurol 2007;6:431-441.
29. Hartung H-P, Gonsette R, Konig N, et al: Mitoxantrone in progressive multiple sclerosis: A placebo-controlled, double-blind, randomised, muticentre trial. Lancet 2002;360:2018-2025.
30. Goodin DS, Arnason BG, Coyle PK, et al: The use of mitoxantrone (Novantrone) for the treatment of multiple sclerosis. Neurology 2003;61:1332-1338.
31. Ghalie R, Edan G, Laurent M, et al: Cardiac adverse effects associated with mitoxantrone (Novantrone) therapy in patients with MS. Neurology 2002;59:909-913.
32. Avasarala JR, Cross AH, Clifford DB, et al: Rapid onset mitoxantrone-induced cardiotoxicity in secondary progressive multiple sclerosis. Mult Scler 2003;9:59-62.
33. Edan G, Brochet B, Clanet M, et al: Safety profile of mitoxantrone in a cohort of 802 multiple sclerosis patients: A 4 year mean follow-up study. Neurology 2004;62;(Suppl5):A493.
34. Brassat D, Recher C, Waubant E, et al: Therapy-related acute myeloblastic leukemia after mitoxantrone treatment in a patient with MS. Neurology 2002;59:954-955.
35. ABN Guidelines for Use of the Licensed MS Disease Modifying Treatments. Association of British Neurologists. 2008. Available at: http://www.theabn.org/downloads/ABN-MS-Guidelines-2007.pdf (accessed on 20 November 2008)
36. The Once Weekly Interferon for MS Study Group: Evidence of interferon beta-1a dose response in relapsing-remitting MS: The OWIMS Study. Neurology 1999;53:679-686.
37. Barbero P, Verdun E, Bergui M, et al: High-dose, frequently administered interferon beta therapy for relapsing-remitting multiple sclerosis must be maintained over the long term: The interferon beta dose-reduction study. J Neurol Sci 2004;222:13-19.
38. Clanet M, Radue EW, Kappos L, et al: A randomized, double-blind, dose-comparison study of weekly interferon beta-1a in relapsing MS. Neurology 2002;59:1507-1517.
39. Koch-Henriksen N, Sorensen PS, Christensen T, et al: A randomized study of two interferon-beta treatments in relapsing-remitting multiple sclerosis. Neurology 2006;66:1056-1060.
40. Mikol DD, Barkhof F, Chang P, et al: The REGARD trial: A randomised assessor-blinded trial comparing interferon beta-1a and glatiramer acetate in relapsing-remitting multiple sclerosis. Presented at the 23rd Congress of the European Committee for the Treatment and Research in Multiple Sclerosis (ECTRIMS), Prague, Czech Republic, October 14, 2007.
41. BEYOND study: Results do not support regulatory filling for Betaferon 500 mcg. Bayer HealthCare Pharmaceuticals, October 29, 2007. Available at: http://www.pharma.bayer.com/scripts/pages/en/news_room/news_room/news_room38.php (accessed October 2008).
42. Combination Therapy in Patients With Relapsing-Remitting Multiple Sclerosis (MS) CombiRx. ClinicalTrials.gov. Available at: http://clinicaltrials.gov/ct2/show/NCT00211887?term=multiple+sclerosis+interferon+glatiramer&rank=1 (accessed October 2008).
43. Kappos L, Traboulsee A, Constantinescu C, et al: Long-term subcutaneous interferon beta-1a therapy in patients with relapsing-remitting MS. Neurology 2006;67:944-953.
44. Noseworthy JH: How much can we learn from long-term extension trials in multiple sclerosis? Neurology 2006;67:930-931.
45. Khan OA, Tselis AC, Kamholz JA, et al: A prospective, open-label treatment trial to compare the effect of IFNbeta-1a (Avonex), IFNbeta-1b (Betaseron), and glatiramer acetate (Copaxone) on the relapse rate in relapsing-remitting multiple sclerosis: Results after 18 months of therapy. Mult Scler 2001;7:349-353.
46. Brown MG, Kirby S, Skedgel C, et al: How effective are disease-modifying drugs in delaying progression in relapsing-onset MS? Neurology 2007;69:1498-1507.
47. Trojano M: Is it time to use observational data to estimate treatment effectiveness in multiple sclerosis? Neurology 2007:69:1478-1479.
48. Pittock SJ, McClelland RL, Mayr WT, et al: Clinical implications of benign multiple sclerosis: A 20-year population-based follow-up study. Ann Neurol 2004;56:303-306.
49. Sayao AL, Devonshire V, Tremlett H: Longitudinal follow-up of "benign" multiple sclerosis at 20 years. Neurology 2007;68:496-500.

50. Ramtahal J, Jacob A, Das K, Boggild M: Sequential maintenance treatment with glatiramer acetate after mitoxantrone is safe and can limit exposure to immunosuppression in very active, relapsing remitting multiple sclerosis. J Neurol 2006;253:1160-1164.
51. Freedman MS, Patry DG, Grand'Maison F, et al: Canadian MS Working Group: Treatment optimization in multiple sclerosis. Can J Neurol Sci 2004;31:157-168.
52. Rudick R, Lee J, Simon J, et al: Defining interferon beta response status in multiple sclerosis patients. Ann Neurol 2004;56:548-555.
53. Rio J, Nos V, Tintore M, et al: Defining the response to interferon-beta in relapsing-remitting multiple sclerosis patients. Ann Neurol 2006;59:344-352.
54. Clerico M, Barbero P, Contessa G, et al: Adherence to interferon-beta treatment and results of therapy switching. J Neurol Sci 2007;259:104-108.
55. Milanese C, La Mantia L, Palumbo R, et al: A post-marketing study on interferon β 1b and 1a treatment in relapsing-remitting multiple sclerosis: Different response in drop-outs and treated patients. J Neurol Neurosurg Psychiatr 2003;74;1689-1692.
56. Ruggieri RM, Settipani N, Viviano L, et al: Long-term interferon-beta treatment for multiple sclerosis. Neurol Sci 2003;24:361-364.
57. Tremlett HL, Oger J: Interrupted therapy: Stopping and switching of the beta-interferons prescribed for MS. Neurology 2003;61:551-554.
58. O'Rourke KE, Hutchinson M: Stopping beta-interferon therapy in multiple sclerosis: An analysis of stopping patterns. Mult Scler 2005;11:46-50.
59. Rio J, Porcel J, Tellez N, et al: Factors related with treatment adherence to interferon beta and glatiramer acetate therapy in multiple sclerosis. Mult Scler 2005;11:306-309.
60. Hemmer B, Stuve O, Kieseier B, et al: Immune response to immunotherapy: The role of neutralising anitbodies to interferon beta in the treatment of multiple sclerosis. Lancet Neurol 2005;4: 403-412.
61. Bertolotto A, Malucchi S, Sala A, et al: Differential effects of three interferon betas on neutralizing antibodies in patients with multiple sclerosis: A follow up study in an independent laboratory. J Neurol Neurosurg Psychiatry 2002;73:148-153.
62. Sorensen PS, Koch-Henriksen N, Ross C, et al: Appearance and disappearance of neutralizing antibodies during interferon-beta therapy. Neurology 2005;65:33-39.
63. Sorensen PS, Tscherning T, Mathiesen HK, et al: Neutralizing antibodies hamper IFNbeta bioactivity and treatment effect on MRI in patients with MS. Neurology 2006;67:1681-1683.
64. Francis GS, Rice GPA, Alsop JC, et al: Interferon β-1a in MS: Results following development of neutralizing antibodies in PRISMS. Neurology 2005;65:48-55.
65. Kappos L, Clanet M, Sandberg-Wollheim M, et al: Neutralizing antibodies and efficacy of interferon β-1a: A 4-year controlled study. Neurology 2005;65:40-47.
66. Giovannini G, Goodman A: Neutralizing anti-IFN-β antibodies: How much more evidence do we need to use them in practice?. Neurology 2005;65:6-8.
67. Goodin DS, Frohman EM, Hurwitz B, et al: Neutralizing antibodies to interferon beta: Assessment of their clinical and radiographic impact. An evidence report: Report of the Therapeutics and Technology Assessment Subcommittee of the American Academy of Neurology. Neurology 2007;68:977-984.
68. Sorensen PS, Deisenhammer F, Duda P, et al: EFNS Task Force on Anti-IFN-beta Antibodies in Multiple Sclerosis: Guidelines on use of anti-IFN-beta antibody measurements in multiple sclerosis: Report of an EFNS Task Force on IFN-beta antibodies in multiple sclerosis. Eur J Neurol 2005;12:817-827.
69. Petersen B, Bendtzen K, Koch-Henriksen N, et al: Persistence of neutralizing antibodies after discontinuation of IFNB therapy in patients with relapsing-remitting multiple sclerosis. Mult Scler 2006;12:247-252.
70. Wingerchuk DM: Current evidence and therapeutic strategies for multiple sclerosis. Semin Neurol 2008;28:56-68.
71. Correale J, Rush C, Amengual A, Goicochea MT: Mitoxantrone as rescue therapy in worsening relapsing-remitting MS patients receiving IFN-beta. J Neuroimmunol 2005;162:173-183.
72. Gladstone DE, Zamkoff KW, Krupp L, et al: High-dose cyclophosphamide for moderate to severe refractory multiple sclerosis. Arch Neurol 2006;63:1388-1393.
73. Fernandez O: Combination therapy in multiple sclerosis. J Neurol Sci 2007;259:95-103.
74. Cohen J, Confavreux C: Combination therapy in multiple sclerosis. In Cohen JA, Rudick RA, (eds): Multiple Sclerosis Therapeutics, 3rd ed. London, Informa Healthcare, 2007, pp 681-697.
75. Pulicken M, Bash CN, Costello K, et al: Optimization of the safety and efficacy of interferon beta 1b and azathioprine combination therapy in multiple sclerosis. Mult Scler 2005;11:169-174.

76. Jeffery DR, Chepuri N, Durden N, Burdette J: A pilot trial of combination therapy with mitoxantrone and interferon beta-1b using monthly gadolinium-enhanced magnetic resonance imaging. Mult Scler 2005;11:296-301.
77. Smith DR, Weinstock-Guttman B, Cohen JA, et al: A randomized blinded trial of combination therapy with cyclophosphamide in patients with active multiple sclerosis on interferon beta. Mult Scler 2005;11:573-582.
78. Le Page E, Leray E, Taurin G, et al: Mitoxantrone as induction treatment in aggressive relapsing remitting multiple sclerosis: Treatment response factors in a 5 year follow-up observational study of 100 consecutive patients. J Neurol Neurosurg Psychiatry 2008;79:52-56.
79. Sorensen PS, Koch-Henrisken N, Ravnborg M, et al: Immunomodulatory treatment of multiple sclerosis in Denmark: A prospective nationwide survey. Mult Scler 2006;12:253-264.
80. Ebers G, Traboulsee A, Li D, et al: Final results from the interferon beta-1b 16-year long-term follow-up study. 22nd Congress of the European Committee for Treatment and Research in Multiple Sclerosis. Spain, Madrid, 2006.
81. O'Rourke K, Walsh C, Antonelli G, Hutchinson M: Predicting beta-interferon failure in relapsing-remitting multiple sclerosis. Mult Scler 2007;13:336-342.
82. European Study Group on Interferon β-1b in Secondary Progressive MS: Placebo-controlled multicentre randomised trial of interferon β-1b in treatment of secondary progressive multiple sclerosis. Lancet 1998;352:1491-1497.
83. Cohen JA, Cutter GR, Fischer JS, et al: IMPACT Investigators: Benefit of interferon β-1a on MSFC progression in secondary progressive MS. Neurology 2002;59:679-687.
84. Secondary Progressive Efficacy Trial of Recombinant Interferon-beta-1a in MS (SPECTRIMS) Study Group: Randomized controlled trial of interferon-beta-1a in secondary progressive MS. Neurology 2001;56:1496-1504.
85. Li D, Zhao G, Paty D, University of British Columbia MS/MRI Analysis Research Group, and the SPECTRIMS Study Group: Randomized controlled trial of interferon beta-1a in secondary progressive MS: MRI results. Neurology 2001;56:1505-1518.
86. The North American Study Group on Interferon beta-1b in Secondary Progressive MS: Interferon beta-1b in secondary progressive MS: Results from a 3-year controlled study. Neurology 2004;63:1788-1795.
87. Hommes OR, Sorenson PS, Fazekas F, et al: Intravenous immune globulin in secondary progressive multiple sclerosis: Randomised placebo-controlled trial. Lancet 2004;364:1149-1156.
88. Kappos L, Weinshenker B, Pozzilli C, et al: Interferon beta-1b in secondary progressive MS: A combined analysis of the two trials. Neurology 2004;63:1779-1787.
89. Cohen JA, Antel JP: Does interferon beta help in secondary progressive MS? Neurology 2004;63:1768-1769.
90. Goodkin DE, Kinkel RP, Weinstock-Guttman B, et al: A phase II study of i.v. methylprednisolone in secondary-progressive multiple sclerosis. Neurology 1998;51:239-245.
91. Goodkin DE, Rudick RA, VanderBrug Medendorp S, et al: Low-dose (7.5 mg) oral methotrexate reduces the rate of progression in chronic progressive multiple sclerosis. Ann Neurol 1995;37:30-40.
92. Wolinsky JS, Narayana PA, O'Connor P, et al: Glatiramer acetate in primary progressive multiple sclerosis: Results of a multinational, multicenter, double-blind, placebo-controlled trial. Ann Neurol 2007;61:14-24.
93. Leary SM, Miller DH, Stevenson VL, et al: Interferon beta-1a in primary progressive MS: An exploratory, randomized, controlled trial. Neurology 2003;60:44-51.
94. Kita M, Cohen JA, Fox RJ, et al: Double blind placebo controlled phase II trial of mitoxantrone in patient with primary progressive multiple sclerosis. Neurology 2004;62(Suppl 5):A99.
95. Montalban X: Overview of European pilot study of interferon beta-Ib in primary progressive multiple sclerosis. Mult Scler 2004;10(Suppl 1):S62.
96. Pohlau D, Przuntek H, Sailer M, et al: Intravenous immunoglobulin in primary and secondary chronic progressive multiple sclerosis: A randomized placebo controlled multicentre study. Mult Scler 2007;13:1107-1117.
97. Karussis D, Biermann LD, Bohlega S, et al: A recommended treatment algorithm in relapsing multiple sclerosis: Report of an international consensus meeting. Eur J Neurol 2007;13:61-71.

16 Management of Aggressive Multiple Sclerosis: Options and Challenges

GILLES EDAN • SEAN P. MORRISSEY

Diagnosis of Menacing Multiple Sclerosis

About 10 years ago, three multiple sclerosis (MS) research groups reported their findings in management of MS in patients who were menaced by development of severe disability within a short time. First, in 1997, Edan and colleagues[1] published their findings of a randomized controlled trial of mitoxantrone in “aggressive” MS. Also in 1997, Weinstock-Guttman and associates[2] published their findings from an open-label trial of cyclophosphamide (CTX) in “fulminant” MS (also called, according to Weinshenker and Rodriquez,[3] “rapidly worsening” MS or “catastrophic MS type II”). Finally, in 1999, Weinshenker and coworkers[4] published the results of a controlled randomized trial of therapeutic plasma exchange (TPE) in MS and other idiopathic inflammatory demyelinating diseases (IIDD) ("catastrophic MS type I"). Those three types of menacing MS should be clearly distinguished from other MS disease courses with lesser clinical activity and/or lesser degree of disability accumulation. Although menacing MS cases are most likely to be rare,[3] their diagnosis and management are true challenges for even experienced MS neurologists. This review focuses on relapsing-remitting MS forms—that is, MS cases in which there is strong clinical evidence, as well as magnetic resonance imaging (MRI) and/or neuropathologic evidence, that rapid and severe clinical deterioration is dominated by a focal neuroinflammatory process.

Before discussing the management of aggressive and catastrophic MS, it is important to briefly recall the definition of MS and the key findings from natural MS history studies concerning mean values of annual relapse rates, relapse duration and severity, time to relapse recovery, and mean times for accumulation of moderate and severe disability. Such findings are helpful because they allow operationalization of the clinical definitions for a heterogeneous and rare subgroup of patients with menacing MS.

MS is defined as an inflammatory-demyelinating disease of the central nervous system with evidence of lesions disseminated in space and time. Symptoms and signs have to be typical for MS, usually based on clinical but also laboratory-supported evidence.[5,6] Natural history studies of acute attacks suggest that, in adult patients, the overall mean annual relapse rate is about 0.5 during the first years.[7] In adults, the mean time from a first neurologic event to clinical recovery in clinically isolated syndromes carrying a high risk for development of MS is about 6 months.[8] In general, however, the mean duration of a relapse is estimated to be about 4 to 6 weeks: improvement leveled after 2 weeks in 50% of patients; and after 8 weeks in 67%.[9] Regarding development of relapse-dependent residual deficit, Lublin and colleagues[10] reported that, after a mean of 64 days after an exacerbation, 42% of patients had residual deficit of at least 0.5, and 28% had residual of 1.0 point or greater on the Extended Disability Status Scale (EDSS). About 50% of MS patients with an acute attack are responsive to steroid treatment, and studies in patients after a severe attack showed recovery in about 45% with steroid treatment.[11] Natural history data from untreated severe MS relapses (most of the patients had a first MS attack) suggested that more than 50% of these patients had no or only insignificant clinical recovery with loss of their ambulatory functions.[12,13] Furthermore, natural history studies in adult MS patients showed that an EDSS score of 3 is reached after a mean of 7.7 years, and EDDS score of 6 after a mean of 15 years.[14]

Malignant MS was already recognized in the 19th century,[15] and the name was originally applied to a disease course that was fatal within a few years after disease onset.[16] Survival in malignant MS ranged from a couple of weeks[17] to 5 years. Early studies[18,19] reported death rates of about 5%, but subsequent studies found no fatal cases within the first 5 years after disease onset,[20,21] almost none (about 1%),[22-25] or approximately 5%.[26] Poser[27] defined malignant MS in patients acquiring an EDSS or DSS score of 7 or more within 5 years of disease duration. Confavreux and colleagues[23] described "hyperacute" MS cases in which patients developed severe disability within the first 5 years; they found a rate of about 8% in the Lyon cohort, somewhere between the findings of two other studies (12%[28] and 3%[27]). More recently, malignant MS was defined by Lublin and Reingold as "a disease with a rapid progressive course leading to significant disability in multiple neurological systems or death in a relatively short time after disease onset."[29]

More general clinical criteria used to distinguish between the two different forms of menacing MS (catastrophic MS types I and II versus aggressive MS), or between menacing MS and other less active MS courses, include the following:

- Disease duration: onset versus shorter duration (<5 or 10 years) versus longer duration
- Relapsing-remitting (RRMS) versus (secondary) progressive (SPMS) forms
- Duration of deterioration period: a few weeks (<3 months) versus 3 to 6 months versus 12 months or longer
- Relapse frequency: usually at least two relapses within the preceding 12 months
- Degree of confirmed (i.e., examined 3 months apart) accumulated disability over the preceding 12 months

These criteria may be applied either in patients with treatment failure (e.g., high-dose steroids, interferon [IFN]-beta, or glatiramer acetate) or in untreated patients. Current laboratory criteria refer basically to MRI lesion activity in the preceding months (new, active, and especially gadolinium-enhancing lesions). Because the MRI variables allow a more quantitative description of aggressive MS, and because preliminary evidence suggests their importance for treatment response in aggressive MS, they are increasingly used in routine research protocols and by regulatory authorities.

Because there is considerable overlap of aggressive MS with catastrophic MS (types I and II) concerning both diagnosis and management, we will discuss the operational criteria in detail, citing from the original publications (Table 16-1). In the following sections, we use an operational definition of aggressive MS based on two studies.[1,30] The term "aggressive" MS is the official one used by the French regulatory authorities that approved mitoxantrone for treatment in this indication, and the definition of "aggressive" RRMS (and SPMS), is based on the protocol of a randomized controlled trial that combined clinical and MRI activity variables.[1]

Aggressive multiple sclerosis is defined as follows:

1. Over a period of 12 months, two relapses, causing residual deficits, and one new gadolinium-enhancing lesion on an MRI scan performed within the preceding 3 months *or*
2. Progression of 2 points on the EDSS during the preceding 12 months and at least one new gadolinium-enhancing lesion on an MRI scan performed within the preceding 3 months.

Based on our experience, especially with long-term follow-up in patients with aggressive RRMS treated with mitoxantrone,[30] we focus here on early and clearly relapsing courses of menacing MS and touch only very briefly on secondary or primary progressive MS.

Use of Therapeutic Plasma Exchange, Cyclophosphamide, and Mitoxantrone in Catastrophic Multiple Sclerosis

USE OF THERAPEUTIC PLASMA EXCHANGE AND MITOXANTRONE IN TYPE I CATASTROPHIC MULTIPLE SCLEROSIS

The Mayo Clinic group performed a pioneering trial design[4] for TPE in type I catastrophic MS.[4,31-34] Eligible patients were between 18 and 60 years of age had either clinically definite or laboratory-supported MS (n = 12) or IIDD (n = 10) with a

TABLE 16–1 Menacing Multiple Sclerosis

Category	Synopsis	References for Full Operational Criteria	Treatment Options
Catastrophic MS			
Type I	A catastrophic acute attack developing over days to weeks with major disability that fails to respond after standard treatment with corticosteroids	3, 4	TPE M/MP
Type II (rapidly worsening MS)	Rapidly worsening disability with or without superimposed relapses over a 3 to 6-mo period	2, 3, 37	M/MP CTX
Aggressive MS			
	In the preceding 12 mo, very active disease (≥2 relapses) or important residual deficit (≥2 EDSS points) plus MRI lesion activity	1, 30, 39, 40	M/MP CTX ALEM

ALEM, alemtuzumab; CTX, cyclophosphamide; EDSS, Extended Disability Status Scale; MS, multiple sclerosis; M/MP, mitoxantrone combined with methylprednisolone; TPE, therapeutic plasma exchange.

Data from Edan G, Miller D, Clanet M, et al: Therapeutic effect of mitoxantrone combined with methylprednisolone in multiple sclerosis: A randomised multicentre study of active disease using MRI and clinical criteria. J Neurol Neurosurg Psychiatry 1997;62:112-118.

recent severe attack (3 weeks to 3 months from onset). IIDD included acute disseminated encephalomyelitis (ADEM), neuromyelitis optica, Marburg's variant of MS, recurrent transverse myelitis, and localized cerebral inflammatory demyelination. Patients were required to have had an acute fulminant neurologic deficit affecting consciousness, language, brainstem function, or spinal cord function and resulting in marked impairment in activities of daily living by virtue of one or more of the following targeted neurologic deficits (TNDs): coma, aphasia, acute severe cognitive dysfunction, hemiplegia, paraplegia, or quadriplegia. There must have been no or only minimal neurologic deficit in the TND before the attack. All included patients were steroid nonresponsive; that is, they had no or only trivial improvement of their symptoms after a course of high dose intravenous (IV) methylprednisolone (MP) (7 mg/kg/day, or equivalent high-dose parenteral corticosteroid treatment) lasting at least 5 days. With regard to neurologic deficit duration, participation required a minimum of 21 days from onset, 14 days from the onset of intravenous MP therapy, or 12 days from onset if the deficit continued to worsen after 5 full days of intravenous steroid treatment. Treatment success was measured as a functionally important change (change in one functional system of EDSS), and not a 1-point EDSS change. In cases in which the EDSS was insensitive to the neurologic deficit (e.g., cognitive dysfunction, aphasia), a global assessment by two masked evaluators was performed. If there was not sufficient clinical evidence for a confident clinical diagnosis of IIDD, or only evidence of a single brain lesion, a brain biopsy was performed.

The mean EDSS score was 7.5 ± 1.8, with an estimated EDSS change of more than 6 points.[4] The majority of the patients had a first demyelinating event (90%), and the rest had RRMS.[31] No MRI inclusion criteria were required. Based on previous experience in MS,[32-34] Weinshenker and colleagues[4] performed a randomized, crossover clinical trial of TPE in these patients with type I catastrophic attacks in MS or IIDD. The primary outcome in this study was moderate to marked (functionally important) improvement in TND, and only patients who failed to improve in TND during the first treatment period were eligible for crossover. Seven treatments of TPE (continuous flow centrifugation) were performed over 14 days, with a TPE every other day (about 1.1 plasma volumes, or 54 mL/kg). For statistical analysis, a z-score approach was performed, with a one-sided rank-sum test to look for differences in the distribution of z-scores between TPE and sham treatment arms.[4]

In the active TPE arm during the first treatment period, 5 of 11 patients improved, compared with 1 of 11 in the sham treatment arm.[4] After crossover, no further improvement was observed in the 6 TPE nonresponders. In the sham exchange group, there were 10 patients for whom the initial treatment failed, of whom 2 died (1 from pulmonary embolus, and 1, who was found to have ADEM on postmortem examination, from progressive intracranial pressure and herniation). After crossover, 5 of the final 8 patients remained in treatment failure, and 3 experienced a moderate to marked clinical improvement. TPE overall was well tolerated, and the most common adverse event was transient (resolving over 1 month) and asymptomatic anemia, which occurred in most patients and was severe (hemoglobin < 8 g/dL) in 4. In a post hoc analysis of 19 TPE-treated and biopsied patients with a "fulminant" attack,[31] 10 were found to be TPE responders. All 10 responders had pattern II MS lesions according to the classification of Lucchinetti and associates,[35] whereas the 3 patients with pattern I and the 6 with pattern III lesions were all nonresponders.

Differences between lesion patterns were recently characterized further by Marik and colleagues,[36] who observed in 8 postmortem cases of catastrophic MS a role of innate immunity in the formation of hypoxia-like demyelinating lesions (pattern III).

A recent French multicenter study[37] used clinical inclusion criteria similar to those proposed by the Mayo Clinic for "catastrophic" MS,[3] but in addition a marker of MRI activity. Thirty patients with catastrophic MS at disease onset were treated with mitoxantrone. Catastrophic MS was defined as either a severe attack (scenario I catastrophic MS according to Weinshenker[3]; $n = 3$) or a rapidly aggressive MS course (Weinshenker's scenario II catastrophic MS, specifying two attacks in 3 months or three attacks in 6 months with severe neurologic deficits; $n = 27$).

USE OF MITOXANTRONE AND CYCLOPHOSPHAMIDE IN RAPIDLY WORSENING MULTIPLE SCLEROSIS WITH OR WITHOUT SUPERIMPOSED RELAPSES (TYPE II CATASTROPHIC MULTIPLE SCLEROSIS)

Experience with Cyclophosphamide

In their prototypical paper, Weinstock-Guttman and coworkers[2] reported on 17 consecutive patients with "fulminant" RRMS not responsive to either steroids or IFN-beta who had a rapid, continuous neurologic decline with EDSS score deterioration of at least 1.5 during 3 to 6 months of observation. They were treated with IV cyclophosphamide (CTX) pulse therapy (500 mg/m^2) combined with 1 g IV methylprednisolone (MP) for 5 days. There were 9 women and 7 men; mean disease duration was 9 ± 7.4 years; all patients had an EDSS score greater than 6 (and 10 of 17 had a score ≥ 8); 16 patients had SPMS and 1 had PPMS. At 12-month follow-up, 4 of the 17 patients were clinically stable, and 9 had clinically improved by 1 EDSS point or better. Five of 10 nonambulatory patients (EDSS score ≥ 8) improved to an EDSS score of 6.5 or better. CTX in general was well tolerated, and the most common adverse events were nausea, leukopenia, and alopecia.

Experience with Mitoxantrone

Our group[37] recently reported on 30 mitoxantrone-treated cases of malignant MS (3 corresponding to type I and 27 to type II catastrophic MS). There were 21 women and 9 men (mean age, 29.6 ± 8 years), with a mean disease duration of 5.7 months (range, 2 weeks to 12 months). Patients who had a clinical presentation compatible with neuromyelitis optica were excluded. Treatment response after high-dose intravenous steroids had to be either absent or negligible, and after steroid treatment the residual neurologic deficit had to be at least EDSS 2. Mitoxantrone had to be considered as the first-line drug within the first 12 months after disease onset. The mean dose of intravenous MP before mitoxantrone treatment was 11.2 ± 6 g (range, 3 to 30 g).

Sixty percent of the patients received six intravenous infusions, 1 month apart, of 20 mg IV mitoxantrone (M) combined with 1 g IV methylprednisolone (MP) (M/MP therapy). Seven patients (23%) had three courses of M/MP, given 1 month apart, followed by monthly mitoxantrone infusions. Five patients (17%) received between three and five monthly infusions of M/MP. The mean cumulative mitoxantrone dose was 107 ± 24 mg. Almost 80% of the patients received a maintenance therapy within 6 months: 19 patients received IFN-beta, 1 CTX, 2 glatiramer acetate, and 1 mycophenolate mofetil. In addition, at least two of the three following MRI features (brain or spinal cord) were present on an MRI scan performed within 4 weeks before initiation of mitoxantrone therapy: (1) at least 10 T2-weighted lesions, (2) presence of large lesions (diameter > 2 cm), and (3) at least 5 gadolinium-enhancing lesions (or one big gadolinium-enhancing lesion).

Regarding the 27 cases of catastrophic MS (type II) with severe relapses, there were 9 patients with at least two severe relapses in the 3-month period before mitoxantrone treatment, 16 with at least three severe relapses in the 6 months prior to the mitoxantrone treatment period, and 2 with two severe relapses in the 4 to 5 months before mitoxantrone treatment. A total of 87 severe relapses in all 30 patients with catastrophic MS (type I or type II) were noted in the 6 months before mitoxantrone treatment began, but in the 12 months after mitoxantrone there were only 10 relapses. Annualized relapse rates were 6.0 ± 2 before mitoxantrone and 0.3 ± 0.7 thereafter. Twenty-four of the 30 patients had no further relapse after mitoxantrone treatment. Mean EDSS scores were 4.8 ± 1.5 (30 of 30 patients) at month 0 (before mitoxantrone treatment) and 2.9 ± 1.6 (29 of 30 patients) after treatment. EDSS scores improved after mitoxantrone treatment in 26 patients, remained stable in 1, and deteriorated despite mitoxantrone treatment in 3. Regarding MRI results, 29 of 30 patients had gadolinium-enhancing lesions: 7 of the 29 (24%) had more than 10, 5 (17%) had between 6 and 10, and 17 (59%) had between 1 and 5 gadolinium-enhancing lesions. After mitoxantrone treatment, 5 patients (17%) continued to have gadolinium-enhancing lesions, compared with 29 patients (97%) before treatment.

Use of Mitoxantrone, Alemtuzumab, and Cyclophosphamide in Aggressive Multiple Sclerosis

USE OF MITOXANTRONE IN AGGRESSIVE MULTIPLE SCLEROSIS

Inclusion criteria for the French-British mitoxantrone trial[1] in patients with "very active/aggressive" RRMS and SPMS required not only clinical evidence (relapse rate and EDSS deterioration in the 12-month before treatment initiation) but also MRI activity at two or more time points prior to study entry. Study inclusion was performed with a two-step selection: first clinically, and then according to MRI criteria. Patients had clinically definite MS by the Poser criteria,[5] were between 18 and 45 years of age, and had a disease duration of less than 10 years. With regard to the clinical activity, they had had either at least two relapses with sequelae within the previous 12 months (RRMS) or progression of 2 points on the EDSS over the same period (SPMS). Definitions of RRMS and SPMS were compatible with those of Lublin and Reingold[29]; all patients had to be ambulant (EDSS ≤ 6). Regarding steroid treatment, at the time of selection RRMS patients had not had "an intensive steroid therapy" for at least 1 month and no immunosuppressive therapy within the past 3 months. There was a 2-month baseline MRI period with three scans (at months −2, −1, and 0) with MRI performed before and after gadolinium injection. During the MRI baseline period, all patients received 1 g MP after the monthly MRI scan. Only patients who developed at least one active MRI lesion during the baseline period were randomized. This approach should increase the chances to recruit selectively those patients with "aggressive" MS who have both clinical and MRI evidence of active focal inflammatory pathology. It is important to note that only about half of the patients satisfying the clinical criteria for "aggressive" MS fulfilled also the required MRI inclusion criteria: 43 (51%) of the 85 patients who fulfilled the clinical inclusion criteria were excluded from the study—36 because they had no new lesion on their baseline MRI and 7 for other reasons (3 for abnormalities on echocardiography, 3 for clinical adverse events before the start of the study, and 1 for severe relapse before start that precluded study participation). Similar inclusion criteria were used in an observational study of 100 consecutive cases of aggressive MS.[30]

Again, the M/MP treatment regimen consisted of intravenous infusions of 20 mg mitoxantrone (M) combined with 1g methylprednisolone (MP) each month for 6 months (total of six infusions and total cumulative dose of 120 mg mitoxantrone). In the British-French trial,[1] a significant treatment effect was observed in regard to the primary end point, the proportion of patients by treatment group without new gadolinium-enhancing MRI lesions (Table 16-2). Treatment benefits were also observed on two secondary end points, the mean number of new gadolinium-enhancing lesions at month 6 ($P < .001$) and the mean number of new T2 lesions from baseline to the end of treatment ($P < .05$). Globally, there was an 85% reduction of new lesions in the M/MP group. Unblinded clinical assessments of the patients

TABLE 16–2 Principal Efficacy Criteria of Mitoxantrone in Patients with Aggressive Multiple Sclerosis*

	Mitoxantrone Group (*n* = 21)	Control Group (*n* = 21)	*P* value	% Reduction in Relation to Controls
Clinical outcome criteria (unblinded)				
Relapse rate	0.33	1.47	<.001	–81
Patients without a relapse (%)	66	33	<.001	
Number of relapses treated with steroids	5	19	<.01	–80
Increase in disability (no. patients)	1	6	<.01	–84
Clinical improvement (no. patients)	12	3	<.01	
Change in EDSS score (points)	–1.1	+0.1	<.05	
MRI outcome criteria (blinded)—primary outcomes of study				
Patients without new lesions at month 6 (%)	90	30	<.001	66
Number of new or enlarging T2-weighted lesions (mean)	1.1	5.5	<.05	80
Cumulative number of gadolinium-enhanced lesions at month 6 (mean)	1.2	5.6	<.001	84
No. gadolinium-enhancing lesions at month 6 (mean)	0.1	2.9	<.001	97

EDSS, Enhanced Disability Status Scale; MRI, magnetic resonance imaging.
*French multicenter study (study duration: 6 mo).
From Edan G, Miller D, Clanet M, et al: Therapeutic effect of mitoxantrone combined with methylprednisolone in multiple sclerosis: A randomised multicentre study of active disease using MRI and clinical criteria. J Neurol Neurosurg Psychiatry 1997;62:112-118.

showed a benefit for mitoxantrone recipients: Improvements in mean EDSS scores from month 0 to months 2 through 6 were significant for mitoxantrone recipients (all $P < .05$); in contrast, the MP recipients generally deteriorated. During the 2-month baseline period, the M/MP and MP recipients had annualized relapse rates of 3.1 and 2.9, respectively, similar to their rates for the 12 months preceding therapy (3.1 and 2.4, respectively). During the treatment period, there were fewer relapses in the M/MP group than in the MP group (7 versus 31 relapses). This effect was even more pronounced during the last 4 months of treatment (1 versus 19 relapses). During the treatment period, the proportion of patients free of exacerbations was 67% in the M/MP group and 33% in the MP group. Regarding adverse events, mitoxantrone was well tolerated overall. Minor and transient alopecia occurred in 7 patients (all in the M/MP group). Eight of 15 women (all in the M/MP group) developed amenorrhea between months 2 and 6. Amenorrhea was transient for 7 of these women and persistent for 1 woman aged 44 years. As expected, all patients in the M/MP group experienced pronounced neutropenia, which began 2 weeks after injection but resolved within a few days. At the next monthly injection, minor leukopenia was noted in 4 patients and did not require a dose adjustment. Nine patients received concomitant treatment for nausea. There was no evidence of cardiotoxicity or serious side effects.

Long-term efficacy of mitoxantrone was assessed in 100 patients with aggressive RRMS who received treatment with mitoxantrone as induction therapy monthly for 6 months and were monitored for up to 5 years.[30] During the first year after mitoxantrone start, the annual relapse rate was reduced by 91%, 78% of patients remained relapse free, MRI activity was reduced by 89%, the mean EDSS score decreased by 1.2 points ($p < .10^{-6}$), and 64% of patients improved by 1 point or more on the EDSS. At a longer term (up to 5 years), the reduction in annual relapse rate was sustained (0.29 to 0.42 relapses), the median time to first relapse was 2.8 years, and disability remained improved. Younger age and lower EDSS score at mitoxantrone start were predictive of better treatment response. Three patients experienced an asymptomatic decrease of the left ventricular ejection fraction (LEVF) less than 50% (1 reversible). One patient was diagnosed with acute myeloid leukemia, underwent successful treatment, and was in remission 5 years after diagnosis. In the French consortium open-label study[38] of 802 (MS) consecutive MS patients treated with mitoxantrone (mean cumulative dose: M = 70 mg/m^2), acute leukemia was diagnosed in 2 patients (0.25% incidence), 20 and 22 months after initiation of mitoxantrone treatment. Over a mean follow-up of 5 ± 1.5 years, 1 patient (a 54-year-old woman) was diagnosed with cardiac heart failure. LVEF was tested at baseline and during follow-up in 789 of the 802 patients and was less than 50% in 35 patients (4.4%). In 20 of these 35 patients, mitoxantrone was stopped, and in 15 of the 35, reduced LEVF developed 9 to 64 months after mitoxantrone cessation.[38]

USE OF ALEMTUZUMAB IN AGGRESSIVE MULTIPLE SCLEROSIS

The Cambridge group[39,40] reported their experience of alemtuzumab (ALEM) in 58 MS patients (36 with SPMS and 22 with RRMS). Of particular interest was the RRMS group and their treatment responsiveness to ALEM. For the 22 RRMS patients, disease duration ranged from 9 months to 12 years (mean, 2.7 ± 2.9 years). Seventeen RRMS patients were drug naïve (disease duration, 9 to 41 months; mean, 1.7 ± 0.9 years). In these 17 patients, the annualized relapse rate was 2.8/year (with a rate of 3.4 relapses per patient in the 12-month period before ALEM start), and their EDSS scores increased by 2.1 ± 2.0 points (range, 0 to 7.5 points) during the 12 months before treatment. The remaining 5 RRMS patients had experienced IFN-beta treatment failure (disease duration, 17 months to 12 years; mean, 6.3 ± 4.9 years). The EDSS increase in this group during the 12 months before ALEM treatment was 2.4 ± 2.3 (range, 0 to 5.5), and the relapse rate was 2.0/patient. Sustained increase in disability was measured and defined as an increase in the EDSS score of at least 1.0 point on consecutive examinations over 6 months for EDSS baseline scores lower than 6.0 (or 0.5 points for baseline scores > 6.0). After treatment with ALEM, the relapse rate dropped by 91% (annualized relapse rate, 0.19/patient), and the annualized EDSS change was reduced by 2.36. At 1 year after treatment, 16 of the 22 RRMS patients had improved their EDSS scores, and 5 were stable. At 2 years, 14 of those patients were re-examined, of whom 13 showed sustained improvement.[40]

USE OF CYCLOPHOSPHAMIDE IN AGGRESSIVE MULTIPLE SCLEROSIS

Khan and co-authors[41] reported findings in 14 patients with rapidly deteriorating RRMS (>3 points EDSS progression during the 12 months before initiation of pulsed CTX therapy) unresponsive to either immunomodulatory drugs or steroids. Reggio and colleagues[42] performed pulsed CTX in 30 patients with active and deteriorating RRMS unresponsive to INF-beta (defined as the occurrence, over the 12 months prior to study entry, of at least two relapses, or a severe relapse with EDSS worsening of >2 points in any functional system, or EDSS deterioration of at least 1.5 points while receiving IFN-beta). MRI activity criteria were reported but were not part of the inclusion criteria. Mean age was 33 ± 8 years, and disease duration was 8 ± 4 years. The EDSS score at study entry was 2.6 ± 1.23, and the duration of prior INF-beta treatment was 60 ± 23 months. Both of these open-label studies[41,42] reported significant clinical improvement in their patients with pulsed CTX treatment (monthly from 500 mg/m^2 to 1500 mg/m^2 for 24 months) regarding both EDSS score and relapse rate.

Conclusion

In determining a management strategy for aggressive MS, one should consider the following:

1. Make sure that the diagnosis of aggressive MS is correct.
2. "Aggressive" MS is defined as either of the following:
   a. Two relapses over the preceding 12 months, both causing residual deficits, and one new gadolinium-enhancing lesion on an MRI scan performed less than 3 months ago.
   b. A 2-point EDSS progression during the preceding 12 months and one new gadolinium-enhancing lesion on an MRI scan performed less than 3 months ago.
3. For type I catastrophic MS, consider TPE as first-line treatment (if there is no response, then consider mitoxantrone); for type II catastrophic MS, consider mitoxantrone as first-line treatment (if no response, then consider CTX).
4. In our experience, the first-line treatment for aggressive MS should be M/MP, consisting of monthly intravenous infusions of mitoxantrone (12 mg/m^2; maximum dose, 20 mg) combined with 1 g MP over a period of 6 months (total of six infusions; total cumulative dose of mitoxantrone, 120 mg); mitoxantrone is approved for this indication in France and for worsening MS in the United States and some European countries.
5. If mitoxantrone fails, consider other off-label treatments, such as ALEM,[39,40] CTX,[2,41,42] or TPE.[33]
6. Once response has been achieved, consider maintenance therapy with IFN-beta or glatiramer acetate.
7. In aggressive MS, 6 months of M/MP treatment had a significant effect on both clinical and MRI activity variables,[1] and 5-year follow-up data on 100 consecutive cases of mitoxantrone-treated aggressive RRMS suggested that mitoxantrone had a sustained long-term beneficial effect.[30]

REFERENCES

1. Edan G, Miller D, Clanet M, et al: Therapeutic effect of mitoxantrone combined with methylprednisolone in multiple sclerosis: A randomised multicentre study of active disease using MRI and clinical criteria. J Neurol Neurosurg Psychiatry 1997;62:112-118.
2. Weinstock-Guttman B, Kinkel R, Cohen J, et al: Treatment of fulminant multiple sclerosis with intravenous cyclophosphamide. Neurologist 1997;3:178-185.
3. Weinshenker BG, Rodriquez M: Treatment of catastrophic multiple sclerosis. In McDonald WI, Noseworthy J, eds: Multiple Sclerosis 2. Blue Book Series. Philadelphia, Butterworth Heinemann, 2001.
4. Weinshenker BG, O'Brien PC, Petterson TM, et al: A randomized trial of plasma exchange in acute central nervous system inflammatory demyelinating disease. Ann Neurol 1999;46:878-886.
5. Poser CM, Paty DW, Scheinberg L, et al: New diagnostic criteria for multiple sclerosis: Guidelines for research protocols. Ann Neurol 1983;13:227-231.
6. Polman CH, Reingold SC, Edan G, et al: Diagnostic criteria for multiple sclerosis: 2005 Revisions to the "McDonald Criteria.". Ann Neurol 2005;58:840-846.
7. Confavreux C, Compston A: The cause and course of multiple sclerosis: The natural history of multiple sclerosis. In Compston A, Confavreaux C, Lassman H, et al (eds): McAlpine's Multiple Sclerosis, 4th ed. London, Churchill Livingstone Elsevier, 2006, pp 183-269.
8. Neuhaus A, Güntner M, Morrissey SP: Risk factors for conversion to multiple sclerosis in patients with a clinically isolated syndrome. Presented at the 23rd Congress of the European Committee for the Treatment and Research in Multiple Sclerosis (ECTRIMS). Prague, Czech Republic, October 2007.
9. O'Connor PW, Goodman A, Willmer-Hulme AJ, et al: Natalizumab Multiple Sclerosis Trial Group: Randomized multicenter trial of natalizumab in acute MS relapses: Clinical and MRI effects. Neurology 2004;62:2038-2043.
10. Lublin FD, Baier M, Cutter G: Effect of relapses on development of residual deficit in multiple sclerosis. Neurology 2003;61:1528-1532.
11. Weinshenker B: Plasma exchange for severe attacks of demyelinating disease of the central nervous system. In Kappos L, Johnson K, Kesselring J, Radu E (eds): Multiple Sclerosis: Tissue Destruction and Repair. London, Martin Dunitz, 2001, pp 267-274.
12. Kurtzke JF: Course of exacerbations of multiple sclerosis in hospitalized patients. AMA Arch Neurol Psychiatry 1956;76:175-184.
13. Kurtzke JF, Beebe GW, Nagler B, et al: Studies on the natural history of multiple sclerosis: 7. Correlates of clinical change in an early bout. Acta Neurol Scand 1973;49:379-395.
14. Weinshenker BG, Bass B, Rice GP, et al: The natural history of multiple sclerosis: A geographically based study. I: Clinical course and disability. Brain 1989;112(Pt 1):133-146.
15. Rindfleisch E: Histologisches Detail zur grauen Degeneration von Gehirn und Rückenmark. Arch Pathol Anat Physiol Klin Med (Virchow) 1863;26:474-483.
16. Marburg O: Die sogenannte "akute Multiple Sklerose" (Encephalomyelitis periaxialis scleroticans). Jahrb Psychiatrie 1906;27:211-312.
17. Guillain G, Alajouanine T: La forme aigue de la sclerose en plaques. Bulletin de l'Académie de la Médecine (Paris) 1928;99:366-376.
18. Müller R: Studies in disseminated sclerosis. Acta Med Scand 1949;133;(Suppl 222):1-214.
19. Kolb LC: The social significance of multiple sclerosis. Res Publ Assoc Res Nerv Ment Dis 1950;28:28-43.
20. Runmarker B, Andersen O: Prognostic factors in a multiple sclerosis incidence cohort with twenty-five years of follow-up. Brain 1993;116(Pt 1):117-134.
21. Poser S, Kurtzke JF, Poser W, et al: Survival in multiple sclerosis. J Clin Epidemiol 1989;42: 159-168.
22. Broman T, Andersen O, Bergmann L: Clinical studies on multiple sclerosis: I. Presentation of an incidence material from Gothenburg. Acta Neurol Scand 1981;63:6-33.
23. Confavreux C, Aimard G, Devic M: Course and prognosis of multiple sclerosis assessed by the computerized data processing of 349 patients. Brain 1980;103:281-300.
24. Percy AK, Nobrega FT, Okazaki H, et al: Multiple sclerosis in Rochester, Minn.: A 60-year appraisal. Arch Neurol 1971;25:105-111.
25. Leray E, Morrissey SP, Yaouanq J, et al: Long-term survival of patients with multiple sclerosis in West France. Mult Scler 2007;13:865-874.
26. Rüiise T, Grønning M, Aarli JA, et al: Prognostic factors for life expectancy in multiple sclerosis analysed by Cox-models. J Clin Epidemiol 1988;41:1031-1036.

27. Poser S: Multiple Sclerosis: An Analysis of 812 Cases by Means of Electronic Data Processing. Berlin, Springer, 1978.
28. Bauer HJ, Firnhaber W, Winkler W: Prognostic criteria in multiple sclerosis. Ann N Y Acad Sci 1965;122:542-551.
29. Lublin FD, Reingold SC: Defining the clinical course of multiple sclerosis: Results of an international survey. National Multiple Sclerosis Society (USA) Advisory Committee on Clinical Trials of New Agents in Multiple Sclerosis. Neurology 1996;46:907-911.
30. Le Page E, Leray E, Taurin G, et al: Mitoxantrone as induction treatment in aggressive relapsing remitting multiple sclerosis: Treatment response factors in a 5 year follow-up observational study of 100 consecutive patients. J Neurol Neurosurg Psychiatry 2008;79:52-56.
31. Keegan M, König F, McClelland R, et al: Relation between humoral pathological changes in multiple sclerosis and response to therapeutic plasma exchange. Lancet 2005;366:579-582.
32. Rodriguez M, Karnes WE, Bartleson JD, et al: Plasmapheresis in acute episodes of fulminant CNS inflammatory demyelination. Neurology 1993;43:1100-1104.
33. Weinshenker BG, Keegan BM: Therapeutic plasma exchange. In Cohen JA, Rudick RA (eds): Multiple Sclerosis Therapeutics. London, Martin Dunitz, 2007, pp 551-567.
34. Weiner HL, Dau PC, Khatri BO, et al: Double-blind study of true vs. sham plasma exchange in patients treated with immunosuppression for acute attacks of multiple sclerosis. Neurology 1989;39:1143-1149.
35. Lucchinetti C, Brück W, Parisi J, et al: Heterogeneity of multiple sclerosis lesions: Implications for the pathogenesis of demyelination. Ann Neurol 2000;47:707-717.
36. Marik C, Felts PA, Bauer J, et al: Lesion genesis in a subset of patients with multiple sclerosis: A role for innate immunity? Brain 2007;130(Pt 11):2800-2815.
37. Ory S, Debouverie M, Le Page E, et al: [Use of mitoxantrone in early multiple sclerosis with malignant disease course: Observational study in 30 patients with clinical and MRI outcomes after one year.] Rev Neurol (Paris) 2008, Jun 9 [Epub ahead of print].
38. Le Page E, Leray E, Brochet B, et al: Long-term safety profile of mitoxantrone in a French cohort of 802 multiple sclerosis patients: Final report. Presented at the 22nd Congress of the European Committee for the Treatment and Research in Multiple Sclerosis (ECTRIMS), Madrid, September 2006.
39. Coles AJ, Wing MG, Molyneux P, et al: Monoclonal antibody treatment exposes three mechanisms underlying the clinical course of multiple sclerosis. Ann Neurol 1999;46:296-304.
40. Coles AJ, Cox A, Le Page E, et al: The window of therapeutic opportunity in multiple sclerosis: Evidence from monoclonal antibody therapy. J Neurol 2006;253:98-108.
41. Khan OA, Zvartau-Hind M, Caon C, et al: Effect of monthly intravenous cyclophosphamide in rapidly deteriorating multiple sclerosis patients resistant to conventional therapy. Mult Scler 2001;7:185-188.
42. Reggio E, Nicoletti A, Fiorilla T, et al: The combination of cyclophosphamide plus interferon beta as rescue therapy could be used to treat relapsing-remitting multiple sclerosis patients: Twenty-four months follow-up. J Neurol 2005;252:1255-1261.

17 Symptomatic Therapy in Multiple Sclerosis

ANJALI SHAH • SCOTT L. DAVIS • ANGELA BATES • GARY E. LEMACK • TERESA C. FROHMAN • ELLIOT M. FROHMAN

Multiple sclerosis (MS) is the most common disabling neurologic disease of young adults.[1] Making the diagnosis of MS is often challenging, but one could argue that the challenge really begins after the diagnosis is established and treatment begins. MS is a complex disease, and patients can experience a wide variety of symptoms that can affect their ability to carry out normal activities of daily living (ADLs). Although a myriad of symptoms can afflict MS patients, the most commonly reported ones involve visual disturbances, fatigue, heat intolerance, spasticity, and bladder dysfunction. Attempts to improve the quality of life of MS patients should incorporate not only disease-modifying therapies but should a course of action for global multidisciplinary management focused on quality of life and functional capabilities.

In this chapter, the most common issues that MS patients face are discussed and recommendations are given for the evaluation and management for each.

The information presented should serve as a useful reference for clinicians in their care of patients and families who live with MS.

Neuro-ophthalmology

VISUAL SYMPTOMS

The disease process in MS has a high predilection for affecting the anterior visual apparatus, producing one of the most characteristic syndromes associated with the disorder, acute inflammatory optic neuritis (ON).[2,3] Rarely, inflammation can also involve the anterior segments of the eye, culminating in various forms of uveitis (anterior, intermediate, and posterior). Involvement of the afferent visual system produces a number of symptoms related to abnormal processing of the information that is ultimately transmitted to the higher cortical centers for visual perception. The efferent visual system is organized for coordination of the two eyes during steady fixation and eye movements. The principal goal of the efferent system is the achievement of foveation, stereoscopy, and depth perception. The disease process in MS often targets central nervous system (CNS) circuitries that disrupt eye movements. Ocular motility disorders in MS are generally the consequence of periventricular inflammation within the brainstem tegmentum (ventral to the fourth ventricle or cerebral aqueduct).[3] In this section, we describe the afferent and efferent neuro-ophthalmologic hallmarks of MS and their associated symptoms. We underscore the various therapeutic interventions that have been used to mitigate what often are perceived by patients as highly stress-provoking and often disabling visual and vestibular concomitants of the MS disease process.

OPTIC NEUROPATHY

Acute ON represents one of the signature clinical syndromes of MS, affecting about two thirds of patients at some point during their clinical history.[2,3] In those with a first clinically isolated demyelinating syndrome, ON is the forme fruste in about 20% to 40% of patients. Patients typically describe the onset symptoms as evolving acutely to subacutely, and they describe diminished vision, which can range from mild changes to complete blindness. As demonstrated in the Optic Neuritis Treatment Trial (ONTT), more than 90% of patients with ON describe pain in the affected side or sides, which can manifest in a variety of ways.[4-7] For instance, the discomfort can be perceived as dull and aching, focally lancinating, or pressure-like, particularly with movement of the globe.

Visual loss from ON can involve compromises in high- and low-contrast acuity and sensitivity, color desaturation, and visual field deficits.[2] An important and conspicuous outcome of the ONTT was the observation that, despite previous and long-held assumptions about the predominant association of specific field abnormalities with acute ON, any field defect can be related to the syndrome.[7] A number of visual illusions can be associated with acute ON and its aftermath, including microsomia and macrosomia, scintillations, phosphenes, and light sensitivity changes.

Optic nerve inflammation in ON typically occurs unilaterally in adults (in approximately 70% of patients), in a retrobulbar distribution.[2] In children, ON is not uncommonly bilateral and anterior in distribution, resulting in funduscopic evidence of disc swelling (also known as papillitis).[8] Bedside examination by the neurologist should include pinhole corrected high-contrast visual acuity, visual fields by confrontation, an attempt to assess color saturation (we use Ishihara plates), assessment of pupillary light reflexes, and an attempt to reveal a relative afferent pupillary defect (RAPD).[2,3] Further, careful funduscopic examination must be completed to exclude other etiologies. The most common finding on fundus examination in a typical case of retrobulbar ON is the presence of normal anatomy; hence, the adage, "The patient sees nothing and the doctor sees nothing." When the distribution of inflammation is more anterior, then acute fundus changes can include disc margin obscuration, disc elevation, hyperemic retinal vasculature, and even retinal hemorrhages.

A fully developed case of anterior ON is referred to as papillitis and can easily mimic the funduscopic features of papilledema (differentiating these two conditions has obvious implications for rendering a correct diagnosis and treatment plan). Chronic fundus changes include pallor of the optic disc (principally from astrogliosis) and atrophy. Studies have confirmed that, after acute ON, most patients lose axons and ganglion cell neurons in the retina (with temporal quadrant predilection) over a period of about 3 to 6 months and that such structural changes are associated with visual deficits (acuity, low-contrast acuity, visual fields, and color).[9-12] Recently, axonal and neurodegenerative processes in the retina have been shown to parallel corresponding changes in brain parenchymal fraction measures (i.e., brain atrophy) within the same patients.[13] There also appears to be a relationship between severity of retinal changes and MS subtypes.[14] Once the diagnosis of acute ON has been confirmed, treatment can be initiated, typically with high-dose corticosteroids.[2,5,15] The ONTT demonstrated that high-dose intravenous methylprednisolone at 1 g daily (i.e., 250 mg IV every 6 hours) for 3 days, followed by an 11-day oral prednisone taper, resulted in reduced pain, hastened visual recovery, and reduced the risk of subsequent demyelinating events (by about 50%) for up to 2 years; however, there has been great controversy concerning the use of other steroid preparations, the appropriate dose, the need for tapering, and the route of administration.[5,15] To date there continues to be little evidence to support the application of one regimen over another, except that there does appear to be consensus concerning the use of high-dose regimens for ON and other acute exacerbations of MS.[15]

After acute ON, many patients experience some persistent, albeit less severe, visual symptoms. Some recognize a difference in acuity or color perception in the affected eye compared with the fellow eye. Patients may describe problems with brightness sensitivity and glare in conditions of high ambient lighting. Chronic pain is rare after acute ON and should prompt a search for an alternative or additional cause.

The goal in treating chronic visual symptoms is primarily to optimize function and reduce discomfort. Therefore, it is important for all patients with persistent visual complaints to be seen by an ophthalmologist or optometrist to ensure that maximum refraction can be achieved. It is helpful to recognize that myopia, emerging presbyopia, astigmatisms, and anisometropia (different corrections across the two eyes) can be corrected, at least partially, if identified. Such corrections not only help to optimize function but also can reduce eye strain–induced headaches (asthenopia). Measures of intraocular pressure and slit-lamp examination should be performed to assess for any evidence of emerging glaucoma and cataracts, two conditions that MS patients are more likely to develop given their not infrequent use of corticosteroids for disease-related exacerbations. For those with light sensitivity and sluggishly reacting pupils, high-quality sunglasses can be very helpful.

In addition to acute ON, most MS patients develop chronic and often occult changes in the retina and optic nerve.[9-14] Such changes occur even in the absence of a history of acute ON, very much analogous to the subclinical lesions and atrophy that develop in the brain of MS patients.[10] At autopsy, axonal and neurodegeneration within the retina can be demonstrated in almost all MS patients.[16,17] Given the insidiously slow course of chronic optic neuropathy, many patients do not perceive any visual deficits or report that "something is not quite right with my vision, but it's hard to describe."

With respect to disease-modifying therapy for optic neuropathies, certainly any agents that can reduce the risk and severity of MS exacerbations will confer potential benefits on the anterior visual system and its high predilection for attack. Recently, natalizumab, a novel treatment for relapsing forms of MS, was shown to exert a potentially neuroprotective effect on vision, compared with placebo, in a phase I randomized controlled trial.[18] This study involved serial measures of low-contrast letter acuity performance, a validated assessment that sensitively reflects visual function. Natalizumab-treated patients performed significantly better over time on this test, compared with placebo-treated patients. We now know that low-contrast letter acuity performance directly predicts the structural integrity of the retinal nerve fiber layer.[10] For instance, for every line of low-contrast visual acuity that is lost, there is a corresponding reduction in the average retinal nerve fiber layer thickness by 4 to 6 μm, as measured by optical coherence tomography.[10]

UVEITIS

In a minority of MS patients, inflammatory mechanisms target the uveal tract (anterior uveitis), vitreous, or retinal vessels (posterior uveitis).[3] In the latter variety, mononuclear cell trafficking leads to perivenular phlebitis. Uveitis can be challenging to confirm at the bedside with the basic ophthalmoscope. Many of the most characteristic lesions tend to be located in the peripheral retina, making confirmation by the examiner using a direct ophthalmoscope a formidable challenge.

EYE MOVEMENT ABNORMALITIES

Eye movement abnormalities produce some of the most frequent and disabling symptoms in MS.[3] The circuitry that is involved in the final integration of signaling pathways for saccades, smooth pursuit, and vestibular ocular reflexes is localized to the tegmentum of the brainstem just ventral to the fourth ventricle (at the medulla and pons) and the cerebral aqueduct (midbrain).[3] These periventricular tract systems are at high risk for being affected by inflammatory demyelination.

The most common abnormality of ocular motility is internuclear ophthalmoparesis (INO), which is characterized by slowing of the adducting eye during horizontal saccades. An INO is the result of a lesion within the medial longitudinal fasciculus (MLF) located in the dorsomedial brainstem tegmentum.[19-21] Saccades are used when gazing at a new visual target (as with reading or scanning a picture) and during fast reset of the eyes after a vestibular ocular reflex (as with head or body turning while walking or driving). Those with INO have a reduced synchronization of binocular movements; this produces a position discrepancy between the eyes that can result in double vision and the illusion of environmental movement (i.e., oscillopsia). The transient loss of coordinated eye movements also compromises accurate foveation (visual processing of information) and depth perception. The abducting eye in patients with INO typically exhibits nystagmus during the horizontal saccade, which also contributes to the symptom of oscillopsia and visual blur.[19,20] When the MLF lesion occurs at a rostral midbrain level, an extreme form of the syndrome can be identified, with the patient exhibiting ocular divergence (exo) of the two eyes in primary position in conjunction with bilateral INO (the so-called wall-eyed bilateral INO, or WEBINO syndrome).[3] Such patients become monocular fixators, because use of both eyes results in persistent diplopia.

Other ocular motor syndromes associated with MS include cranial nerve palsies (VI > III > IV), skew deviation (supranuclear vertical misalignment of the eyes secondary to otolithic dysfunction), all forms of nystagmus (e.g., gaze-evoked, primary position, pendular), and saccadic intrusions (e.g., square wave jerks, saccadic oscillations, flutter, and even opsoclonus in rare cases).[3] All of these abnormalities result in displacement of objects of visual interest off the fovea centralis of the macula, thereby producing "retinal slip" and a corresponding degradation in visual acuity.

Perhaps the most disabling eye movement abnormality in patients with MS is acquired pendular nystagmus.[3] This disturbance is characterized by a constant to-and-fro movement of the eyes in a number of possible planes (horizontal, vertical, rotary, or elliptical). Pendular nystagmus is variable with respect to the frequency and amplitude of the movements, but it almost always results in poor vision and reduced ability to read, as well as impairment in a number of ADLs (e.g., driving, walking, reaching for objects) and in work performance.

When ocular motor syndromes first appear in patients with relapsing MS, the primary treatment strategy is to intervene with high-dose corticosteroids.[15] With visual recovery from ON, the treatment does not appear to ultimately affect final outcome, but our experience with ocular motility disorders in MS has been quite the opposite. Rapid intervention with anti-inflammatory treatments (corticosteroids and intensive chemotherapy in those with monumental syndromes or highly disseminated and active lesions) has much more commonly aborted syndrome progression and residual PVR deficits than watchful waiting. In those with predominantly progressive MS disease, we have also observed the insidious and essentially occult evolution of these syndromes without a corresponding acute exacerbation (according to the patient). In such cases, we have not been impressed with the efficacy of corticosteroid treatment intervention to mitigate the symptoms nor to change the final disposition of the clinical signs; late treatment here is likely to be too late indeed. Once an ocular motor disturbance such as INO has persisted for a longer term (perhaps 6 months or more), the abnormality tends to be recalcitrant.[20]

When ocular motor syndromes and their associated clinical signs become chronic, we are faced with a challenging treatment dilemma. There are few therapeutic tools to apply to these often disabling syndromes. In the situation of a cranial nerve palsy or skew deviation, we can consider consulting our ophthalmology colleagues for prismatic correction to help facilitate interocular coregistration (for the primary position of gaze). However, this approach should be considered only after there is evidence to suggest that the motility defect is relatively stable (i.e., minimal worsening or recovery). In the interim, many patients with significant diplopia will use an eye patch (alternating sides to promote use of the affected eye). On occasion, we have found the use of compounded 4-aminopyridine to be beneficial in those with significant ocular slowing or limitation, particularly if the symptoms are exaggerated by exercise or exposure to heat. This agent, a potassium channel blocker that prolongs duration of the axonal action potential, is currently under intensive study for treatment of a variety of MS-related symptoms.

Nystagmus is among the most difficult symptoms to treat in MS. Over time, many patients develop compensation mechanisms that can either dampen the amplitude of the eye movement, or identify a head position (null zone) that mitigates the often-associated oscillopsia.

Among the myriad forms of nystagmus that can occur in MS, the pendular type has been, in our experience, the most disabling. The constant oscillating movements result in retinal slip and poor vision with oscillopsia of various degrees of severity. Convergence, as with near vision, can effectively reduce the amplitude and frequency of these movements in many patients, but it is not a sufficient strategy for most visual circumstances (such as eccentric or distance viewing). Prismatic corrections have been attempted to bring the eyes into some degree of convergence based on these observations. However, we have not found this to be a useful approach in most of our patients.

The most effective therapy for pendular nystagmus has been the use of memantine (10 to 20 mg three times daily as tolerated) or gabapentin (100 to 2000 mg three times daily as tolerated).[22,23] Although we have used a multitude of other membrane stabilizers (some of which do work in individual patients), these two agents have been the most effective. Although recent studies suggested that 4-aminopyridine is effective in some forms of nystagmus, particularly downbeat,[24] we have not been impressed with the application of this therapy for any form of MS-related nystagmus.

In rare circumstances, some patients have a profound misalignment of the eyes secondary to MS; we individualize the consideration for eye muscle surgery and refer such patients to specialized centers with extensive experience in those procedures.

Vestibular Dysfunction

Vestibular dysfunction is common in patients with MS. Nystagmus is often a derivative of the disease process that targets brainstem and cerebellar vestibular pathways, resulting in a variety of types of intrusion on steady gaze (whether in primary or eccentric eye positions). In many patients with nystagmus, the illusion of self or environmental (oscillopsia) movement is a reflection of true vertigo. A mismatch between centrally projecting signals (originating from the inner ear) in the brainstem results in a bias that produces a vestibular slow phase eye movement punctuated by a saccadic reset (hence, the slow and fast phases of most forms of nystagmus).

Notwithstanding the common occurrence of vestibular dysfunction related to the primary histopathology of MS, the most likely cause of vertigo in such patients is in fact the most common cause of vertigo in any clinic: benign paroxysmal positioning vertigo.[25] This syndrome relates to the dislocation of utricular macular otoconia (calcium carbonate crystals) into one of the semicircular canals (most commonly the posterior), rendering it gravity sensitive with change in head or body position. Such changes lead to migration of the otoconia within the canal and result in depolarization of neurons from the involved canal, through the eighth cranial nerve to the brainstem, and ultimately to the ocular motor nuclei innervated by the respective canal. This sequence of events results in a highly characteristic nystagmus that can be easily identified at the bedside with a number of provocative techniques (e.g., the Dix-Hallpike maneuver); it is treated effectively by attempting to reposition the otoconial mass onto the macular membrane (e.g., with the Epley maneuver).[26] The purpose of underscoring the role of benign paroxysmal positioning vertigo in MS is to highlight the selective treatment intervention for this pathophysiology in comparison to the application of corticosteroids for inflammatory demyelination.

The second most common cause of vertigo in MS is related to the development of demyelinating plaques, most commonly identified in one of two anatomic localizations—the medullary tegmentum (in the vicinity of the vestibular apparatus) and the root entry zone of cranial nerve VIII at the pontomedullary junction.[25,26] In such cases, the rapid application of high-dose corticosteroids is highly appropriate treatment. Despite the involvement of cranial nerve VIII at the root entry zone by demyelination, hearing loss is very uncommon in MS.

Neurogenic Bowel

It has been reported that between 43% and 66% of MS patients have bowel dysfunction[27-29] compared with only 2% to 15% of the general population.[30] Although bowel dysfunction is frequently experienced in our patients, it has been infrequently studied systematically. A review of this subject reported that, among some 18,000 papers published about MS over the previous 3 decades, only 30 articles pertained to bowel dysfunction.[31]

Similar to bladder dysfunction, bowel dysfunction is characterized as disorders of storage or elimination. The reduced incidence of bowel dysfunction compared with bladder dysfunction in MS patients suggests that it may be less influenced by the distribution of CNS lesions, or it may be under-recognized or under-reported, or both. In our MS clinic, constipation is the most common bowel dysfunction, followed by poor evacuation and incontinence.

The pathophysiology of constipation in MS patients is poorly understood. The gut is influenced by neural, endocrine, and luminal input and coordination. The neural system is composed of the intrinsic and extrinsic nervous systems. The intrinsic nervous system contains Meissner's and Auerbach's plexi. Although it is well recognized that neurotransmitters play a role in this process, the physiologic role of each is still unclear.[32] The extrinsic nervous system is responsible for innervations of the gut through signals from the sympathetic and parasympathetic systems.

Sympathetic innervation consists of the T5-L2 spinal levels and is largely inhibitory through noradrenergic input. Parasympathetic input is from the vagus and sacral nerves. Stimulation of the parasympathetic nervous system promotes peristalsis, blood flow to the gut, and intestinal secretion. The external sphincter receives innervations from the pudendal nerve (S2-S4). These same spinal levels are responsible for perineal sensation.

Colonic mass movements cause movement of fecal matter from the colon to the rectum via the rectosigmoid colon. Distal colon distention stimulates signals indicating the need to defecate. If it is appropriate to defecate, a series of steps occur to initiate a bowel movement. Valsalva movements increase the intra-abdominal pressure, leading to pelvic floor drop and relaxation of both the internal and external anal sphincters. Defecation then begins. If defecation is deemed inappropriate, contraction of the external anal sphincter decreases the sensation to void.

CONSTIPATION

A patient who states "I am constipated" is frequently referring to straining, hard stools, or inability to have a bowel movement.[33] Constipation is defined as fewer than three bowel movements in a week. However, stool frequency alone does not define constipation. The Rome I and Rome II classifications (Table 17-1) were developed to help standardize the definition. Stool consistency and form are described using the Bristol Stool Scale.[34]

Constipation can be caused by several factors. A review of diet and fluid intake is recommended as a first-line evaluation. Patients may limit fluid intake because

TABLE 17–1 Rome Classifications for Constipation*

Rome I Criteria (Two or more of the following present for at least 3 mo)	Rome II Criteria (Two or more of the following present in least 12 wk, which need not be consecutive, during the preceding 12 mo)
1. Straining with >1 of 4 defecations 2. Lumpy or hard stools with >1 of 4 defecations 3. Sensation of incomplete evacuation with >1 of 4 defecations 4. Two or fewer bowel movements in a week	1. Straining with >1 of 4 defecations 2. Lumpy or hard stools with >1 of 4 defecations 3. Sensation of incomplete evacuation with >1 of 4 defecations 4. Sensation of anorectal obstruction or blockage with >1 of 4 defecations 5. Manual maneuvers to facilitate evacuation with >1 of 4 defecations (e.g., digital evacuation, support of the pelvic floor) 6. <3 defecations per week
Abdominal pain is not required, loose stools are not present, and there are insufficient criteria for IBS.	Loose stools are not present, and there are insufficient criteria for IBS.

IBS, irritable bowel syndrome.

*Note: These criteria may not apply when the patient is taking laxatives.

Data from Whitehead WE, Wald A, Diamant NE, et al: Functional disorders of the anus and rectum. Gut 1999;45(Suppl 2):II55-II59, and Drossman DA: The functional gastrointestinal disorders and the Rome II process. Gut 1999;45(Suppl 2):II1-II5.

of bladder dysfunction or dysphagia. The causes may be iatrogenic, secondary to drugs used to treat spasticity, paresthesias, pain, or bladder dysfunction. Decreased physical activity and mobility can greatly affect the frequency of bowel movements. Secondary medical causes that may or may not be related to MS require screening. Evaluations for symptoms of psychiatric disorders, physical or sexual abuse, pelvic surgery, and thyroid dysfunction may be required, because these conditions have been implicated as causative factors in constipation.[35]

Several agents are available to address the various physiologic causes of constipation. Adequate treatment for constipation frequently involves a combination of modalities. Also, as the disease course changes, bowel patterns may also change, so periodic reassessment is recommended.

- *Bulking agents:* Common forms include psyllium (from the ispaghula husk), bran, and calcium polycarbophil. Fiber supplementation is necessary, but excessive amounts can cause gastrointestinal discomfort such as abdominal bloating or gas. Recommended amounts of fiber intake range from 4 to 20 g/day.[4]
- *Osmotic agents:* These commonly contain magnesium and are available as magnesium oxide and magnesium sulfate. Magnesium oxide is primarily used in mild to moderately severe constipation; it is dosed at 15 to 30 mL/day and typically causes a bowel movement in 8 hours. Magnesium sulfate is dosed similarly but can cause a more explosive bowel movement with liquid-like consistency. Magnesium sulfate should be avoided in the elderly.
- *Poorly absorbed sugars:* Lactulose, polyethylene glycol (PEG), and sorbitol are effective in patients with more chronic constipation. Lactulose is dosed at 15 to 30 mL/day and often takes 2 to 3 days for effect. Sorbitol dosing ranges from 5 to 20 mg and has been reported to be equally as efficacious as lactulose with less cost. Nausea is a common side effect of both lactulose and sorbitol. Also, lactulose has a bitter taste, whereas PEG is tasteless and odorless and therefore more tolerable. PEG is now available over the counter (MiraLax) and is approved for use in children. Dosing ranges from 17 to 36 g/day. It is provided in a powder form and can be mixed with noncarbonated beverages. The most common adverse effect with PEG is abdominal cramping.
- *Stimulants:* These agents increase intestinal motility and secretions. Common agents include senna, cascara, and castor oil. The recommended dose of senna is 187 mg in tablet or powder form per day. It works rapidly and can occasionally lose its effect if abused. Senna is generally preferred over the other stimulant agents because of better tolerability.[35]
- *Stool softeners:* Docusate sodium is dosed at two 100-mg tablets daily. Docusate sodium in combination with a stimulant (senna) quite effectively treats mild to moderate constipation in MS patients in our clinic.
- *Prokinetic agents:* Lubiprostone is a fatty acid in the prostone class. It is a chloride channel activator and increases intestinal fluid secretion. Studies of patients with chronic idiopathic constipation report that it slows gastric emptying but does improve small bowel and colonic transit times.[36,37] Lubiprostone increased the number of spontaneous bowel movements, reduced straining, and increased quality of patient satisfaction with bowel habits compared to placebo.[38] Tegaserod is a 5-hydroxytryptamine 4 ($5HT_4$) partial agonist that improves gastric emptying and colonic emptying times.[37] It was

well tolerated and effective for many patients. However, it was removed from the market in 2007 after being associated with increased risk of coronary and cerebrovascular events. Tegaserod was released for limited use in approved patients with no history of cardiovascular disease in July 2007.

- *Enemas, suppository:* Tap, saline, and soapsud enemas work quickly and effectively to soften stool and assist in expelling the contents of the rectum. Saline enemas are reported to be the safest[35] of the three. Several types of enemas are available, and physicians are encouraged to monitor which type a patient is using and with what frequency, to prevent electrolyte imbalance. A unique device combines liquefied glycerin and docusate into a small, convenient, and effective minidose enema (Enemeez). For those with rectal pain, a similar formulation that also includes the local anesthetic benzocaine (Enemeez Plus) may be used. Rectal pain can also be effectively treated by the use of belladonna and opium (B&O) Supprettes. These small, suppository-like devices are highly effective rectal analgesic agents. Bisacodyl and glycerin suppositories stimulate the rectal wall through stretch mechanisms. They are safe and effective in patients suffering from symptoms of dysphagia, nausea, or vomiting.
- Behavioral techniques or defecation training has been used in conjunction with anorectal biofeedback to reduce dependence on medications. Compliance has been limited in defecation training; however, biofeedback was effective in a small group of MS patients.[39] Patients are guided through various relaxation techniques that are aimed at increased perception of the gut in order to reduce discoordination of the various gastrointestinal signals.
- Surgery may be indicated in refractory cases, to ease caregiver burden of care or for severely debilitated patients. Often, quality of life does improve in those with colostomies, because constipation can cause pain, discomfort, and embarrassment to patients.
- If possible, physical activity is encouraged. For the patient with limited leg movement, upper or lower body ergometry is recommended. Upper body ergometry is useful in patients with limited lower limb strength. Aerobic training in the form of bicycle ergometry improved bowel function in MS patients.[40]

FECAL INCONTINENCE

Patients with bowel incontinence may be more reluctant to report symptoms to their physician than patients with constipation, because of discomfort or feelings of humiliation. About 51% of MS patients reported at least one instance of bowel incontinence is the preceding 3 months.[41] It is necessary for the clinician not only to screen for constipation but to also ask about bowel continence during routine clinical visits.

Fecal incontinence is defined as an involuntary loss of stool per rectum,[42] usually caused by reduced anal squeeze pressures. A diet and fluid history should be evaluated in the incontinent patient. As with constipation, problems with spasticity, fatigue, weakness, and impaired mobility can cause bowel continence issues.[31] Secondary causes unrelated to MS, such as infection, trauma, rectal prolapse, thyroid disorders, or severe fecal impaction, should be screened for in each patient. Consultation with a gastroenterologist is frequently necessary for further testing and evaluation. Digital rectal examination is recommended, but additional testing is frequently necessary.[31] Anal and rectal manometry, electromyography, and radiologic studies (magnetic resonance imaging, defecography, anal ultrasonography) are often required to accurately determine the cause in persistent cases.

Treatment is directed at the underlying cause. Drug therapy with loperamide can be used in patients who have chronic diarrhea with fecal incontinence. This is not recommended for patients with symptoms of diarrhea and constipation. Biofeedback training is used to improve pelvic floor muscles and rectal sensory perception. Transanal electrostimulation activates the anal canal on a fixed schedule and theoretically strengthens the pelvic floor muscles.[43,44]

Surgical repair is indicated for trauma and for medically refractory cases. Several techniques are available, including pelvic floor muscle repair, formation of a new external anal sphincter via muscle transposition, and even development of a "false" anal sphincter with the use of hydraulic rings. Fecal diversion with colostomy is used if these options fail or are not feasible.

Bowel dysfunction is a common and treatable disorder in MS patients. There remains a huge void in the MS literature regarding optimal management bowel dysfunction. The clinician is encouraged to screen, educate, assess, and counsel the patient with bowel dysfunction for maximum satisfaction with treatment.

Neurogenic Bladder

Bladder dysfunction affects between 63% and 90%.[27,28,45] of MS patients. The North American Research Committee on Multiple Sclerosis (NARCOMS) reported that patients with relapsing-remitting MS are more likely to develop bladder symptoms than those with primary progressive or secondary progressive forms.[45] Neurogenic bladder dysfunction has been reported to correlate with increased sexual dysfunction,[46-48] and also with increasing disability.[45]

The upper urinary tract consists of the ureters and renal parenchyma. Upper urinary tract abnormalities are present in about 17% of MS patients, although, in most cases, the abnormalities are subtle and likely of limited clinical impact.[49] The bladder, urethra, and urethral sphincters comprise the lower urinary tract. Continence is maintained through maintenance of a low-pressure, compliant bladder and a functioning sphincteric mechanism, all sustained by intact cerebral and spinal input via the parasympathetic, sympathetic, and somatic pathways.[50]

Voiding disorders occur as a result of lesions at the suprapontine, suprasacral, or sacral levels of the spinal cord. Common disorders in MS patients include neurogenic detrusor overactivity (NDO) and detrusor sphincter dyssynergia (DSD). Detrusor hyporeflexia, or failure to empty, has been associated with brainstem/pontine lesions, and DSD has been associated with the presence of cervical cord lesions.[51]

SCREENING

The initial evaluation of an MS patient with bladder symptoms includes a history, physical examination, urinalysis, and uroflowmetry with measurement of a post-void residual (PVR). The patient should be questioned regarding urinary frequency, urgency, urge incontinence, nocturia, and history of urinary tract calculi and urinary tract infections. A voiding diary (at least 2 days) is strongly recommended. Total fluid intake before going to bed should be discussed, because nocturia is a common complaint among MS patients with lower urinary tract symptoms, and limiting fluids during the 2 to 3 hours before bedtime can help reduce the likelihood of nocturnal voids.

It is important for the MS clinician to include bladder function in the system review, because some patients may not realize that urinary or bowel dysfunction can be well managed. One study looked at MS patients' self-reported analysis of bladder and bowel dysfunction and compared patient perceptions with objective measurements of PVR. The objective measurements were found to correlate poorly with subjective assessments,[52] suggesting that all MS patients may benefit from urinary screening and evaluation.

The physical examination can include evaluation of the bulbocavernosus reflex (assesses S2-S4 levels), sensory testing of the perineal region, and assessment of anal sphincter tone. In men, a prostate evaluation is recommended. Women should be evaluated for prolapse, because treatable prolapse conditions may be associated with urinary symptoms very similar to those typically reported by patients with MS. A urinalysis is used to screen for disorders such as diabetes and infection. Uroflowmetry records urinary flow, time to void, and volume voided as well as the overall flow pattern. A bell-shaped pattern of flow is expected, indicating a peak urinary flow at midstream. An interrupted flow pattern suggests either DSD or Valsalva voiding (a sign of detrusor underactivity) and may necessitate further assessment and treatment. The PVR evaluation assesses the amount of urine in the bladder wall after urination and can be performed by catheterization or, preferably, by diagnostic ultrasonography (with the use of a bladder scan machine). Typical bladder storage capacity is 200 to 500 mL, and after voiding there should be less than 50 mL of volume detectable in the bladder.[50] The significance of elevated PVR volumes is not always clear, although certainly those patients with high volumes who are found to have recurrent infections, persistent small-volume incontinence, and difficulty voiding might benefit from efforts to reduce the residual.

The evaluations described here can often be done quickly in the physician's office and provide pertinent and valuable information. If no distinct pattern is ascertained, referral to a neurourologist is recommended. The urologist may proceed with additional tests such as cystoscopy, urodynamics, and imaging of the upper or lower tracts.

The site of central lesions may help in determining of the type of bladder and urethral sphincter dysfunction.[51] A review of lesion sites and urodynamic dysfunction found that brainstem lesions often resulted in NDO and cervical cord lesions often resulted in DSD.

TREATMENT

Before initiating pharmacologic management, MS patients should be encouraged to perform timed voiding. For patients who complain of some difficulty with stream initiation, the use of gentle Valsalva or Credé maneuver (placement of abdominal pressure) may be effective.[50] Pelvic floor exercises (e.g., Kegel's) have also been reported to be an effective intervention in male and female MS patients with lower urinary tract symptoms.[53] A trial comparing the use of pelvic floor muscle training, electromyography biofeedback, and neuromuscular electrical stimulation demonstrated that all three treatments, used in combination, reduced lower urinary tract dysfunction, including urinary urgency, frequency, hesitation, and involuntary leakage of urine.[54]

MS patients with failure-to-store disorders (typically NDO) often complain of urgency, frequency, and nocturia and have small-volume bladders with a spastic detrusor muscle pattern on urodynamic testing. Treatment includes use of antimuscarinics, anticholinergics, mixed agents (e.g., oxybutynin), and the tricyclic antidepressant, imipramine. Controlled-release medication formulations usually have a reduced side effect profile (less constipation and dry mouth) and are typically easier to tolerate than immediate-release formulations. Also, the reduced dose frequency allows for improved compliance. Oxybutynin, which has been available for several decades in immediate-release formulation, is thought to be associated with more frequent cognitive side effects. Several new agents are available, each with its possible niche in the treatment of overactive bladder. Currently, tolterodine, darifenacin, solifenacin, and trospium all have once-daily formulations, but head-to-head trials have not been conducted in patients with neurogenic overactive bladder. Therefore, choosing which medication might work best or might be best tolerated is difficult for any individual patient. Ensuring an adequate trial (in general at least 2 to 4 weeks of therapy) is perhaps the most relevant approach when considering the multitude of antimuscarinic agents currently available.[55]

Patients with nocturia or nocturnal enuresis should be advised to empty the bladder before going to bed and to decrease fluid intake 2 to 3 hours before bedtime. This can be challenging for patients who have medications that are dosed in the evening. Spicy foods, caffeinated products, and acidic foods can also result in bladder irritation and subsequent urinary frequency. Similarly, alcoholic beverages frequently have a diuretic effect and should be avoided before bedtime. If behavioral strategies are not effective, nocturia can be effectively managed with oral desmopressin (DDAVP). Dosage ranges are available from 0.1-mg to 0.6-mg tablets that should be administered in the evening. Patients should be educated to consume less than 8 ounces of water at night while taking desmopressin. The nasal form is no longer indicated for nocturnal enuresis because of reports of hyponatremia-related seizures occurring with this formulation. A baseline sodium level should be checked and monitored every 3 to 6 months. Desmopressin should not be used in patients with known hyponatremia or renal failure or dysfunction, or in those with significant edema or known congestive heart failure.

Failure to empty is commonly caused by an outlet disorder or a hyporeflexic or areflexic bladder. Patients may complain of frequency, slow initiation of stream (hesitation), slow stream, prolonged voiding time, and dribbling of urine. Failure to empty due to DSD may be managed with the α-antagonist class of medications (prazosin, terazosin, doxazosin, tamsulosin), although long-term studies on their use in neurogenic populations are lacking. In some cases, clean intermittent catheterization may need to be instituted for patients with severely impaired emptying.

Intravesical instillation of capsaicin and resiniferatoxin has been studied for use in medically refractory cases of NDO.[56] Both substances desensitize C-fiber axons which are believed to trigger detrusor overactivity.[57] Resiniferatoxin demonstrates

1000-fold greater potency than capsaicin.[58] Also, capsaicin's tolerance is limited to pain and discomfort with instillation. Resinferatoxin has demonstrated improved bladder capacities in patients with NDO. Intravesical injections of botulinum toxin are gaining popularity for treatment of failure-to-store and failure-to-empty bladder disorders with favorable results.[59] Clinical trials of the use of botulinum toxin are ongoing, and it remains an investigational use of the drug.

Cannabinoid treatment has been studied in patients with advanced MS.[60] A nasal spray containing 2.5 mg of active delta-9-tetrahydrocannabinol (THC) and cannabidiol per spray (Sativex) significantly reduced urinary urgency, frequency, and nocturia in a group of 15 MS patients. Secondary outcomes with significant improvement included spasticity, pain, and quality of sleep.

Surgical options may need to be considered for patients with severe urinary incontinence unresponsive to medical therapies and for those who have recurrent infections resulting in MS exacerbations. For patients with incontinence related to overactive bladder, sacral neuromodulation (InterStim) has been found to be a very effective treatment alternative, although traditionally its use has been limited to patients with idiopathic overactive bladder.[61] Augmentation cystoplasty, ileovesicostomy, and ileal conduit urinary diversion are all complex surgical procedures in which bowel is used to either augment or replace the function of the bladder, and each may have a role in severely affected patients.

Routine screening and evaluation for neurogenic bladder can provide benefit in reducing long-term complications such as infection, dependence on catheterization, sexual dysfunction, and disability.

Sexual Dysfunction

Sexual dysfunction (SD) is a common symptom in MS patients. It is reported to affect approximately 45% to 56%[62-64] of female and 66% to 78%[27,63] of male patients. Although its importance and potentially adverse implications on relationships are generally recognized, SD is infrequently discussed in the clinical setting. In one study, as many as 94% of women reported that sexuality had never been discussed in the context of their office visits.[28] Similarly, clinicians often report reluctance to "pry" into this domain of history taking, and they often feel ill equipped to provide counseling for these formidably challenging issues.[65] SD is linked to a reduced quality of life and is a principal cause of marital instability and other relationship problems.[64] Not surprisingly, relationship partners may not fully recognize or fully understand the link between their partner's fatigue or decreased libido and the MS disease process.

PATHOGENESIS

The neurophysiology of SD has been evaluated in a few studies. One study performed somatosensory evoked potential (SSEP) measurements of the pudendal nerve in a group of men[66] and women[67] with MS. The disruption of pudendal nerve SSEP response correlated highly with SD in men and women.

An Israeli group took a novel approach, using quantitative sensory testing (QST), and evaluated the effects of vibration and temperature stimuli in the female perineal region to determine its relevance to female SD.[62] Each participant underwent a neurologic examination and completed the Female Sexual Function Index (FSFI).[68] The FSFI is a validated test in the general population and is often used in clinical trials. A decrease in clitoral vibration effect correlated with SD with 89% sensitivity and 59% specificity. The other parameters tested, including thermal changes to the vagina and clitoris and the vibratory effect on the vagina, did not demonstrate any correlation with SD. Interestingly, cerebellar dysfunction consistently correlated with SD in the realms of difficulty in achieving orgasm and overall sexual function. Cerebellar function is not commonly thought to play a role in the sexual cycle, but the authors suggested that the cerebellum may play a role in the organization of the various steps of the cycle (e.g., arousal, tachycardia, tachypnea, sweating, vaginal secretions, clitoral engorgement). A cerebellar disruption may cause disorganization of this process and may ultimately play a role in delay or inability to climax.

CHARACTERIZING SYMPTOMS

Common symptoms of SD in women with MS include difficulty achieving orgasm/climax, decreased sexual libido, increased or decreased vaginal sensation, lack of sufficient lubrication, and dyspareunia.[27,46,64,66,67,69,70] Common male symptoms of SD include erectile dysfunction (ED), loss of early-morning erection, ejaculatory and/or orgasmic dysfunction, reduced penile sensation, and reduced libido. There is no consensus on the effects of age, disease duration, disability, and education level on SD.[64,71]

SCREENING

SD is often multifactorial in origin. Foley and Iverson[71] devised a conceptual model of sexual problems in MS and divided them among three categories (Table 17-2):

- *Primary:* MS related CNS dysfunction that *directly* impairs sexual feelings or responsiveness
- *Secondary:* MS-related physical changes that *indirectly* impair sexual response
- *Tertiary:* Disability related to psychological, emotional, social, or cultural influences

Whereas clinicians may express reluctance in discussing sexual function with patients, it has been shown that patients believe it is appropriate to address these issues during their office visits.[72] In setting up a discussion with a patient concerning SD, it is strategically useful to inform the patient that a substantial percentage of the MS population are afflicted with this problem and that in many cases it is a derivative of the disease process affecting the physiology of sexual functioning. Further, we have found that a series of objective and targeted questions can facilitate open and honest discussion of SD. These include questions such as the following:

- Describe changes in your sexual interest and desires that have occurred since your diagnosis.
- Are you having difficulty with sexual arousal or difficulty achieving orgasm?
- Male-specific: Are you having difficulty achieving or maintaining erection or difficulty with ejaculation?
- Female-specific: Are you having difficulty with painful sex or with lubrication?

TABLE 17–2 Sexual Problems in Multiple Sclerosis

Primary	Secondary	Tertiary
Altered genital sensation	Fatigue	Altered self-image
Decreased libido	Muscle weakness	Lowered self-esteem
Difficulty with arousal	Spasticity	Depression
Difficulty achieving orgasm	Ambulation/mobility	Anger
Decreased lubrication	Tremor	Fear of rejection by partner
Difficulty achieving or maintaining an erection	Ataxia	Guilt
	Sphincteric difficulty	Change in gender roles in the family
	Cognitive difficulty	Feelings of dependency
	Nongenital sensory changes	

Data from Foley F, Iverson J: Multiple Sclerosis and the Family. New York, Demos, 1992.

Once SD is established, the clinician is encouraged to rule out potential underlying medical causes. Review of cardiovascular, endocrine, and other neurologic disorders and screening for thyroid function, fasting glucose, and glycated hemoglobin (Hgb A1) are recommended. Testosterone levels have been studied in the general population. Low levels of testosterone are not consistently correlated with SD in men or women.[73] Testosterone levels decline with age in women,[4] which makes it difficult to assess whether declines are age or disease related. Also, testosterone levels in women should be measured in the middle third of their menstrual cycle and in the morning hours only. Diagnosis and treatment are recommended to be done in conjunction with a neurourologist, endocrinologist, or gynecologist.

Each patient should be screened for depression.[74] The selective serotonin reuptake inhibitor (SSRI) class of antidepressants, although very effective, frequently cause decreased libido as a side effect. Bupropion is an antidepressant that is being studied for its effect on improving libido and orgasm enhancement. For patients with depression well controlled with an SSRI, when reduced libido is reported, we often add a daytime dose of bupropion to counteract these effects. Many of our patients subsequently indicate important restoration of libido and sexual satisfaction. A patient's cultural or religious background may influence attitudes about sex and should be taken into consideration.[72]

The Multiple Sclerosis Intimacy and Sexuality Questionnaire-19, a 19-question self-report scale developed by Sanders and Foley,[75] is a validated instrument used to specifically assess for sexual function in MS patients. Time to completion is about 15 minutes. Patients can complete the scale ahead of time or while waiting to see the provider. The questionnaire can help the provider determine whether the patient's SD is related to the primary, secondary, or tertiary causes.

Zorzon and coworkers evaluated MS patients with and without SD and the presence and location of pathologic lesions on magnetic resonance imaging.[70] Patients reporting SD had relative pontine atrophy compared with MS patients with no self-reported SD. No significance differences were identified with respect to total brain, frontal, or pontine T1 or T2 lesion load. There was also an association between the presence of bladder dysfunction, depression, and SD. In a 2-year follow-up study of the same patients, there was no significant difference in the proportion of patients expressing SD. However, the number of symptoms that patients reported did increase over time, more commonly in men than in women. Men had an increased inability to ejaculate and greater orgasmic dysfunction. Bladder dysfunction continued to be strongly correlated with SD.[48]

DIAGNOSTIC TESTING

Although urodynamic studies may not be predictive, the presence of bladder dysfunction has consistently been found to be correlated with SD.[27,46-48,63] The similar anatomic underpinnings for genitourinary physiology have been proposed as a possible reason for the connection. Urodynamic studies revealed no consistent pattern (detrusor-external sphincter dyssynergia, detrusor hyperreflexia with impaired contractility, detrusor hyporeflexia, or detrusor areflexia) associated with SD.[27] No significant differences in tibial nerve SSEPs were present in patients with SD compared to those without SD.

The presence of spasticity (particularly in the lower extremities) has been reported to be significantly associated with SD.[63] Whether SD improves with treatment of spasticity and/or bladder dysfunction remains to be studied.

TREATMENT

Treatment of SD has been studied in the context of counseling, behavioral modification, and pharmacologic intervention.

General treatment recommendations applicable for both sexes include adequate treatment of neuropathic or visceral pain and spasticity, because either condition can impede sexual performance and cause fatigue. Also, energy-conserving positions are recommended. Assessment and treatment of neurogenic bladder and bowel dysfunction is crucial. Patients with bladder dysfunction or retention should be advised to empty the bladder with the use of a Foley catheter before engaging in sexual activities. Sexual activities may need to occur in the morning, because MS patients may have disabling fatigue late in the day.

One study involving couples with SD included weekly counseling for 3 months with a trained psychologist.[76] Each session addressed education, symptom management, and sensate focus training. Sensate focus is a form of cognitive behavioral therapy and body mapping exercise. Partners are encouraged to pay attention to various parts of their own bodies, which allows them to understand what else brings them pleasure, and then they try the sensate focusing on their partner's body. Significant improvement was found in marital satisfaction, problem-solving communication, and effective communication in MS patients and their partners. This study highlighted the importance and benefits of counseling and communication between partners as an effective means to improve relationships.

The introduction of sildenafil has revolutionized the treatment of ED in the male population. In a double-blind, placebo-controlled study on the effects of sildenafil versus placebo in male MS patients, 90% of patients experienced improved erections, compared with 24% of those on placebo.[77] Newer, longer-lasting agents, including vardenafil and tadalafil, have emerged but have not been specifically studied in MS patients.[30] Other agents currently being studied for ED include vibrator use, fispemifene, DA-8159, SK3530, and UK-369.003.

Other treatments for men with ED include vacuum pump devices (not accepted by most), injection therapy (with intracavernosal alprostadil), and implantation of penile prostheses.[30,56] For these interventions to be effective, some degree of manual dexterity is required by the patient or his partner. It is important to remember that ED is just one of several possible symptoms of SD in men. The clinician is encouraged to screen for decreased libido or ejaculatory problems.

Sildenafil in female MS patients with SD resulted in significant improvement in lubrication but not in other domains of SD, including desire and ability to achieve orgasm.[60] Hormone replacement treatment (HRT) can aid in lubrication. For those patients who cannot take HRT, water-soluble lubricants are recommended (Astroglide, Lubrens, KY). Decreased sensation or difficulty in achieving orgasm can be aided with the use of vibrators. Over the years, we have found the Eroscillator to be among the most effective of these. In general, effective vibrator stimulation involves high-intensity, high-frequency, wall-powered devices that are applied to the region just above the clitoris in women or to the ventral aspect of the penile corona in men. Other types of treatment being studied include various forms of cognitive behavioral therapy, testosterone transdermal patch treatment, and medications including tadalafil, ropinirole, and Wellbutrin XL.

Clinicians have generally been reluctant to ask about the presence of SD, because many are not sure how to address these issues. Some providers may believe it is personally intrusive to discuss a patient's sexual history. However, a professional discussion concerning SD can be therapeutic and enlightening and can allow the patient to discuss a potentially sensitive and important symptom. Germane to the discussion of SD is recognition that many patients have a low self-image, which may serve to intensify SD and represents an obstacle to opening discussion and addressing this important topic. Reinforcement of the fact that many patients experience similar complaints can optimize the physician-patient alliance and facilitate partner-to-partner communication about their sexual relationship.

Fatigue

Fatigue has been identified as one of the most common symptoms for patients with MS. As many as 90% of MS patients complain of fatigue as their primary symptom.[78] There is no universally accepted definition for fatigue, and many of its underlying mechanisms remain uncertain. MS-related fatigue is typically defined as a "sense of physical tiredness and lack of energy" distinct from sadness or weakness. Another definition was proposed in the Multiple Sclerosis Council for Clinical Practice Guidelines: "a subjective lack of physical and/or mental energy that is perceived by the individual or caregiver to interfere with usual or desired activities."[79] It is important to differentiate this state from fatigability, which is a generalized sense of exhaustion, not present at rest, that affects the patient after a few minutes of physical activity and disappears after rest. It is possible for fatigue and fatigability to exist concurrently in the same patient. However, the two problems probably represent different types of pathophysiology. Fatigability predominantly affects the lower limbs and is frequently associated with motor involvement.[80]

Fatigue may occur at any stage of MS, and worsening fatigue is often the first symptom of an acute exacerbation. It can occur intermittently or be constant in nature. In one report, 40% of patients were fatigued every day across a 30-day period.[29] It is unclear whether transient and chronic fatigue patterns are different or whether they share a common pathophysiology.

PATHOGENESIS OF FATIGUE

Many aspects of fatigue suggest that it may be related to the underlying demyelinating pathology. Demyelination causes slowing and desynchronization of nerve transmission and may even result in complete conduction block. Experts have explored peripheral causes of fatigue by repetitive nerve stimulation and electromyographic measurements in paretic lower extremities. Some studies have showed that reduced muscular force may serve as another source for fatigue, suggesting that it may be caused by a transformation of fatigue-resistant fibers into fatigable ones.[80]

Fatigue may result because of an inability to sustain the central drive to spinal motor neurons (i.e., central fatigue), and it is often demonstrated in complaints related to difficulties in mental performance. Impairment of the volitional drive to the descending motor pathways has also been suggested as another central mechanism for fatigue.[80] Functional MRI studies suggest that the cumulative effect of neuronal and axonal damage can lead to recruitment of expanded pools of cortical neurons in order to protect specific abilities which may unmask latent pathways.[79] Impaired interactions between functionally related cortical and subcortical areas entail excessive use of neuronal pools and could potentially represent one explanation for central fatigue.

Increased fatigue has also been observed in individuals during acute viral or bacterial infections, a process that may be related to the induced released of proinflammatory cytokines. Both human and animal studies have found an association between MS fatigue and particular cytokines, including tumor necrosis factor-α and interleukin 1.[80] MS patients treated with interferon agents commonly complain of increased fatigue, especially during the initial period (weeks to months) of treatment.

SECONDARY FACTORS

There are many additional factors that may worsen fatigue for patients with MS. Heat commonly worsens fatigue and is related to the instability of signal conduction in demyelinated nerves. Increased body temperature can induce conduction block in vulnerable axons, resulting in deterioration of neurologic functioning, commonly known as Uhthoff's phenomenon.

Depression may also increase fatigue and has a high prevalence, occurring in approximately 50% of MS patients.[79] Depression may be a secondary reaction to living with a chronic debilitating condition, or it may occur in the context of an endogenous mood disorder such as depression or bipolar disease. Regardless of the cause, it is important to identify and treat mood symptoms with an appropriate antidepressant medication. Further, it is often necessary to combine medication treatment with psychotherapy in order to obtain optimal results.

Many MS patients with fatigue also complain of sleep difficulties. Previous studies using polysomnographic studies demonstrated normal sleep latency without clear associations with nocturnal hypoxia or associated sleep fragmentation.[80] Sleep difficulties may be secondary to intractable pain, spasticity, or nocturnal bladder dysfunction. Studies in this area remain limited, and further research is needed to gain a better understanding of the underlying mechanisms associated with MS sleep disturbances and fatigue.

Other general medical conditions may also play a role in exacerbating fatigue. Infections, most commonly urinary tract or upper respiratory tract infections, can often worsen fatigue. Metabolic causes including thyroid disease, liver dysfunction, and anemia (iron, drug-related, vitamin B_{12}, or folate deficiencies) should also be excluded in the evaluation of a patient with fatigue.

It is also important to review the patient's medication profile for potential offending agents, because many medications are known to be associated with increasing fatigue. Medications that frequently cause fatigue-related side effects include antispasticity agents (baclofen or tizanidine), narcotic analgesics, sedative-hypnotics, and anticonvulsant agents. Patients often report increased fatigue as a result of interferon therapy. This may be minimized by pretreatment with nonsteroidal anti-inflammatory drugs before, and often after, interferon injection. We have observed the greatest success using a buffered, long-acting formulation of naproxen (Naprelan). For postinterferon injection headaches, we have found the most success using triptans at the time of the interferon injection.

MS patients frequently avoid physical activity because of concerns about symptom deterioration with elevated body temperature or prolonged exertion. Lack of physical activity worsens weakness and fatigue and may lead to other health issues such as decreased cardiovascular, endocrine, and pulmonary functioning. Additionally, limited mobility plays a substantial role in the worsening of spasticity and constipation and may also contribute to loss of bone mineral density. In exercise studies, people with MS were shown to have decreased peak oxygen levels during maximal incremental exercise, compared with healthy subjects.[81] This finding suggests that MS patients may have reduced cardiovascular fitness as a result of deconditioning. Insufficient activity in MS patients is linked to muscle changes that occur independently of the CNS damage (i.e., lowered oxidative capacity, lowered muscle dynamic properties, increased muscle fatigue, impaired metabolic responses of muscles to load, and impaired excitation-contraction coupling).[82] Therefore, there may be an imbalance between the increased metabolic need of MS patients and lowered supply characteristics of the cardiovascular system. In one study, maximum exercise tolerance improved after patients completed 8 weeks of aerobic exercise and neurorehabilitation; there was a significant improvement in walking capacity after aerobic training.[81] Several studies showed clear benefit for MS patients in improving fitness levels and quality-of-life measures.[81-85]

TREATMENT

It is important that the treatment of fatigue include a global approach with both nonpharmacologic and pharmacologic agents. Because confounding factors such as depression or hypothyroidism can often exacerbate fatigue, it is important to exclude other conditions or optimize their current management if necessary. Nonpharmacologic therapies include the use of local cooling devices, energy management strategies, and focused rehabilitation. Rehabilitation has been demonstrated to lead to improvement in fatigue, better quality of life, and lower rates of physical decline in MS patients.[86] Also, immunologic studies comparing normal controls to MS patients undergoing similar exercise routines concluded that changes in heart rate, lactate, and immune markers for Th1 and Th2 were similar across all groups.[87] Several medications have been found to be beneficial for reducing the severity of fatigue (Table 17-3).

MS-related fatigue can often be a severe problem interfering with the patient's ability to work or continue other daily activities. It is important to evaluate and address any potential confounding factors that may worsen fatigue. A combination of pharmacologic intervention and an individually tailored physical activity plan is recommended for each MS patient. Finally, MS patients should be encouraged to engage in physical activity, not only because it provides general improvements that apply to all individuals, but because it is safe and allows for greater function at later stages of the disease process.

Heat Intolerance

It is well described that the majority of MS patients are subject to reversible and often stereotypic symptoms that can be provoked by a number of factors, including increases in ambient or core body temperature. It is estimated that 60% to 80% of the MS population experiences transient increases in the frequency or severity of clinical signs and symptoms as a result of elevated body temperature.[88] Both physical functions (e.g., walking, running, driving, writing, reading) and cognitive functions (e.g., memory retrieval, processing speed, multitasking) can be impaired by heat exposure, greatly affecting overall patient safety as well as the ability of individuals with MS to perform routine ADLs.[40]

PATHOGENESIS

The precise mechanisms for impaired neural function in demyelinated axons due to increases in temperature are not completely understood but are likely to be related to structural and physiologic changes within the axon itself.[88] With the myelin removed, increases in temperature may profoundly affect the mechanisms that generate action potentials, influencing the threshold of current necessary to excite an axon, the rate at which current is generated, and the total amount of current available.[89-91] Increased temperature may also influence the electrical properties of the nerve fiber by increasing the rate of recovery processes (partly mediated by potassium channel activation and sodium channel inactivation), which surpass the action potential generating processes (sodium channel activation).[92] Individuals with MS may be susceptible to impairments in neural conduction with relatively small increases in core body temperature (as little as 0.5° C).[93,94] The likelihood that neural conduction will be affected at a demyelinated site is related to the magnitude of myelin loss and the time since demyelination occurred, suggesting that individuals with more severe and longer duration of MS may be more susceptible to conduction impairments.[95]

TABLE 17–3 **Medications Used for the Treatment of Multiple Sclerosis–Related Fatigue**

Medication	Effects in Improving Fatigue	Mechanism of Action	Side Effects
Amantadine	Widely used and moderately effective	Effect on fatigue is unclear, but known to have monoaminergic, cholinergic, and glutaminergic effects[79]	Neuromalignant syndrome Nausea Dizziness Sleep disturbance
Modafinil	Evaluated in several studies with varying results[79] but commonly used in clinical settings with good results	α_1-Adrenergic properties; widely used as a wake-promoting agent for the treatment of narcolepsy	Headache Nausea Dizziness Elevated blood pressures Tachycardia Sleep disturbance
Acetyl L-carnitine	Found in a small study to be better tolerated and more effective than amantadine[144]	Carnitine is a cellular component involved in energy metabolism	Abdominal discomfort
4-aminopyridine (4-AP)	Shown to be effective in reducing fatigue and may also improve weakness and heat sensitivity	Potassium channel blocker intended to improve conduction in demyelinated pathways	May increase serum potassium level ECG changes observed in clinical trials but not felt to be significant[145] Seizures

ECG, electrocardiographic.

Compounding temperature-related nerve conduction problems, individuals with MS may have impaired neural control of autonomic and endocrine functions.[96] Areas of the sympathetic nervous system (hypothalamic area and interomediolateral columns of the spinal cord) that control thermoregulatory functions are susceptible to demyelination in individuals with MS.[97] Conduction slowing and blockade secondary to increases in core body temperature may culminate in a decrease or halting of neural signaling to the cutaneous vasculature and sweat glands, thereby impairing appropriate thermoregulatory responses (increases in skin blood flow and sweating). Diminished sweating was previously described in MS patients.[98-100] Using a cholinergic analog to evaluate and quantify peripheral sweat gland function independent of CNS control, Davis and colleagues[101] demonstrated that diminished sweat function observed in individuals with MS is caused by reduced sweat gland output rather than diminished sweat gland

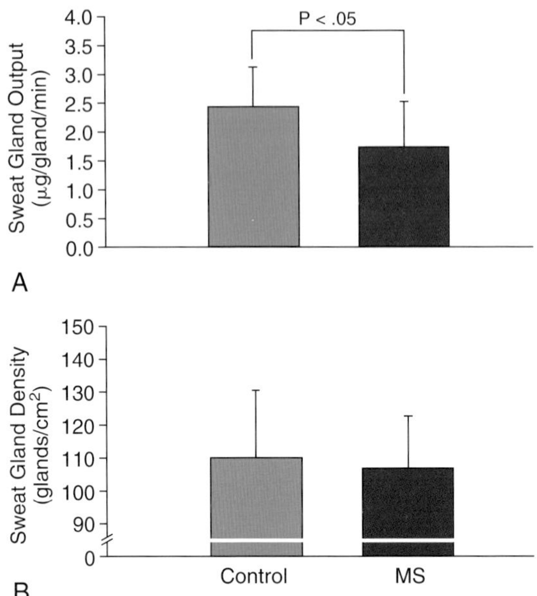

Figure 17–1 **A,** Data from patients with multiple sclerosis (MS) showing decreased gland output per sweat gland ($P < .05$) compared with matched, healthy controls after iontophoresis of pilocarpine, a cholinergic agent. **B,** No differences were observed in the number of sweat glands recruited between healthy controls and patients with MS. Data are expressed as mean ± SD. (Data from Davis SL, Wilson TE, Vener JM, et al: Pilocarpine-induced sweat gland function in individuals with multiple sclerosis. J Appl Physiol 2005;98:1740-1744.)

recruitment (Fig. 17-1). This diminished sweat function, although peripheral in origin, may be suggestive of CNS impairments causing conduction abnormalities or even neuronal loss within the descending sudomotor pathways due to the disease process.[97,100] Impaired sweat function appears to occur more frequently in patients with more severe cases of MS disease.[98]

The temporary worsening of neurologic signs and symptoms of MS in response to heat exposure can compromise ADLs and other functional capabilities of patients, even in mildly affected individuals.[102] In the past, physicians instructed MS patients to minimize their exposure to high ambient temperatures and to avoid exercise or intense physical work in order to avoid the exaggeration of these symptoms. However, lack of exercise often results in deconditioning, reduced functional capabilities, less weight-bearing exercise with consequences on bone and mineral metabolism, and greater risk of injury.[102,103] Evidence now indicates that exercise is beneficial to individuals with MS, because it improves fitness and sense of well-being, reduces fatigue in some, and increases strength.[40]

TREATMENT

To reduce the potentially detrimental effects of heat sensitivity, several treatment strategies have been employed to enhance the ability of individuals with MS to execute a number of daily activities that may have been abandoned, including regular exercise. Simple behavioral strategies are used to minimize heat exposure, such as performing work or exercise outdoors during the early morning or late evening, when temperatures are cooler. A small number of studies have reported potential benefits of cooling strategies that are convenient methods available to

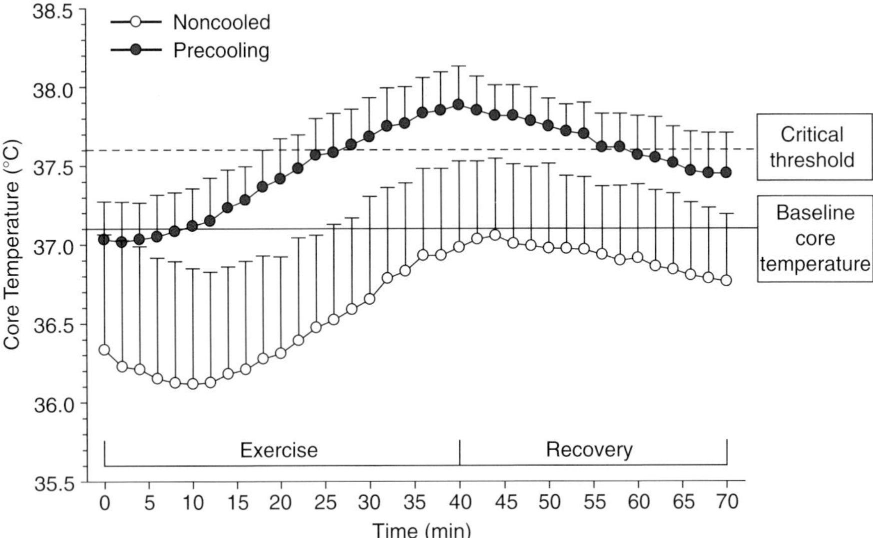

Figure 17–2 Core body temperatures responses during 30 minutes of aerobic exercise and subsequent recovery after a noncooled trail (*open circles*) and a precooled trial (*closed circles*). Core body temperature in the precooled trial remained below baseline values during exercise and recovery, whereas core temperature during the noncooled trail exceeded the critical threshold (0.5° C) for potential increases in symptom worsening. Data are expressed as mean ± SD. (Data from White AT, Wilson TE, Davis SL, Petajan JH: Effect of precooling on physical performance in multiple sclerosis. Mult Scler 2000;6:176-180.)

most MS patients, such as cold showers, application of ice packs, use of regional cooling devices, and cold beverages.[104-107]

Precooling (cooling before heat exposure or exercise) presents another option for minimizing heat stress in MS patients. White and colleagues[108] demonstrated that water-immersion precooling (cooling the lower limbs in 20° C water for 30 minutes before physical activity) was effective in preventing gains in core temperature during physical work and may minimize heat-induced conduction difficulties (Fig. 17-2). Precooling in this study allowed heat-sensitive individuals with MS to perform exercise with greater physical comfort and fewer side effects. The heat load during exercise was reduced most effectively by precooling the greatest body mass while minimizing thermogenic responses (i.e., shivering).[109] The beneficial effects of cooling can last for several hours, depending on the intensity of the activities performed after precooling.

Investigations have examined the use of commercially available cooling garments as a strategy to combat heat-induced worsening of symptoms in MS patients.[106,110-117] These garments have been recommended because they can be comfortably worn during heat exposure or exercise. Use of cooling garments resulted in improvements in neurologic function (motor performance and visual acuity) as well as perceived subjective benefits (feeling less fatigued) in thermally sensitive MS patients.[110-113,115,117] A number of factors can influence the ability of these garments to provide effective cooling, including closeness of fit of the garment and characteristics of the individuals wearing the suit, such as body size and percentage of body fat.[88] The cooling garment may increase metabolic demand and decrease efficiency for patients with disabilities during the performance of physical work because of the weight of the garment and associated accessories. The cost of these garments also my limit accessibility and availability to individuals with MS.

Drugs, such as the potassium channel blocker 4-aminopyridine, have been prescribed by physicians to treat heat sensitivity in MS patients. Anecdotal evidence suggests that this drug may limit the worsening of MS symptoms during heat exposure or exercise. Investigations are currently underway to determine whether pharmaceutical interventions such as 4-aminopyridine can protectively modulate axonal channels and improve neural function in individuals with MS during a thermal stress.

Worsening of clinical symptoms during heat exposure is typically reversible when the core body temperature is lowered. Individuals with MS should stop exercising, find an environment with a cooler ambient temperature, and ingest ice-cold liquids. If symptoms do not subside within several hours, they should contact their physician.

Pain

Pain is common in patients with MS and affects both physical and emotional well-being. Pain can substantially interfere with the ability to work, maintain relationships, and enjoy life. Estimates of the prevalence of pain in MS have ranged from 29% to 86%.[118] Patients with MS are more likely to have moderate or severe pain, to require analgesic use, and to describe pain as interfering with their ADLs, compared with individuals without MS. Risk factors associated with a greater likelihood for developing pain with MS include older age, greater disease severity, and longer disease duration. Men and women appear to have a comparable risk for developing pain, and patients with relapsing-remitting forms may have less risk for experiencing pain than those with more progressive forms of the disease. Greater perceived pain severity has been associated with increased disability, female gender, increased age, depression, and an unstable disease course.[118]

TYPES OF PAIN

Several different pain conditions are associated with MS. One category of pain is central neuropathic pain, which is defined as pain in a neurologic distribution with altered sensation and no history or clinical evidence of peripheral neuropathy.[118] The most common central neuropathic pain conditions are extremity pain, trigeminal neuralgia, and Lhermitte's phenomenon.

Extremity pain is usually a chronic form of pain and is often described as "burning" pain in one or both lower extremities. The discomfort can be perceived by patients as shooting, lancinating, electrical, or vibrating. The pain is often worse at night and is exacerbated by physical activity. Demyelination resulting in central hyperexcitability and disruption of the spinothalamic pathways may be a source of central extremity pain. Although many MS-related syndromes result in a compromise or loss of neurologic function, pain syndromes are thought to signify a gain of function secondary to exuberant ephaptic electrical discharges in central tract systems.

Trigeminal neuralgia is relatively common in MS. It is roughly 20 times more prevalent in MS patients compared with the general population.[118] There is often a higher proportion of bilateral involvement (albeit not typically concomitantly) in MS patients. MRI and autopsy findings support the conclusion that MS lesions at the trigeminal nerve root entry zone may account for some of the cases of trigeminal neuralgia in MS patients.

Lhermitte's phenomenon is a transient, short-lasting electrical sensation triggered by neck movement that is generally felt in the neck or lower back. It has been associated with cervical lesions involving the posterior columns and is speculated to be related to hypersensitivity of demyelinated sensory axons to stretching.[118] Typically, symptoms resolve after the acute event, but they can recur intermittently, especially during acute exacerbations. We have also been impressed with the number of patients who have an equivalent sign localized to the thoracic and lumbosacral spinal cord, with similar discharges provoked by trunk or leg movements.

TREATMENT

It is important to determine whether pain is primarily neuropathic or non-neuropathic in etiology, in order to direct the most effective therapeutic intervention. Whereas MS patients commonly have neuropathic pain, they may have pain associated with an underlying musculoskeletal or inflammatory pathology. Pain may be associated with sensory disturbances or related to predominantly motor symptoms (i.e., spasticity). Many of the pharmacologic approaches for MS neuropathic pain are based on studies of other neuropathic pain conditions, such as post-stroke and spinal cord injury pain. Gabapentin, pregabalin, lamotrigine, and tricyclic antidepressants have each been recommended for the treatment of central pain based on efficacy in randomized control trials.[118] Carbamazepine (in its various formulations) is generally considered the first-line agent for the treatment of trigeminal neuralgia. Surgical neurovascular decompression can also play a role; it may be effective for decreasing pain that is refractory to pharmacologic treatments. Several studies have explored the role of oral synthetic delta-9-tetrahydrocannabinol (THC), or dronabinol, in reducing MS-related pain and spasticity, and it was suggested to reduce spasticity-related pain.[119] There is anecdotal evidence that patients whose pain is refractory to many traditional neuropathic agents have had excellent relief with judicious use of methadone.

Pain is a common problem among MS patients, and it results in impairments in physical and emotional functioning that can have a profound impact on a patient's quality of life. It can also compound other problems, such as fatigue, depression, and insomnia. Therefore, it is important to frequently assess for the presence of pain in MS patients and to identify its underlying etiology, so as to provide the most effective therapeutic benefit for the patient.

Spasticity

Spasticity is a disorder that involves increased resistance of a muscle or group of muscles to an externally imposed stretch, often with more resistance to rapid stretch. In MS, this can be caused by lesions in the brain, spinal cord, or both.[120] Spasticity is a component of the upper motor neuron syndrome, which also includes increased spinal reflexes, muscle overactivity, flexor spasms, extensor plantar responses, and disordered motor control. Although the pathophysiology remains a subject of debate, spasticity appears to occur as a result of spinal, supraspinal, or cerebral dysfunction. The result is an imbalance between classic inhibitory (dorsal reticulospinal) and excitatory (mostly arising from bulbopontine tegmentum) pathways.[121-124] The clinical presentation is largely dependent on the anatomic site of injury or insult. A cross-sectional study of spasticity prevalence in MS patients reported that lower limb spasticity is almost twice as prevalent as upper limb spasticity (97% versus 50%).[125]

Up to 84% of MS patients have some degree of spasticity.[126] The most immediate consequence is decreased activity with an increasing cost of energy, particularly associated with movement. Spasticity is functionally significant because it can cause ambulation difficulty, decreased ability to complete ADLs, worse fatigue, and increased burden of care for the caretaker. Additionally, it can negatively affect cardiovascular, sexual, endocrine, and pulmonary functions. If it is left untreated, a vicious cycle of inactivity begets more inactivity, and eventually the patient is at high risk for development of joint contractures, deep venous thrombosis, and decubitus ulcers. However, spasticity frequently is not adequately treated.[125] Its high prevalence in MS patients and its potentially debilitating long-term consequences makes its inclusion as part of the routine office visit evaluation vital. The Consortium of Multiple Sclerosis Centers (CMSC) Clinical Guidelines for the treatment of spasticity recommend that spasticity be screened for regardless of whether MS patients complain about it.[120]

ASSESSMENT

The evaluation of spasticity involves observation (particularly with movements), physical examination, and possibly the use of measurement devices. Patients should be examined both while seated and dynamically. For example, for shoulder/arm spasticity, the patient should be asked to extend and reach for an object in various planes. If the lower limb is involved, the patient's gait should be observed, taking into consideration how varying surfaces (carpet, tile, and grass) and elevations (stairs, hills) may influence gait mechanics. The Ashworth,[127] Modified Ashworth,[128] and Spasm Frequency Scales[129] are the most commonly used tools in the clinical assessment (Tables 17-4, 17-5, and 17-6).

Noxious stimuli usually worsen spasticity. The clinician is encouraged to screen for urinary tract infections, impacted bowels, pressure ulcers, fatigue, psychological stress, increased pain, and poorly fitting wheelchairs as causative factors.[120,121] Some MS-specific reasons for the presence or worsening of spasticity include MS exacerbations, disease progression, and interferon-beta therapy.[130,131]

TREATMENT

Not all patients exhibiting spasticity require treatment. There are instances in which spasticity is importantly utilized to benefit patients in ambulating or performing other voluntary movements, particularly in those with severe weakness. As such, the treatment of spasticity should be undertaken with caution in all patients. Often, mild cases of spasticity are managed sufficiently without medication.

TABLE 17–4 Ashworth Scale

Score	Description
0	Normal tone
1	Slight hypertonus, a "catch" when limb is moved
2	Mild hypertonus, limb moves easily
3	Moderate hypertonus, passive limb movement difficult
4	Severe hypertonus, limb rigid

From Ashworth B: Preliminary trial of carisoprodol in multiple sclerosis. Practitioner 1964;192: 540-542.

TABLE 17–5 Modified Ashworth Scale

Score	Description
0	No increase in tone
1	Slight increase in tone, manifested by a catch and release or by minimal resistance at the end of the EOM when the affected part is moved in flexion or extension
1+	Slight increase in muscle tone, manifested by a catch followed by minimal resistance throughout the remainder (less than half) of the ROM
2	More marked increase in muscle tone through most of the ROM, but affected part easily moved
3	Considerable increase in muscle tone, passive movement difficult
4	Affected part rigid in flexion or extension

ROM, range of motion.

From Bohannon RW, Smith MB: Interrater reliability of a modified Ashworth scale of muscle spasticity. Phys Ther 1987;67:206-207.

TABLE 17–6 Spasm Frequency Scale

Score	No. of Spasms per Day
0	None
1	≤1
2	1-5
3	5-9
4	≥10

Modified from Snow BJ, Tsui JK, Bhatt MH, et al: Treatment of spasticity with botulinum toxin: A double-blind study. Ann Neurol 1990;28:512-515.

For mild spasticity, patients should be encouraged to stretch as frequently as possible. The National Multiple Sclerosis Society (NMSS) website (http://www.nationalmssociety.org [accessed October 2008]) has a free online manual on proper stretching techniques and positioning for patients. It is vital to recommend stretching before the development of any increased muscle tone. Stretching of the upper and lower limbs with a focus on the hamstring and ankle plantarflexors, performed daily for 5 to 10 minutes, is highly encouraged in all of our clinic patients. Illustration of these simple techniques in the clinic is helpful for patients and their family members. Studies have demonstrated that worsening spasticity is strongly correlated with increased levels of disability.[126]

Both physical and occupational therapists can educate and assist patients to develop a proper routine of stretching and positioning of the lower limbs. For severe joint spasticity or contracture, serial casting, either alone or in combination with other spasticity treatments, may be beneficial. The therapist applies a plantar cast around the involved joint or joints that is changed one to two times weekly. Each casting involves increasing the stretch on the tendon and involved joint. Occupational therapists also assist with education on the treatment of spasticity by providing custom-fitted splints to prevent elbow or hand contractures.

Both physical and occupational therapists use cryotherapy (topical cold therapy) and transcutaneous electrical nerve stimulation (TENS) to inhibit or diminish stretch reflexes. Cryotherapy can be in the form of cold-water baths (24° C), cooling vests, or local cold applications (see earlier discussion). Local cold application and aquatic therapy in cool pools (80° to 82° F) are the most effective modalities to treat spasticity and build or maintain endurance.[120] Heat therapy is generally not recommended, because it can worsen symptoms (albeit transiently) in most patients. Nevertheless, there are certainly exceptions, and some patients find mild heating pad therapy helpful for muscle relaxation without corresponding symptoms. High-frequency (100-Hz) TENS application for 20 minutes a day for 4 weeks significantly reduced spasticity and improved ambulation in a pilot study.[132] The long-term effects of TENS units on spasticity in MS patients is unknown.

Several oral medications are available to treat spasticity. Table 17-7 presents a full list of medications, dosages, indications, and side effects. Oral baclofen is reported to be most commonly prescribed drug in MS patients with spasticity.[126] Because the effect of each medication on an individual patient is unique, a slow titration on or off each drug is essential. A combination of medications is often necessary for optimal control of spasticity, particularly when both tonic and phasic components are present.

Chemodenervation in the form of botulinum toxin and phenol injections is another modality of therapy for spasticity. Only botulinum toxin types A and B are approved for use in humans. Despite not being approved by the U.S. Food and Drug Administration (FDA) for use in spasticity, botulinum toxin has gained popularity because of its focal action and lack of sedating side effects.[121,133] Two randomized controlled trials demonstrated effectiveness of botulinum toxin for hip adductor spasticity in MS patients.[129,134] Botulinum toxin injections generally work within 72 hours of injection and last for up to 12 weeks. The injections are intramuscular, and, from our clinic's experience, they often work best in conjunction with a focused physical or occupational therapy program. Side effects are minimal and

TABLE 17–7 Spasmolytic Medications

Medication	Recommended Daily Dosage	Half-life	Metabolism	Site of Action	Laboratory Monitoring	Side Effects	Notes
Baclofen	10-80 mg (in 3-4 divided doses)	2-6 hr	Kidney, liver	CNS, GABA-B inhibition	LFT q6 mo	Somnolence, fatigue, constipation, nausea, vomiting	Only generic form is available
Cannabis	5-20 mg (in 2-4 divided doses)	19-36 hr	Liver, kidney	Unknown		Nausea, vomiting, somnolence, increased appetite	
Clonazepam	0.125-3 mg (maximum, 3 mg/day); often dosed at night only	12 hr	Liver	Benzodiazepine	LFT q 6 mo	Drowsiness, sedation, ataxia	Preferred in phasic spasms, myoclonic movements, or RLS
Clonidine	0.1-0.4 mg oral/ transdermal patch	5-19 hr	Liver, kidney	Central α_2-agonist		Bradycardia, depression, syncope, fatigue, hypotension	
Cyproheptadine	4-16 mg (in 1-2 divided doses)		Kidney	Serotonergic antagonist		Increased appetite, weight gain	Also helpful for patients with myoclonic movements or RLS

Table continued on following page

TABLE 17–7 Spasmolytic Medications (Continued)

Medication	Recommended Daily Dosage	Half-life	Metabolism	Site of Action	Laboratory Monitoring	Side Effects	Notes
Dantrolene	25-100 mg (in 4 divided doses)	4-15 hr (after oral dose)	Liver	Inhibits calcium release at sarcoplasmic reticulum	LFT q3-6 mo	Most hepatotoxic, postural instability, slurred speech, diarrhea	No blood–brain barrier passage
Diazepam	2-40 mg (in 2-4 divided doses)	20-80 hr	Liver	CNS, facilitates GABA-A agonist	Patient should not consume alcohol when using diazepam	Sedating, memory impairment	Used to treat oral and intrathecal baclofen withdrawal symptoms
Fampridine-SR	10-30 mg (in 3 divided doses)			Potassium channel blocker; may increase central motor conduction	LFT q6 mo	Can cause seizures if stopped abruptly; nausea, tingling, distal artery vasospasm, hepatotoxicity	
Gabapentin	300-3600 mg (in 3-4 divided doses)	5-7 hr	Excreted unchanged in urine	GABA analog		Somnolence, dizziness, ataxia, fatigue	Safe for those with hepatic dysfunction

TABLE 17–7 Spasmolytic Medications (Continued)

Medication	Recommended Daily Dosage	Half-life	Metabolism	Site of Action	Laboratory Monitoring	Side Effects	Notes
Levetiracetam	25-3000 mg (in 1-3 divided doses)	7 hr	Kidney	Unknown; believed to work through GABA and glycine channels		Loss of appetite, mood disorder, fatigue, headache	
Piracetam	12-24 g (in 1-3 divided doses)	5-6 hr	Excreted unchanged in urine	GABA derivative; nootropic agent	LFT q6 mo	Nausea, flatulence	
Tizanidine (capsule and tablet form)	2-36 mg (in 1-3 divided doses); slow titration is recommended	2.5 hr	Liver	Central α_2-agonist, glycine facilitator	LFT q6 mo	Orthostatic hypotension, drowsiness, dry mouth, dizziness, MS patient prone to muscle weakness	Recommend initiating at night

Data from references 121 and 146 through 155.
CNS, central nervous system; GABA, γ-aminobutyric acid; LFT, liver function testing; MS, multiple sclerosis; RLS, restless leg syndrome; SCI, spinal cord injury.

include some local muscle tenderness and bruising. The cost of the medication and the lack of FDA approval make access to botulinum toxin limited to selected patients.

Phenol injections are useful in patients who are largely bed bound and have joint contractures that make dressing, bathing, and grooming difficult, as well as those whose spasticity predisposes them to develop pressure ulcers. The recommended concentration is 3% to 6%.[50,135] The onset of effect is immediate, and effects last up to 36 weeks.[136] Intramuscular phenol injection therapy for MS has not been reported in the literature. Phenol injections have demonstrated equal or better effects on gait and tolerance in pediatric compared with adult cerebral palsy patients.[137,138] Despite the potential benefits, the application of phenol injection therapy is limited by the frequent occurrence of painful dysesthesias.[50] The treatment should be given by a clinician who had had formal training in the administration of these injections, as well as experience in the use of electrical stimulation and advanced knowledge of anatomic spasticity patterns. Injections into inappropriate muscles or nerves can lead to debilitating consequences.

Patients exhibiting profound spasticity that is not sufficiently managed with oral, chemodenervation, or combinations of therapy may benefit from an intrathecal baclofen (ITB) pump. ITB therapy was approved for use in spasticity of spinal origin in 1992, and that of cerebral origin in 1996.[139] Baclofen is delivered into the intrathecal space, and the dosage can be precisely adjusted with the use of transabdominal telemetry. A significant reduction in spasticity with ITB therapy has been reported in several studies.[140,141] In one study, MS patients reported most satisfaction with ITB therapy compared to oral medications.[126] Respiratory function and sleep continuity appear to be superior with ITB therapy compared to oral baclofen in patients with intractable spasticity.[142] Surgical complications are rare but can include catheter kinks, disconnection, incisional pain, and pump malfunction.[120,140] An ITB pump trial is highly recommended to allow the patient to experience the effect of the medication, monitor for any adverse events, and to ensure proper patient selection. Selection of patients for ITB therapy is crucial, because baclofen withdrawal is a potentially fatal emergency. The patient must adhere to a schedule of follow-up appointments. The Synchromed II device lasts approximately 6 years and has a larger medication reservoir than its predecessor, the Synchromed I.

Severe spasticity that manifests in the form of joint contractures may require neurosurgical or orthopedic surgical interventions.[50,120] Neurosurgical procedures include myelotomy, rhizotomy, or intrathecal nerve blocks with alcohol or phenol, and are often performed when the previously described interventions are ineffective or to specifically alleviate severe pain associated with spasticity. Orthopedic procedures are used when painful joint contractures impede ambulation, ADLs, and caregiving and to lessen pain.

The clinician is reminded to address spasticity as a common symptom of MS. Early identification and treatment is beneficial for the patient and caregivers. Because each patient's MS disease is unique, the treatment of spasticity must be individualized to optimize muscle relaxation while attempting to maximize function and safety.

Conclusion

The ability to recognize and manage the multitude of symptoms with which MS patients are faced can have a significant and beneficial impact on their quality of life. Clinicians should actively screen for, address, and educate MS patients, their families, and caregivers regarding the myriad of ways in which disease affects the individual and the potential therapeutic strategies to address them.

REFERENCES

1. Sadovnick AD, Ebers GC: Epidemiology of multiple sclerosis: A critical overview. Can J Neurol Sci 1993;20:17-29.
2. Balcer LJ: Clinical practice: Optic neuritis. N Engl J Med 2006;354:1273-1280.
3. Frohman EM, Frohman TC, Zee DS, et al: The neuro-ophthalmology of multiple sclerosis. Lancet Neurol 2005;4:111-121.
4. Optic Neuritis Study Group: Visual function 15 years after optic neuritis: A final follow-up report from the Optic Neuritis Treatment Trial. Ophthalmology 2008;115:1078-1082, e5.
5. Beck RW, Cleary PA, Anderson MM Jr, et al: A randomized, controlled trial of corticosteroids in the treatment of acute optic neuritis. The Optic Neuritis Study Group. N Engl J Med 1992;326:581-588.
6. Beck RW, Trobe JD, Moke PS, et al: High- and low-risk profiles for the development of multiple sclerosis within 10 years after optic neuritis: Experience of the optic neuritis treatment trial. Arch Ophthalmol 2003;121:944-949.
7. Keltner JL, Johnson CA, Spurr JO, Beck RW: Baseline visual field profile of optic neuritis: The experience of the optic neuritis treatment trial. Optic Neuritis Study Group. Arch Ophthalmol 1993;111:231-234.
8. Brady KM, Brar AS, Lee AG, et al: Optic neuritis in children: Clinical features and visual outcome. J AAPOS 1999;3:98-103.
9. Costello F, Coupland S, Hodge W, et al: Quantifying axonal loss after optic neuritis with optical coherence tomography. Ann Neurol 2006;59:963-969.
10. Fisher JB, Jacobs DA, Markowitz CE, et al: Relation of visual function to retinal nerve fiber layer thickness in multiple sclerosis. Ophthalmology 2006;113:324-332.
11. Trip SA, Schlottmann PG, Jones SJ, et al: Retinal nerve fiber layer axonal loss and visual dysfunction in optic neuritis. Ann Neurol 2005;58:383-391.
12. Frohman E, Costello F, Zivadinov R, et al: Optical coherence tomography in multiple sclerosis. Lancet Neurol 2006;5:853-863.
13. Gordon-Lipkin E, Chodkowski B, Reich DS, et al: Retinal nerve fiber layer is associated with brain atrophy in multiple sclerosis. Neurology 2007;69:1603-1609.
14. Pulicken M, Gordon-Lipkin E, Balcer LJ, et al: Optical coherence tomography and disease subtype in multiple sclerosis. Neurology 2007;69:2085-2092.
15. Frohman EM, Shah A, Eggenberger E, et al: Corticosteroids for multiple sclerosis: I. Application for treating exacerbations. Neurotherapeutics 2007;4:618-626.
16. Ikuta F, Zimmerman HM: Distribution of plaques in seventy autopsy cases of multiple sclerosis in the United States. Neurology 1976;26:26-28.
17. Toussaint D, Perier O, Verstappen A, Bervoets S: Clinicopathological study of the visual pathways, eyes, and cerebral hemispheres in 32 cases of disseminated sclerosis. J Clin Neuro-ophthalmol 1983;3:211-220.
18. Balcer LJ, Galetta SL, Calabresi PA, et al: Natalizumab reduces visual loss in patients with relapsing multiple sclerosis. Neurology 2007;68:1299-1304.
19. Frohman TC, Galetta S, Fox R, et al: The medical longitudinal fasciculus (MLF) in ocular motor physiology. Neurology 2008;70:e57-e67.
20. Frohman EM, Frohman TC, O'Suilleabhain P, et al: Quantitative oculographic characterisation of internuclear ophthalmoparesis in multiple sclerosis: The versional dysconjugacy index Z score. J Neurol Neurosurg Psychiatry 2002;73:51-55.
21. Frohman EM, Zhang H, Kramer PD, et al: MRI characteristics of the MLF in MS patients with chronic internuclear ophthalmoparesis. Neurology 2001;57:762-768.

22. Starck M, Albrecht H, Pollmann W, et al: Drug therapy for acquired pendular nystagmus in multiple sclerosis. J Neurol 1997;244:9-16.
23. Strupp M, Brandt T: Pharmacological advances in the treatment of neuro-otological and eye movement disorders. Curr Opin Neurol 2006;19:33-40.
24. Kalla R, Glasauer S, Buttner U, et al: 4-Aminopyridine restores vertical and horizontal neural integrator function in downbeat nystagmus. Brain 2007;130:2441-2451.
25. Frohman EM, Zhang H, Dewey RB, et al: Vertigo in MS: Utility of positional and particle repositioning maneuvers. Neurology 2000;55:1566-1569.
26. Frohman EM, Kramer PD, Dewey RB, et al: Benign paroxysmal positioning vertigo in multiple sclerosis: Diagnosis, pathophysiology and therapeutic techniques. Mult Scler 2003;9:250-255.
27. Zivadinov R, Zorzon M, Locatelli L, et al: Sexual dysfunction in multiple sclerosis: A MRI, neurophysiological and urodynamic study. J Neurol Sci 2003;210:73-76.
28. Hulter BM, Lundberg PO: Sexual function in women with advanced multiple sclerosis. J Neurol Neurosurg Psychiatry 1995;59:83-86.
29. Chia YW, Fowler CJ, Kamm MA, et al: Prevalence of bowel dysfunction in patients with multiple sclerosis and bladder dysfunction. J Neurol 1995;242:105-108.
30. DasGupta R, Fowler CJ: Bladder, bowel and sexual dysfunction in multiple sclerosis: Management strategies. Drugs 2003;63:153-166.
31. Wiesel PH, Norton C, Glickman S, Kamm MA: Pathophysiology and management of bowel dysfunction in multiple sclerosis. Eur J Gastroenterol Hepatol 2001;13:441-448.
32. Winge K, Rasmussen D, Werdelin LM: Constipation in neurological diseases. J Neurol Neurosurg Psychiatry 2003;74:13-19.
33. Sandler RS, Drossman DA: Bowel habits in young adults not seeking health care. Dig Dis Sci 1987;32:841-845.
34. Heaton KW, Radvan J, Cripps H, et al: Defecation frequency and timing, and stool form in the general population: A prospective study. Gut 1992;33:818-824.
35. Feldman M. Friedman LS, Brandt LT: Sleisenger and Fordtran's Gastrointestinal and Liver Disease, 8th ed. Philadelphia, Saunders Elsevier, 2006.
36. Rivkin A, Chagan L: Lubiprostone: Chloride channel activator for chronic constipation. Clin Ther 2006;28:2008-2021.
37. Prather CM, Camilleri M, Zinsmeister AR, et al: Tegaserod accelerates orocecal transit in patients with constipation-predominant irritable bowel syndrome. Gastroenterology 2000;118:463-468.
38. Camilleri M, Bharucha AE, Ueno R, et al: Effect of a selective chloride channel activator, lubiprostone, on gastrointestinal transit, gastric sensory, and motor functions in healthy volunteers. Am J Physiol 2006;290:G942-G947.
39. Wiesel PH, Norton C, Roy AJ, et al: Gut focused behavioural treatment (biofeedback) for constipation and faecal incontinence in multiple sclerosis. J Neurol Neurosurg Psychiatry 2000;69:240-243.
40. Petajan JH, Gappmaier E, White AT, et al: Impact of aerobic training on fitness and quality of life in multiple sclerosis. Ann Neurol 1996;39:432-441.
41. Hinds JP, Eidelman BH, Wald A: Prevalence of bowel dysfunction in multiple sclerosis: A population survey. Gastroenterology 1990;98:1538-1542.
42. Whitehead WE, Wald A, Diamant NE, et al: Functional disorders of the anus and rectum. Gut 1999;45(Suppl 2):II55-II59.
43. Osterberg A, Graf W, Eeg-Olofsson K, et al: Is electrostimulation of the pelvic floor an effective treatment for neurogenic faecal incontinence? Scand J Gastroenterol 1999;34:319-324.
44. Leroi AM, Karoui S, Touchais JY, et al: Electrostimulation is not a clinically effective treatment of anal incontinence. Eur J Gastroenterol Hepatol 1999;11:1045-1047.
45. Hadjimichael OC: Bladder Symptoms Among Registry Participants, NARCOMS Project, Yale Center for Multiple Sclerosis Treatment and Research, West Haven, CT, 2002. United Spinal Association, Multiple Sclerosis Quarterly Report Online. Available at: http://www.unitedspinal.org/publications/msqr/2002/07/ (accessed October 2008).
46. Borello-France D, Leng W, O'Leary M, et al: Bladder and sexual function among women with multiple sclerosis. Mult Scler 2004;10:455-461.
47. Nortvedt MW, Riise T, Frugard J, et al: Prevalence of bladder, bowel and sexual problems among multiple sclerosis patients two to five years after diagnosis. Mult Scler 2007;13:106-112.
48. Zorzon M, Zivadinov R, Monti Bragadin L, et al: Sexual dysfunction in multiple sclerosis: A 2-year follow-up study. J Neurol Sci 2001;187:1-5.

49. Lemack GE, Hawker K, Frohman E: Incidence of upper tract abnormalities in patients with neurovesical dysfunction secondary to multiple sclerosis: Analysis of risk factors at initial urologic evaluation. Urology 2005;65:854-857.
50. Braddom R: Physical Medicine and Rehabilitation, 3rd ed. Philadelphia, Saunders, 2005.
51. Araki I, Matsui M, Ozawa K, et al: Relationship of bladder dysfunction to lesion site in multiple sclerosis. J Urol 2003;169:1384-1387.
52. Kragt JJ, Hoogervorst EL, Uitdehaag BM, Polman CH: Relation between objective and subjective measures of bladder dysfunction in multiple sclerosis. Neurology 2004;63:1716-1718.
53. Vahtera T, Haaranen M, Viramo-Koskela AL, Ruutiainen J: Pelvic floor rehabilitation is effective in patients with multiple sclerosis. Clin Rehabil 1997;11:211-219.
54. McClurg D, Ashe RG, Marshall K, Lowe-Strong AS: Comparison of pelvic floor muscle training, electromyography biofeedback, and neuromuscular electrical stimulation for bladder dysfunction in people with multiple sclerosis: A randomized pilot study. Neurourol Urodyn 2006;25:337-348.
55. Woderich R, Fowler CJ: Management of lower urinary tract symptoms in men with progressive neurological disease. Curr Opin Urol 2006;16:30-36.
56. Litwiller SE, Frohman EM, Zimmern PE: Multiple sclerosis and the urologist. J Urol 1999;161: 743-757.
57. Watanabe T, Yokoyama T, Sasaki K, et al: Intravesical resiniferatoxin for patients with neurogenic detrusor overactivity. Int J Urol 2004;11:200-205.
58. Kim JH, Rivas DA, Shenot PJ, et al: Intravesical resiniferatoxin for refractory detrusor hyperreflexia: A multicenter, blinded, randomized, placebo-controlled trial. J Spinal Cord Med 2003;26:358-363.
59. Cruz F, Silva C: Botulinum toxin in the management of lower urinary tract dysfunction: Contemporary update. Curr Opin Urol 2004;14:329-334.
60. Brady CM, DasGupta R, Dalton C, et al: An open-label pilot study of cannabis-based extracts for bladder dysfunction in advanced multiple sclerosis. Mult Scler 2004;10:425-433.
61. Wallace PA, Lane FL, Noblett KL: Sacral nerve neuromodulation in patients with underlying neurologic disease. Am J Obstet Gynecol 2007;197:96 e91-e95.
62. Gruenwald I, Vardi Y, Gartman I, et al: Sexual dysfunction in females with multiple sclerosis: Quantitative sensory testing. Mult Scler 2007;13:95-105.
63. Valleroy ML, Kraft GH: Sexual dysfunction in multiple sclerosis. Arch Phys Med Rehabil 1984;65:125-128.
64. Mattson D, Petrie M, Srivastava DK, McDermott M: Multiple sclerosis: Sexual dysfunction and its response to medications. Arch Neurol 1995;52:862-868.
65. Rubin R: Communication about sexual problems in male patients with multiple sclerosis. Nurs Stand 2005;19:33-37.
66. Yang CC, Bowen JD, Kraft GH, et al: Physiologic studies of male sexual dysfunction in multiple sclerosis. Mult Scler 2001;7:249-254.
67. Yang CC, Bowen JR, Kraft GH, et al: Cortical evoked potentials of the dorsal nerve of the clitoris and female sexual dysfunction in multiple sclerosis. J Urol 2000;164:2010-2013.
68. Rosen R, Brown C, Heiman J, et al: The Female Sexual Function Index (FSFI): A multidimensional self-report instrument for the assessment of female sexual function. J Sex Marital Ther 2000;26:191-208.
69. Chancellor MB, Blaivas JG: Urological and sexual problems in multiple sclerosis. Clin Neurosci 1994;2:189-195.
70. Zorzon M, Zivadinov R, Bosco A, et al: Sexual dysfunction in multiple sclerosis: A case-control study. I: Frequency and comparison of groups. Mult Scler 1999;5:418-427.
71. Foley F, Iverson J: Multiple Sclerosis and the Family. New York, Demos, 1992.
72. Schmidt EZ, Hofmann P, Niederwieser G, et al: Sexuality in multiple sclerosis. J Neural Transm 2005;112:1201-1211.
73. Traish AM, Goldstein I, Kim NN: Testosterone and erectile function: From basic research to a new clinical paradigm for managing men with androgen insufficiency and erectile dysfunction. Eur Urol 2007;52:54-70.
74. Beck AT, Ward CH, Mendelson M, et al: An inventory for measuring depression. Arch Gen Psychiatry 1961;4:561-571.
75. Sanders AS, Foley FW, LaRocca NG, Zemon V: The Multiple Sclerosis Intimacy and Sexuality Questionnaire-19 (MSISQ-19). Sex Disabil 2000;18:3-26.
76. Christopherson JM, Moore K, Foley FW, Warren KG: A comparison of written materials vs. materials and counselling for women with sexual dysfunction and multiple sclerosis. J Clin Nurs 2006;15:742-750.

77. Green BG, Martin S: Clinical assessment of sildenafil in the treatment of neurogenic male sexual dysfunction: After the hype. NeuroRehabilitation 2000;15:101-105.
78. Crenshaw SJ, Royer TD, Richards JG, Hudson DJ: Gait variability in people with multiple sclerosis. Mult Scler 2006;12:613-619.
79. Lapierre Y, Hum S: Treating fatigue. Int MS J 2007;14:64-71.
80. Comi G, Leocani L, Rossi P, Colombo B: Physiopathology and treatment of fatigue in multiple sclerosis. J Neurol 2001;248:174-179.
81. Rampello A, Franceschini M, Piepoli M, et al: Effect of aerobic training on walking capacity and maximal exercise tolerance in patients with multiple sclerosis: A randomized crossover controlled study. Phys Ther 2007;87:545-555; discussion 555-549.
82. Rasova K, Brandejsky P, Havrdova E, et al: Spiroergometric and spirometric parameters in patients with multiple sclerosis: Are there any links between these parameters and fatigue, depression, neurological impairment, disability, handicap and quality of life in multiple sclerosis? Mult Scler 2005;11:213-221.
83. Newman MA, Dawes H, van den Berg M, et al: Can aerobic treadmill training reduce the effort of walking and fatigue in people with multiple sclerosis: A pilot study. Mult Scler 2007;13:113-119.
84. Rasova K, Havrdova E, Brandejsky P, et al: Comparison of the influence of different rehabilitation programmes on clinical, spirometric and spiroergometric parameters in patients with multiple sclerosis. Mult Scler 2006;12:227-234.
85. Schulz KH, Gold SM, Witte J, et al: Impact of aerobic training on immune-endocrine parameters, neurotrophic factors, quality of life and coordinative function in multiple sclerosis. J Neurol Sci 2004;225:11-18.
86. Di Fabio RP, Soderberg J, Choi T, et al: Extended outpatient rehabilitation: Its influence on symptom frequency, fatigue, and functional status for persons with progressive multiple sclerosis. Arch Phys Med Rehabil 1998;79:141-146.
87. Heesen C, Gold SM, Hartmann S, et al: Endocrine and cytokine responses to standardized physical stress in multiple sclerosis. Brain Behav Immun 2003;17:473-481.
88. Syndulko K, Jafari M, Woldanski A, et al: Effects of temperature in multiple sclerosis: A review of literature. J Neurol Rehabil 1996;10:23-34.
89. Davis FA: Pathophysiology of multiple sclerosis and related clinical implications. Mod Treat 1970;7:890-902.
90. Davis FA: Axonal conduction studies based on some considerations of temperature effects in multiple sclerosis. Electroencephalogr Clin Neurophysiol 1970;28:281-286.
91. Schauf CL, Davis FA: Impulse conduction in multiple sclerosis: A theoretical basis for modification by temperature and pharmacological agents. J Neurol Neurosurg Psychiatry 1974;37: 152-161.
92. Huxley AF: Ion movements during nerve activity. Ann N Y Acad Sci 1959;81:221-246.
93. Rasminsky M: The effects of temperature on conduction in demyelinated single nerve fibers. Arch Neurol 1973;28:287-292.
94. Davis SL, Frohman TC, Crandall CG, et al: Modeling Uhthoff's phenomenon in MS patients with internuclear ophthalmoparesis (INO). Neurology 2008;70(13 Pt 2):1098-1106.
95. Smith KJ, McDonald WI: The pathophysiology of multiple sclerosis: The mechanisms underlying the production of symptoms and the natural history of the disease. Philos Trans R Soc B Biol Sci 1999;354:1649-1673.
96. Huitinga I, De Groot CJ, Van der Valk P, et al: Hypothalamic lesions in multiple sclerosis. J Neuropathol Exp Neurol 2001;60:1208-1218.
97. Andersen EB, Nordenbo AM: Sympathetic vasoconstrictor responses in multiple sclerosis with thermo-regulatory dysfunction. Clin Autonom Res 1997;7:13-16.
98. Cartlidge NE: Autonomic function in multiple sclerosis. Brain 1972;95:661-664.
99. Noronha MJ, Vas CJ, Aziz H: Autonomic dysfunction (sweating responses) in multiple sclerosis. J Neurol Neurosurg Psychiatry 1968;31:19-22.
100. Vas CJ: Sexual impotence and some autonomic disturbances in men with multiple sclerosis. Acta Neurol Scand 1969;45:166-182.
101. Davis SL, Wilson TE, Vener JM, et al: Pilocarpine-induced sweat gland function in individuals with multiple sclerosis. J Appl Physiol 2005;98:1740-1744.
102. Petajan JH, White AT: Recommendations for physical activity in patients with multiple sclerosis. Sports Med 1999;27:179-191.
103. White LJ, Dressendorfer RH: Exercise and multiple sclerosis. Sports Med 2004;34:1077-1100.
104. Bassett SW, Lake BM: Use of cold applications in the management of spasticity: Report of three cases. Phys Ther Rev 1958;38:333-334.

105. Boynton BL, Garramone PM, Buca JT: Observations on the effects of cool baths for patients with multiple sclerosis. Phys Ther Rev 1959;39:297-299.
106. Scherokman BJ, Selhorst JB, Waybright EA, et al: Improved optic nerve conduction with ingestion of ice water. Ann Neurol 1985;17:418-419.
107. Watson CW: Effect of lowering of body temperature on the symptoms and signs of multiple sclerosis. N Engl J Med 1959;261:1253-1259.
108. White AT, Wilson TE, Davis SL, Petajan JH: Effect of precooling on physical performance in multiple sclerosis. Mult Scler 2000;6:176-180.
109. White AT, Davis SL, Wilson TE: Metabolic, thermoregulatory, and perceptual responses during exercise after lower vs. whole body precooling. J Appl Physiol 2003;94:1039-1044.
110. Beenakker EA, Oparina TI, Hartgring A, et al: Cooling garment treatment in MS: Clinical improvement and decrease in leukocyte NO production. Neurology 2001;57:892-894.
111. Capello E, Gardella M, Leandri M, et al: Lowering body temperature with a cooling suit as symptomatic treatment for thermosensitive multiple sclerosis patients. Ital J Neurol Sci 1995;16: 533-539.
112. Flensner G, Lindencrona C: The cooling-suit: A study of ten multiple sclerosis patients' experiences in daily life. J Adv Nurs 1999;29:1444-1453.
113. Kinnman J, Andersson T, Andersson G: Effect of cooling suit treatment in patients with multiple sclerosis evaluated by evoked potentials. Scand J Rehabil Med 2000;32:16-19.
114. Kinnman J, Andersson U, Wetterquist L, et al: Cooling suit for multiple sclerosis: Functional improvement in daily living? Scand J Rehabil Med 2000;32:20-24.
115. Ku YT, Montgomery LD, Lee HC, et al: Physiologic and functional responses of MS patients to body cooling. Am J Phys Med Rehabil 2000;79:427-434.
116. Meyer-Heim A, Rothmaier M, Weder M, et al: Advanced lightweight cooling-garment technology: Functional improvements in thermosensitive patients with multiple sclerosis. Mult Scler 2007;13:232-237.
117. Schwid SR, Petrie MD, Murray R, et al: A randomized controlled study of the acute and chronic effects of cooling therapy for MS. Neurology 2003;60:1955-1960.
118. O'Connor AB, Schwid SR, Herrmann DN, et al: Pain associated with multiple sclerosis: Systematic review and proposed classification. Pain 2008;137:96-111.
119. Lienau FS, Fullgraf H, Moser A, Feuerstein TJ: Why do cannabinoids not show consistent effects as analgetic drugs in multiple sclerosis? Eur J Neurol 2007;14:1162-1169.
120. Haselkorn JK, Balsdon Richer C, Fry Welch D, et al: Overview of spasticity management in multiple sclerosis: Evidence-based management strategies for spasticity treatment in multiple sclerosis. J Spinal Cord Med 2005;28:167-199.
121. Satkunam LE: Rehabilitation medicine: 3. Management of adult spasticity. Can Med Assoc J 2003;169:1173-1179.
122. Nielsen JB, Crone C, Hultborn H: The spinal pathophysiology of spasticity: From a basic science point of view. Acta Physiol (Oxf) 2007;189:171-180.
123. Sheean G: The pathophysiology of spasticity. Eur J Neurol 2002;9(Suppl 1):3-9; discussion 53-61.
124. Ivanhoe CB, Reistetter TA: Spasticity: The misunderstood part of the upper motor neuron syndrome. Am J Phys Med Rehabil 2004;83:S3-S9.
125. Barnes MP, Kent RM, Semlyen JK, McMullen KM: Spasticity in multiple sclerosis. Neurorehabil Neural Repair 2003;17:66-70.
126. Rizzo MA, Hadjimichael OC, Preiningerova J, Vollmer TL: Prevalence and treatment of spasticity reported by multiple sclerosis patients. Mult Scler 2004;10:589-595.
127. Ashworth B: Preliminary trial of carisoprodol in multiple sclerosis. Practitioner 1964;192:540-542.
128. Bohannon RW, Smith MB: Interrater reliability of a modified Ashworth scale of muscle spasticity. Phys Ther 1987;67:206-207.
129. Snow BJ, Tsui JK, Bhatt MH, et al: Treatment of spasticity with botulinum toxin: A double-blind study. Ann Neurol 1990;28:512-515.
130. Frese A, Bethke F, Ludemann P, Stogbauer F: Enhanced spasticity in primary progressive MS patients treated with interferon beta-1b. Neurology 1999;53:1892-1893.
131. Bramanti P, Sessa E, Rifici C, et al: Enhanced spasticity in primary progressive MS patients treated with interferon beta-1b. Neurology 1998;51:1720-1723.
132. Armutlu K, Meric A, Kirdi N, et al: The effect of transcutaneous electrical nerve stimulation on spasticity in multiple sclerosis patients: A pilot study. Neurorehabil Neural Repair 2003;17: 79-82.

133. Francisco GE: Botulinum toxin: Dosing and dilution. Am J Phys Med Rehabil 2004;83:S30-S37.
134. Hyman N, Barnes M, Bhakta B, et al: Botulinum toxin (Dysport) treatment of hip adductor spasticity in multiple sclerosis: A prospective, randomised, double blind, placebo controlled, dose ranging study. J Neurol Neurosurg Psychiatry 2000;68:707-712.
135. Cullu E, Ozkan I, Culhaci N, Alparslan B: A comparison of the effect of doxorubicin and phenol on the skeletal muscle: May doxorubicin be a new alternative treatment agent for spasticity? J Pediatr Orthop 2005;14:134-138.
136. Patel DR, Soyode O: Pharmacologic interventions for reducing spasticity in cerebral palsy. Ind J Pediatr 2005;72:869-872.
137. Gooch JL, Patton CP: Combining botulinum toxin and phenol to manage spasticity in children. Arch Phys Med Rehabil 2004;85:1121-1124.
138. Wong AM, Chen CL, Chen CP, et al: Clinical effects of botulinum toxin A and phenol block on gait in children with cerebral palsy. Am J Phys Med Rehabil 2004;83:284-291.
139. Rawlins PK: Intrathecal baclofen therapy over 10 years. J Neurosci Nurs 2004;36:322-327.
140. Coffey JR, Cahill D, Steers W, et al: Intrathecal baclofen for intractable spasticity of spinal origin: Results of a long-term multicenter study. J Neurosurg 1993;78:226-232.
141. Parke B, Penn RD, Savoy SM, Corcos D: Functional outcome after delivery of intrathecal baclofen. Arch Phys Med Rehabil 1989;70:30-32.
142. Bensmail D, Quera Salva MA, Roche N, et al: Effect of intrathecal baclofen on sleep and respiratory function in patients with spasticity. Neurology 2006;67:1432-1436.
143. Drossman DA: The functional gastrointestinal disorders and the Rome II process. Gut 1999;45(Suppl 2):II1-II5.
144. Tomassini V, Pozzilli C, Onesti E, et al: Comparison of the effects of acetyl L-carnitine and amantadine for the treatment of fatigue in multiple sclerosis: Results of a pilot, randomised, double-blind, crossover trial. J Neurol Sci 2004;218:103-108.
145. Romani A, Bergamaschi R, Candeloro E, et al: Fatigue in multiple sclerosis: Multidimensional assessment and response to symptomatic treatment. Mult Scler 2004;10:462-468.
146. Zafonte R, Lombard L, Elovic E: Antispasticity medications: Uses and limitations of enteral therapy. Am J Phys Med Rehabil 2004;83:S50-S58.
147. Barbeau H, Richards C, Bedard P: Action of cyproheptadine in spastic paraparetic patients. J Neurol Neurosurg Psychiatry 1982;45:923-926.
148. Tacconi MT, Wurtman RJ: Physiological disposition of oral piracetam in Sprague-Dawley rats. J Pharm Pharmacol 1984;36:659-662.
149. Bass B, Weinshenker B, Rice GP, et al: Tizanidine versus baclofen in the treatment of spasticity in patients with multiple sclerosis. Can J Neurol Sci 1988;15:15-19.
150. Dunevsky A, Perel AB: Gabapentin for relief of spasticity associated with multiple sclerosis. Am J Phys Med Rehabil 1998;77:451-454.
151. Feldman RG, Kelly-Hayes M, Conomy JP, Foley JM: Baclofen for spasticity in multiple sclerosis: Double-blind crossover and three-year study. Neurology 1978;28:1094-1098.
152. Hawker K, Frohman E, Racke M: Levetiracetam for phasic spasticity in multiple sclerosis. Arch Neurol 2003;60:1772-1774.
153. Hudgson P, Weightman D: Baclofen in the treatment of spasticity. Br Med J 1971;4:15-17.
154. Maritz NG, Muller FO: Pompe van Meerdervoort HF: Piracetam in the management of spasticity in cerebral palsy. South Afr Med J 1978;53:889-891.
155. Mueller ME, Gruenthal M, Olson WL, Olson WH: Gabapentin for relief of upper motor neuron symptoms in multiple sclerosis. Arch Phys Med Rehabil 1997;78:521-524.

18 Unconventional Medicine and Multiple Sclerosis: The Role of Conventional Health Providers

ALLEN C. BOWLING

Many patients with multiple sclerosis (MS) use complementary and alternative medicine (CAM), yet many MS health professionals, including neurologists, may not be knowledgeable about these therapies and may not even be aware of which CAM therapies are being used by their patients. CAM therapies may be beneficial or harmful and may interact with conventional MS medications. Therefore, the quality of care that is provided to MS patients may be improved if neurologists and other clinicians have the knowledge and skills, when appropriate, to offer objective CAM information to patients, guiding them away from therapies that may be harmful or ineffective and toward those that are of low risk and possibly effective.

The aim of this review is to provide knowledge and skills to practicing clinicians so that they will be able to guide and inform their MS patients about CAM.

To this end, it provides primarily basic efficacy and safety information about CAM therapies that are likely to be encountered in day-to-day interactions with MS patients. This information is provided in a format that should familiar and accessible to conventional medicine practitioners. In addition, information and strategies that may be especially practical in patient interactions are provided in the sections entitled, "Application to Clinical Practice." This is *not* intended to be an extensive review of all of the available MS-relevant CAM therapies or to provide an in-depth critique of CAM clinical studies; reviews with broader scope and more detailed analysis may be found elsewhere.[1-5]

Definitions

Different definitions and terms are used in the area of unconventional medicine. One definition of unconventional medicine is that it refers to forms of medicine that are not taught widely in medical schools or generally available in hospitals.[6] The National Institutes of Health (NIH) has proposed a classification scheme for unconventional medical practices that includes biologically based therapies, alternative medical systems, mind–body interventions, manipulative and body-based methods, and energy therapies (Table 18-1).[7] Unconventional medical therapies may be used in an *alternative* or *complementary* manner; alternative use indicates that they are used instead of conventional medicine, and complementary use means that they are used in conjunction with conventional medicine. A term that includes both of these approaches is *complementary and alternative medicine*, or CAM. *Integrative medicine* refers to the combined use of conventional and unconventional medical practices.

Multiple Sclerosis: Conventional and Unconventional Medicine

Over the past decade, there have been remarkable advances in understanding the pathology of MS and in treating the disease. There are now multiple effective therapies for MS-related symptoms, and there are disease-modifying therapies that decrease the relapse rate, reduce magnetic resonance imaging (MRI) activity, and slow progression of disability.

TABLE 18–1 National Institutes of Health Classification Scheme for Complementary and Alternative Medicine

Category	Examples
Biologically based therapies	Herbs, diets, dietary supplements, bee venom therapy
Alternative medical systems	Traditional Chinese medicine, homeopathy, Ayurveda
Mind–body interventions	Guided imagery, meditation, hypnosis
Manipulative and body-based methods	Chiropractic medicine, massage
Energy therapies	Therapeutic touch, magnets

Despite this remarkable progress, the treatment options that are currently available to MS patients have significant limitations. Disease-modifying and symptomatic therapies may produce side effects and may be only partially effective.[8] Also, proven therapies may be limited in number or nonexistent, especially for patients with progressive forms of MS[9] and for some symptoms, such as weakness, limb ataxia, and gait disorders.[8]

Because of the limitations of conventional medicine, and for other reasons, many people with MS are interested in, and use, unconventional medical therapies. In studies conducted in the United States,[10-12] Canada,[13] Australia,[14] Germany,[15] and Denmark,[16] it has been reported that one half to three fourths of people with MS use some form of CAM. Comparable studies in the United States found that 40% to 50% of the general population use some form of CAM.[6,17] Studies of people with MS, as well as those of the general population, indicate that most of those who use CAM use it in combination with conventional medicine.[6,10]

CAM INFORMATION SOURCES AND CONVENTIONAL HEALTH PROVIDERS

With a large number of people with MS using CAM, there is a need for detailed, MS-relevant CAM information. However, some of the information that is available to people with MS is biased, inaccurate, and not evidence based. One survey of 50 lay books on CAM found that MS was sometimes defined incorrectly; five or six therapies, on average, were recommended; no two books had the same recommendations; and few books discouraged the use of any CAM therapies.[7] Vendors of CAM products may exaggerate claims, and CAM practitioners and product vendors may have limited MS-specific information and experience. Moreover, by definition, most conventional health providers have little or no knowledge of, or experience with, CAM therapies. Given the lack of reliable MS-specific information in this area, conventional health providers who are willing to become knowledgeable about CAM can provide an important service to MS patients by providing objective CAM information and by referring patients to reputable CAM information resources.

EVIDENCE: CONVENTIONAL AND UNCONVENTIONAL MEDICINE

There are limitations in both the quality and quantity of information in the area of CAM. It is important for conventional health providers to recognize that, because treatment options may be limited, people with MS may be willing to make treatment decisions with limited information.[7] Also, it is important to acknowledge that, like some unconventional therapies, some conventional MS therapies and practices have limitations and may not be entirely evidence based. For example, conventional therapies for MS symptoms and disease modification may be only partially effective, and the use of these therapies may be limited by side effects.[8,18] In addition, no conventional therapies are available to treat some MS symptoms. Finally, conventional medical therapies and practices are sometimes recommended and used with little or no evidence; arbitrary clinical and MRI criteria may be used to determine whether disease-modifying therapies are effective[19], and various "combination" immune therapies may be used for patients who have disease activity on monotherapy.[20]

TABLE 18–2 Levels of Involvement in Complementary and Alternative Medicine (CAM)

"Don't ask, don't tell."
Refer patients to reliable sources of CAM information.
Provide CAM information to patients.
Make recommendations about CAM therapies.
Practice CAM therapies.

LEVELS OF INVOLVEMENT IN CAM

Conventional health providers may interact with patients in several different ways regarding CAM (Table 18-2).[7] The lowest level of involvement is a "Don't ask, don't tell" approach, in which CAM therapies are simply not discussed by health providers or by patients. Clinicians who use this approach have made the choice to be uninvolved with CAM. This choice may not be helpful and may, in fact, be dangerous to patients who are considering CAM and want objective information about the possible benefits and risks of specific therapies. Beyond this uninvolved approach, there are progressively increasing levels of involvement. A simple and helpful measure is to refer patients to reliable lay sources of information on MS and CAM.[1,4] Conventional health providers may go one step further by becoming knowledgeable and providing CAM information themselves. Finally, health providers may become even more involved by actually recommending or practicing CAM therapies; in either case, *caution* must be exercised, because this level of involvement potentially raises important licensing and liability issues.

CATEGORIZING AND REVIEWING MULTIPLE SCLEROSIS–RELEVANT CAM THERAPIES

The remainder of this review provides evidence-based information about MS-relevant CAM therapies and describes how this information may be used in day-to-day clinical encounters with MS patients. To provide structure, focus, and a conceptual framework within this vast and ever-changing subject area, we generally consider those therapies that are relatively popular and for which there is some published evidence. These therapies are presented in a format that indicates whether they are typically used for disease-modifying or symptomatic effects. This framework should make the information accessible to clinicians and may be useful for discussing CAM therapies with patients. As will be noted, it is important to determine why a particular CAM therapy is being considered (e.g., for a disease-modifying effect or a specific symptomatic effect) and then to evaluate the therapy for that specific indication. Also, the "Application to Clinical Practice" sections provide information and strategies for conveying MS-relevant CAM information to patients.

Disease-Modifying Effect

For disease-modifying effects, many CAM therapies are *claimed*, often erroneously, to be effective. CAM therapies with the potential for disease-modifying effects are of great interest to people with MS. Therefore, this area is likely to be encountered frequently by health providers, and it is one in which health providers may provide objective information that can be very helpful to patients.

APPLICATION TO CLINICAL PRACTICE

Importantly, many of the CAM therapies that are claimed to have disease-modifying effects in MS are biologically based therapies, such as dietary supplements (see Table 18-1). These therapies, especially those that have undergone limited investigation, could possibly have beneficial effects in MS, but they could also have no therapeutic effect, or they could even worsen MS or antagonize the effects of conventional disease-modifying medications. These concerns may not be provided with lay information about CAM therapies and may not be readily apparent to people with MS who are considering using biologically based CAM therapies for disease-modifying effects. Conventional health providers can provide this information to MS patients.

POLYUNSATURATED FATTY ACID–ENRICHED DIETS AND OTHER DIETS

On the basis of scientific, epidemiologic, animal model, and clinical trial studies, there is suggestive evidence for a disease-modifying effect of diets that are low in saturated fats and high in polyunsaturated fatty acids (PUFAs), which include ω-6 and ω-3 fatty acids.[1-5]

Among the clinical trial studies, a diet that is low in saturated fat and high in PUFAs was developed by Swank and Dugan and was reported to produce therapeutic effects in MS.[21,22] Importantly, the significance of these results is not known because this study was not controlled, randomized, or blinded.

There have been three randomized controlled trials of ω-6 fatty acids in people with relapsing-remitting MS.[23-25] Two of them reported a statistically significant decrease in attack severity and duration.[23,24] The available data from the three prospective linoleic acid studies were later pooled, reanalyzed, and showed beneficial effects on disability progression in those with mild disease at the start of the trial.[26]

There have been several studies of ω-3 fatty acids. The most rigorous of these was a large, randomized, double-blind, controlled trial.[27] There was no statistically significant treatment effect. However, for progression of disability, there was a trend that favored the treatment group ($P < .07$). Another small (32 patients) randomized study evaluated ω-3 fatty acids as a treatment in combination with interferons or glatiramer acetate.[28] There was a trend for improved emotional and physical functioning in those taking ω-3 fatty acids.

Supplementation with modest doses of ω-3 and ω-6 fatty acids is usually well tolerated. In the United States, the Food and Drug Administration (FDA) has classified fish oil as "generally regarded as safe." The long-term safety of supplementation with other ω-3 fatty acids and all ω-6 fatty acids is not known. Some ω-3 and ω-6 fatty acids may have mild anticoagulant effects. The ω-6 fatty acids may raise triglyceride levels. Some ω-6 fatty acids may rarely provoke seizures. Because supplementation with PUFAs (ω-3 or ω-6) can cause vitamin E deficiency, supplementation with modest doses of vitamin E may be indicated.[3-5]

Other diets have been claimed to be effective MS therapies. For many of these dietary approaches, there is no clear underlying rationale and no scientific or clinical evidence to support their use in MS. Diets for MS that are not supported by a strong rationale or clinical data include allergen-free diets, gluten-free diets, pectin- and fructose-restricted diets, severely sugar-restricted diets, and diets that reduce or eliminate processed foods.[2]

Application to Clinical Practice

The use of dietary approaches is a relatively common CAM strategy among MS patients. At this time, of all of the CAM therapies (including dietary and other approaches), the one with the best evidence for a disease-modifying effect in MS is a PUFA-enriched diet.[2,5] For patients who are considering the use of CAM therapies for a disease-modifying effect, it may be helpful for clinicians to state that the best available evidence for a disease-modifying effect in MS is that for a PUFA-enriched diet.

If patients choose to use a PUFA-enriched diet, then conventional health providers may review the available information about effectiveness and safety. Precautions may need to be taken for those with hypertriglyceridemia, seizure disorders, coagulopathies, antiplatelet or anticoagulant medication use, or upcoming surgery. Supplementation with modest doses of vitamin E may be indicated. Importantly, the evidence concerning PUFA-enriched dietary approaches in MS is not definitive. Consequently, patients should be aware that the exact effect of these approaches on the disease is not known, and the safety and effectiveness of these approaches in combination with disease-modifying medications are not known.

If a specific diet is followed, it is important for patients to maintain a well-balanced intake of nutrients. Some extreme dietary approaches that focus on one specific aspect of the diet may actually create problems by causing nutrient deficiencies.

ANTIOXIDANTS

It has been proposed that free radicals play a role in MS and therefore that antioxidants may have a disease-modifying effect MS.[1-4,29] Commonly used antioxidant supplements include selenium and vitamins A, C, and E. Other antioxidant compounds, some of which are marketed specifically to MS patients, include α-lipoic acid, inosine, uric acid, coenzyme Q10, grape seed extract, pycnogenol, and oligomeric proanthocyanidins (known as "OPCs").[1-4]

There is conflicting information about free radicals and antioxidants in MS.[2,3,7] For years, it has been proposed that free radicals may play a role in the pathogenesis of MS. There is evidence that free radical–induced oxidative damage is increased in MS patients and that oxidative damage plays a role in both myelin injury and axonal damage. These findings suggest that antioxidants could be beneficial in MS. On the other hand, since some antioxidants activate T cells and macrophages, these antioxidants pose theoretical risks in MS. These compounds could worsen MS or antagonize the effects of immune-suppressing and immune-modulating medications.

Studies of antioxidants in demyelinating disease, especially human clinical trials, are limited but generally have demonstrated that antioxidants are well tolerated and do not appear to have adverse effects. In one study, 18 people with MS were treated with multiple antioxidants for 5 weeks.[30] No worsening of disease was noted, but this study was too small and too short to provide any definitive results about the safety and effectiveness of antioxidants in MS.

More recent antioxidant studies in experimental autoimmune encephalomyelitis (EAE) and MS have produced promising results. In EAE, several different antioxidants, including α-lipoic acid[31] and uric acid precursors,[32] were shown to decrease disease severity. In small human clinical studies, inosine (a uric acid precursor)[33] and α-lipoic acid[34] were well tolerated. Studies of several antioxidants in MS are currently being conducted.

Application to Clinical Practice

MS patients may be informed of the limited information that is available about antioxidants and MS. Until more evidence is obtained, it may be best for MS patients to use antioxidants with care. For those patients who are aware of the information in this area and want to increase their antioxidant intake, the most conservative approach is to increase consumption of fruits and vegetables.[1] If supplements are taken, it may be best to take modest doses of vitamins A, C, and E.[1] At this time, it is not clear whether more aggressive (and more expensive) antioxidant supplements such as α-lipoic acid, inosine, coenzyme Q10, pycnogenol, and OPCs have any therapeutic effects in MS.

ECHINACEA AND OTHER "IMMUNE-STIMULATING" SUPPLEMENTS

In some books on alternative medicine, it is stated erroneously that MS is an immune disease and that people with MS should take echinacea and other dietary supplements that are known to activate T cells and macrophages. This is misleading and potentially dangerous information. Ingestion of compounds that activate T cells and macrophages, especially in large amounts or over long periods, could potentially worsen MS or antagonize the therapeutic effects of conventional disease-modifying medications.

The evidence for immune system activation by dietary supplements is generally based on in vitro or animal model studies. There is a case report of a patient who developed acute disseminated encephalomyelitis (ADEM) after intramuscular administration of a mixture of herbs that included echinacea.[35] Because of the limited evidence in this area, the precautions about using these supplements should be viewed as theoretical risks. In addition to echinacea,[3,4,36] other dietary supplements that have been shown to activate T cells or macrophages[3,4] include the herbs alfalfa, ashwagandha (*Withania somnifera*), Asian ginseng, astragalus, cat's claw, garlic, maitake mushroom, mistletoe, shiitake mushroom, Siberian ginseng, and stinging nettle, as well as zinc, the hormone melatonin, and the antioxidant vitamins and minerals discussed earlier.

Application to Clinical Practice

Dietary supplements are widely used by MS patients. Because these supplements may be obtained without a prescription, it is important for health providers to determine which ones are being taken and to provide MS-relevant information. Based on some lay CAM literature, some MS patients may have the incorrect belief that they should be activating their immune system. Educating patients and guiding them away from "immune-stimulating" supplements that pose theoretical risks in MS, especially when taken in high doses or for long periods of time, may improve the quality of care and decrease out-of-pocket expenses for patients.

VITAMIN B_{12}

It is sometimes claimed that vitamin B_{12} supplements are effective for treating MS. However, there are no studies to support the widespread use of these supplements in MS patients.

For MS patients generally, there is no convincing evidence that vitamin B_{12} supplementation provides clinically significant beneficial effects. One small, 6-month study of high-dose vitamin B_{12} supplementation in six patients with progressive MS found that the level of disability was stable or worsened.[37] In another study of 138 MS patients over 24 weeks, vitamin B_{12} monotherapy was compared with the "Cari Loder regime" (vitamin B_{12} along with phenylalanine and lofepramine).[38,39] After 2 weeks of treatment, both groups showed mild neurologic improvement. The group treated with the Cari Loder regime showed some additional mild neurologic improvement and mild relief of some MS symptoms, but the clinical significance of the small therapeutic effects observed in this study is not clear.

A small fraction of MS patients have vitamin B_{12} deficiency.[1,3,40] Supplementation is recommended for these patients.

Application to Clinical Practice

Because some MS patients may have vitamin B_{12} deficiency and vitamin B_{12} deficiency may mimic MS, all patients with MS should have vitamin B_{12} testing. If the level is normal, then there is no convincing evidence that vitamin B_{12} supplementation is beneficial. If the level is low, then additional testing may be indicated, intramuscular or oral vitamin B_{12} should be administered, and follow-up vitamin B_{12} testing should be done periodically.[3]

Disease-Modifying and Symptomatic Effect

Some CAM therapies are claimed to have both disease-modifying and symptomatic effects in MS.

APPLICATION TO CLINICAL PRACTICE

As noted earlier for disease-modifying approaches, it is important for practitioners and patients to recognize that, because of uncertain effects on disease activity and on conventional disease-modifying medications, biologically based CAM approaches need to be used with caution for disease-modifying effects. This consideration may not be readily apparent to patients and should be discussed directly and clearly with them.

VITAMIN D AND CALCIUM

Two actions of vitamin D and calcium are relevant in MS. First, in terms of symptomatic effects, MS patients are at risk for developing osteoporosis and osteopenia.[41] Vitamin D and calcium play critical roles in maintaining bone density.

In addition, vitamin D exerts immune-modulating effects that could have a disease-modifying effect in MS.[42] In EAE, disease severity is worsened by vitamin D deficiency and improved by vitamin D supplementation.[43] Epidemiologic studies indicate that the use of vitamin D supplements and high vitamin D levels are associated with a decreased risk of developing MS.[44,45] At this time, there are very limited clinical trial data concerning vitamin D in MS. A preliminary report of a small, short-term study of 11 MS patients found that treatment with a vitamin D analog, known as "19-nor," did not produce significant benefits on the basis of MRI or clinical outcome measures.[46] Another small study of 15 MS patients found that the active form of vitamin D, calcitriol, was safe and well tolerated for up to 1 year.[47] Further studies are needed to determine whether vitamin D prevents or delays the onset of MS and also whether vitamin D has disease-modifying effects in those with an established diagnosis of MS.

The adequate intake (AI) of vitamin D is 200 to 600 IU daily, and that of calcium is 1000 to 1200 mg daily. The tolerable upper intake level (UL) of vitamin D is 2000 IU daily, and that of calcium is 2500 mg daily. High doses of vitamin D may cause fatigue, abdominal cramps, nausea, vomiting, renal damage, high blood pressure, and multiple other effects.[1,3,4]

Application to Clinical Practice

As noted, vitamin D and calcium are relevant in MS for two reasons. First, for bone density considerations, MS patients who are at risk for osteoporosis should have bone densitometry performed. Those with osteoporosis or osteopenia should be considered for vitamin D and calcium supplementation as well as other measures, including increased weight-bearing activity, osteoporosis medications, and minimizing or eliminating risk factors. For disease-modifying considerations, the information on vitamin D is too limited at this time to make any specific recommendations. It is not known whether intake of vitamin D and calcium has any disease-modifying effect on MS or any effects on the efficacy of conventional disease-modifying medications. If MS patients choose to take vitamin D or calcium supplements, they should be aware of the AI and UL values for these supplements (listed in the previous paragraph).

MARIJUANA (CANNABIS)

Marijuana is a quintessential CAM topic. Some MS clinical studies have produced suggestive results, the pharmacology is intriguing, and important issues are raised about the roles of patients, healthcare providers, and the law in clinical decision making. Marijuana, which is also known as cannabis, contains compounds known as cannabinoids (CBs), which include tetrahydrocannabinol (THC). Through neuronal receptors, CBs suppress excessive neuronal activity and therefore could play a role in some MS symptoms, such as spasticity and pain. Also, through neuroprotective and immune-modulating effects, CBs could have disease-modifying effects in MS.[1,2,4,48,49]

Although some studies suggest that marijuana has both symptomatic and disease-modifying actions in MS, these findings are not definitive. In EAE, CBs have produced symptomatic and disease-modifying effects.[47] In 2003, the first large, rigorous clinical trial of cannabis in MS reported that CBs produced subjective, but not objective, evidence for symptom relief.[50] A 12-month follow-up to this study showed that THC had a small treatment effect on muscle spasticity and a possible therapeutic effect on disability.[51] Studies of an orally administered form of cannabis (Sativex) showed beneficial effects on multiple MS symptoms, including pain, spasticity, and sleeping difficulties.[52] In the United Kingdom, the Cannabinoid Use in Progressive Inflammatory Brain Disease (CUPID) study is evaluating the effects of oral THC on approximately 500 people with progressive MS.

Marijuana has many possible side effects. It may cause nausea, vomiting, sedation, increased risk of seizures, poor pregnancy outcomes, impaired driving, decreased coordination, decreased lung function, and increased risk of cancer of the lung, head, and neck.[1-4]

Application to Clinical Practice

For MS patients who are interested in using marijuana, objective safety and efficacy information may be provided. As noted, marijuana has produced suggestive, but not definitive, effects in MS studies. The possible side effects of marijuana, some of which could be severe, may be discussed with patients. Patients should also be aware that marijuana is illegal in many states and countries.

GINKGO BILOBA

Ginkgo biloba is an extract that is derived from the leaf of the *Ginkgo biloba* tree. It is one of the most extensively studied and most popular herbs.[1-4]

In theory, ginkgo could have disease-modifying as well as symptomatic effects in MS. Ginkgo, which contains platelet-activating factor (PAF) antagonists and flavonoids, has both anti-inflammatory and anti-oxidant effects.[1-4] In EAE, some, but not all, studies indicate that ginkgo decreases disease severity.[53] Ginkgo does not appear to be effective for treating attacks in MS patients[54] and has never been studied for preventing attacks. In small MS clinical studies, ginkgo was shown to improve cognition[55] and decrease fatigue.[56]

Gingko may cause side effects. Because of its PAF antagonist action, ginkgo has anticoagulant effects. Also, it may rarely provoke seizures. Other possible side effects include dizziness, rashes, headaches, nausea, vomiting, diarrhea, and flatulence.[3]

Application to Clinical Practice

Patients who are interested in ginkgo may be given information about its effectiveness and safety in MS. Health professionals may clarify why patients are interested in taking ginkgo and review other available disease-modifying or symptomatic therapies. Patients may be informed that the effects of ginkgo on the course of disease and on conventional disease-modifying medications is not known. Because of its side effect profile, ginkgo should be avoided or used with caution in those patients who have seizure disorders or coagulopathies, take antiplatelet or anticoagulant medications, or are undergoing surgery.

BEE VENOM THERAPY

Bee venom therapy (BVT) involves using bee stings to produce therapeutic effects in MS and other conditions.[1,4] Some chemical constituents in bee venom could have anti-inflammatory effects and other actions that, in theory, could be beneficial for MS.[1,4] However, it is not known whether any of these effects are clinically relevant. Actual clinical studies of BVT in MS are limited. In the highest quality study to date, 26 patients with relapsing-remitting or progressive MS were evaluated in a randomized, controlled, crossover study of placebo versus BVT.[57] BVT did not produce therapeutic effects on attack rate, disability progression, MRI measures, fatigue, or quality of life.

BVT is usually well tolerated. Some lay publications recommend that BVT be given periorbitally for optic neuritis, but periorbital bee stings may actually *cause* optic neuritis.[58] Very rarely, bee stings cause anaphylaxis.[1,4]

Application to Clinical Practice

Patients who are interested in BVT may be informed that there is no evidence of BVT efficacy for disease-modifying or symptomatic effects in MS. It may be helpful to provide information about therapies for which safety and efficacy studies have been performed. Because of the risk of optic neuritis, periorbital BVT should be avoided. Patients may be told that BVT can rarely cause side effects, including anaphylaxis. Because of possible allergic reactions, patients who choose to use BVT should have an epinephrine kit available and should know how to use it.

HYPERBARIC OXYGEN

Hyperbaric oxygen (HBO) is sometimes claimed to be an effective therapy for MS and many other diseases.[1,4] HBO is indeed a recognized medical therapy, but only for a limited number of conditions, including burns, severe infections, decompression sickness, radiation-induced tissue injury, and carbon monoxide poisoning.[1,4] In MS, one study in the 1980s found that HBO was effective,[59] but multiple subsequent studies did not generally find beneficial effects. Two independent reviews of the various studies of HBO in MS concluded that HBO has no consistent therapeutic effect in MS and that HBO should not be used to treat MS patients.[60,61]

Although it is often well tolerated, HBO can cause side effects. Mild visual symptoms may occur. Rare side effects include pneumothorax, seizures, pressure injury to the ear, and cataracts. In addition, HBO is expensive.[1,4]

Application to Clinical Practice

HBO is sometimes marketed specifically to MS patients. Patients who are considering HBO should be given information about the lack of efficacy of this therapy in MS. Unlike some CAM therapies which have undergone little or no investigation in MS, HBO has actually been extensively studied in MS and has *not* been found to be effective. In addition, HBO may rarely cause side effects and is expensive.

LOW-DOSE NALTREXONE

It has been claimed that low doses of oral naltrexone, an opiate antagonist, are effective for relieving MS symptoms, slowing disability progression, and preventing attacks.[1] It has been hypothesized that low-dose naltrexone (LDN) therapy could be therapeutic for MS through excitotoxic and antioxidant mechanisms.[1,62] At this time, several studies of LDN in MS are being conducted, but there have been no published studies of this therapy in EAE or MS. In addition, the safety of LDN use in MS and in the general population has not been well studied.[1]

Application to Clinical Practice

Because it is claimed to be effective for both disease-modifying and symptomatic effects in MS, LDN is of interest to some MS patients. Those who are interested in this therapy may be told that, at this time, there is no objective safety or efficacy information about LDN in MS. Without any clinical studies, it is not known whether this therapy is beneficial, harmful, or without effect in MS. Patients who are interested in LDN may be given information about other conventional or CAM therapies for which there is evidence.

Symptomatic Effect

A vast array of CAM therapies are claimed to have beneficial effects on multiple MS symptoms.

APPLICATION TO CLINICAL PRACTICE

For some MS patients, the cautious use of CAM for symptomatic therapy may be reasonable. As noted, disease-modifying CAM strategies, especially those that are biologically based and poorly studied in MS, are risky because they could worsen disease or antagonize disease-modifying medications, leading to irreversible central nervous system injury. In contrast, symptomatic CAM therapies that are possibly effective and of low risk may be reasonable for some patients, because irreversible harm is unlikely. For example, CAM therapies could be considered for mild symptoms such as mild spasticity or mild fatigue. Also, CAM therapies may be reasonable for symptoms for which conventional medical therapy is partially effective or nonexistent. CAM should not be used initially or exclusively for severe symptoms such as disabling spasticity or intractable pain; in some of these situations, however, it may be reasonable for patients to use CAM along with conventional medical therapies.

YOGA

Yoga, which was developed in India thousands of years ago, is widely practiced but has undergone limited clinical investigation.[1,4] One well-designed, controlled trial in MS found that, relative to a control group, both yoga and conventional exercise produced significant improvement in fatigue.[63] Yoga is usually safe. In the study of yoga in MS, there were no serious adverse effects.[63]

Application to Clinical Practice

Yoga may be therapeutic for MS fatigue. For patients who are interested in CAM approaches, yoga is a low-risk procedure that may provide symptomatic relief. Yoga may be modified for those with disabilities.[1] Difficult postures or vigorous exercise should be avoided or done with caution by pregnant women and by patients with fatigue, heat sensitivity, gait instability, or significant heart, lung, or bone conditions.[1,3]

TAI CHI

Tai chi, a martial art that has been practiced for centuries in China, has undergone limited investigation in MS.[1,4] Small, nonblinded studies of tai chi in MS have produced suggestive beneficial effects on walking, spasticity, and social and emotional functioning.[64,65] Further studies are needed. Tai chi is usually well tolerated but may cause mild side effects, such as strained muscles and joints.[1,4] Although the exercises may be modified for patients with disabilities, there is a risk of falling while doing tai chi.

Application to Clinical Practice

Tai chi is a therapy for which there is limited efficacy information in MS. However, it is a low-risk therapy and in some situations may be reasonable for symptomatic treatment. Because of the risk of falls, it should be avoided or used with caution by those patients with severe osteoporosis, acute low back pain, significant joint injuries, or bone fractures.[1,4]

HERBAL MEDICINE: CRANBERRY, KAVA-KAVA, ST. JOHN'S WORT, VALERIAN

Some herbal therapies may produce therapeutic effects for symptoms that occur with MS. However, they may also have possible side effects.[1,3,4] These herbal therapies include the following:

- *Cranberry:* This herb, possibly through a novel mechanism of action, may be effective for preventing urinary tract infections (UTIs), especially in women with normal bladder function.[3,66,67] Cranberry may increase the coagulant effect of warfarin (Coumadin),[68] and its long-term use in high doses may increase the risk of kidney stones.[69]
- *Kava-kava:* This herb contains compounds that, like benzodiazepines, interact with γ-aminobutyric acid (GABA)-A receptors, and it may be effective for treating mild anxiety.[1,4,69,70] However, there have been more than 50 cases of liver toxicity associated with kava-kava, some of which have led to liver transplantation or death.[71] Kava-kava is now banned in Canada and Europe, but it is still available in the United States.
- *St. John's wort:* This herb may be effective for treating mild to moderate depression.[1,3,69,72] It is usually well tolerated but may cause fatigue and photosensitivity.[1,3,73] Because it induces cytochrome P-450 enzymes, it may alter levels of many drugs, including anticonvulsants, warfarin (Coumadin), antidepressants, and oral contraceptives.[3,69,73]
- *Valerian:* In studies of variable quality, valerian has been shown to be beneficial for insomnia.[3,74] It is sometimes claimed to be effective for anxiety, depression, and spasticity, but it has not been well studied for these conditions. Valerian is generally well tolerated but may cause sedation.[3]

Application to Clinical Practice

Patients who are interested in these herbal therapies may be informed of the efficacy information that is available, which is limited but suggestive for some MS symptoms. In the case of cranberry, it may be reasonable for some patients to use this herb for UTI prevention. However, cranberry should not be used to treat known UTIs. For St. John's wort, even if patients choose to use this herb, they should be told not to self-diagnose and self-treat for depression. For all of these herbs, patients may be made aware of the side effects. Because of the possible severe side effects of kava-kava, this herb should not be used. Because St. John's wort and valerian may cause fatigue, they may worsen MS fatigue or increase the sedating effect of some medications.

Conclusion

The study of CAM in MS is an evolving field. At this time, there is some information about the effectiveness and safety of these therapies. Because these therapies are used frequently by MS patients, neurologists and other health professionals may improve the quality of care of MS patients by providing objective CAM information to patients.

Acknowledgment

The author would like to thank the MS foundation for a grant that supported this work.

REFERENCES

1. Bowling AC: Complementary and alternative medicine and multiple sclerosis. New York, Demos Medical Publishing, 2007.
2. Bowling AC, Stewart TM: Current complementary and alternative therapies of multiple sclerosis. Curr Treatment Options Neurol 2003;5:55-68.
3. Bowling AC, Stewart TM: Dietary Supplements and Multiple Sclerosis: A Health Professional's Guide. New York, Demos Medical Publishing, 2004.
4. Polman CH, Thompson AJ, Murray TJ, et al: Multiple Sclerosis: The Guide to Treatment and Management. New York, Demos Medical Publishing, 2006, pp 117-179.
5. Stewart TM, Bowling AC: Polyunsaturated fatty acid supplementation in MS. Int MS J 2005;12:88-93.
6. Eisenberg D, Davis R, Ettner S, et al: Trends in alternative medicine use in the United States, 1990-1997. JAMA 1998;280:1569-1575.
7. Bowling AC, Ibrahim R, Stewart TM: Alternative medicine and multiple sclerosis: An objective review from an American perspective. Int J MS Care 2000;2:14-21.
8. Kesselring J: Complications of multiple sclerosis. In McDonald WI, Noseworthy JH: Multiple Sclerosis 2. Philadelphia, Butterworth Heinemann, 2003, pp 217-227.
9. Thompson A: Treatment of progressive multiple sclerosis. In McDonald WI, Noseworthy JH: Multiple Sclerosis 2. Philadelphia, Butterworth Heinemann, 2003, pp 341-359.
10. Berkman C, Pignotti M, Cavallo P, et al: Use of alternative treatments by people with multiple sclerosis. Neurorehab Neural Repair 1999;13:243-254.
11. Nayak S, Matheis RJ, Schoenberger NE, et al: Use of unconventional therapies by individuals with multiple sclerosis. Clin Rehabil 2003;17:181-191.
12. Shinto L, Yadav V, Morris C, et al: Demographic and health-related factors associated with complementary and alternative medicine (CAM) use in multiple sclerosis. Mult Scler 2006;12:94-100.
13. Page SA, Verhoef MJ, Stebbins RA, et al: The use of complementary and alternative therapies by people with multiple sclerosis. Chronic Dis Can 2003;24:75-79.
14. Hooper KD, Pender MP, Webb PM, et al: Use of traditional and complementary medical care by patients with multiple sclerosis in South-East Queensland. Int J MS Care 2001;3:13-28.
15. Apel A, Greim B, Konig N, et al: Frequency of current utilisation of complementary and alternative medicine by patients with multiple sclerosis. J Neurol 2006;253:1331-1336.

16. Stenager E, Stenager EN, Knudsen L, et al: The use of non-medical/alternative treatment in multiple sclerosis: A 5 year follow-up study. Acta Neurol Belg 1995;95:18-22.
17. Barnes PM, Powell-Griner E, McFann K, et al: Complementary and alternative medicine use among adults: United States, 2002. Adv Data 2004;343:1-20.
18. Noseworthy J: Treatment of relapses and relapsing remitting multiple sclerosis. In McDonald WI, Noseworthy JH: Multiple Sclerosis 2. Philadelphia, Butterworth Heinemann, 2003, pp 169-191.
19. Bashir K, Buchwald L, Coyle P, et al: Optimizing immunomodulatory therapy for MS patients: An integrated management model. J Neurol Sci 2002;201:89-90.
20. Kaufman M: Combining therapies with interferon beta for relapsing and early progressive MS: A review. Int J MS Care 2002;4:50-65.
21. Swank R: Multiple sclerosis: Twenty years on low fat diet. Arch Neurol 1970;23:460-474.
22. Swank R, Dugan B: Effect of low saturated fat diet in early and late cases of multiple sclerosis. Lancet 1990;336:37-39.
23. Millar J, Zilkha K, Langman M, et al: Double-blind trial of linoleate supplementation of the diet in multiple sclerosis. Br Med J 1973;1:765-768.
24. Bates D, Fawcett P, Shaw D, et al: Polyunsaturated fatty acids in treatment of acute remitting multiple sclerosis. Br Med J 1978;2:1390-1391.
25. Paty D: Double-blind trial of linoleic acid in multiple sclerosis. Arch Neurol 1983;40:693-694.
26. Dworkin R, Bates D, Millar J, et al: Linoleic acid and multiple sclerosis: A reanalysis of three double-blind trials. Neurology 1984;34:1441-1445.
27. Bates D, Cartlidge N, French J, et al: A double-blind controlled trial of long chain n-3 polyunsaturated fatty acids in the treatment of multiple sclerosis. J Neurol Neurosurg Psychiatry 1989;52:18-22.
28. Weinstock-Guttman B, Baier M, Park Y, et al: Low fat dietary intervention with omega-3 fatty acid supplementation in multiple sclerosis patients. Prostaglandins Leukot Essent Fatty Acids 2005;73:392-404.
29. van Meeteren ME, Teunissen CE, Dijkstra A, et al: Antioxidants and polyunsaturated fatty acids in multiple sclerosis. Eur J Clin Nutr 2005;59:1347-1361.
30. Mai J, Sorenson P, Hansen J: High dose antioxidant supplementation to MS patients: Effects on glutathione peroxidase, clinical safety, and absorption of selenium. Biol Trace Elem Res 1990;24:109-117.
31. Scott GS, Spitsin SV, Kean RB, et al: Therapeutic intervention in experimental allergic encephalomyelitis by administration of uric acid precursors. Proc Natl Acad Sci U S A 2002;99:16303-16308.
32. Marracci GH, Jones RE, McKeon GP, et al: Alpha lipoic acid inhibits T cell migration into the spinal cord and suppresses and treats experimental autoimmune encephalomyelitis. J Neuroimmunol 2002;131:104-114.
33. Spitsin S, Hooper DC, Leist T, et al: Inactivation of peroxynitrite in multiple sclerosis patients after oral administration of inosine may suggest possible approaches to therapy of the disease. Mult Scler 2001;7:313-319.
34. Yadav V, Marracci G, Lovera J, et al: Lipoic acid in multiple sclerosis: A pilot study. Mult Scler 2005;11:159-165.
35. Schwarz S, Knauth M, Schwab S, et al: Acute disseminated encephalomyelitis after parenteral therapy with herbal extracts: A report of two cases. J Neurol Neurosurg Psychiatry 2000;69:516-518.
36. Percival SS: Use of echinacea in medicine. Biochem Pharmacol 2000;60:155-158.
37. Kira J, Tobimatus S, Goto I: Vitamin B12 metabolism and massive-dose methyl vitamin B12 therapy in Japanese patients with multiple sclerosis. Int Med 1994;33:82-86.
38. Loder C, Allawi J, Horrobin DF: Treatment of multiple sclerosis with lofepramine, L-phenylalanine, and vitamin B-12: Mechanism of action and clinical importance. Roles of the locus coeruleus and central noradrenergic systems. Med Hypotheses 2002;59:594-602.
39. Wade DT, Young CA, Chaudhuri KR, Davidson DLW: A randomized placebo controlled exploratory study of vitamin B-12, lofepramine, and L-phenylalanine (the "Cari Loder regime") in the treatment of multiple sclerosis. J Neurol Neurosurg Psychiatry 2002;73:246-249.
40. Goodkin D, Jacobsen D, Galvez N, et al: Serum cobalamin deficiency is uncommon in multiple sclerosis. Arch Neurol 1994;51:1110-1114.
41. Weinstock-Guttman B, Gallagher E, Baier M, et al: Risk of bone loss in men with multiple sclerosis. Mult Scler 2004;10:170-175.
42. Cantorna M, Humpal-Winter J, DeLuca H: In vivo upregulation of interleukin-4 is one mechanism underlying the immunoregulatory effects of 1,25-dihydroxyvitamin D3. Arch Biochem Biophys 2000;377:135-138.
43. Cantorna M, Hayes C, DeLuca H: 1, 25-Dihydroxyvitamin D3 reversibly blocks the progression of relapsing encephalomyelitis, a model of multiple sclerosis. Proc Natl Acad Sci U S A 1996;93: 7861-7864.

44. Munger KL, Zhang SM, O'Reilly E, et al: Vitamin D intake and incidence of multiple sclerosis. Neurology 2004;62:60-65.
45. Munger KL, Levin LI, Hollis BW, et al: Serum 25-hydroxyvitamin D levels and risk of multiple sclerosis. JAMA 2006;296:2832-2838.
46. Fleming JO, Hummel AL, Beinlich BR, et al: Vitamin D treatment of relapsing-remitting multiple sclerosis (RRMS): A MRI-based pilot study. Neurology 2000;54: A338.
47. Wingerchuk DM, Lesaux J, Rice GPA, et al: A pilot study of oral calcitriol (1,25-dihydroxyvitamin D3) for relapsing-remitting multiple sclerosis. J Neurol Neurosurg Psychiatry 2005;76:1294-1296.
48. Bowling AC: Worthless weed or pot of gold? Int J MS Care 2003;5:138,166.
49. Bowling AC: Cannabinoids in MS: Are we any closer to knowing how best to use them? Mult Scler 2006;12:523-525.
50. Zajicek J, Fox P, Sanders H, et al: Cannabinoids for treatment of spasticity and other symptoms related to multiple sclerosis (CAMS study): Multicentre randomized placebo-controlled trial. Lancet 2003;362:1517-1526.
51. Zajicek J, Sanders HP, Wright DE, et al: Cannabinoids in multiple sclerosis (CAMS) study: Safety and efficacy data for 52 weeks follow-up. J Neurol Neurosurg Psychiatry 2005;76:1664-1669.
52. Barnes MP: Sativex: Clinical efficacy and tolerability in the treatment of symptoms of multiple sclerosis and neuropathic pain. Expert Opin Pharmacother 2006;7:607-615.
53. Braquet P, Esanu A, Buisine E, et al: Recent progress in ginkgolide research. Med Res Rev 1991;11:295-355.
54. Brochet B, Guinot P, Orgogozo J, et al: Double-blind, placebo controlled, multicentre study of ginkgolide B in treatment of acute exacerbations for multiple sclerosis. The Ginkgolide Study Group in Multiple Sclerosis. J Neurol Neurosurg Psychiatry 1995;58:360-362.
55. Lovera J, Bagert B, Smoot K, et al: Ginkgo biloba for the improvement of cognitive performance in multiple sclerosis: A randomized, placebo-controlled trial. Mult Scler 2007;13:376-385.
56. Johnson SK, Diamond BJ, Rausch S, et al: The effect of Ginkgo biloba on functional measure in multiple sclerosis: A pilot randomized controlled trial. Explore (NY) 2006;2:19-24.
57. Wesselius T, Heersema DJ, Mostert JP, et al: A randomized crossover study of bee sting therapy for multiple sclerosis. Neurology 2005;65:1764-1768.
58. Song H-S, Wray SH: Bee sting optic neuritis. J Clin Neuro-ophthalmol 1991;11:45-49.
59. Fischer BH, Marks M, Reich T: Hyperbaric oxygen treatment of multiple sclerosis: A randomized, placebo-controlled, double-blind study. N Engl J Med 1983;308:181-186.
60. Kleijnen J, Knipschild P: Hyberbaric oxygen for multiple sclerosis: Review of controlled trials. Acta Neurol Scand 1995;91:330-334.
61. Bennett M, Heard R: Hyperbaric oxygen therapy for multiple sclerosis. Cochrane Database Syst Rev 2004, (1):CD003057.
62. Agrawal YP: Low dose naltrexone therapy in multiple sclerosis. Med Hypotheses 2005;64:721-724.
63. Oken BS, Kishiyama S, Zajdel D, et al: Randomized controlled trial of yoga and exercise in multiple sclerosis. Neurology 2004;62:2058-2064.
64. Husted C, Pham L, Hekking A, et al: Improving quality of life for people with chronic conditions: The example of t'ai chi and multiple sclerosis. Altern Ther 1999;5:70-74.
65 Mills M, Allen J: Mindfulness of movement as a coping strategy in multiple sclerosis: A pilot study. Gen Hosp Psychiatry 2000;22:425-431.
66. Linsenmeyer T, Harrison B, Oakley A, et al: Evaluation of cranberry supplement for reduction of urinary tract infections in individuals with neurogenic bladders secondary to spinal cord injury: A prospective, double blinded, placebo-controlled, crossover study. J Spinal Cord Med 2004;27:29-34.
67. Waites KB, Canupp KC, Armstrong S, et al: Effect of cranberry extract on bacteriuria and pyuria in persons with neurogenic bladder secondary to spinal cord injury. J Spinal Cord Med 2004;27:35-40.
68. Suvarna R: Possible interaction between warfarin and cranberry juice. Br Med J 2003;327:1454.
69. Jellin JM, Gregory PJ, Batz F, et al: Pharmacist's Letter/Prescriber's Letter Natural Medicines Comprehensive Database, 8th ed. Stockton, California, Therapeutic Research Faculty, 2006.
70. Russo E: Handbook of Psychotropic Herbs: A Scientific Analysis of Herbal Remedies for Psychiatric Conditions. New York, Haworth Herbal Press, 2001, pp 160-179.
71. Clouatre DL: Kava kava: Examining new reports of toxicity. Toxicol Lett 2004;150:85-96.
72. Werneke U, Horn O, Taylor DM: How effective is St. John's wort? The evidence revisited. J Clin Psychol 2004;65:611-617.
73. Izzo AA: Drug interactions with St. John's wort (*Hypericum perforatum*): Review of the clinical evidence. Int J Clin Pharmacol Ther 2004;42:139-148.
74. Mischoulon D, Rosenbaum JF: Natural Medications for Psychiatric Disorders: Considering the Alternatives. Philadelphia, Lippincott Williams & Wilkins, 2002, pp 132-146.

19 Is Multiple Sclerosis a Neurodegenerative Disorder?

RANJAN DUTTA • BRUCE D. TRAPP

Multiple sclerosis (MS), an inflammatory demyelinating disease of the central nervous system (CNS), affects more than 2 million people worldwide[1-3] and is the leading cause of nontraumatic neurological disability in young adults in North America and Europe. The cause of MS is unknown, and the clinical disease course is variable and unpredictable. MS is a chronic disease afflicting twice as many females as males.

The majority (about 85%) of MS patients have a biphasic disease course, which is initially characterized by alternating episodes of neurologic disability and recovery. This phase of the disease, termed relapsing-remitting multiple sclerosis (RRMS), can last years or decades.[1,2] Within 25 years, approximately 90% of RRMS patients exhibit a secondary progressive disease course (SPMS) characterized by steadily increasing permanent neurological disability.[2,4] Approximately 10% of MS patients experience primary progressive disease (PPMS) characterized by a steady decline in neurologic function from disease onset without recovery. A small percentage (about 5%) of MS patients also exhibit a progressive relapsing course (PRMS), which is characterized by steady progressive neurological decline punctuated by well-demarcated acute attacks with or without recovery.

The diversity of clinical course and patterns of disease progression have generated significant interest in the underlying pathologic processes that are responsible for reversible and permanent disability in MS patients. An important question is whether RRMS and PPMS are the same disease. If the answer is yes, one could argue that inflammation is secondary to an underlying neurodegenerative disease process. Although the age at onset and number of relapses vary significantly in RRMS and PPMS, these two MS cohorts reach permanent disability milestones at similar ages.[5,6] One interpretation of these epidemiological findings is that all MS patients have a similar rate of primary neurodegeneration with variable secondary inflammatory demyelinating lesions. The relapses result in earlier diagnosis of MS, but they have marginal effect on the progression of permanent neurologic disability.

The purpose of this chapter is to discuss the role of axonal transection and neurodegeneration in MS. Both play significant roles in MS disease progression, and the possibility that MS may be a primary neurodegenerative disease with secondary inflammatory demyelination is discussed.

Neurologic Disability in Relapsing-Remitting Multiple Sclerosis

The pathologic hallmark of MS is the presence of inflammatory demyelinated lesions of brain and spinal cord white matter. These lesions cause the rapid-onset and reversible neurologic disability of RRMS. New lesion areas can be delineated by brain imaging. Those that enhance with gadolinium (GAD) are considered to be "new" and reflect breakdown of the blood brain barrier, infiltration of hematogenous leukocytes, demyelination, and oligodendrocyte death. The edema associated with "MS lesions" is a major contributor to the neurological relapses, because it blocks the conduction of action potentials. Demyelination is another contributor to the transient disability.

Why is the disability transient? The brain employs a number of adoptive mechanisms that restore function to demyelinated white matter. These work in the environment of the demyelinated area and in more generalized network plasticity. The axon responds to loss of the insulating myelin by distributing its voltage-gated sodium (Na^+) channels along the demyelinated axolemma.[7] These axons slowly regain the ability to conduct axon potentials, albeit at a reduced velocity. With time, the edema that induced conduction block resolves. In some lesions, the demyelinated axons are remyelinated, and nerve conduction is restored. From a system neuroscience point of view, recent functional magnetic resonance imaging (MRI) studies have identified cortical areas of brain that are activated after a white matter lesion. This activation can be transient and may reflect recovery of function within the lesion.[8,9]

The scenarios described are the logical and accepted explanation for the neurologic disability associated with relapse and remission. Current MS therapies focus on reducing the occurrence of inflammatory demyelinated lesions by inhibiting the immune system. Although current immune therapies delay the relapsing-remitting phase of the disease process, they do not stop the disease, and they appear to have marginal effect on slowing the progressive stages of MS (SPMS or PPMS). Are these different diseases, or are there other pathologic targets in MS brains? We do not know if we are dealing with one or multiple disease etiologies in the MS patient cohort. We do know, however, that myelin and white matter are not the only targets of the MS disease process. It is generally accepted that axonal degeneration is the major cause of the irreversible neurologic disability associated with SPMS and PPMS. In addition, the gray matter is a significant target of the MS disease process, and recent studies support the notion that gray matter demyelination may exceed white matter demyelination in some MS patients. The remainder of this chapter focuses on axonal and neuronal pathology in MS brain.[10,11]

AXONAL TRANSECTION DURING INFLAMMATORY DEMYELINATION

A series of papers in the late 1990s described a variety of axonal changes in actively demyelinating lesions observed in postmortem MS brains. Most of these changes involve alterations in the axonal cytoskeleton or the accumulation of proteins that are transported down the axon. Ferguson and colleagues[12] described axonal accumulations of the amyloid precursor protein (APP) in acutely demyelinated axons. APP is present at undetectable levels in normally myelinated axons, but it can accumulate at detectable levels following demyelination. APP is not specific for altered fast axonal transport in MS lesions, because any fast axonally transported protein will accumulate.[12] The pore-forming subunits of N-type calcium channel[13] and metabotrophic glutamate receptors[14] also accumulate in acutely demyelinated axons[15] and, if inserted into the axolemma, may contribute to axonal dysfunction and transection. Alterations in the cytoskeleton of acutely demyelinated axons are expected, as one of the functions of myelin is to stabilize the axonal cytoskeleton so as to maximize transport to presynaptic terminals.

One of the best-characterized myelin-induced axonal changes is the phosphorylation of axonal neurofilaments.[16] Phosphorylation increases the extension of sidearms from the neurofilaments, which in turn increases interfilament spacing and axonal diameter. We used antibodies against nonphosphorylated neurofilaments to examine axonal changes in demyelinated MS lesions. As expected, many demyelinated axons contained a dramatic increase in nonphosphorylated neurofilament epitopes.[17] In addition, a striking number of nonphosphorylated neurofilament positive ovoids were present in acute MS lesions.[17] Using confocal microscopy and three-dimensional reconstructions, we established that many of the ovoids were transected ends of axons. How was this done and why was it important? If you transect a CNS axon, the axonal segment distal to the transection will degenerate. The part of the axon still connected to the neuronal cell body can survive and mend the cut. Axonal transport continues in this axon, but the mended end cannot handle the transported material, which accumulates and forms an ovoid (Fig. 19-1). Three-dimensional reconstruction of the ovoids established that most of the ovoids were connected to a single axon and therefore represented the cut ends of the transected axons. This observation is important for two reasons. First, when a CNS axon is cut, the function of that axon is lost forever. Second, the number of transected axons in acute MS lesions was very abundant, exceeding 11,000 per cubic millimeter of lesion area. Transected axons were identified and quantified in MS lesions from patients with disease durations ranging from 2 weeks to 27 years, using antibodies to nonphosphorylated neurofilaments.[17] The identification of significant axonal transection in patients with short disease duration when inflammatory demyelination is predominant established the concept that axonal loss occurs at disease onset in MS. Positive correlations between inflammatory activity of MS lesions and axonal damage suggests that inflammation modulates axonal pathology in MS patients.[12-15,17,18]

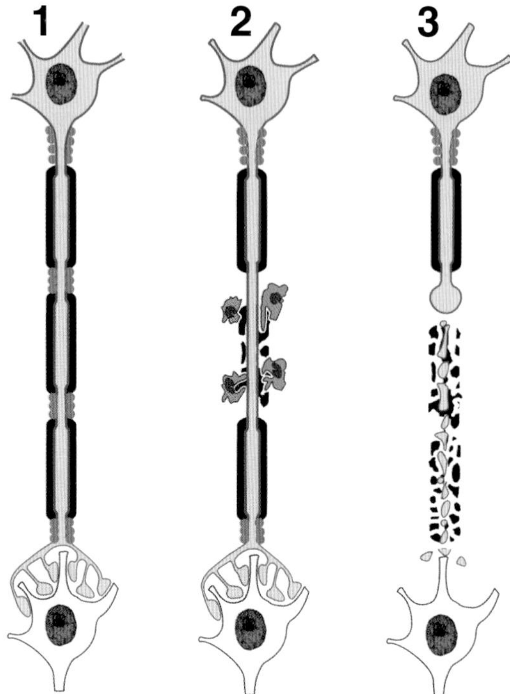

Figure 19–1 Axonal transection during inflammatory demyelination. **1**, Normal cell. **2**, Demyelination is an immune-mediated process that can lead to axonal transection. **3**, After the axon is transected, its distal end rapidly degenerates while the proximal end connected to the neuronal cell body survives. The neuron continues to transport molecules and organelles down the transected axon, and they accumulate at the transaction site and form an ovoid (**3**). (From Trapp BD, Nave K-A: Multiple sclerosis: An immune or neurodegenerative disorder? Ann Rev Neurosci 2008;31:247-269.)

With all this axonal loss occurring in acute MS lesions, why are relapses reversible? The human brain has a remarkable ability to compensate for neuronal loss. For example, it has been estimated that patients with Parkinson's disease loose more than 70% of their dopaminergic neurons before they show clinical signs.[19,20] In addition, most demyelinated axons survive the acute demyelinating environment. If it takes a 60% to 70% loss of neurons or axons to produce irreversible neurologic disability, an acute demyelinated lesion is unlikely to generate this much axonal loss.[21] The only data that address this issue is a case report that estimated less than 22% axonal loss at sites distal to a fatal brainstem lesion.[21] Therefore, axonal loss does not have an immediate clinical readout during early stages of RRMS. With time and additional lesions, however, axonal loss can drive the clinical aspects of MS. The conversion of RRMS to SPMS is therefore thought to occur when the brain exhausts its capacity to compensate for further axonal loss.[22] Axonal loss in MS patients is supported by variety of analyses, including whole brain atrophy[23-25] and reductions in the neuronal-specific amino acid, *N*-acetyl aspartate acid (NAA).[27-29]

IMMUNE-MEDIATED AXONAL LOSS

Axonal pathology and the number of transected axons correlate with the degree of inflammatory activity (number of immune cells) in acute MS lesions.[20,15,17] Axonal transection, therefore, is thought to result from nonspecific damage caused by the inflammatory process. In other words, demyelinated axons are vulnerable to the inflammatory environment of an actively demyelinating white matter lesion. Activated immune and glial cells release a plethora of substances, including proteolytic enzymes, matrix metalloproteases, cytokines, oxidative products, and free radicals, that can damage axons.[30] Inducible nitric oxide synthase (iNOS), a key enzyme required for synthesis of nitric oxide (NO), is significantly increased in acute MS lesions.[31,32] NO and its derivative, peroxynitrite, can inhibit mitochondrial respiration, modify the activity of ion channels, and reduce axonal survival. Activated immune cells, axons, and astrocytes are potential sources for excessive levels of glutamate in acute MS lesions,[33,34] and magnetic resonance spectroscopy studies of MS brains have detected elevated glutamate levels in acute MS lesions.[35] Activation of α-amino-3-hydroxy-5-methyl-4-isoxazole propionate (AMPA) and/or kainate (but not *N*-methyl-D-aspartate [NMDA]) glutamate receptors can damage axons, and AMPA/kainate receptor antagonists can be axon-protective under hypoxic/ischemic conditions.[36,37] It is possible, therefore, that demyelinated axons are vulnerable to excitotoxic damage by glutamate.

Another possible mechanism of axonal degeneration in MS is a specific immunologic attack on the axon. Immune-mediated axonal transection is suggested by the strong correlation between inflammation and axonal transection. The terminal axonal ovoids are often surrounded by macrophages and activated microglia in acute MS lesions.[17] Whether these cells are directly attacking axons, protecting axons, or removing debris remains to be determined. Direct immunologic targeting of axons is not without precedence. Primary immune-mediated attack against gangliosides on peripheral nervous system axons has been identified as a cause of axonal degeneration in the autoimmune disease acute motor axonal neuropathy (AMAN), a variant of Guillain-Barré syndrome (GBS).[38] Unlike AMAN, antibodies to axonal components in the CNS have not been localized to MS lesions.[38,39] Additionally, as most axons survive the acute demyelinating process, it seems unlikely that there is a specific immunologic attack against axons. Cytotoxic CD8-positive T cells have been identified as possible mediators of axonal transection in MS lesions,[40,41] in EAE mice,[42] and in vitro.[43,44] Further, some reports indicate that axonal subpopulations may be targeted by immune-mediated mechanisms.[45-47] Despite the current paucity of direct evidence supporting a specific immunologic attack on axons in MS, we should not ignore the possibility of cell-mediated mechanisms of axon loss.

Neurologic Disability in Secondary Progressive Multiple Sclerosis

Although new inflammatory demyelinating lesions may contribute to disability in SPMS, many SPMS patients continue to decline neurologically without evidence of new inflammatory demyelinating lesions as measured by MRI. Most importantly, SPMS patients do not respond to anti-inflammatory therapies. One logical and accepted explanation for the continuous neurologic decline in SPMS is degeneration of chronically demyelinated axons. Although this hypothesis is intuitively attractive, it is difficult to unequivocally prove such a phenomenon, as one would have to sample and quantify demyelinated axons in the same location at multiple time points, which is impossible. However, there are a convincing number of correlations and "proof of principle" studies that support a continuous loss of chronically demyelinated axons in MS brain.

AXONAL LOSS DUE TO LOSS OF MYELIN-DERIVED TROPHIC SUPPORT

Proof of principle for the degeneration of chronic demyelinated axons is derived from mice that lack individual myelin proteins. These mice were created to investigate the role of myelin proteins during the process of myelination, including the myelin-associated glycoprotein (MAG), 2′,3′-cyclic nucleotide 3′-phosphodiesterase (CNP), and proteolipid protein (PLP). Surprisingly, each of these myelin proteins could be removed from oligodendrocytes without major effects on the process of myelination.[48-50] All three lines of mice, however, developed a late-onset, slowly progressing axonopathy and axonal degeneration. These studies established that, in addition to axonal insulation, myelin/oligodendrocytes provide trophic support that is essential for long-term axonal survival. Furthermore, the role of myelin proteins in axonal support could be separated from their role in myelin formation. The axonal pathology that preceded axonal degeneration is different in the MAG-null mice compared with the PLP-null and CNP-null mice. In the MAG-deficient mice, the reduction in axonal caliber was most prominent in paranodal regions of the myelin internodes and was due in part to reduced phosphorylation on neurofilaments.[48] In the PLP- and CNP-null mice, axonal swelling precedes axonal degeneration. These swelling occurred most often at distal paranodes, suggesting a defect in retrograde axonal transport at nodes of Ranvier.[49,51] Compared with PLP-null mice, the CNP-null mice had a more severe axonal phenotype.[50] PLP-null mice also exhibit alterations in compact myelin membrane spacing, and when their compact myelin phenotype was rescued by the peripheral myelin protein P_0.[52] Although the role of oligodendrocytes in myelin formation and axonal survival are segregated in MAG- and CNP-null mice, the mechanisms by which these proteins provide such support are currently unknown.

If removal of single myelin proteins can cause axonal degeneration without affecting the structure of myelin, it should not be surprising that loss of myelin as it occurs in MS can cause axonal degeneration. Several findings support axonal loss during the later stages of MS. The MS brain undergoes continuous atrophy when new inflammatory demyelinating lesions are rare.[20] Pathologic studies have identified transected axons and axoplasmic changes that render the axon dysfunctional and at risk of degenerating. Postmortem studies have identified axonal retraction bulbs, the histologic hallmark of transected axons, in chronic inactive lesions.[18] Although their numbers are small, these ovoids are transient structures, and the accumulative degeneration of chronically demyelinated axons over decades would be substantial. How many axons are lost in chronic MS lesions? Estimates of total axonal loss in spinal cord, corpus callosum, and optic nerve lesions approach 70%.[44,46,53] Moreover, as discussed in detail later, the 30% of demyelinated axons that remain in these chronic lesions have significant structural and molecular changes that are detrimental to normal function and survival.[28,53,55] These observations implicate axonal degeneration as a cause of irreversible neurologic impairment during chronic progressive stages of MS.

DEGENERATION OF CHRONICALLY DEMYELINATED AXONS

Indirect evidence supports general mechanisms by which chronically demyelinated axons degenerate. Few of these mechanisms have been directly tested because of a paucity of animal models in which demyelinated axons persist for extended periods. The central hypotheses involve an imbalance between energy demand and energy supply. In normal myelinated fibers, Na^+ channels are concentrated at the nodes of Ranvier, allowing the action potential to rapidly jump from node to node. When Na^+ enters nodal axoplasm, it is rapidly exchanged for extracellular K^+ by the sodium-potassium adenosine triphosphatase (Na^+,K^+-ATPase). This continuous energy-dependent ion exchange is required for maintenance of axonal polarization to support the repetitive axonal firing that is essential for many neuronal functions. Therefore, myelination not only promotes rapid nerve conduction but also conserves energy.

Although loss of myelin per se may not kill axons, it renders them more vulnerable to physiologic stress and degeneration by substantially increasing the energy requirement for nerve conduction. Following demyelination, Na^+ channels become diffusely distributed along the denuded axolemma. This supports depolarization of the demyelinated axonal segment and permits less efficient, nonsaltatory action potential propagation at the cost of increased energy required to restore transaxolemmal Na^+ and K^+ gradients. If axonal Na^+ rises above its nominal concentration of approximately 20 mmol/L,[56] the Na^+/Ca^{2+} exchanger, which exchanges axoplasmic Ca^{2+} for extracellular Na^+, will operate in the reverse Ca^{2+}-import mode. With increasing electrical traffic, axoplasmic Ca^{2+} rises, and eventually a Ca^{2+}-mediated degenerative response is initiated. An underlying mechanism of Ca^{2+}-mediated axonal degeneration is reduced axoplasmic production of adenosine triphosphate (ATP). This impairs Na^+,K^+-ATPase function, which causes axoplasmic ionic imbalances and leads to Ca^{2+}-mediated injury. Excessive axoplasmic Ca^{2+} accumulation results in a vicious cycle of impaired mitochondrial operation, reduced energy production, and compromised axonal transport.

This vulnerability to degeneration is compounded by several additional factors. The mitochondria that reach chronically demyelinated axoplasm are likely to be compromised and to have a reduced capacity for ATP production as a result of decreased neuronal transcription of nuclear-encoded mitochondrial genes.[57] In microarray comparisons[57] of control and MS motor cortex, 26 nuclear-encoded mitochondrial genes were found to be decreased, and the function of mitochondrial complexes I and III was reduced by 40% to 50% in mitochondrial-enriched preparations from MS motor cortex. Localization and quantification of mitochondrial gene transcripts by in situ hybridization, as well as microarray comparisons of control and MS white matter, support decreased mitochondrial gene transcripts in neurons but not in glia in chronic MS brains.[57] Neurons in chronic MS brains are likely to be sending defective mitochondria to chronically demyelinated axons. Reduced ATP production can render neurons less susceptible to stress.[58] Reduced neuronal ATP production may protect neurons in chronic MS brains, but at the expense of putting their demyelinated segments at risk for degeneration due to low ATP production.

Additional support for degeneration of chronically demyelinated axons comes from ultrastructural studies of chronically demyelinated spinal cord lesions.[57] In the same lesions that averaged 70% axonal loss, 50% of the remaining demyelinated axons contained fragmented neurofilaments and dramatically reduced numbers of mitochondria and microtubules.

Another feature of the chronic MS lesions is axonal swelling. Histologic comparison of axons in normal-appearing white matter, acute MS lesions, and chronic MS lesions detected a statistically significant increase in axonal diameters in chronic MS lesions.[59] In addition, axonal swelling correlated with T1 and magnetization transfer ratio (MTR) changes on MRI (but not T2 MRI changes).[59] Altered T1 and MTR sequences identify chronic lesions with severe axonal loss and swelling, whereas T2-only changes correlated with breakdown of the blood–brain barrier, with or without acute demyelination. Axoplasmic swelling, therefore, is a pathologic hallmark of chronically demyelinated CNS axons that is likely to reflect, in part, increased axoplasmic Ca^{2+}.

Recent studies also support the notion that chronically demyelinated axolemma eventually loose critical molecules that are essential for propagation of action potentials. Thus, many chronically demyelinated axons may be dysfunctional prior to degeneration because they lack voltage-gated Na^+ channels[60] or Na^+,K^+-ATPase or both.[61] In addition, a linear correlation was reported between the percentages of demyelinated axons with and without Na^+,K^+-ATPase and both T1 contrast ratio ($P < .0006$) and MTR ($P < .0001$).[61] In acutely demyelinated lesions, Na^+,K^+-ATPase was detectable on demyelinated axolemma, whereas 58% of chronic lesions contained less than 50% Na^+,K^+-ATPase–positive demyelinated axons. Chronically demyelinated axons that lack Na^+,K^+-ATPase cannot exchange axoplasmic Na^+ for K^+ and are incapable of nerve transmission. Reduced exchange of axonal Na^+ for extracellular K^+ also increases the axonal Na^+ concentration, which, in turn, reverses the Na^+/Ca^{2+} exchanger, leading to increased axonal Ca^{2+} and contributing to Ca^{2+}-mediated axonal degeneration (Fig. 19-2).

These data support the concept that many chronically demyelinated axons are nonfunctional before degeneration. Loss of axonal Na^+ channels and/or Na^+,K^+-ATPase, therefore, is likely to be a contributor to continuous neurologic decline observed in chronic stages of MS, and the quantitative MRI may provide a valuable predictor of this process in longitudinal studies of MS patients.

Neuronal Compensation

A number of adaptive and neuroprotective mechanisms repress or delay the neuronal degeneration and neurological decline that occurs in MS patients. As mentioned earlier, functional MRI studies have identified the activation of cortical areas that compensate for functional loss caused by new MS lesions. Other mechanisms of neuronal compensation operate at the cellular level and include alterations in neuronal gene expression. These gene changes were first identified by unbiased comparisons of 33,000 messenger RNA (mRNA) transcripts in motor cortices from control and MS patients. Among the 555 significantly altered transcripts, 488 were decreased and 67 were increased in MS cortex.[57,62]

Altered genes, when grouped into ontology-based biologic processes, showed decreases in two gene families, oxidative phosphorylation and synaptic transmission. Reduction in mRNA and protein levels was confirmed by reverse transcriptase polymerase chain reaction (RT-PCR) and Western blots. Of the

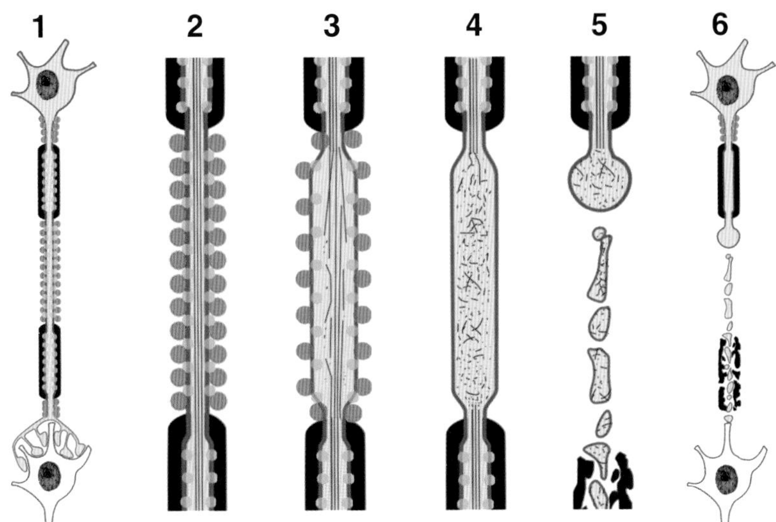

Figure 19–2 Degeneration of chronically demyelinated axons. After demyelination (**1**), sodium (Na^+) channels (•) redistribute along the demyelinated axolemma (**2**). With time, the demyelinated axon becomes swollen (**2**), and the neurofilaments (•) become disorganized. Na^+ channels and sodium-potassium adenosine triphosphatase (Na^+,K^+-ATPase) (•) are eventually lost from the axonal surface, neurofilaments become fragmented (**3,4**), and the axon eventually undergoes degeneration (**5,6**).

103 nuclear-encoded mitochondrial genes, 26 were decreased in MS cortices. In addition, mitochondria isolated from MS cortex had reduced function of respiratory chain complexes I and III. As reduced ATP production can protect cells from noxious stress and reduce apoptosis, reduction of mitochondrial gene expression may be a part of a neuroprotective response. The neurotransmitter changes were restricted to presynaptic and postsynaptic components of inhibitory neurotransmitters. Reduced inhibitory input into neurons has been associated with upregulation of neuroprotective pathways.[63]

Of the 67 genes increased in MS cortex, 9 were members of the ciliary neurotrophic factor (CNTF) family (Fig. 19-3A). CNTF is a proven neurotrophic factor that enhances neuronal survival during development and in disease. Translational and transcriptional products of CNTF-related genes were quantified and localized in control and MS cortices.[62] CNTF, the tripartite CNTF receptor complex, and downstream CNTF signaling molecules including the anti-apoptotic molecule Bcl2 were increased in neurons in MS cortex. An active and functionally significant role of CNTF in MS patients is supported by the report that MS patients with CNTF-null mutations have an earlier disease onset and a more aggressive disease course.[64]

These gene changes were present in myelinated motor cortices, where they represent part of the endogenous defense mechanisms mounted by the MS brain to maintain neurons and combat progressive neurologic decline. The gray matter of MS patients is not immune to demyelination, and cortical MS lesions are a prominent but underappreciated feature of the disease.

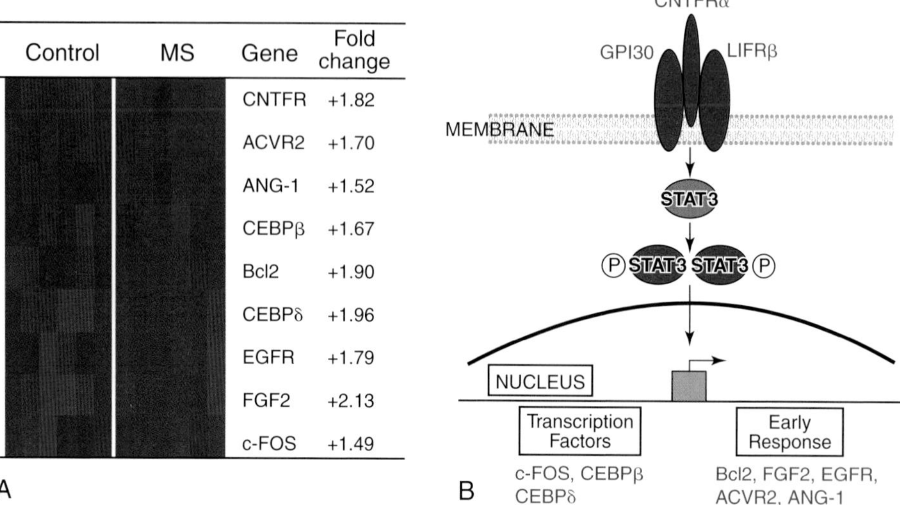

Figure 19–3 Upregulation of a ciliary neurotrophic factor (CNTF)-mediated neuroprotection in motor cortex of patients with multiple sclerosis (MS). **A,** Messenger RNA (mRNA) encoding CNTF and multiple members of the CNTF signaling pathway are increased in MS cortex. **B,** Schematic representation shows the CNTF signaling pathway members that were increased in MS cortex (denoted by red color). ACVR2, activin type 2 receptor; ANG-1, angiopoietin-1; CEBP, CCAAT/enhancer binding protein; CNTFRα, CNTF receptor α; EGFR, epidermal growth factor receptor; FGF2, fibroblast growth factor 2; GP130, glycoprotein 130; LIFRβ, leukemia-inhibitory factor receptor β; P, phosphorus; STAT3, signal transducer and activator of transcription 3. (From Dutta R, McDonough J, Chang A, et al, Activation of the ciliary neurotrophic factor (CNTF) signalling pathway in cortical neurons of multiple sclerosis patients. Brain 2007;130:2566-2576, by permission of Oxford University Press.)

Cortical Demyelination

In addition to the commonly described white matter locations, demyelination also occurs in the gray matter of MS patients.[65-68] Cortical demyelination can be extensive and may exceed white matter demyelination in some MS patients. The full extent of gray matter demyelination, however, is unknown, as gray matter lesions are not routinely detected by MRI analyses. Current knowledge is derived from histologic analysis of postmortem brains, which has described three patterns of demyelination (see Fig. 19-4A). Type I lesions occur at the leukocortical junction, demyelinating both white matter and cortex. Type II lesions are small, perivascular, demyelinated lesions that are restricted to the cortex. Type III lesions are strips of demyelination that extended into the cortex from the pial surface; they can traverse several gyri and often stop at cortical layer 4 or 5. They can extend to the white matter, but at present there is no indication that they demyelinate axons in the white matter. All three cortical lesion types are detected in the same MS brain. Type II lesions do not significantly contribute to the cortical lesion load, and it appears from limited analysis that types I and III lesions contribute equally to the total cortical lesion load. No single cortical lesion type appears to predominate in individual patients. However, it is unknown whether subgrouping

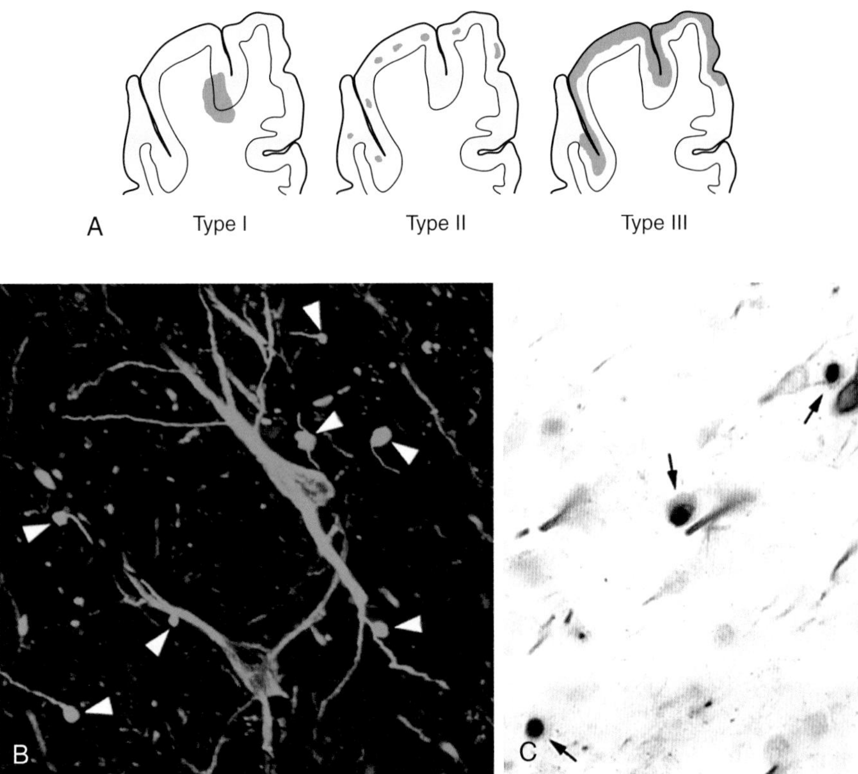

Figure 19–4 Cortical demyelination in brains of patients with multiple sclerosis (MS). **A,** Three patterns of cortical demyelination *(orange areas)* occur in MS brains. Type I lesions occur at the leukocortical junction and demyelinate both white and gray matter. Type II lesions are small, perivascular lesions. Type III lesions extended into the cortex from the pial surface and often involve multiple gyri. Transected neurites (axons and dendrites) (**B,** *arrowheads*) and tunnel-positive apoptotic neurons (**C,** *arrows*) are present in cortical lesions. (**A,** Peterson JW, Trapp BD: Neuropathobiology of multiple sclerosis. Neurol Clin 2005;23:107-129; **B** and **C,** Peterson JW, Bo L, Mork S, et al: Transected neurites, apoptotic neurons and reduced inflammation in cortical multiple sclerosis lesions. Ann Neurol 2001;50:389-400. © 2001 American Neurological Association. Reprinted with permission of John Wiley & Sons, Ltd.)

of patients with variable pathogenesis[69] can identify patients with particular cortical lesion subtypes. Mechanisms of demyelination and characteristics of the immune response or demyelinating inflammatory environment may be different for each cortical lesion subtype.

HOW COMMON ARE CORTICAL LESIONS?

An immunocytochemical study prospectively quantified the area of demyelination in the cingulated gyrus and frontal, parietal, and temporal cortices of 20 postmortem MS brains. Approximately 27% of the cortical area analyzed was demyelinated in the 80 brain sections studied.[68] The extent of cortical demyelination varied among patients (2% to 78%), and the cingulate gyrus had significantly more demyelination than other cortical areas examined. Because so few brain areas have been systematically analyzed for demyelination, it is impossible at present to draw conclusions regarding the extent of cortical demyelination in MS brains. However, there are some trends that may prove important in elucidating the underlying mechanisms of cortical demyelination. For example, type III lesions appear to be more prominent in brain regions with deep sulci. Deep sulci usually contain large vessels and expanded Virchow-Robin spaces. These expanded cerebrospinal fluid compartments often harbor foci of immune cells that may contribute to subpial demyelination. Cortical demyelination is prominent in most, but not all, MS brains, and cortical lesion load may exceed white matter lesion load in some MS patients.

WHY ARE CORTICAL LESIONS NOT SEEN ON MAGNETIC RESONANCE IMAGING?

Standard MRI sequences measure alterations in tissue water. Breakdown of the blood brain barrier and infiltration of leukocytes are the hallmarks of new gadolinium (GAD) enhanced white matter lesions. Cortical lesions are not detected by routine MRI sequences because demyelination occurs without breakdown of the blood brain barrier and without significant infiltration of hematogenous leukocytes.[10,68] Gray matter lesions are hard to detect macroscopically in postmortem brain because they do not change color. Microscopically, they are not hypercellular because of the paucity of immune cells and therefore are often missed on routine cellular stains such as hematoxylin and eosin. Demyelination without significant participation of immune cells from the blood questions the basic premises of MS pathogenesis. Is it possible that the immune response is secondary to a primary demyelinating process? It is also possible that mechanisms have evolved to inhibit cortical inflammation and thus protect neurons from destruction.

Despite the paucity of immune cells from blood, neuronal and axonal pathology are prominent features of cortical lesions. In cortical regions of acute type I lesions, transected neurites (axons and dendrites) (see Fig. 19-4B) averaged more than 3000/mm^3 of lesion area. Apoptotic neurons (see Fig. 19-4C) were increased in cortical lesions compared to myelinated cortex in the same sections, and, in contrast to white matter lesion areas, cortical lesion areas did not contain perivascular cuffs or phagocytic macrophages.[10]

CORTICAL LESIONS MUST CONTRIBUTE TO DISEASE BURDEN IN MULTIPLE SCLEROSIS

Neuronal damage to motor and sensory cortex would affect ambulatory decline in MS patients. In addition to motor and sensory deficits, gray matter lesions may provide the pathologic correlate for the cognitive and executive dysfunction that arises in 40% to 70% of MS patients.[70,72] Recent studies have also raised the possibility of a global cortical pathology in MS patients, which may be independent of demyelination. These studies used brain imaging techniques to measure cortical thickness and raised the possibility that cortical thinning is an early event in MS pathogenesis, is independent of white matter lesion load, and is different from the brain atrophy patterns observed in normal aging.[72] Cortical regions with cortico-cortico connections were reported to have more thinning than primary sensory or motor cortices. If these conclusions stand up to larger prospective studies using more sensitive imaging techniques, we will have to consider the possibility that cortical pathology precedes white matter lesions in MS.

Future Challenges

The major challenge for MS researchers is to develop therapies that stop or prevent MS. To do this, we need to elucidate and understand the cause of the disease. As MS is not inherited, gene linkage studies will not identify a causative gene or altered cellular pathway, as has been the case for neurodegenerative diseases with inherited forms. It is fundamentally important to determine whether inflammatory demyelination is primary or secondary in the MS disease process. Are RRMS and PPMS the same disease with different clinical presentations? One can argue that the concept of MS as an autoimmune disease induced by molecular mimicry has little direct support despite decades of searching for the initiating environmental agent. Recently, there has been renewed interest in the role of the axon and axon-myelin interactions in the pathogenesis of MS. It is possible that this interaction is the key to understanding the cause of MS, and it is possible that MS is a primary neurodegenerative disease with secondary inflammatory demyelination. Regardless of the cause of MS, axons and neurons are important therapeutic targets in MS.

CAN WE PREVENT AXONAL DEGENERATION IN MULTIPLE SCLEROSIS?

Persistent demyelinated axonal Na^+ accumulation that increases with depolarization[73] is thought to contribute to Ca^{2+}-mediated axonal degeneration in MS brain. Inhibition of Na^+ channel and Ca^{2+}-mediated activators are thus logical therapeutic targets that may delay axonal degeneration and permanent neurologic disability in MS patients. In animal models of MS, systemic administration of the class I anti-arrhythmic flecainide[74] or Na^+ channel-blocking anticonvulsants (lamotrigine, phenytoin, carbamazepine)[75-77] reduced neurologic disability, prompting phase I trials of Na^+ channel blocking agents in MS patients.

One of the best-characterized axon protective mechanisms in myelin disease is remyelination. Repair of the myelin restores conduction and prevents axonal degeneration. Some MS lesions are successfully remyelinated, and production of new oligodendrocytes that remyelinate MS lesions is the best-characterized and most abundant adult human brain repair phenomenon. Current remyelination therapies focus on transplantation of oligodendrocyte-producing cells and manipulation of endogenous remyelination.[78,79] Studies are also beginning to unravel the molecular mechanisms by which myelin-forming cells provide trophic support to axons (for review, see Nave and Trapp[80]). A small-molecule therapy that mimics the axonal trophic support of myelin could delay axonal degeneration independent of immunosuppressive or regenerative strategies.

Summary

Is MS a neurodegenerative disease? The answer is "yes." The most convincing evidence demonstrating the degenerative aspect of MS is the unprecendented brain atrophy of some patients with end-stage MS. Neurodegeneration is a fundamental aspect of MS pathogenesis, and loss of axons, dendrites, and neurons is the major cause of permanent neurologic disability in MS patients. The important question is whether the neurodegeneration is primary to the inflammatory demyelination. Current hypotheses support primary inflammatory demyelination as the underlying cause of axonal loss in MS. The transition from RRMS to SPMS is thought to occur when a threshold of axonal loss is reached and the compensatory capacity of the CNS is surpassed, resulting in steady progression of permanent neurologic symptoms. Although immunomodulatory therapies can delay the progression of MS, they have not succeeded in preventing neurological decline. Elucidation of the molecular mechanisms responsible for neuronal injury and determining whether axonal or neuronal pathology precedes demyelination are essential for the development of therapies that will stop neurologic decline in MS patients. This represents a significant challenge to the MS research community. Multidisciplinary approaches, new animal models, a better understanding of the natural history of MS, and a mindset to look for novel aspects of MS pathogenesis will aid in this important endeavor.

Acknowledgments

This work was supported by NIH PO1 NS38667 to B.D.T. The authors would like to thank Dr. Grahame Kidd for assistance with figures.

REFERENCES

1. Weinshenker BG: Epidemiology of multiple sclerosis. Neurol Clin 1996;14:291-308.
2. Noseworthy JH, Lucchinetti C, Rodriguez M, Weinshenker BG: Multiple sclerosis. N Engl J Med 2000;343:938-952.
3. Hauser S, Oksenberg JR: The neurobiology of multiple sclerosis: Genes, inflammation, and neurodegeneration. Neuron 2006;52:61-76.
4. Weinshenker BG, Bass B, Rice GP, et al: The natural history of multiple sclerosis: A geographically based study. I: Clinical course and disability. Brain 1989;112:133-146.
5. Confavreux C, Vukusic S: Age at disability milestones in multiple sclerosis. Brain 2006;129 (Pt 3):595-605.
6. Kremenchutzky M, Rice GP, Baskerville J, et al: The natural history of multiple sclerosis: A geographically based study. 9: Observations on the progressive phase of the disease. Brain 2006;129 (Pt 3):584-594.
7. Waxman SG: Ions, energy and axonal injury: Towards a molecular neurology of multiple sclerosis. Trends Mol Med 2006;12:192-195.
8. Reddy H, Narayanan S, Arnoutelis R, et al: Evidence for adaptive functional changes in the cerebral cortex with axonal injury from multiple sclerosis. Brain 2000;123(Pt 11):2314-2320.
9. Pantano P, Iannetti GD, Caramia F, Mainero C, Di Legge S, et al: Cortical motor reorganization after a single clinical attack of multiple sclerosis. Brain 2002;125:1607-1615.
10. Peterson JW, Bo L, Mork S, et al: Transected neurites, apoptotic neurons and reduced inflammation in cortical MS lesions. Ann Neurol 2001;50:389-400.
11. Kutzelnigg A, Lucchinetti CF, Stadelmann C, et al: Cortical demyelination and diffuse white matter injury in multiple sclerosis. Brain 2005;128(Pt 11):2705-2712.

12. Ferguson B, Matyszak MK, Esiri MM, Perry VH: Axonal damage in acute multiple sclerosis lesions. Brain 1997;120:393-399.
13. Kornek B, Storch MK, Bauer J, et al: Distribution of a calcium channel subunit in dystrophic axons in multiple sclerosis and experimental autoimmune encephalomyelitis. Brain 2001;124: 1114-1124.
14. Geurts JJ, Wolswijk G, Bo L, et al: Altered expression patterns of group I and II metabotropic glutamate receptors in multiple sclerosis. Brain 2003;126(Pt 8):1755-1766.
15. Bitsch A, Schuchardt J, Bunkowski S, et al: Acute axonal injury in multiple sclerosis: Correlation with demyelination and inflammation. Brain 2000;123:1174-1183.
16. Sanchez I, Hassinger L, Paskevich PA, et al: Oligodendroglia regulate the regional expansion of axon caliber and local accumulation of neurofilaments during development independently of myelin formation. J Neurosci 1996;16:5095-5105.
17. Trapp BD, Peterson J, Ransohoff RM, et al: Axonal transection in the lesions of multiple sclerosis. N Engl J Med 1998;338:278-285.
18. Kornek B, Storch MK, Weissert R, et al: Multiple sclerosis and chronic autoimmune encephalomyelitis: A comparative quantitative study of axonal injury in active, inactive, and remyelinated lesions. Am J Pathol 2000;157:267-276.
19. Lloyd KG: CNS compensation to dopamine neuron loss in Parkinson's disease. Adv Exp Med Biol 1977;90:255-266.
20. Trapp BD, Ransohoff RM, Fisher E, Rudick RA: Neurodegeneration in multiple sclerosis: Relationship to neurological disability. Neuroscientist 1999;5:48-57.
21. Bjartmar C, Kinkel RP, Kidd G, et al: Axonal loss in normal-appearing white matter in a patient with acute MS. Neurology 2001;57:1248-1252.
22. Trapp BD, Ransohoff R, Rudick R: Axonal pathology in multiple sclerosis: Relationship to neurologic disability. Curr Opin Neurol 1999;12:295-302.
23. Fisher E, Rudick RA, Cutter G, et al: Relationship between brain atrophy and disability: An 8-year follow-up study of multiple sclerosis patients. Mult Scler 2000;6:373-377.
24. Fisher E, Rudick RA, Simon JH, et al: Eight-year follow-up study of brain atrophy in patients with MS. Neurology 2002;59:1412-1420.
25. Stevenson VL, Miller DH: Magnetic resonance imaging in the monitoring of disease progression in multiple sclerosis. Mult Scler 1999;5:268-272.
26. De Stefano N, Guidi L, Stromillo ML, et al: Imaging neuronal and axonal degeneration in multiple sclerosis. Neurol Sci 2003;24(Suppl 5):S283-S286.
27. Narayana PA, Doyle TJ, Lai D, Wolinsky JS: Serial proton magnetic resonance spectroscopic imaging, contrast-enhanced magnetic resonance imaging, and quantitative lesion volumetry in multiple sclerosis. Ann Neurol 1998;43:56-71.
28. Matthews PM, De Stefano N, Narayanan S, et al: Putting magnetic resonance spectroscopy studies in context: Axonal damage and disability in multiple sclerosis. Semin Neurol 1998;18:327-336.
29. Arnold DL: Magnetic resonance spectroscopy: Imaging axonal damage in MS. J Neuroimmunol 1999;98:2-6.
30. Hohlfeld R: Biotechnological agents for the immunotherapy of multiple sclerosis: Principles, problems and perspectives [invited review]. Brain 1997;120:865-916.
31. Bo L, Dawson TM, Wesselingh S, et al: Induction of nitric oxide synthase in demyelinating regions of multiple sclerosis brains. Ann Neurol 1994;36:778-786.
32. Liu JS, Zhao ML, Brosnan CF, Lee SC: Expression of inducible nitric oxide synthase and nitrotyrosine in multiple sclerosis lesions. Am J Pathol 2001;158:2057-2066.
33. Matute C, Alberdi E, Domercq M, et al: The link between excitotoxic oligodendroglial death and demyelinating diseases. Trends Neurosci 2001;24:224-230.
34. Steinman L: Multiple sclerosis: A two-stage disease. Nat Immunol 2001;2:762-764.
35. Srinivasan R, Sailasuta N, Hurd R, et al: Evidence of elevated glutamate in multiple sclerosis using magnetic resonance spectroscopy at 3 T. Brain 2005;128(Pt 5):1016-1025.
36. Tekkok SB, Goldberg MP: Ampa/kainate receptor activation mediates hypoxic oligodendrocyte death and axonal injury in cerebral white matter. J Neurosci 2001;21:4237-4248.
37. Li S, Stys PK: Mechanisms of ionotropic glutamate receptor-mediated excitotoxicity in isolated spinal cord white matter. J Neurosci 2000;20:1190-1198.
38. Ho TW, McKhann GM, Griffin JW: Human autoimmune neuropathies. Annu Rev Neurosci 1998;21:187-226.
39. Hafer-Macko C, Hsieh S-T, Li CY, Ho TW, Sheikh KA: Acute motor axonal neuropathy: An antibody-mediated attack on axolemma. Ann Neurol 1996;40:635-644.

40. Babbe H, Roers A, Waisman A, et al: Clonal expansions of CD8(+) T cells dominate the T cell infiltrate in active multiple sclerosis lesions as shown by micromanipulation and single cell polymerase chain reaction. J Exp Med 2000;192:393-404.
41. Skulina C, Schmidt S, Dornmair K, et al: Multiple sclerosis: Brain-infiltrating CD8+ T cells persist as clonal expansions in the cerebrospinal fluid and blood. Proc Natl Acad Sci U S A 2004;101:2428-2433.
42. Huseby ES, Liggitt D, Brabb T, et al: A pathogenic role for myelin-specific CD8(+) T cells in a model for multiple sclerosis. J Exp Med 2001;194:669-676.
43. Medana I, Martinic MA, Wekerle H, Neumann H: Transection of major histocompatibility complex class I-induced neurites by cytotoxic T lymphocytes. Am J Pathol 2001;159:809-815.
44. Giuliani F, Goodyer CG, Antel JP, Yong VW: Vulnerability of human neurons to T cell-mediated cytotoxicity. J Immunol 2003;171:368-379.
45. Ganter P, Prince C, Esiri MM: Spinal cord axonal loss in multiple sclerosis: A post-mortem study. Neuropathol Appl Neurobiol 1999;25:459-467.
46. Lovas G, Szilagyi N, Majtenyi K, et al: Axonal changes in chronic demyelinated cervical spinal cord plaques. Brain 2000;123:308-317.
47. Evangelou N, Konz D, Esiri MM, et al: Size-selective neuronal changes in the anterior optic pathways suggest a differential susceptibility to injury in multiple sclerosis. Brain 2001;124 (Pt 9):1813-1820.
48. Yin X, Crawford TO, Griffin JW, et al: Myelin-associated glycoprotein is a myelin signal that modulates the caliber of myelinated axons. J Neurosci 1998;18:1953-1962.
49. Klugmann M, Schwab MH, Puhlhofer A, et al: Assembly of CNS myelin in the absence of proteolipid protein. Neuron 1997;18:59-70.
50. Lappe-Siefke C, Goebbels S, Gravel M, et al: Disruption of Cnp1 uncouples oligodendroglial functions in axonal support and myelination. Nat Genet 2003;33:366-374.
51. Griffiths I, Klugmann M, Anderson T, et al: Axonal swellings and degeneration in mice lacking the major proteolipid of myelin. Science 1998;280:1610-1613.
52. Yin X, Baek RC, Kirschner DA, et al: Evolution of a neuroprotective function of central nervous system myelin. J Cell Biol 2006;172:469-478.
53. Bjartmar C, Kidd G, Mork S, et al: Neurological disability correlates with spinal cord axonal loss and reduce *N*-acetyl aspartate in chronic multiple sclerosis patients. Ann Neurol 2000;48:893-901.
54. De Stefano N, Matthews PM, Fu L, et al: Axonal damage correlates with disability in patients with relapsing-remitting multiple sclerosis: Results of a longitudinal magnetic resonance spectroscopy study. Brain 1998;121:1469-1477.
55. Gonen O, Catalaa I, Babb JS, et al: Total brain N-acetylaspartate: A new measure of disease load in MS. Neurology 2000;54:15-19.
56. Stys PK, Lehning E, Saubermann AJ, Lopachin RM Jr: Intracellular concentrations of major ions in rat myelinated axons and glia: Calculations based on electron probe X-ray microanalyses. J Neurochem 1997;68:1920-1928.
57. Dutta R, McDonough J, Yin X, et al: Mitochondrial dysfunction as a cause of axonal degeneration in multiple sclerosis patients. Ann Neurol 2006;59:478-489.
58. Horiguchi T, Kis B, Rajapakse N, et al: Opening of mitochondrial ATP-sensitive potassium channels is a trigger of 3-nitropropionic acid-induced tolerance to transient focal cerebral ischemia in rats. Stroke 2003;34:1015-1020.
59. Fisher E, Chang A, Fox R, et al: Imaging correlates of axonal swelling in chronic multiple sclerosis brains. Ann Neurol 2007;62:219-228.
60. Black JA, Newcombe J, Trapp BD, Waxman SG: Sodium channel expression within chronic multiple sclerosis plaques. J Neuropathol Exp Neurol 2007;66:828-837.
61. Young EB, Fowler CD, Kidd GJ, et al: Imaging correlates of decreased axonal Na^+/K^+ ATPase in chronic MS lesions. Ann Neurol 2008;63:428-435.
62. Dutta R, McDonough J, Chang A, et al: Activation of the ciliary neurotrophic factor (CNTF) signalling pathway in cortical neurons of multiple sclerosis patients. Brain 2007;130(Pt 10):2566-2576.
63. Hardingham GE, Fukunaga Y, Bading H: Extrasynaptic NMDARs oppose synaptic NMDARs by triggering CREB shut-off and cell death pathways. Nat Neurosci 2002;5:405-414.
64. Giess R, Maurer M, Linker R, et al: Association of a null mutation in the CNTF gene with early onset of multiple sclerosis. Arch Neurol 2002;59:407-409.

65. Brownell B, Hughes JT: Distribution of plaques in the cerebrum in multiple sclerosis. J Neurol Neurosurg Psychiatry 1962;25:315-320.
66. Lumsden CE: The neuropathology of multiple sclerosis. In Vinken PJ, Bruyn GW (eds): Handbook of Clinical Neurology, vol. 9: Multiple Sclerosis and Other Demyelinating Diseases. Amsterdam: North-Holland, 1970, pp 217-309.
67. Kidd D, Barkhof F, McConnell R, et al: Cortical lesions in multiple sclerosis. Brain 1999;122: 17-26.
68. Bo L, Vedeler CA, Nyland HI, et al: Subpial demyelination in the cerebral cortex of multiple sclerosis patients. J Neuropathol Exp Neurol 2003;62:723-732.
69. Lucchinetti C, Bruck W, Parisi J, et al: Heterogeneity of multiple sclerosis lesions: Implications for the pathogenesis of demyelination. Ann Neurol 2000;47:707-717.
70. Rao SM, Leo GJ, Bernardin L, Unverzagt F: Cognitive dysfunction in multiple sclerosis: I. Frequency, patterns, and prediction. Neurology 1991;41:685-691.
71. Beatty WW, Paul RH, Wilbanks SL, et al: Identifying multiple sclerosis patients with mild or global cognitive impairment using the Screening Examination for Cognitive Impairment (SEFCI). Neurology 1995;45:718-723.
72. Charil A, Dagher A, Lerch JP, et al: Focal cortical atrophy in multiple sclerosis: Relation to lesion load and disability. Neuroimage 2007;34:509-517.
73. Smith MR, Smith RD, Plummer NW, et al: Functional analysis of the mouse Scn8a sodium channel. J Neurosci 1998;18:6093-6102.
74. Bechtold DA, Kapoor R, Smith KJ: Axonal protection using flecainide in experimental autoimmune encephalomyelitis. Ann Neurol 2004;55:607-616.
75. Lo AC, Saab CY, Black JA, Waxman SG: Phenytoin protects spinal cord axons and preserves axonal conduction and neurological function in a model of neuroinflammation in vivo. J Neurophysiol 2003;90:3566-3571.
76. Black JA, Shujun L, Hains Bryan C, et al: Exacerbation of experimental autoimmune encephalomyelitis after withdrawal of phenytoin and carbamazepine. Ann Neurol 2007;62:21-33.
77. Bechtold DA, Miller SJ, Dawson AC, et al: Axonal protection achieved in a model of multiple sclerosis using lamotrigine. J Neurol 2006;253:1542-1551.
78. Miller RH, Mi S: Dissecting demyelination. Nat Neurosci 2007;10:1351-1354.
79. Gallo V, Armstrong RC: Myelin repair strategies: A cellular view. Curr Opin Neurol 2008;21: 278-283.
80. Nave K-A, Trapp BD: Axon-glial signaling and the glial support of axon function. Annu Rev Neurosci 2008;31:535-561.

20

Lessons from the Past and Future Approaches for Immunologic Therapies in Multiple Sclerosis

HEINZ WIENDL • NICO MELZER •
CHRISTOPH KLEINSCHNITZ • SVEN G. MEUTH

The therapeutic advances in multiple sclerosis of recent years are impressive and the future perspectives for immune therapy hold several promises. However, one should not forget that the number of approved therapies for multiple sclerosis at present is opposed by numerous examples of failed trials in the past. Those trials imply several lessons to be learned, because they were based on a convincing rationale, had positive results from animal models, but failed in larger trials or were stopped due to unexpected adverse events. This chapter gives examples of lessons from the past, looking for reasons why those therapeutic approaches failed and what these failures could mean to our concepts of pathogenesis and trial design. Future therapeutic approaches are also discussed, and the most important examples are listed and named, including pathogenetically oriented immune therapies, immunosuppressants and immunomodulators, novel immunomodulatory agents, and autologous stem cell transplantation. The tables provide examples from the past (Table 20-1) as well as the most important samples from future approaches for therapy (Table 20-2).

Lessons from the Past

MODIFICATION OF THE CYTOKINE PATTERN

Tumor Necrosis Factor-α Antagonists

Tumor necrosis factor-α (TNF-α), initially characterized for its tumoricidal activity, plays an important role in acute and chronic inflammation.[1,2] TNF-α, mainly produced by T cells and macrophages, activates the vascular endothelium and increases its permeability. Together with interferon-γ (IFN-γ), TNF-α stimulates the release of glutamate and the production of nitric oxide, reactive oxygen derivates, interleukin 1 (IL-1), and many other cytokines as well as all metabolites of arachidonic acid. TNF-α belongs to a large (≥10 members) ligand family that activates a corresponding family of structurally related receptors.[3] The receptors trigger diverse signals for cell proliferation and apoptosis, depending on the cellular context, which play an important role in development and immune response.

TNF-α proved to be an essential pathogenetic factor in various models of experimental autoimmune encephalomyelitis (EAE) and multiple sclerosis (MS). The elimination of TNF-producing macrophages, antagonization with TNF antibodies, administration of therapeutic drugs affecting TNF-α production (e.g., thalidomide, pentoxifylline, rolipram), as well as doses of soluble TNF receptor (lenercept) all showed clear positive effects on pathogenesis in animal models.[4,5] Furthermore, a series of studies in MS patients showed a correlation of TNF levels in blood, serum, or cerebrospinal fluid (CSF) with the clinical course and disease activity.[6-12]

In an open phase I study, two patients with a severe secondary chronic progressive form of MS (SPMS) were treated with a monoclonal antibody against TNF-α (infliximab, cA2).[13] Inflammatory activity as measured by magnetic resonance imaging (MRI), CSF lymphocytic pleocytosis, and immunoglobulin G (IgG) index was clearly increased after the infusions were administered and dropped back to its initial level after 2 to 3 weeks.

In a phase II study in patients with mainly relapsing-remitting MS (RRMS), the effect of the soluble TNF receptor–immunoglobulin fusion protein lenercept on the development of new lesions in MRI was examined.[14] MRI showed no significant difference between lenercept and placebo with respect to the cumulative number of new active lesions. However, in the lenercept group, the number of clinical exacerbations was significantly higher, exacerbations occurred earlier, duration of relapses was longer, time to clinical exacerbations was shortened, and neurologic deficits appeared to be more serious.

The unexpected and surprising negative results for infliximab and lenercept require careful analysis, particularly because they question present concepts of MS pathogenesis. In the lenercept study, the increase in the clinical exacerbation rate was overt, whereas MRI findings showed only a trend toward increased activity during therapy, and the number of new lesions did not differ significantly from that in the placebo group. The MRI scans were taken prior to each intravenous infusion. In contrast, in the infliximab study, where increased MRI activity appeared, examinations were conducted shortly after antibody infusions. After 2 to 3 weeks, MRI activity dropped back to its initial level. In almost all patients, antibodies against the TNF receptor construct were generated. Although they did

TABLE 20–1 Examples of Treatment Trials in Multiple Sclerosis that Failed, were Halted Prematurely, or Were Associated with Unexpected Adverse Effects

Agent	(Assumed) Mechanism of Action	Characteristics/ Trial Design	Disease Course	Outcome: MRI	Outcome: Clinical/ Side Effects	Further or Ongoing Trials	Comment
Immunosuppressants							
Linomide (Roquinimex)	Synthetic immunomodulator: inhibition of IFN-γ and TNF-α	Three multicentric phase III studies in 715, 350, and 501 pts, terminated early	RRMS, SPMS	Positive	Positive	—	Cardiopulmonary toxicity
Sulfasalazine	Anti-inflammatory and immunomodulatory properties	Clinical study in 199 pts, 36 mo	PPMS, RRMS, SPMS	No sustained effect	No sustained effect	—	Initially positive effect, absence of long-term benefit
Deoxyspergualine (DSG, Gusperimus)	Interaction with intracellular heat-shock protein (HSP70) and activation of NF-κB	Multicentric clinical study in 236 pts, 12 mo	RRMS, SPMS	No effect	No effect	—	Overall effects unconvincing
Cladribine (chlorodeoxyadenosine, 2-CdA)	Adenosindeaminase-resistant purine nucleoside: induction of long-lasting lymphopenia	Multicentric clinical study in 159 pts, 12 mo	PPMS, SPMS				
Cytokine Modulators							
Lenercept (RO-452081)	Soluble TNF-receptor p55: inhibition of TNF-α-functions	**Phase II** study in 168 pts (10, 50, or 100 mg every 4 wk for up to 12 mo	RRMS	No effect	Worsening	—	Paradoxical effect of TNF-α; discrepancy between MRI and clinical effects
Infliximab (cA2)	TNF-α neutralizing antibody; human/murine chimeric IgG1: inhibition of TNF-α functions	Open **phase I** study in 2 pts, 2 mo	SPMS	Worsening	No effect on EDSS	—	Paradoxical effect of TNF-α

TABLE 20–1 Examples of Treatment Trials in Multiple Sclerosis that Failed, were Halted Prematurely, or Were Associated with Unexpected Adverse Effects (Continued)

Agent	(Assumed) Mechanism of Action	Characteristics/ Trial Design	Disease Course	Outcome: MRI	Outcome: Clinical/ Side Effects	Further or Ongoing Trials	Comment
Cytokine Modulators (Continued)							
TGF-β2	Immune suppression, pleiotropic growth factor	Open dose escalation study in 11 pts, 6 mo	SPMS	No effect	No effect	—	Bioavailability in the CNS?; nephrotoxicity
IL-10	Recombinant cytokine: inhibition of macrophage APC function, upregulation of Th2 cells	Open dose escalation study, terminated	RRMS, SPMS	—	—	—	Insufficient efficacy, possible induction of exacerbations
IL-4, BAY 36-1677	Recombinant cytokine: mutein with 2 AA exchanges and selectivity for T cells, B cells, and monocytes, upregulation of Th2 cells	(terminated)	—	—	—	—	Insufficient efficacy
Inducers of Remyelination							
IVIG (Gamimune N)	Diverse immunomodulatory effects; in addition, promotion of remyelination in animal model	Randomized, double-blind study in 55 pts, 12 mo	SDON	Not done	No overall effect	—	Remyelination potential may depend on disease activity, time point, dose, and duration of treatment
		Randomized, double-blind study in 67 pts, 6 mo	RRMS, SPMS (TND)	No effect	No effect		
		Randomized, double-blind study in 10 pts, 6 wk	RRMS	Not done	No effect		

Table continued on following page

TABLE 20–1 Examples of Treatment Trials in Multiple Sclerosis that Failed, were Halted Prematurely, or Were Associated with Unexpected Adverse Effects (Continued)

Agent	(Assumed) Mechanism of Action	Characteristics/ Trial Design	Disease Course	Outcome: MRI	Outcome: Clinical/ Side Effects	Further or Ongoing Trials	Comment
Antigen-Derived Therapies							
Oral myelin (Myloral; AI-100)	Bovine MBP; induction of systemic tolerance via stimulation of antigen-specific regulatory (Th2, Th3) cells	**Phase II** study in 30 pts, 12 mo	RRMS	Not done	Possible	—	Inappropriate dose?; individual importance of the antigen?
		Multicentric **phase III** study in 515 pts, 24 mo	RRMS	Not documented	No effect		
APL (CGP77116; NBI-5788)	APL peptide analog of human MBP 83-99	**Phase II** study in 8 pts, 50 mg/wk, terminated; maximum, 9 mo	RRMS	Worsening	Worsening	—	Interindividual differences in target epitopes (e.g., "epitope spreading")?; unexpected effects on different T-cell populations; allergic reactions
		Phase II study in 142 pts (5, 20, or 50 mg/wk), terminated, 4 mo planned	RRMS	Positive	No effect		
DR2:MBP$^{84\text{-}102}$ (AG284)	Soluble HLA-DR2 with a single noncovalently bound MBP peptide	**Phase I** trial in 33 pts, 3 mo	SPMS	No effect	No effect	—	Short observation time
TCR-Directed Therapies							
T-cell vaccination	Attenuated autologous MBP-reactive T-cell clones, induction of anticlonotypic T-cell responses	**Pilot study** in 8 pts, 22-38 mo	RRMS	Mixed	Mixed	—	Small no. of pts; complexity and diversity of human autoimmune T cells; role of MBP in MS pathogenesis?

TABLE 20–1 Examples of Treatment Trials in Multiple Sclerosis that Failed, were Halted Prematurely, or Were Associated with Unexpected Adverse Effects (Continued)

Agent	(Assumed) Mechanism of Action	Characteristics/ Trial Design	Disease Course	Outcome: MRI	Outcome: Clinical/ Side Effects	Further or Ongoing Trials	Comment
TCR-Directed Therapies (Continued)							
TCR peptide vaccination	TCR Vβ5.2 (residues 38-58), induction of anti-TCR regulatory effects	**Pilot study** in 23 pts, all HLA-DRB1*1501 positive, 12 mo	PPMS, SPMS	Not done	No effect	—	Small no. of pts; marginal effect on disease progression; heterogeneity and individuality of TCR repertoire and antigen specificity
T-cell Inactivation							
Extracorporeal photopheresis (PTX)	Direct or indirect induction of apoptosis on circulating T cells	Randomized, placebo-controlled study in 16 pts, 18 mo	SPMS	No effect	No effect	—	Quantities of peripheral CNS-antigen reactive T cells in chronic MS? Relevance of CNS specific milieu for perpetuation of immune response in chronic MS

Table continued on following page

TABLE 20–1 Examples of Treatment Trials in Multiple Sclerosis that Failed, were Halted Prematurely, or Were Associated with Unexpected Adverse Effects (Continued)

Agent	(Assumed) Mechanism of Action	Characteristics/ Trial Design	Disease Course	Outcome: MRI	Outcome: Clinical/ Side Effects	Further or Ongoing Trials	Comment
Costimulatory Molecules							
CTLA-4-Ig (abatacept, RG2077)	Negative regulator of T-cell function; effects on $CD4^+CD25^+$ regulatory cells	**Pilot study** in 16 pts, single infusions (2, 10, 20, or 35 mg/kg) or multidose of 10 mg/kg	RRMS	—	No major adverse effect	Finished	Reason for worse outcome in treated group: probable randomization failure; the clinical effectiveness in MS remains unclear
		330 pts, double-blind, placebo-controlled multicenter **phase II** trial (2 or 10 mg/kg infusions on days 1, 15, and 29, then every 4 wk until day 197)	RRMS	Accumulation of inflam matory MRI activity (low-dose group); fewer new Gd-enhancing T1 lesions in 10 mg/kg group	Accumulation of relapses in low-dose group; fewer relapses in 10 mg/kg group	Study prematurely halted	
Anti-CD40L (anti-CD154, IDEC-131)	Antibody interacting with the co-stimulatory pathway CD40-CD40L	**Pilot study** (IDEC-131) in 15 pts	RRMS	Positive	No relapses for at least 6 mo	Finished	Potential interference with the thrombocyte system
		46 pts, double-blind, placebo-controlled **phase II** trial (15 mg/kg IV for 5 wk, then every 1 mo for 3 mo)	RRMS	—	MS study halted, because 1 pt developed thromboembolism in a study of Crohn's disease (later: 2 more pts)	Stopped, although all pts had preexisting risk factors for clotting	

TABLE 20–1 Examples of Treatment Trials in Multiple Sclerosis that Failed, were Halted Prematurely, or Were Associated with Unexpected Adverse Effects (Continued)

Agent	(Assumed) Mechanism of Action	Characteristics/ Trial Design	Disease Course	Outcome: MRI	Outcome: Clinical/ Side Effects	Further or Ongoing Trials	Comment
Anti-adhesion Molecules							
Anti-LFA1 (CD11/CD18, Hu23F2G)	LFA1/ICAM-antagonist, inhibition of cell adhesion between leukocytes and vascular endothelial cells	Open phase I study (24 pts) and a subsequent phase II study (169 pts) with humanized anti-LFA1 (Hu23F2G)	SPMS PPMS	Negative	Negative	Finished	So far no report about beneficial effects in MS
Chemotaxis							
CCR1 antagonist (BX-471)	CCR antagonist, reduces transmigration of autoreactive T cells to the CNS	600 mg **orally, phase II**	RRMS	Negative	Negative	Finished; trials on other CCR antagonists (CCR2: 2 phase I and 1 phase II; CCR5: phase II and III trial in HIV) planned or ongoing	Complexity of the cytokine system, "ligand issue"

Table continued on following page

TABLE 20–1 Examples of Treatment Trials in Multiple Sclerosis that Failed, were Halted Prematurely, or Were Associated with Unexpected Adverse Effects (Continued)

Agent	(Assumed) Mechanism of Action	Characteristics/ Trial Design	Disease Course	Outcome: MRI	Outcome: Clinical/ Side Effects	Further or Ongoing Trials	Comment
Novel Immunomodulators							
PDE inhibitors (ibudilast, rolipram)	Downregulation of inflammatory responses by changing levels of cAMP and cGMP; shifting the cytokine milieu to Th2-driven responses	**Open-label, crossover** study of 18 pts (rolipram)	RRMS, SPMS	—	Negative	Terminated due to lack of clinical efficacy; dose-dependent side effects (e.g., nausea, emesis)	Regarded as immunomodulator treatment; first generation of PDE inhibitors with problems concerning side effects; second generation compounds are improved concerning side effects
PPAR-γ agonists: TZDs (pioglitazone, rosiglitazone)	Inhibition of T-cell activation, reduction of proinflammatory cytokines	**Phase I/II proof-of-principle study**, 22 pts taking IFN-beta-1a using pioglitazone; observation period: 1 yr	RRMS	Positive	—	Finished	Clinical potential in MS unclear, broad experience in other disease entities, candidate for continuation
Hydrolytic enzymes	Increase the specific hydrolytic activity on putative ingested (auto)antigens in the serum	**Oral drug** (90 mg bromelain + 48 mg trypsin + 100 mg rutosid), phase III	RRMS	Negative	Negative	Finished	Hopes are raised based on single observations; no proof of efficacy

TABLE 20–1 Examples of Treatment Trials in Multiple Sclerosis that Failed, were Halted Prematurely, or Were Associated with Unexpected Adverse Effects (Continued)

Agent	(Assumed) Mechanism of Action	Characteristics/ Trial Design	Disease Course	Outcome: MRI	Outcome: Clinical/ Side Effects	Further or Ongoing Trials	Comment
Hematopoetic Stem Cell Transplantation							
HSCT	"Resetting" of the immune system	~250 pts with MS have undergone HSCT, variable outcomes; based on the different study protocols throughout the trials, comparability is constricted	RRMS, SPMS, PPMS	Variable outcome	Variable outcome, superior responses in RRMS or active SPMS compared with PPMS	Finished trials are available, further trials are running (e.g., ASTIMS)	Variable outcome in clinical and MRI readout parameters; differences in pt selection and treatment protocols in different studies; further trials are warranted
Anti-infectious Therapies							
Antiviral agents (acyclovir, valacyclovir)	Treatment of a suggested infectious component of the disease	**Double-blind, placebo-controlled trial,** acyclovir (800 mg) for 2 yr, 60 pts	RRMS	Not used	Tendency (not significant) for fewer exacerbations during treatment	Finished	Negative or marginally positive reports; whether specific elimination of viruses would effect MS lesion pathogenesis remains questionable
		Phase II, valacyclovir for 24 wk, randomized, double-blind, placebo-controlled, 70 pts	RRMS	Beneficial effect for pts with high level of MRI disease activity	Negative	Finished	
Antibiotics (rifampicin, azithromycin)	Treatment of a suggested infectious component of the disease	**Pilot study** of rifampicin (300 mg) and azithromycin (500 mg every other day) over 6 mo, 8 pts	RRMS	Positive	Negative	Finished	Causal role of bacteria in MS is discussed controversially; positive effects of antibiotics are most likely not directly related to their antimicrobial properties

Table continued on following page

TABLE 20–1 Examples of Treatment Trials in Multiple Sclerosis that Failed, were Halted Prematurely, or Were Associated with Unexpected Adverse Effects (Continued)

Agent	(Assumed) Mechanism of Action	Characteristics/ Trial Design	Disease Course	Outcome: MRI	Outcome: Clinical/ Side Effects	Further or Ongoing Trials	Comment
Neuroprotection and Neurorepair							
Riluzole	Inhibition of glutamate release, modulation of glutamate receptors, inhibition of TREK-1 channels	Small treatment study in 16 pts (50 mg bid) over 1 yr	PPMS	No effect on new lesions, but reduction of cervical cord atrophy and development of T1-hypointense lesions	Negative	Finished	Data suffer from several limitations, including small pt no., pt selection, and length of observation
Xaliproden	Modulation of 5-HT1a	Multicenter, randomized, **phase II trial**	—	Results still pending	Results still pending	—	Results still pending
Neurotrophic factors (BDNF, IGF-1)	Reversal of neuronal and axonal damage, promotion of remyelination, acting via specific receptors (e.g., TrkR)	**Open-label study**, 7 pts, SC recombinant IGF-1 (50 mg), 6 mo	RRMS	Negative	Negative	Finished	Clinical potential in MS unclear, only one trial in 7 pts

AA, amino acid; APC, antigen-presenting; APL, altered peptide ligand; ASTIMS, Autologous Stem cell Transplantation International Multiple Sclerosis; BDNF, brain-derived neurotrophic factor; cAMP, cyclic adenosine monophosphate; cGMP, cyclic guanosine monophosphate; CCR, chemokine receptor; CNS, central nervous system; CTLA, cytotoxic T lymphocyte–associated antigen; EDSS, Enhanced Disability Status Scale; Gd, gadolinium; HIV, human immunodeficiency virus; HLA, human leukocyte antigen; HSCT, hematopoietic stem cell transplantation; 5-HT1a, 5-hydroxytryptamine 1a; ICAM, intercellular adhesion molecule; IDEC-131, humanized anti-CD154 antibody; IGF, insulin-like growth factor; IFN, interferon; Ig, immunoglobulin; IL, interleukin; IVIG, intravenous immune globulin; LFA1, lymphocyte function-associated antigen 1; MBP, myelin basic protein; MRI, magnetic resonance imaging; MS, multiple sclerosis; NF-κB, nuclear factor-κB; PDE, phosphodiesterase; PML, progressive multifocal leukoencephalopathy; PPAR, peroxisome proliferator–activated receptor; PPMS, primary progressive multiple sclerosis; pts, patients; RRMS, relapsing remitting multiple sclerosis; SDON, stable deficit after optic neuritis; SPMS, secondary progressive multiple sclerosis; TCR, T-cell receptor; TGF, transforming growth factor; TND, targeted neurologic deficits; TNF, tumor necrosis factor; TREK, TWIK-related K^+ channel; TrkR, tyrosine kinase receptor; TZDs, thiazolidinediones; VLA, very late antigen.

not inhibit the binding of TNF, they accelerated drug elimination and thereby may have shortened the duration of the drug's effect. On the other hand, it has been suggested that anti-TNF antibodies that bind TNF may, themselves, act as a "TNF sink", releasing the TNF later and inducing exacerbation of disease. Moreover, it is becoming increasingly clear that TNF exhibits potent immunosuppressive properties in addition to its well-established pro-inflammatory effects; this might be an explanation for the immune and disease-activating effects of anti-TNF treatment of MS. For example, in TNF-deficient mice, myelin-specific T-cell reactivity failed to regress, and the expansion of activated/memory T cells was abnormally prolonged, leading to exacerbated EAE.[15]

Transforming Growth Factor-β2

Transforming growth factor-β is a multifunctional polypeptide growth factor. Three highly homologous isoforms exist in mammalians (TGF-β1, TGF-β2, and TGF-β3).[16] Depending on cell type and growth conditions, isoforms differ in their potential efficacy and their biologic activity. Almost all cells express all three types of TGF-β receptors. In general, TGF-β has a stimulatory effect on cells of mesenchymal origin and an inhibitory effect on cells of epithelial or neuroectodermal origin.

An inhibitory effect of TGF-β1 or TGF-β2 on the development of EAE has been shown in several investigations. On the other hand, neutralizing antibodies against TGF-β1 worsened the disease progress.[17-22]

In an open dose escalation and toxicity study, no significant effect on either Enhanced Disability Status Scale (EDSS) score or MRI lesion load was shown for TGF-β2. However, consistent with the observation that TGF-β is able to block cell adhesion and migration into the central nervous system (CNS),[22] a trend toward reduction of CSF pleocytosis could be observed during the treatment period. The cytokine immune deviation with TGF-β2 in SPMS did not lead to a slower disease progression or to reduction of lesion load in the CNS. It is not clear whether local TGF-β2 bioavailability in the CNS is sufficient for exertion of antiinflammatory effects. However, direct renal toxicity at the doses applied limits the use of TGF-β2 in humans. Furthermore, application for longer periods increases the danger of extended tissue fibrosis and deposition of extracellular matrix.

Commentary on Cytokine Modulators

Our initial hope that the success of IFN-beta would usher in a multitude of cytokine therapies has faded. None of the other cytokines tested so far in pilot trials was truly promising. Clinical trials testing the effects of cytokines or cytokine inhibitors in MS patients have often been derived from studies involving the EAE model. However, it is also important to consider findings from transgenic animal studies in designing therapeutic approaches for MS.[24] Furthermore it is important to state if EAE experiments better represent RRMS or SPMS. Most EAE-directed therapies affect the clonal expansion of T cells, the first immune cells to enter the CNS.[24] Several examples have now shown that cytokines represent a part of a

TABLE 20–2 Future Approaches in Multiple Sclerosis Therapy: Assumed Targets, Examples, and Rationale

(Assumed) Drug Target	Example Agents	Therapeutic Rationale
CNS antigens	Oral myelin, MBP8298, soluble MBP/HLA-D2 complex, DNA-plasmids of MBP	Induction of immune tolerance via bystander suppression, T-cell anergy
	APLs	Same as above
T cells and TCR	T cell, TCR, and DNA vaccines	Attenuation of autoaggressive T cells, stimulation of counter-regulatory immune mechanisms
	Antibodies against T-cell differentiation molecules: Anti-CD3 (muromab), anti-CD4 (priliximab, cM-T412), anti-CD52 (alemtuzumab [Campath-1H])	T-cell suppression/depletion
	Antibodies against and/or peptide antagonists of costimulatory molecules: CTLA4-Ig (abatacept [BMS188667; RG2077]); anti-CD40L (IDC131); anti-IL-2 receptor (daclizumab)	Inhibition of T-cell proliferation/activation
B cells and antibodies	Plasma exchange, IVIG, anti-CD20 (B-cell) antibody (rituximab)	Removal of autoantibodies/pathogenic humoral factors
Th1/Th2 balance	Antibodies against and/or antagonists of pro-inflammatory cytokines: Anti-TNF-α (infliximab, etanercept); anti-IL-12 (ABT-874, CNTO-1275); anti-TGF-β	Shift toward Th2-mediated (anti-inflammatory) immune response, inhibition of immune cell proliferation/activation
	Administration/increased production of anti-inflammatory cytokines: IL-10; IL-4; fumarate (BG12)	
	Phosphodiesterase inhibitors: Mesopram, rolipram, ibudilast	
	Thiazolidinedions: Pioglitazone, rosiglitazone	
Adhesion molecules	Antibodies against and/or antagonists of adhesion molecules on T cells/endothelial cells: Anti-$\alpha_4\beta_1$-integrin (VLA-4) (natalizumab); oral VLA-4 antagonists (SB683699, CDP 323); anti-LFA-1 (CD11a) (Hu23F2G, efalizumab)	Prevention of autoaggressive T-cell transmigration into the CNS
Chemokines/CCRs	Antibodies against and/or antagonists of CCRs on T cells/endothelial cells: CCR1 inhibitor (BX-471: ZK811752); CCR2 inhibitor; CCR5 inhibitor	Disruption of chemotactic gradients, prevention of autoaggressive T-cell transmigration into the CNS

TABLE 20–2 Future Approaches in Multiple Sclerosis Therapy: Assumed Targets, Examples, and Rationale (Continued)

(Assumed) Drug Target	Example Agents	Therapeutic Rationale
Blood–brain barrier tissue transmigration	Matrix metalloproteinase inhibitors: Minocycline, α-lipoic acid, ω-3 fatty acid	Extracellular matrix preservation, prevention of autoaggressive T-cell transmigration into the CNS
Proliferating cells including pathogenetic relevant immune cells	Anthracenediones: Mitoxantrone, pixantrone Alkylating agents: Cyclophosphamide, treosulfan Antimetabolites: Azathioprine, methotrexate, mycophenolate mofetil, cladribine, teriflunomide Antiproliferatives: Sirolimus, temsirolimus, laquinimod Calcineurin inhibitors: Cyclosporine	Various mechanisms of action: T- and B-cell depletion, induction of apoptosis, inhibition of T- and B-cell activation/proliferation, reduced antibody formation, anti-inflammatory cytokine shift
Circulating lymphocytes, homing of lymphocytes	Lymphocyte sphingosine 1-phosphate receptor agonist: FTY720	Increased lymphocyte homing to secondary lymphatic organs, prevention of autoaggressive T-cell transmigration into the CNS
Various inflammatory and immune pathways	Statins: Simvastatin, atorvastatin	Various mechanisms of action: Inhibition of T- and B-cell activation/proliferation; downregulation of chemokine receptors, adhesion molecules, and costimulatory factors; inhibition of MHC class II expression; anti-inflammatory cytokine shift
Sex hormone balance	Estriol Testosterone	Shift toward Th2-mediated (anti-inflammatory) immune response

Table continued on following page

TABLE 20–2 Future Approaches in Multiple Sclerosis Therapy: Assumed Targets, Examples, and Rationale (Continued)

(Assumed) Drug Target	Example Agents	Therapeutic Rationale
Free radicals	Uric acid precursors	Reduced CNS tissue damage
Infectious pathogens	Antivirals: Acyclovir, valacyclovir Antibiotics: Rifampicin, azithromycin	Elimination of pathogens that induce or trigger MS (e.g., EBV, HHV-6, CP)
Ion channels (Na^+, K^+, Ca^{2+})	Na^+ channel blockers: Phenytoin, flecainide Ca^{2+} channel blockers: Nitrendipine, bepridile K^+ channel blockers: shk-Dap(22), TRAM-34-α1	Reduction of direct axonal and neuronal damage; decreased Ca^{2+} overload; reduced proliferation of immune cells
Various neuroprotective pathways on neurons, axons, glia cells; glutamate receptors	Neurotrophic factors: IGF-1, CNTF, LIF, BDNF Cannabinoids: Δ9-THC, cannabis extract Hematopoietic growth factors: Erythropoietin, G-CSF Glutamate transmission: MK-801, NBQX, riluzole	Various mechanisms of action: Increased neuronal and glial survival, reduced axonal damage, excitotoxicity and invasion of immune cells, anti-inflammatory cytokine shift
Remyelination and repair	Stem cells: Neuronal/oligodendroglial precursors	Replacement of damaged neurons, glia cells, and myelin
	HSCT	Ablation and rebooting of the immune system, definite disease cure
	IVIG	Supporting endogenous remyelination

APL, altered peptide ligand; BNDF, brain-derived neurotrophic factor; CCR, chemokine receptor; CNS, central nervous system; CNTF, ciliary neurotrophic factor; CTLA, cytotoxic T lymphocyte–associated antigen; EBV, Epstein-Barr virus; G-CSF, granulocyte colony-stimulating factor; HHV-6, human herpes virus 6; HLA, human leukocyte antigen; HSCT, hematopoietic stem cell transplantation; Ig, immunoglobulin; IGF, insulin-like growth factor; IL, interleukin; IVIG, intravenous immune globulin; LFA, leukocyte function antigen; LIF, leukemia inhibitory factor; MBP, myelin basic protein; MHC, major histocompatibility complex; MS, multiple sclerosis; TCR, T-cell receptor; TGF, transforming growth factor; THC, tetrahydrocannabinol; TNF, tumor necrosis factor; VLA, very late antigen.

complex network.[25] Therapeutic application of any one of the cytokines or their respective inhibitory components could be expected to disturb this balance in a complicated way. Additionally, it has to be assumed that, in contrast to animal models, there is great heterogeneity in the immunopathology, the clinical phenotype, and the therapeutic response of MS patients.[26] Similar considerations also apply to the increasing family of chemokines and their possible use as therapeutic targets.[27] Theoretically, cytokine/anticytokine and also chemokine/antichemokine therapies seem more suitable for treatment of acute exacerbations than for long-term therapy.

CHEMOTAXIS

Active MS is characterized by the presence of inflammatory foci disseminated in the CNS. The cellular composition of these inflammatory infiltrates is determined partly by the local spectrum of secreted chemokines, which are key contributors to the directional movement of leukocytes.[28,29] Various studies have underlined the importance of chemokine/chemokine-receptor interactions in EAE and MS pathogenesis. For example, certain chemokines and/or their respective receptors are up-regulated in MS and EAE.[30-33] A variety of experimental studies have demonstrated that genetic ablation of chemokines has the potential to prevent or ameliorate CNS inflammation.[34-37] Pharmacologic interference with the chemokine network has therefore been regarded as a promising strategy for effective treatment in MS.[38]

Chemokine Receptor Antagonists: BX-471

BX-471 (ZK811752) is a recently developed oral chemokine receptor 1 (CCR1) antagonist. Positive results from phase I trials in autoimmune diseases including MS have been reported.[39] However, a double-blind, placebo-controlled phase II study failed to demonstrate efficacy on primary or secondary outcome parameters.[40] Several further studies addressing chemokine receptor antagonists (e.g., CCR2, CCR5) are currently underway.[34] One has to take into consideration that the chemokine system, like the complex cytokine network, is characterized by its large redundancy. Therefore, a definite assessment of the extent to which blockade of a solitary chemokine or chemokine receptor mediates significant clinical effects remains difficult. Large controlled trials are warranted to further address this therapeutic approach.

IMMUNOSUPPRESSANTS

Roquinimex (Linomide)

Roquinimex (Linomide) is a synthetic immunomodulator that has been successfully applied in animal models of various autoimmune diseases. Its primary effects are thought to be mediated by inhibition of IFN-γ and TNF-α release from natural killer (NK) cells and macrophage activity.[41] Linomide inhibits development of acute EAE for as long as 7 days after disease induction[42] and is capable of blocking spontaneous and induced attacks in chronic EAE.[43]

In two phase II studies, Linomide reduced the number of active lesions on MRI and improved the clinical end points (EDSS) in SPMS and RRMS.[44,45] These encouraging data resulted in multicentric phase III studies in RRMS and SPMS. However, trials had to be terminated 1 month after patients became fully enrolled due to unanticipated serious cardiopulmonary toxicities, pancreatitis, and death.[46] The trial duration was too short to determine unequivocally any clinical (EDSS change) or paraclinical (MRI) benefits.[47] These results emphasize the importance of designing well-structured and large phase III studies with high numbers of patients for the identification of rather rare adverse events in a given disease.[48] The substance was promising in animal experiments and showed convincing beneficial effects with relatively low prevalence of side effects in the phase II studies, which led to enthusiastic expectations. It failed in the large phase III studies because of species-specific side effects on the cardiopulmonary system.

Sulfasalazine

Sulfasalazine is an orally applicable, well-known drug, mainly used in rheumatology, with an anti-inflammatory and immunomodulatory efficacy. Its multifaceted effects work on B-cell proliferation, synthesis of immunoglobulins, chemotaxis for neutrophilic granulocytes, release of TNF-α, and reduction of pro-inflammatory lipoxygenase products and thromboxane. It induces immunosuppressive prostaglandins, reduces synthesis of reactive oxygen compounds, and binds radicals. It also stabilizes lipid membranes of the cell. Sulfasalazine was also shown to be beneficial in EAE.[49,50]

In the study of the Mayo Clinic Canadian Cooperative Sulfasalazine Study Group,[51] patients with primary progressive MS (PPMS), RRMS, or SPMS received either oral sulfasalazine or placebo for at least 3 years. During the first 18 months, sulfasalazine reduced the relapse rate, inhibited disease progression, and increased the time until the first relapse. The number of relapse-free patients was increased, and positive modifications in MRI were observed. Surprisingly, these initial effects were not continued into the second phase of the study. After 3 years, sulfasalazine showed no effect on MS disease progression. The reasons underlying the observed early (but statistically not significant) benefit and the later lack of effect of sulfasalazine are not clear. However, the study underscores the importance of long-term observation periods for the assessment of positive therapeutic effects.[52,53] Short- or middle-term improvements in clinical parameters do not always allow conclusions concerning a long-term benefit for disease progression.

REMYELINATION

Intravenous Immunoglobulin

As a result of multifaceted mechanisms, human intravenous immune globulins (IVIG) modulate mainly humoral but also cellular immune responses.[54] However, polyclonal IgG and several IgM monoclonal antibodies can also promote remyelination[55] by binding to oligodendrocytes.[56]

A successful pilot study in patients with stable deficit after optic neuritis that did not respond to a corticosteroid treatment showed a tendency toward improved visual acuity with the use of IVIG.[57] However, this finding could not be confirmed in a larger consecutive study.[58] IVIG was also tested for its ability to reverse permanent motor neurologic deficits in MS.[59] Treatment showed no effect on the primary end point (isometric muscle strength) after 6 months, and the study was terminated. In another trial, patients with RRMS and stable clinical deficits were treated with IVIG.[60] No significant differences were observed in central motor conduction time or in EDSS score, neurologic rating scale, or manual muscle testing within 6 weeks after treatment.

These trial data may reflect the observation that polyclonal immunoglobulins have no influence on proliferation, differentiation or migration of oligodendrocytic precursor cells.[61] However, a secondary analysis of the IVIG in an optic neuritis trial showed that IVIG may enhance or worsen visual function, depending on the degree of clinical disease activity during the first year after administration.[58] This finding is consistent with experimental evidence that immunoglobulins may induce remyelination in animals with stable advanced demyelination but have no remyelinating effect in animals with ongoing inflammatory demyelination. Therefore, their remyelination potential may depend on disease activity, time point, dose, and duration of treatment.

ANTIGEN-DERIVED THERAPIES

Oral Tolerance: Myloral (AI-100)

The systemic application of an antigen induces T-cell anergy, immune deviation, or clonal deletion. The idea of oral tolerance (or "mucosal tolerance") refers to the observations that ingestion of an antigen induces an antigen-specific hyporesponsiveness in T cells and that activity of inflammatory reactions is downregulated by so-called bystander effects.[62] After antigen contact, specific mucosal lymphatic cells induce CD4- and CD8-positive regulatory cells (Th2, Th3, or others), leading to an antigen-specific suppression at the site of inflammation via secretion of IL-10, TGF-β, and IL-4. These effects depend on dosage and nature of the antigen (peptide or protein) as well as on the optimal administration (with or without adjuvant, orally, nasally, or intrabronchially). Higher antigen doses induce regulatory cells that are believed to induce clonal anergy in antigen-specific cells; lower doses induce regulatory cells that suppress the antigen-specific response.

Oral administration of putative autoantigens led to a diminution or suppression of clinical symptoms in a disease-specific as well as an antigen-specific manner in a series of experimental model systems (EAE and others).[62] Bystander suppression has been shown in EAE, where tolerance induction with myelin basic protein (MBP) inhibited the development of a proteolipid protein (PLP)-induced disease.[63] Oral tolerance has been tested clinically in a series of diseases (rheumatoid arthritis, uveitis, juvenile diabetes).

Oral bovine myelin (Myloral, AI-100) showed a significant clinical effect in a small phase II study.[64] This could not be confirmed in a subsequent multicentric, double-blind, placebo-controlled phase III study (516 patients with RRMS), in which the observed reduction of relapse rate did not differ significantly between the myelin-treated group and the placebo group. MRI scans also showed no treatment effect.[65,66] The trial data showed no significantly positive effects for oral bovine myelin on disease progression or MRI activity in MS. Nevertheless, the concept of autoantigen-based therapy in MS still remains attractive, mainly because of the huge logistic advantages of oral administration. However, transfer from animal data to therapy of human disease largely depends on the optimized influence of five crucial parameters[67]: (1) the chosen antigen (e.g., protein, peptide, neoantigen), (2) dosage, (3) duration of therapy, (4) mode of administration (orally, nasally, or intrabronchially), and (5) stage of disease (the potential for induction of regulatory cells by antigens typically decreases with disease progression).

Altered Peptide Ligands

Altered peptide ligands (APLs) are analogs of immunogenic peptides that differ by one or two amino acids from the original peptide that induces a full immune response. These mutant peptides bind to the same T-cell receptor/major histocompatibility complex (TCR/MHC), but with different affinity and kinetics, and therefore do not elicit a complete immune response.[68] APLs may modulate the cytokine pattern of T cells[69] and can induce T-cell anergy.[70] Administration of APLs led to disease inhibition in EAE models,[71,72] and several clinical trials with altered peptides have been initiated in MS. In a phase II study using a soluble human MBP 83-99 peptide,[73] high-dose therapy (50 mg/week) led to clinical exacerbation with high MRI inflammatory activity, unusually large lesions, or involvement of the peripheral nervous system. This was accompanied by an increase of up to 1000-fold in precursor frequencies of MBP(83-99)-specific T cells in peripheral blood and CSF cross-reacting with the administered APL.[73] In a larger, placebo-controlled study using the same APL (5, 20, or 50 mg human MBP 83-99 peptide versus placebo), exacerbations could not be observed either clinically or on MRI.[74]

Commentary on Antigen-Derived Therapies

The prototype of an autoantigen-directed, autoantigen-derived selective agent is glatiramer acetate (GA, Copaxone, copolymer-1), a standardized polypeptide mixture historically modeled after MBP. Except for GA, none of the putatively antigen-selective therapies has so far proved to provide a truly convincing clinical benefit to MS patients. On the contrary, the two phase II trials of an APL derived from MBP peptide 83-99 had to be halted prematurely because of allergic reactions.[73,74] Furthermore, in one of the studies, a tendency to trigger exacerbations was observed.[73] These inadvertent effects indicate that, in certain patients, the APL can cross-stimulate and activate encephalitogenic, MBP(83-99)-specific T cells. It may be that the autoimmune reaction eventually evades the effects of the APL therapy, for example, by epitope spreading. The results of the second, multicenter trial indicated that low-dose APL treatment induces a shift of the T-cell response from Th1 to Th2,[74] which is reminiscent of the immunologic effect of GA.[75-77]

In the end, the T-cell response in the human system toward various CNS-candidate autoantigens is much more complex and diverse than in the EAE-model using inbred animal strains. The heterogeneity and individuality of the TCR repertoire implies that a selective immune therapy will only work if the therapy can be individualized or tailored by the development of specific APL “cocktails” for individual patients or groups of patients with similar immunologic features. Therefore, attempts to develop more potent and more selective immunomodulators have failed so far, despite the apparently promising immunologic effects of the APLs.

CONCLUDING REMARKS ON FAILED TRIAL EXAMPLES

Despite the tremendous progress in MS therapy over the last years, the number of therapeutic strategies that (1) failed to show benefit for MS patients, (2) demonstrated a critical risk-benefit ratio despite obvious therapeutic efficacy, or (3) raised controversies in terms of their assumed efficacy or practicability is considerable. Lessons to be learned from the most prominent examples are the following:

1. Promising agents may paradoxically increase disease activity (TNF-α antagonists).
2. It is difficult to predict true therapeutic efficacy in humans from successful trials in animal models (TNF-α blockers, oral tolerance, remyelinating effect of IVIG, CCR1 antagonist).
3. Short-term favorable effects may be reversed on prolonged follow-up (sulfasalazine).
4. Effective drugs may be associated with unforeseen adverse effects (e.g., Linomide, CD40L).
5. Selectivity of immune interference is not necessarily associated with higher effectiveness but may possibly increase the risk of unexpected adverse effects (e.g., APLs).

Nonetheless, all of the examples mentioned here have added tremendously to our growing understanding of the cross-talk between the nervous and immune systems in MS, and their importance for scientific progress should not be underestimated.[78]

Future Therapies

According to the American National MS Society, a huge number of trials in MS are in progress or have recently been completed (information available at http://nationalmssociety.org [accessed October 2008]). Table 20-2 exemplifies and summarizes the most important substances currently under development and highlights the possible sites of drug action. Major groupings of agents or strategies are described in the following sections. For more detailed information on agents or strategies of interest, the reader is referred to recent review articles (e.g., Kleinschnitz and colleagues[79]).

PATHOGENETICALLY ORIENTED IMMUNE THERAPIES

Leukocyte Differentiation Molecules

Anti-CD52 Antibody: Alemtuzumab (Campath-1)

Among the biologic agents used in the treatment of autoimmune disorders, monoclonal antibodies (mABs) are considered to be especially promising candidates. Initially, the goal of antibody treatment was to deplete certain subsets of immune cells that were suspected to be pathogenetically relevant. Therefore, early studies in MS targeted T-cell differentiation molecules such as CD3 and CD4 (for review, see Hohlfeld and Wekerle[80]).

Alemtuzumab (Campath-1) is a humanized mAb directed against the CD52 antigen, which is commonly expressed on T and B cells, monocytes, and eosinophils. The antibody causes rapid and persisting lymphocyte depletion. Application in SPMS demonstrated an interesting dissociation between (1) the observed suppression of T cells and inflammatory lesions and (2) the progressive CNS tissue loss and patient disability.[81,82] At least in subjects with SPMS, this might indicate that nonspecific T-cell downregulation is ineffective. It also raises the possibility that Campath-1 treatment triggers increased antibody-mediated CNS damage by augmenting B-cell activity. For unknown reasons, about one third of patients treated with Campath-1 patients develop antibodies against the thyreotropin receptor and subsequent carbimazole-responsive autoimmune hyperthyroidism (Graves' disease).[82,83] A phase II clinical trial designed to compare the safety and efficacy of alemtuzumab with that of IFN-beta-1a in RRMS showed highly impressive effects on relapse rate and disease progression.[84] The trial was suspended (but later relaunched) because there was evidence of severe toxicity (idiopathic thrombocytopenic purpura), including one death. Currently, two phase III trials have been launched to evaluate clinical efficacy and long-term safety for potential approval.

Therapeutic approaches targeting leukocyte differentiation molecules decisively depend on the expression of the aimed-for target. However, newer immunologic knowledge concerning the in vivo effects of mAbs and the differential influences of certain mAbs on various immune cell subsets sharing the same leukocyte differentiation molecules has opened new views (and risks). In general, it might be assumed that antibodies aiming at widely distributed leukocyte antigens would have a high potential for serious side effects and that the risk of compromising immune defense mechanisms might counteract their efficacy. However, it is conceivable that intelligent combinations of antibodies might induce a lasting state of self-tolerance in T cells, provided that they are applied at an optimal time point of the course of the disease.

Costimulatory Molecules

T and B cells require two distinct types of signal for effective activation. One signal originates from ligation of the TCR complex and its coreceptors (CD4 and CD8) to an antigenic peptide bound to the presenting MHC molecule (known as the "trimolecular complex"). The second signal depends on either soluble factors such as IL-2 or ligation of cell surface molecules that provide essential costimulatory signals complementary to TCR engagement.[85] It is assumed that costimulatory signals are critically relevant for the regulation of T-cell activation as well as for keeping the balance between differentiation of Th1 and Th2 T helper cells.[86] Therefore, therapeutic blockade of costimulation as a treatment for autoimmune disorders has attracted considerable attention.[87]

Anti-CD25 (IL-2 Receptor) Antibody: Daclizumab

The interaction of IL-2 and its receptor CD25 mediates a pivotal signal for T-cell activation and proliferation. In general, anti-CD25 treatment aims to limit T-cell proliferation by blocking IL-2 signaling via its high-affinity receptor. The IL-2 receptor (IL-2R) antagonist, daclizumab, is a humanized mAb that interferes with the α-chain of the IL-2R.

Three open-label studies in MS have been published. They showed that daclizumab is well tolerated and leads to a significant reduction in MRI activity and improvement in several clinical outcome measures.[88-90] On first glance, the positive results of the first phase II study (designated "CHOICE") might seem surprising or even paradoxical, because CD25 is expressed not only on activated (pathogenic) T cells, but also on suppressor T cells.[91] This could imply a (theoretical) risk of further compromise to the CD25 suppressor system, which is believed to be dysregulated in MS.[92-94] However, the network of putative regulatory cells is complex and probably includes other subtypes of inhibitory cells. A phase IIb study is currently recruiting patients to test the safety and efficacy of daclizumab in a placebo-controlled, double-blind manner.[95] Results of this study are not yet available in published form (January 2009).

B Cells and Antibody Formation

There is increasing evidence that B cells play a decisive role in the development and perpetuation of MS.[96] In so-called pattern II MS lesions, antibodies and complement are found in vast amounts in parallel to T cell and monocyte/macrophage invasion. Therefore, inhibition of autoreactive B cells is a logical therapeutic aim. Especially certain MS variants such as neuromyelitis optica (NMO) are predominantly mediated by humoral mechanisms,[97-100] thus making them preferentially accessible to plasma exchange or immunoglobulin administration.[101,102]

Anti-CD20 Antibody: Rituximab

Rituximab (MabThera) is a genetically engineered chimeric murine/human mAb against CD20, a differentiation antigen that is found on normal and malignant pre-B and mature B lymphocytes but is absent on hematopoietic stem cells, on activated B cells (plasma cells), and in normal tissues. CD20 is vital for the regulation of cell cycle initiation and differentiation.

In an open pilot study in patients with NMO, administration of rituximab led to an impressive reduction in relapse frequency.[103] A number of case series or case reports describing the use of rituximab in "classic" MS are also available.[104-106] Two trials have investigated the potential use of rituximab in MS: the "OLYMPUS" trial of rituximab in PPMS, which is a phase II/III trial, and a phase I/II study involving RRMS patients, the results of which were recently published.[107] Compared with placebo, rituximab resulted in significantly reduced activity on MRI (primary end point: newly occurring gadolinium-enhancing lesions) as well as reduced relapses for about 1 year. This finding was in line with a phase I open study using rituximab, which also showed beneficial effects in reducing MRI and clinical activity.[108] It is interesting to note that the onset of clinical benefit was faster than could be expected simply from depletion or reduction of putatively pathogenic antibodies. This clearly points toward effects of anti-CD20 therapy other than reduction of antibody production, such as effects on the antigen-presenting function of B cells.[108]

Other B Cell–Oriented Therapeutic Approaches

B cells may be targeted directly, for example via agents directed toward CD19, CD20, CD21, or CD22 antigens expressed on the B-cell surface, or indirectly, for example, by disruption of the T-cell/B-cell interaction with inhibitors of costimulatory molecules such as B cell–activating factor (BAFF) (for review, see Dorner and Lipsky[109]). Directly targeted B-cell therapies that are currently being evaluated in autoimmune disorders include rituximab (MabThera/Rituximab), a chimeric monoclonal antibody specific for human CD20 cell surface antigen; ofatumumab (HuMax-CD20), a fully humanized anti-CD20 monoclonal antibody; epratuzumab, a humanized anti-CD22 monoclonal antibody; and ocrelizumab, a second-generation humanized anti-CD20 monoclonal antibody. Indirectly targeted B-cell therapies in development include belimumab (LymphoStat-B), a fully human monoclonal antibody that inhibits BAFF; BR3-Fc, a fusion protein of the BR3 BAFF receptor; and atacicept, a recombinant fusion protein containing the cytokine receptor TACI, which binds to and inhibits BAFF and a proliferation-inducing ligand of B cells (APRIL).

Anti-adhesion Molecules

Leukocyte recruitment to the CNS is regulated by cell adhesion molecules on endothelial cells and chemokines that are released from the site of inflammation.[34] As a first step, the velocity of leukocytes in the bloodstream is focally reduced ("rolling") as they loosely attach to endothelial cells via selectins (E-selectin, P-selectin, L-selectin). Then, firm adhesion of leukocytes to the endothelium is mediated by integrin interactions. Integrins comprise the $\alpha_4\beta_1$, $\alpha_5\beta_1$, and $\alpha_6\beta_1$ isoforms—also known as very late antigen 4 (VLA-4), VLA-5, and VLA-6, respectively—and leukocyte function antigen 1 (LFA-1), which is also a costimulatory molecule in T-cell activation. Whereas leukocytes constitutively express the ligands (LFA-1, VLA-4) on their surface, the corresponding counter-receptors such as intercellular adhesion molecule 1 (ICAM-1), ICAM-2, ICAM-3, and vascular cell adhesion molecule 1 (VCAM-1) on the endothelial cells require specific induction and thereby determine the location of leukocyte/endothelial cell interaction.[110] Antibodies directed against single adhesion molecules can potently inhibit crucial steps in the pathogenesis of MS, especially leukocyte migration. Interestingly, "rolling" is not observed at the blood–brain barrier; rather, encephalitogenic T cells are immediately "captured," by a mechanism in which integrins are pivotally involved.[111]

Anti-$\alpha_4\beta_1$ Integrin (VLA-4) Antibody: Natalizumab

The most promising candidate derived from this substance class is natalizumab. This monoclonal humanized antibody targets $\alpha_4\beta_1$ integrin (VLA-4) on the surface of lymphocytes. It is composed of a human IgG4 framework at the complementarity-determining region (CDR), which is linked to a murine antibody clone to reduce immunogenicity.[111,112] Experiments in EAE established that treatment with anti-α4 mAbs inhibits the interaction between the $\alpha_4\beta_1$ integrin expressed on leukocytes and its ligands on brain endothelium, thereby preventing the accumulation of leukocytes in the CNS.[113,114]

Although a preliminary phase I/II study applying natalizumab in MS patients suggested beneficial effects,[115] the clear proof of the concept was demonstrated in a three-armed, randomized, double-blind phase II trial in RRMS and active SPMS.[115] Treatment significantly reduced the number of new MS brain lesions on monthly gadolinium-enhanced MRI as well as the relapse frequency. Two phase III trials were completed recently.[115,116] The AFFIRM trial tested natalizumab as a monotherapy versus placebo in MS patients who had not received any immunotherapy in the preceding 6 months; 96% of subjects in the treatment arm had no new gadolinium-enhancing lesions, compared with 68% on those in the placebo arm. The rate of clinical relapse was reduced by 67%, and natalizumab also significantly delayed the progression of disability after 2 years.[115] In the SENTINEL study, the combination of natalizumab with the intramuscular formulation of IFN-beta-1a was tested against IFN-beta-1a alone. The combination therapy group had a 54% reduced relapse rate compared with IFN-beta-1a alone, as well as significantly fewer MRI lesions and a markedly higher proportion of relapse-free patients[116]. The most frequent adverse events in both studies included anaphylactoid reactions, increased risk of infections, rash, arthralgia, and headache. Approximately every 10th patient receiving natalizumab developed antibodies, and there was a clear negative impact on therapeutic efficacy in subjects who remained persistently antibody positive (e.g. on second testing).

Based on the positive interim analysis of both phase III trials after 1 year of therapy, natalizumab was approved via fast track by the U.S. Food and Drug Administration for the treatment of "relapsing forms of MS" in November 2004. However, in February 2005, the approval was suspended, and ongoing clinical trials were stopped, because two patients receiving natalizumab in combination with IFN-beta-1a had developed progressive multifocal leukoencephalopathy (PML), a severe opportunistic JC virus infection of the CNS. One of these MS patients later died.[117,118] In addition, a third person enrolled in a study of Crohn's disease was reassessed as having PML on the basis of a histopathologic reexamination that was primarily classified as an astrocytoma. This subject, who also died, had been treated with various additional immunosuppressive and immunomodulatory agents (except IFN) before and in parallel to natalizumab therapy.[119]

As a consequence, an extensive re-examination of all patients who had received natalizumab in clinical trials was performed, and the safety profile of natalizumab was collected and reviewed.[120]

1. No additional cases of PML were identified among more than 3000 patients exposed to natalizumab at that time.
2. Very specific plans for close monitoring of patients receiving natalizumab were developed, and various prerequisites must now be fulfilled before natalizumab administration (information available at: http://www.fda.org and http://www.fda.gov/cder/drug/infopage/natalizumab)
3. The available efficacy data indicate that natalizumab is a very effective drug and MS is a devastating disease with limited treatment options.

Anti-LFA1 (CD11/CD18) Antibody: Hu23F2G and Efalizumab

The LFA-1/ICAM interaction pathway is another key mediator of cell adhesion between leukocytes and vascular endothelial cells. This engagement is mechanistically targeted by Hu23F2G, a humanized anti-LFA1 (CD11/CD18) antibody. Application of this drug in an open phase I study in 24 patients with MS led to a high saturation of LFA-1 on circulating lymphocytes with in vivo inhibition of leukocyte migration.[122] However, a subsequent phase II study enrolling 169 MS patients could not demonstrate beneficial effects on MRI activity and clinical outcomes.[122]

Efalizumab is a recombinant humanized IgG1 ϰ isotype mAb against the CD11a molecule.[123] Efalizumab selectively targets the α chain (CD11a) of LFA-1 and is approved for the treatment of moderate to severe psoriasis.[124] Experience with 19,000 patients allows the conclusion that treatment with efalizumab (administered as a weekly subcutaneous injection) is remarkably safe. However, fatal cases with PML have recently been reported in association with Efalizumab.[125, 126] Treatment with monoclonal anti-CD11a antibodies also protected rats from EAE[126] and reduced the severity of the disease in mice, further supporting this approach as attractive for the treatment of human MS.

Chemotaxis

Blood–Brain Barrier Disruption and Transmigration: Matrix Metalloproteinase Inhibitors

There is increasing evidence that various members of the matrix metalloproteinase (MMP) family mediate fundamental steps in the development of inflammatory demyelinating disorders, such as cell migration, disruption of the blood–brain barrier, demyelination, and cytokine activation.[128-130] Various MMPs were detected in postmortem tissue samples from patients with MS,[131,132] and in particular MMP-7 and MMP-9 seem to play key roles in the pathogenesis of CNS inflammation. Both proteases were found to be increased during EAE, and peak expression levels correlated with maximum disease activity.[132,133] Selective MMP inhibitors prevented or ameliorated inflammatory CNS demyelination when applied in EAE models,[134,135] suggesting that MMPs are suitable targets for the treatment of MS.

Based on their chelating properties, tetracyclines (or certain chemically modified isoforms) are capable of blocking MMP activity. Minocycline, a tetracycline, has attracted increasing interest for the treatment of various neurologic diseases.[136] Minocycline is capable of inhibiting MMP activity independent from its antimicrobial activity,[136] and it exhibited potent synergistic effects with GA and with IFN-beta in animal models of MS.[137,138] A small, open-label trial in 10 patients with MS revealed an impressive reduction in the mean total number of active MRI lesions, implying that minocycline inhibits MMPs and permits transmigration of autoreactive T cells across the blood–brain barrier.

IMMUNOSUPPRESSANTS AND IMMUNOMODULATORS

The concept of using immunosuppression to treat autoimmune disorders has recently attracted considerable reattention, although it becomes increasingly difficult to separate agents labeled "immunosuppressants" from "immunomodulatory" or "immune-specific" substances. The resurrection of this very classic concept is meaningful for a number of reasons:

1. The heterogeneity and complexity of disease mechanisms, including interindividual differences in MS
2. The lack of a definitely identified (auto)antigen in most autoimmune disorders
3. The failures of highly antigen-specific immune therapies
4. The availability of novel (oral) drugs with good safety profiles and potential for long-term use.

Novel Immunosuppressants

Cladribine

Cladribine is an adenosine deaminase–resistant nucleoside analog with selective lymphotoxic specificity. After phosphorylation into the active triphosphate deoxy-nucleotide, the substance accumulates in lymphocytes and monocytes, causing DNA damage and subsequent cell death.[139,140] Its long-lasting lymphocytotoxic activity suggests that it could be useful in modulating conditions involving lymphocyte abnormalities. Therefore, cladribine has been extensively tested for the treatment of lymphoid neoplasms and autoimmune disorders, especially MS.

Evidence on the efficacy of cladribine in delaying disease progression comes mainly from smaller, placebo-controlled trials in chronic progressive MS[141,142] and RRMS.[143,144] The clinical observations were underlined by remarkable MRI effects, such as nearly complete elimination of gadolinium-enhanced T1 lesions and stabilization of T2 lesion volume.[145,146] Although phase I and II studies raised high expectations, a multicenter, double-blind, placebo-controlled study of cladribine in patients with SPMS and PPMS failed to show significant clinical benefit after 1 year.[146] In addition, no effects on whole brain volume or T1 "black holes" were observed.[146,147] Because cladribine reduced the number and volume of gadolinium-enhanced T1-weighted brain lesions and the overall T2 lesion load, there was a discrepancy between those MRI end points and the observed clinical effects.[146] Evaluation of the MRI data led to the conclusion that cladribine triggers strong and prolonged anti-inflammatory effects by MRI criteria but may not influence the mechanisms of continuous tissue destruction and neurodegeneration.[146,147] The substance is available as an oral formulation, and a randomized, double-blind, placebo-controlled phase III study in active inflammatory RRMS has been completed (Cladribine Tablets Treating MS Orally, or CLARITY). Results are expected in 2009.

Treosulfan

Treosulfan (dihydroxybusulfane) is a cytostatic alkylating agent that is approved for the treatment of advanced ovarian cancer. Treosulfan was successfully applied in myelin oligodendrocyte glycoprotein (MOG)-induced EAE.[148] Both severity of acute EAE and long-term disease outcome parameters were improved with a prophylactic and/or therapeutic treatment approach. Furthermore, treosulfan induced concentration-dependent apoptosis in human peripheral blood lymphocytes in vitro.[148] A recent study demonstrated superior immunosuppressive and myeloablative properties of treosulfan compared with cyclophosphamide and busulfan.[149] A small phase I pilot trial investigated the safety and efficacy of treosulfan in active SPMS. Overall, treosulfan was well tolerated. Nine of 11 patients remained on treatment and showed clinical stabilization or improvement on the EDSS and the Multiple Sclerosis Functional Composite (MSFC), and no corticosteroid-requiring relapses were observed. Treosulfan reduced MRI activity and stabilized measures of disease burden.[150] A phase II trial was interrupted due to recruitment problems.

Mycophenolate Mofetil

Another interesting immunosuppressant is mycophenolate mofetil.[150,151,152] It belongs to the antimetabolite group and is a prodrug of the active metabolite, mycophenolic acid. The drug is applied orally, is generally well tolerated, and is therefore convenient for the patient. Its use in neuroimmunologic autoimmune disorders is becoming increasingly popular, although almost all applications are "off label."[151] Very few reports or open-label studies of mycophenolate mofetil in MS exist. Two small trials using mycophenolate mofetil as monotherapy in various progressive MS cases suggested efficacy in this patient population, and application seems safe.[153] Patients with RRMS were enrolled in an open-label phase II clinical trial testing the combination of mycophenolate mofetil with IFN-beta-1a; preliminary efficacy data implied that the combination might be effective concerning clinical and MRI data.[154,155] To finally estimate the role of mycophenolate mofetil, either as a monotherapy or in combination with other MS treatments, controlled and larger studies are clearly warranted.

Pixantrone

Pixantrone (BBR2778) is a novel analog derived from mitoxantrone. Structurally, the 5,8-dihydroxyphenyl ring of mitoxantrone, which has been suspected of causing cardiotoxicity, was replaced by a pyridine ring.[156] In animal experiments and clinical pilot studies of cancer, intravenous pixantrone did not reveal toxic effects on cardiac tissue, and the pharmacokinetic and immunosuppressive properties were similar to those of mitoxantrone.[156-159] Because the substance has proved to be as effective as mitoxantrone in MS animal models, an open-label safety study in 20 RRMS patients has been initiated.[159]

Novel Immunomodulatory Agents

Teriflunomide

Teriflunomide is an analog of leflunomide, which is known from the treatment of rheumatoid arthritis. Teriflunomide belongs to the group of malononitrilamide agents which block the mitochondrial enzyme dihydro-orotate dehydrogenase and inhibit proliferation of T and B cells.[160,161] The oral prodrug is rapidly converted to its active metabolite, A771726. Teriflunomide has been found to suppress EAE in Lewis rats, probably via the suppression of TNF-α and IL-2 production.[162,163] The results from a clinical phase II study testing teriflunomide versus placebo in patients with RRMS and SPMS were published in 2006.[164] Subjects receiving teriflunomide had significantly less active MS lesions and reduced numbers of new lesions on MRI; in addition, EDSS progression was delayed, and a trend toward reduction in relapses was observed. The safety and efficacy of the drug in MS is being further investigated in an ongoing phase III trial. Given that teriflunomide is able to document superior or, at least not inferior, safety and efficacy, this compound could represent an important complement to the available armamentarium of drugs in MS therapy.

Laquinimod

Laquinimod (ABR-215062) is a novel immunomodulator that, at least in EAE, is approximately 20 times more potent than its progenitor, roquinimex (Linomide).[165] The synthetic compound has an excellent oral bioavailability and serves as an immunoregulatory drug without general immunosuppressive properties. Its sustained inhibitory activity on the immune system has been demonstrated in several animal models mimicking autoimmune or inflammatory diseases.[166-168]

Linomide efficiently reduced active MRI lesions in phase II clinical studies of MS[169] but a phase III trial had to be stopped prematurely due to unexpected severe inflammatory side effects such as serositis and myocardial infarction.[169]

Two clinical phase I trials with laquinimod demonstrated that the drug is well tolerated by healthy volunteers and patients with MS. A double-blind, randomized, multicenter, proof-of-concept study in patients with RRMS[169] showed a significant difference between laquinimod and placebo with respect to the mean cumulative number of active MRI lesions. However, clinical outcome parameters (relapse rate, disability) were not different between the two groups. The overall safety profile was favorable, with no signs of undesired tissue inflammation. Laquinimod, therefore, has considerable potential to become a safe and effective oral treatment in MS and is currently being tested in a large phase III trial.

FTY720

The compound FTY720 is derived from the fungus *Isaria sinclairii* and exhibits profound and unique immunoregulatory effects.[170,171] After in vivo phosphorylation, FTY720 forms FTY720P, a high-affinity, nonselective mimetic of the sphingosine 1-phosphate receptor 1 (S1P1). The mechanisms underlying FTY action remain somewhat controversial. Two alternative hypotheses have been proposed, involving different modes and sites of action. The "functional antagonism" hypothesis postulates that some agonists directly bind to S1P1 receptors on lymphocytes. This would cause receptor internalization and degradation, thus preventing lymphocyte egress from lymph nodes along an endogenous chemotactic gradient of S1P.[172] In this scenario, FTY720 would entrap $CD4^+$ and $CD8^+$ T cells and B cells in secondary lymphatic organs, preventing them from being recruited to possible sites of inflammation.[173,174] This "entrapped" homing of lymphocytes critically seems to depend on the expression of various chemokines.[174,175] The second hypothesis assumes that ligand binding to S1P1 receptors on endothelial cells in lymph nodes alters endothelial barrier functions, resulting in blockade of lymphocyte transmigration from the medullary parenchyma of a lymph node to the draining sinuses.[175,176] According to this hypothesis, S1P1 agonism on endothelial cells, but not on lymphocytes, is the crucial mechanism leading to lymphocyte sequestration within the nodes. (For a review on S1P and its receptors, refer to Rosen and Goetzl.[176]) Because of its mechanism of action, FTY720 induces a marked lymphopenia in the peripheral blood but does not provoke general immunosuppression, because the activation of T cells and the responses of memory T and B cells are not impaired.

The therapeutic potency of this agent has been demonstrated in various EAE models.[177,178] In an international, double-blind, placebo-controlled, phase II study of oral FTY720 involving subjects with active RRMS,[179] the total number of enhancing MS lesions on monthly MRI scans (primary outcome) was significantly reduced, and the volumes of enhancing lesions and new T2-weighted lesions were significantly diminished. In addition, a significantly higher proportion of patients receiving FTY720 remained relapse-free, compared with placebo (86% versus 70%). The relapse rate with FTY720 treatment was reduced by 53% to 55%. Two large phase III studies of FTY720 in MS are currently launched. One study is testing the safety and efficacy of two doses against placebo; the other is assessing the efficacy of FTY720 in a head-to-head design against IFN-beta-1a as an active comparator.

FTY720 is clearly one of the most interesting novel immunomodulatory agents currently under investigation, both from an "immune-mechanistic" point of view and as a practical option (oral drug). However, a number of caveats must be taken into account. Phase III studies will demonstrate whether FTY720 is able to document long-term efficacy and, even more important, safety in larger numbers of patients. It is unpredictable at the moment how chronic interference with lymphocyte homing and migration might affect immune surveillance of parenchymal organs, including the CNS, during long-term application.

Fumaric Acid

Another recent approach to induce beneficial immune deviation by enhancing Th2-driven responses in MS is the oral application of fumaric acid esters (BG00012, fumarate). An exploratory, prospective, open-label study of fumaric acid esters was conducted in patients with RRMS. In this small trial (10 subjects), a reduction of relapse rate and reduced volume of gadolinium-enhancing lesions as assessed by MRI was observed after 12 weeks.[180] However, 3 patients discontinued treatment during the first 3 weeks of the study, and several experienced mild to moderate gastrointestinal discomfort.

Kappos and colleagues[181] recently presented the results from a randomized, double-blind, placebo-controlled trial in 257 RRMS patients treated with three different doses of fumarate (BG00012). The highest dose of BG00012 (720 mg/day) significantly reduced the mean number of new gadolinium-enhancing lesions on MRI (primary end point) compared with placebo. The most common adverse effects included flushing, headache, nasopharyngitis, and nausea.[182] The authors concluded that BG00012 is safe and effective in RRMS, at least over the study period of 24 weeks. Two large phase III studies have been initiated.

AUTOLOGOUS STEM CELL TRANSPLANTATION

Given that the ultimate goal of MS treatment should be a cure for the disease, the immunologic rationale of resetting the "deviated" and "misprogrammed" immune system by autologous hematopoietic stem cell transplantation (HSCT) has attracted increasing interest but has also raised several controversies. Conceivably, intensive immune depletion can eliminate autoreactive immune cells regardless of their antigenic specificity, and subsequent regeneration of the immune system from hematopoietic precursors can re-establish immune tolerance. The idea of "resetting" a dysregulated immune system in autoimmune diseases has long appealed immunologists. For autologous HSCT, the patient's immune cells are eradicated ("ablated") by aggressive chemotherapy and are replaced by autologous HSCs that were isolated from the patient's bone marrow or blood before immune ablation. The hopes underlying this procedure are that it permanently removes autoimmune effector cells, is less toxic than conventional immunosuppressive therapies (because the immune system recovers), and offers the chance of permanent cure because the immune system is replenished with "healthy" stem cells.[183-186]

In HSCT, the ablated immune cells can be replaced by transplanted autologous (obtained from the patient), allogenic (obtained from a genetically matched donor), or syngenic (obtained from a twin) HSCs. Although there is no need for chronic immunosuppression after autologous transplantation, the risk of disease relapse seems higher than with allogenic transplants.[185] Experiments in animal models of autoimmune disorders provided the rationale for the current clinical studies of HSCT, which address a variety of severe, inflammatory diseases including MS.[183,186] It remains unclear whether the positive effects on disease course are mediated by the depletion of autoreactive lymphocytes or by the regeneration of the immune repertoire. One study[184] demonstrated that numeric recovery of leukocytes was accompanied by an average doubling of the frequency of naïve CD4+ T cells, at the expense of memory T cells. Importantly, post-transplantational T cells displayed broader clonal diversity and increased specificities compared with those obtained before HSCT. These findings demonstrated that immunologic mechanisms triggered by HSCT go far beyond mere immune ablation.

Although patient databases and the number of studies using HSCT in MS are growing, the approach remains highly controversial. So far, approximately 250 patients with MS have undergone HSCT, with variable outcomes. Comparisons between groups are difficult, because eligibility and technical procedures vary considerably. Two studies demonstrated significant suppression of MRI activity and stabilization of clinical disease after HSCT.[187,188] Most notably, HSCT induced superior responses in RRMS or active SPMS, compared with PPMS.

A phase II trial of autologous HSCT was conducted using clinical and MRI parameters in patients with all common forms of MS and rapid progression in preceding years.[189] Of 19 patients, 18 experienced stabilization or clinical improvement after transplantation; the progression-free survival rate was 95% at 6 years, and MRI lesion load was dramatically reduced. In contrast, another study[190] reported that intense T-cell depletion followed by autologous HSCT failed to prevent clinical progression in patients with rapidly progressive SPMS, although no gadolinium-enhanced lesions were seen on post-treatment MRIs of either the brain or spinal cord. Controlled trials of HSCT are currently underway, including the Autologous Stem cell Transplantation International Multiple Sclerosis (ASTIMS) trial, which is a multicenter, prospective, randomized, single-blinded, phase III study comparing the efficacy of high-dose immunoablation and autologous HSCT with mitoxantrone therapy for the treatment of patients with severe and progressive MS.

One has to critically take into account that the theoretical advantages and reported positive clinical experiences with this strategy are accompanied by a number of open questions and unresolved concerns. The most important of these is undoubtedly the significant risk of treatment-related mortality, which ranged between 5% and 8% in early studies of HSCT, a level that is not acceptable in a primary nonfatal disease such as MS. This drew attention to the essential need for standardized guidelines and selection criteria regarding autologous HSCT in MS,[186] and it was recommended that treatment should take place only in accredited bone marrow transplantation units, that patients should not exceed 50 years of age, and that they should be demonstrated to have highly active RRMS that is resistant to approved immunomodulatory or immunosuppressive therapies.

Conclusion

A substantial number of pivotal and preliminary reports continue to demonstrate encouraging new evidence that advances are being made in the care of MS patients. Despite the disappointments from a number of large pivotal trials, there is an auspicious array of novel agents and upcoming strategies. At present, it is not possible to foresee which, if any, of the new treatment strategies will supersede or complement the currently approved therapies in the near future. Clearly, in addition to immunologic approaches, strategies to enhance repair and promote neuroprotection are of immense importance. It is hoped that the next years will demonstrate how theoretical concepts, existing experimental data, or already available agents can be successfully transferred into everyday MS therapy. The approach of combining different agents or strategies remains promising. At present, however, all of theses approaches are still at an "experimental" state. Except for statements on safety and tolerability, none of them has yet achieved the level necessary for any recommendation or even approval on the basis of study evidence.

Even the latest generation of "humanized" mAbs is clearly immunogenic, because they can induce the production of anti-idiotypic antibodies. Such antibodies can neutralize the desired therapeutic effects and induce allergic reactions, pointing to the need for close monitoring of anti-antibody development. In addition, mAbs may induce a systemic inflammatory response by activating inflammatory cells and mediators after binding to their target. The systemic release of pro-inflammatory cytokines and other soluble mediators is most likely responsible for these reactions. Finally, apart from the effects derived from the postulated mechanism of action, numerous "off-target" effects may be expected or anticipated. It should be noted that many of the so-called immunomodulatory or immunoselective mAbs in fact act as nonselective immunosuppressants, even though their molecular targets are precisely known. Therefore, as in the case of conventional chemical immunosuppressive drugs, these agents might trigger serious adverse events, most notably infections and tumors, again highlighting the issue of risk-benefit profile considerations and appropriate patient selection. Furthermore, totally unexpected side effects cannot be definitely predicted from animal models or early clinical studies, and, although the molecular targets of many biologic agents are precisely known, the exact consequences of inhibition or stimulation of these targets cannot be predicted in the complex organism of a living human being.

Nevertheless, meaningful preclinical studies in animal models are indispensable to develop and verify (or discard) rational therapeutic concepts in the future. This is strikingly underlined by the remarkable number of promising agents initially derived from such preclinical experiments that are now under phase II/III clinical testing. Some of these agents will surely fulfill the key requirements in the treatment of a nonfatal disorder: convenience of drug administration and long-term efficacy plus safety. It is to be expected within the next few years that some of the new candidate biotechnological agents (mAbs, daclizumab, rituximab, alemtuzumab) and novel oral immunomodulatory or immunosuppressive agents (fumaric acid, FTY720, laquinimod, cladribine, teriflunomide) will become available for the treatment of MS to complement the currently available armamentarium.

Acknowledgments

H.W. received honoraria for lecturing and travel expenses for attending meetings and received financial research support from Bayer, Biogen Idec/Elan, Sanofi-Aventis, Schering, Serono, and Teva Pharmaceuticals. HW has served or serves as consultant for Serono, Medac, Sanofi-Aventis/TEVA, Biogen Idec, and Schering.

N.M. has nothing to disclose. C.K. received honoraria for lecturing and travel expenses for attending meetings from Biogen Idec/Elan, Schering, Serono, Bayer, and Sanofi-Aventis. S.G.M. received honoraria for lecturing and travel expenses for attending meetings from Biogen Idec/Elan, MerckSerono, Bayer HealthCare and Sanofi-Aventis.

Parts of this manuscript were published previously (Wiendl H and Hohlfeld R, Therapeutic approaches in multiple sclerosis: lessons from failed and interrupted treatment trials. Bio drugs 2002;16(3):183-200. Kleinschnitz C, Meuth SG, Kieseier BC, Wiendl H, Immunotherapeutic approaches in MS: update on pathophysiology and emerging agents of strategies 2006; Endocr Metab Immune Disord Drug Targets. 2007;7(10):35-63.)

All authors would like to thank Anke Bauer for her help with editing this manuscript.

REFERENCES

1. Aggarwal BB, Natarjan K: Tumor necrosis factor: Developments during the last decade. Eur Cytokine Netw 1996;7:93-124.
2. Beutler BA: The role of tumor necrosis factor in health and disease. J Rheumatol 1999;26(Suppl 57):16-21.
3. Locksley RM, Killeen N, Lenardo MJ: The TNF and TNF receptor superfamilies: Integrating mammalian biology. Cell 2001;104:487-501.
4. Klinkert WEF, Kojima K, Lesslauer W, et al: TNF-alpha receptor fusion protein prevents experimental auto-immune encephalomyelitis and demyelination in Lewis rats: An overview. J Neuroimmunol 1997;72:163-168.
5. Körner H, Lemckert FA, Chaudhri G, et al: Tumor necrosis factor blockade in actively induced experimental autoimmune encephalomyelitis prevents clinical disease despite activated T cell infiltration to the central nervous system. Eur J Immunol 1997;27:1973-1981.
6. Beck J, Rondot P, Catinot L, et al: Increased production of interferon gamma and tumor necrosis factor preceds clinical manifestation in multiple sclerosis: Do cytokines trigger off exacerbations? Acta Neurol Scand 1988;78:318-323.
7. Sharief MK, Hentges R: Association between tumor necrosis factor alpha and disease progression in patients with multiple sclerosis. N Engl J Med 1991;325:467-472.
8. Chofflon M, Juillard C, Juillard P, et al: Tumor necrosis factor alpha production as a possible predictor of relapse in patients with multiple sclerosis. Eur Cytokine Netw 1992;3:523-531.
9. Rudick RA, Ransohoff RM: Cytokine scretion by multiple sclerosis monocytes: Relationship to disease activity. Arch Neurol 1992;49:265-270.
10. Imamura K, Suzumura A, Hayashi F, Marunouchi R: Cytokine production by peripheral blood monocytes/macrophages in multiple sclerosis patients. Acta Neurol Scand 1993;87:281-285.
11. Rieckmann P, Albrecht M, Kitze B, et al: Tumor-necrosis-factor-alpha messenger-RNA expression in patients with relapsing-remitting multiple-sclerosis is associated with disease-activity. Ann Neurol 1995;37:82-88.
12. Van Oosten BW, Barkhof F, Scholten PET, et al: Increased production of tumor necrosis factor alpha, and not of interferon gamma, preceding disease activity in patients with multiple sclerosis. Arch Neurol 1998;55:793-798.
13. van Oosten BW, Barkhof F, Truyen L, et al: Increased MRI activity and immune activation in two multiple sclerosis patients treated with the monoclonal anti-tumor necrosis factor antibody cA2. Neurology 1996;47:1531-1534.
14. Arnason BGW, Jacobs G, Hanlon M: TNF neutralization in MS: Results of a randomized, placebo-controlled multicenter study. The Lenercept Multiple Sclerosis Study Group and The University of British Columbia MS/MRI Analysis Group. Neurology 1999;53:457-465.
15. Kassiotis G, Kollias G: Uncoupling the proinflammatory from the immunosuppressive properties of tumor necrosis factor (TNF) at the p55 TNF receptor level: Implications for pathogenesis and therapy of autoimmune demyelination. J Exp Med 2001;193:427-434.
16. Johns LD, Flanders KC, Ranges GE, Sriram S: Successful treatment of experimental allergic encephalomyelitis with transforming growth factor-β1. J Immunol 1991;147:1792-1796.

17. Kuruvilla AP, Shah R, Hochwald GM, et al: Protective effect of transforming growth factor-β1 on experimental autoimmune diseases in mice. Proc Natl Acad Sci U S A 1991;88:2918-2921.
18. Racke MK, Bonomo A, Scott DE, et al: Cytokine-induced immune deviation as a therapy for inflammatory autoimmune disease. J Exp Med 1994;180:1961-1966.
19. Stevens DB, Gould KE, Swanborg RH: Transforming growth factor-β1 inhibits tumor necrosis factor-alpha/lymphotoxin production and adoptive transfer of disease by effector cells of autoimmune encephalomyelitis. J Neuroimmunol 1994;51:77-83.
20. Fabry Z, Topham DJ, Fee D, et al: TGF-β2 decreases migration of lymphocytes in vitro and homing of cells into the central nervous system in vivo. J Immunol 1995;155:325-332.
21. Calabresi PA, Fields NS, Maloni HW, et al: Phase 1 trial of transforming growth factor beta 2 in chronic progressive MS. Neurology 1998;51:289-292.
22. Wahl SM: Transforming growth factor β: The good, the bad, and the ugly. J Exp Med 1994; 180:1587-1590.
23. Moore KW, de Waal Malefyt R, Coffman RL, O'Garra A: Interleukin-10 and the interleukin-10 receptor. Annu Rev Immunol 2001;19:683-765.
24. Owens T, Wekerle H, Antel J: Genetic models for CNS inflammation. Nat Med 2001;7:161-166.
25. Townsend MJ, McKenzie AN: Unravelling the net? Cytokines and diseases. J Cell Sci 2000;113 (Pt 20):3549-3550.
26. Lassmann H, Bruck W, Lucchinetti C: Heterogeneity of multiple sclerosis pathogenesis: Implications for diagnosis and therapy. Trends Mol Med 2001;7:115-121.
27. Arimilli S, Ferlin W, Solvason N, et al: Chemokines in autoimmune diseases. Immunol Rev 2000;177:43-51.
28. Engelhardt B, Ransohoff RM: The ins and outs of T-lymphocyte trafficking to the CNS: Anatomical sites and molecular mechanisms. Trends Immunol 2005;26:485-495.
29. Gordon EJ, Myers KJ, Dougherty JP, et al: Both anti-CD11a (LFA-1) and anti-CD11b (MAC-1) therapy delay the onset and diminish the severity of experimental autoimmune encephalomyelitis. J Neuroimmunol 1995;62:153-160.
30. Columba-Cabezas S, Serafini B, Ambrosini E, et al: Induction of macrophage-derived chemokine/CCL22 expression in experimental autoimmune encephalomyelitis and cultured microglia: Implications for disease regulation. J Neuroimmunol 2002;130:10-21.
31. Sorensen TL, Trebst C, Kivisakk P, et al: Multiple sclerosis: A study of CXCL10 and CXCR3 co-localization in the inflamed central nervous system. J Neuroimmunol 2002;127:59-68.
32. Omari KM, John GR, Sealfon SC, Raine CS: CXC chemokine receptors on human oligodendrocytes: Implications for multiple sclerosis. Brain 2005;128(Pt 5):1003-1015.
33. Omari KM, John G, Lango R, Raine CS: Role for CXCR2 and CXCL1 on glia in multiple sclerosis. Glia 2006;53:24-31.
34. Charo IF, Ransohoff RM: The many roles of chemokines and chemokine receptors in inflammation. N Engl J Med 2006;354:610-621.
35. Sorensen TL, Tani M, Jensen J, et al: Expression of specific chemokines and chemokine receptors in the central nervous system of multiple sclerosis patients. J Clin Invest 1999;103:807-815.
36. Ubogu EE, Cossoy MB, Ransohoff RM: The expression and function of chemokines involved in CNS inflammation. Trends Pharmacol Sci 2006;27:48-55.
37. Gaupp S, Pitt D, Kuziel WA, et al: Experimental autoimmune encephalomyelitis (EAE) in CCR2(-/-) mice: Susceptibility in multiple strains. Am J Pathol 2003;162:139-150.
38. Fox RJ, Ransohoff RM: New directions in MS therapeutics: Vehicles of hope. Trends Immunol 2004;25:632-636.
39. Elices MJ: BX-471 Berlex. Curr Opin Investig Drugs 2002;3:865-869.
40. Zipp F, Hartung HP, Hillert J, et al: Blockade of chemokine signaling in patients with multiple sclerosis. Neurology 2006;67:1880-1883.
41. Gonzalo J, Gonzalez-Garcia A, Kalland T, et al: Linomide, a novel immunomodulator that prevents death in four models of septic shock. Eur J Immunol 1993;23:2372-2374.
42. Karussis DM, Lehmann D, Slavin S, et al: Inhibition of acute, experimental autoimmune encephalomyelitis by the synthetic immunomodulator Linomide. Ann Neurol 1993;34:654-660.
43. Karussis DM, Lehmann D, Slavin S, et al: Treatment of chronic relapsing experimental autoimmune encephalomyelitis with the synthetic immunomodulator Linomide (quinoline-3-carboxamide). Proc Natl Acad Sci U S A 1993;90:6400-6404.
44. Karussis DM, Meiner Z, Lehmann D, et al: Treatment of secondary progressive multiple sclerosis with the immunomodulator linomide: A double-blind, placebo-controlled pilot study with monthly magnetic resonance imaging evaluation. Neurology 1996;47:341-346.

45. Andersen O, Lycke J, Tollesson PO, et al: Linomide reduces the rate of active lesions in relapsing-remitting multiple sclerosis. Neurology 1996;47:895-900.
46. Noseworthy JH, Wolinsky JS, Lublin FD, et al: Linomide in relapsing and secondary progressive MS: Part I. Trial design and clinical results. North American Linomide Investigators [see comments]. Neurology 2000;54:1726-1733.
47. Wolinsky JS, Narayana PA, Noseworthy JH, et al: Linomide in relapsing and secondary progressive MS: Part II. MRI results. MRI Analysis Center of the University of Texas-Houston, Health Science Center, and the North American Linomide Investigators [see comments]. Neurology 2000;54:1734-1741.
48. Schwid SR, Noseworthy JH: Targeting immunotherapy in multiple sclerosis: A near hit and a clear miss. Neurology 1999;53:444-445.
49. Prosiegel M, Neu I, Ruhenstroth-Bauer G, et al: Suppression of experimental autoimmune encephalitis by sulfasalazine. N Engl J Med 1989;321:545-546.
50. Prosiegel M, Neu I, Vogl S, et al: Suppression of experimental autoimmune encephalomyelitis by sulfasalazine. Acta Neurol Scand 1990;81:237-238.
51. Noseworthy JH, O'Brien P, Erickson BJ, et al: The Mayo-Clinic Canadian Cooperative trial of sulfasalazine in active multiple sclerosis. Neurology 1998;51:1342-1352.
52. Kappos L: Multiple sclerosis trials [letter; comment]. Lancet 1999;353:2242-2243.
53. Rudge P: Are clinical trials of therapeutic agents for MS long enough? [see comments]. Lancet 1999;353:1033-1034.
54. Stangel M, Hartung HP, Marx P, Gold R: Intravenous immunoglobulin treatment of neurological autoimmune disorders. J Neurol Sci 1998;153:203-214.
55. Rodriguez M, Lennon VA: Immunoglobulins promote remyelination in the central nervous system. Ann Neurol 1990;27:12-17.
56. Warrington AE, Asakura K, Bieber AJ, et al: Human monoclonal antibodies reactive to oligodendrocytes promote remyelination in a model of multiple sclerosis. Proc Natl Acad Sci U S A 2000;97:6820-6825.
57. Van Engelen BG, Hommes OR, Pinckers A, et al: Improved vision after intravenous immunoglobulin in stable demyelinating optic neuritis [letter]. Ann Neurol 1992;32:834-835.
58. Noseworthy JH, O'Brien PC, Petterson TM, et al: A randomized trial of intravenous immunoglobulin in inflammatory demyelinating optic neuritis. Neurology 2001;56:1514-1522.
59. Noseworthy JH, Rodriguez M, Petterson T, et al: Multiple sclerosis (MS) disease activity may determine whether immunoglobulin (IVIg) administration enhances or worsens visual function in patients with severe, stable optic neuritis (SDON). Neurology 2000;54;(7 Suppl 3):A258.
60. Stangel M, Boegner F, Klatt CH, et al: Placebo controlled pilot trial to study the remyelinating potential of intravenous immunoglobulins in multiple sclerosis. J Neurol Neurosurg Psychiatry 2000;68:89-92.
61. Stangel M, Compston A, Scolding MJ: Polyclonal immunoglobulins for intravenous use do not influence the behaviour of cultured oligodendrocytes. J Neuroimmunol 1999;96:228-233.
62. Weiner HL, Friedmann A, Miller A, et al: Oral tolerance: Immunologic mechanisms and treatment of animal and human organ-specific autoimmune diseases by oral administration of autoantigens. Ann Rev Immunol 1994;12:809-837.
63. Chen Y, Kuchroo VK, Inobe J-I, et al: Regulatory T cell clones induced by oral tolerance: Suppression of autoimmune encephalomyelitis. Science 1994;265:1237-1240.
64. Weiner HL, Mackin GA, Matsui M, et al: Double-blind pilot trial of oral tolerization with myelin antigens in multiple sclerosis. Science 1993;259:1321-1324.
65. Francis G, Evans A, Panitch H: MRI results of a phase III trial of oral myelin in relapsing-remitting multiple sclerosis. Ann Neurol 1997;42:467.
66. Panitch H, Francis G; the Oral Myelin Study Group: Clinical results of a phase III trial of oral myelin in relapsing-remitting multiple sclerosis. Ann Neurol 1997;42:459.
67. Tian J, Olcott A, Hanssen L, et al: Antigen-based immunotherapy for autoimmune disease: From animal models to humans? Immunol Today 1999;20:190-195.
68. Sloan-Lancaster J, Evavold BD, Allen PM: Induction of T-cell anergy by altered T-cell-receptor ligand on live antigen-presenting cells. Nature 1993;363:156-159.
69. Windhagen A, Scholz C, Höllsbert P, et al: Modulation of cytokine patters of human autoreactive T cell clones by a single amino acid substitution of their peptide ligand. Immunity 1995;2:373-380.
70. Sloan-Lancaster J, Allen PM: Altered peptide ligand induced partial T cell activation: Molecular mechanisms and role in T cell biology. Ann Rev Immunol 1996;14:1-27.

71. Smilek DE, Wraith DC, Hodgkinson S, et al: A single amino acid change in a myelin basic protein peptide confers the capacity to prevent rather than induce experimental autoimmune encephalomyelitis. Proc Natl Acad Sci U S A 1991;88:9633-9637.
72. Nicholson LB, Greer JM, Sobel RA, et al: An altered peptide ligand mediates immune deviation and prevents autoimmune encephalomyelitis. Immunity 1995;3:397-405.
73. Bielekova B, Goodwin B, Richert N, et al: Encephalitogenic potential of the myelin basic protein peptide (amino acids 83-99) in multiple sclerosis: Results of a phase II clinical trial with an altered peptide ligand. Nat Med 2000;6:1167-1175.
74. Kappos L, Comi G, Panitch H, et al: Induction of a non-encephalitogenic type 2 T helper-cell autoimmune response in multiple sclerosis after administration of an altered peptide ligand in a placebo-controlled, randomized phase II trial. The Altered Peptide Ligand in Relapsing MS Study Group. Nat Med 2000;6:1176-1182.
75. Neuhaus O, Farina C, Yassouridis A, et al: Multiple sclerosis: Comparison of copolymer-1-reactive T cell lines from treated and untreated subjects reveals cytokine shift from T helper 1 to T helper 2 cells. Proc Natl Acad Sci U S A 2000;97:7452-7457.
76. Duda PW, Schmied MC, Cook SL, et al: Glatiramer acetate (Copaxone) induces degenerate, Th2-polarized immune responses in patients with multiple sclerosis. J Clin Invest 2000;105: 967-876.
77. Gran B, Tranquill LR, Chen M, et al: Mechanisms of immunomodulation by glatiramer acetate. Neurology 2000;55:1704-1714.
78. Hohlfeld R, Wiendl H: The ups and downs of multiple sclerosis therapeutics. Ann Neurol 2001;49:281-284.
79. Kleinschnitz C, Meuth SG, Kieseier BC, Wiendl H: Immunotherapeutic approaches in MS: Update on pathophysiology and emerging agents or strategies 2006. Endocr Metab Immune Disord Drug Targets 2007;7:35-63.
80. Hohlfeld R, Wekerle H: Autoimmune concepts of multiple sclerosis as a basis for selective immunotherapy: From pipe dreams to (therapeutic) pipelines. Proc Natl Acad Sci U S A 2004:14599-14606.
81. Paolillo A, Coles AJ, Molyneux PD, et al: Quantitative MRI in patients with secondary progressive MS treated with monoclonal antibody Campath 1H. Neurology 1999;53:751-757.
82. Coles AJ, Wing M, Smith S, et al: Pulsed monoclonal antibody treatment and autoimmune thyroid disease in multiple sclerosis. Lancet 1999;354:1691-1695.
83. Coles AJ, Wing MG, Molyneux P, et al: Monoclonal antibody treatment exposes three mechanisms underlying the clinical course of multiple sclerosis. Ann Neurol 1999;46:296-304.
84. Coles AJ, Compston DA, Selmaj KW, et al: Alemtuzumab vs. interferon beta-1a in early multiple sclerosis. CAMMS223 Trial Investigators. N Engl J Med 2008;359(17):1786-1801.
85. Frauwirth KA, Thompson CB: Activation and inhibition of lymphocytes by costimulation. J Clin Invest 2002;109:295-299.
86. Kobata T, Azuma M, Yagita H, Okumura K: Role of costimulatory molecules in autoimmunity. Rev Immunogenet 2000;2:74-80.
87. Howard LM, Kohm AP, Castaneda CL, Miller SD: Therapeutic blockade of TCR signal transduction and co-stimulation in autoimmune disease. Curr Drug Targets Inflamm Allergy 2005;4:205-216.
88. Bielekova B, Richert N, Howard T, et al: Humanized anti-CD25 (daclizumab) inhibits disease activity in multiple sclerosis patients failing to respond to interferon beta. Proc Natl Acad Sci U S A 2004;101:8705-8708.
89. Rose JW, Watt HE, White AT, Carlson NG: Treatment of multiple sclerosis with an anti-interleukin-2 receptor monoclonal antibody. Ann Neurol 2004;56:864-867.
90. Rose JW, Burns JB, Bjorklund J, et al: Daclizumab phase II trial in relapsing and remitting multiple sclerosis: MRI and clinical results. Neurology 2007;69:785-789.
91. Sakaguchi S: Naturally arising Foxp3-expressing CD25+CD4+ regulatory T cells in immunological tolerance to self and non-self. Nat Immunol 2005;6:345-352.
92. Baecher-Allan C, Hafler DA: Suppressor T cells in human diseases. J Exp Med 2004;200:273-276.
93. Viglietta V, Baecher-Allan C, Weiner HL, Hafler DA: Loss of functional suppression by CD4+CD25+ regulatory T cells in patients with multiple sclerosis. J Exp Med 2004;199:971-979.
94. Haas J, Hug A, Viehover A, et al: Reduced suppressive effect of CD4+CD25 high regulatory T cells on the T cell immune response against myelin oligodendrocyte glycoprotein in patients with multiple sclerosis. Eur J Immunol 2005;35:3343-3352.
95. Bielekova B, Catalfamo M, Reichert-Scrivner S, et al: Regulatory CD56(bright) natural killer cells mediate immunomodulatory effects of IL-2Ralpha-targeted therapy (daclizumab) in multiple sclerosis. Proc Natl Acad Sci U S A 2006;103:5941-5946.

96. Lucchinetti C, Bruck W, Parisi J, et al: Heterogeneity of multiple sclerosis lesions: Implications for the pathogenesis of demyelination. Ann Neurol 2000;47:707-717.
97. Lennon VA, Kryzer TJ, Pittock SJ, et al: IgG marker of optic-spinal multiple sclerosis binds to the aquaporin-4 water channel. J Exp Med 2005;202:473-477.
98. Lucchinetti CF, Mandler RN, McGavern D, et al: A role for humoral mechanisms in the pathogenesis of Devic's neuromyelitis optica. Brain 2002;125(Pt 7):1450-1461.
99. Bruck W, Lucchinetti C, Lassmann H: The pathology of primary progressive multiple sclerosis. Mult Scler 2002;8:93-97.
100. Scolding N: Devic's disease and autoantibodies. Lancet Neurol 2005;4:136-137.
101. Keegan M, Konig F, McClelland R, et al: Relation between humoral pathological changes in multiple sclerosis and response to therapeutic plasma exchange. Lancet 2005;366:579-582.
102. Wingerchuk DM, Weinshenker BG: Neuromyelitis optica. Curr Treat Options Neurol 2005;7: 173-182.
103. Cree BA, Lamb S, Morgan K, et al: An open label study of the effects of rituximab in neuromyelitis optica. Neurology 2005;64(7):1270-1272.
103. Monson NL, Cravens PD, Frohman EM, et al: Effect of rituximab on the peripheral blood and cerebrospinal fluid B cells in patients with primary progressive multiple sclerosis. Arch Neurol 2005;62:258-264.
104. Stuve O, Cepok S, Elias B, et al: Clinical stabilization and effective B-lymphocyte depletion in the cerebrospinal fluid and peripheral blood of a patient with fulminant relapsing-remitting multiple sclerosis. Arch Neurol 2005;62:1620-1623.
105. Petereit HF, Rubbert A: Effective suppression of cerebrospinal fluid B cells by rituximab and cyclophosphamide in progressive multiple sclerosis. Arch Neurol 2005;62:1641-1642. author reply 1642.
106. Hauser SL, Waubant E, Arnold DL, et al: B-cell depletion with rituximab in relapsing-remitting multiple sclerosis. N Engl J Med 2008;358:676-688.
107. Bar-Or A, Calabresi PA, Arnlod D, et al: Rituximab in relapsing-remitting multiple sclerosis: A 72-week, open-label, phase I trial. Ann Neurol 2008;63:395-400.
108. McFarland HF: The B cell: Old player, new position on the team. N Engl J Med 2008;358: 664-665.
109. Dorner T, Lipsky PE: B-cell targeting: A novel approach to immune intervention today and tomorrow. Expert Opin Biol Ther 2007;7:1287-1299.
110. Engelhardt B, Briskin MJ: Therapeutic targeting of alpha 4-integrins in chronic inflammatory diseases: Tipping the scales of risk towards benefit? Eur J Immunol 2005;35:2268-2273.
111. Keeley KA, Rivey MP, Allington DR: Natalizumab for the treatment of multiple sclerosis and Crohn's disease. Ann Pharmacother 2005;39:1833-1843.
112. Steinman L: Blocking adhesion molecules as therapy for multiple sclerosis: Natalizumab. Nat Rev Drug Discov 2005;4:510-518.
113. Rice GP, Hartung HP, Calabresi PA: Anti-alpha4 integrin therapy for multiple sclerosis: Mechanisms and rationale. Neurology 2005;64:1336-1342.
114. Tubridy N, Behan PO, Capildeo R, et al: The effect of anti-alpha 4 integrin antibody on brain lesion activity in MS. Neurology 1999;53:466-472.
115. Polman CH, O'Connor PW, Havrdova E, et al: A randomized, placebo-controlled trial of natalizumab for relapsing multiple sclerosis. N Engl J Med 2006;354:899-910.
116. Rudick RA, Stuart WH, Calabresi PA, et al: Natalizumab plus interferon beta-1a for relapsing multiple sclerosis. N Engl J Med 2006;354:911-923.
117. Kleinschmidt-DeMasters BK, Tyler KL: Progressive multifocal leukoencephalopathy complicating treatment with natalizumab and interferon beta-1a for multiple sclerosis. N Engl J Med 2005;353:369-374.
118. Langer-Gould A, Atlas SW, Green AJ, et al: Progressive multifocal leukoencephalopathy in a patient treated with natalizumab. N Engl J Med 2005;353:375-381.
119. Van Assche G, Van Ranst M, Sciot R, et al: Progressive multifocal leukoencephalopathy after natalizumab therapy for Crohn's disease. N Engl J Med 2005;353:362-368.
120. Yousry TA, Major EO, Ryschkewitsch C, et al: Evaluation of patients treated with natalizumab for progressive multifocal leukoencephalopathy. N Engl J Med 2006;354:924-933.
121. Simmons DL, Buckley CD: Some new, and not so new, anti-inflammatory targets. Curr Opin Pharmacol 2005;5:394-397.
122. Lublin F: A phase II trial of anti-CD11/CD18 monoclonal antibody in acute exacerbations of MS. Neurology 1999;52(Suppl 2): A290.

123. Marecki S, Kirkpatrick P: Efalizumab. Nat Rev Drug Discov 2004;3:473-474.
124. Lebwohl M, Tyring SK, Hamilton TK, et al: A novel targeted T-cell modulator, efalizumab, for plaque psoriasis. N Engl J Med 2003;349:2004-2013.
125. Scheinfeld N: Efalizumab: A review of events reported during clinical trials and side effects. Expert Opin Drug Saf 2006;5:197-209.
126. Willenborg DO, Staykova MA, Miyasaka M: Short term treatment with soluble neuroantigen and anti-CD11a (LFA-1) protects rats against autoimmune encephalomyelitis: Treatment abrogates autoimmune disease but not autoimmunity. J Immunol 1996;157:1973-1980.
127. Sellebjerg F, Sorensen TL: Chemokines and matrix metalloproteinase-9 in leukocyte recruitment to the central nervous system. Brain Res Bull 2003;61:347-355.
128. Hartung HP, Kieseier BC: The role of matrix metalloproteinases in autoimmune damage to the central and peripheral nervous system. J Neuroimmunol 2000;107:140-147.
129. Yong VW: Metalloproteinases: Mediators of pathology and regeneration in the CNS. Nat Rev Neurosci 2005;6:931-944.
130. Maeda A, Sobel RA: Matrix metalloproteinases in the normal human central nervous system, microglial nodules, and multiple sclerosis lesions. J Neuropathol Exp Neurol 1996;55: 300-309.
131. Lindberg RL, De Groot CJ, Montagne L, et al: The expression profile of matrix metalloproteinases (MMPs) and their inhibitors (TIMPs) in lesions and normal appearing white matter of multiple sclerosis. Brain 2001;124(Pt 9):1743-1753.
132. Clements JM, Cossins JA, Wells GM, et al: Matrix metalloproteinase expression during experimental autoimmune encephalomyelitis and effects of a combined matrix metalloproteinase and tumour necrosis factor-alpha inhibitor. J Neuroimmunol 1997;74:85-94.
133. Kieseier BC, Clements JM, Pischel HB, et al: Matrix metalloproteinases MMP-9 and MMP-7 are expressed in experimental autoimmune neuritis and the Guillain-Barre syndrome. Ann Neurol 1998;43:427-434.
134. Brundula V, Rewcastle NB, Metz LM, et al: Targeting leukocyte MMPs and transmigration: Minocycline as a potential therapy for multiple sclerosis. Brain 2002;125(Pt 6):1297-1308.
135. Popovic N, Schubart A, Goetz BD, et al: Inhibition of autoimmune encephalomyelitis by a tetracycline. Ann Neurol 2002;51:215-223.
136. Yong VW, Wells J, Giuliani F, et al: The promise of minocycline in neurology. Lancet Neurol 2004;3:744-751.
137. Giuliani F, Fu SA, Metz LM, Yong VW: Effective combination of minocycline and interferon-beta in a model of multiple sclerosis. J Neuroimmunol 2005;165:83-91.
138. Giuliani F, Metz LM, Wilson T, et al: Additive effect of the combination of glatiramer acetate and minocycline in a model of MS. J Neuroimmunol 2005;158:213-221.
139. Sipe JC: Cladribine for multiple sclerosis: Review and current status. Expert Rev Neurother 2005;5:721-727.
140. Beutler E: Cladribine (2-chlorodeoxyadenosine). Lancet 1992;340:952-956.
141. Sipe JC, Romine JS, Koziol JA, et al: Cladribine in treatment of chronic progressive multiple sclerosis [see comments]. Lancet 1994;344:9-13.
142. Beutler E, Sipe JC, Romine JS, et al: The treatment of chronic progressive multiple sclerosis with cladribine. Proc Natl Acad Sci U S A 1996;93:1716-1720.
143. Sipe JC, Romine JS, Koziol J, et al: Cladribine improves relapsing-remitting MS: A double blind placebo controlled study. Neurology 1997;48(Suppl 2):A340.
144. Romine JS, Sipe JC, Koziol JA, et al: A double-blind, placebo-controlled, randomized trial of cladribine in relapsing-remitting multiple sclerosis. Proc Assoc Am Physicians 1999;111:35-44.
145. Rice GP, Filippi M, Comi G: Cladribine and progressive MS: Clinical and MRI outcomes of a multicenter controlled trial. Cladribine MRI Study Group. Neurology 2000;54:1145-1155.
146. Filippi M, Rovaris M, Rice GP, et al: The effect of cladribine on T(1) 'black hole' changes in progressive MS. J Neurol Sci 2000;176:42-44.
147. Filippi M, Rovaris M, Iannucci G, et al: Whole brain volume changes in patients with progressive MS treated with cladribine. Neurology 2000;55:1714-1718.
148. Weissert R, Wiendl H, Pfrommer H, et al: Action of treosulfan in myelin-oligodendrocyte-glycoprotein-induced experimental autoimmune encephalomyelitis and human lymphocytes. J Neuroimmunol 2003;144:28-37.
149. Wiendl H, Kieseier BC, Weissert R, Mylices HA, Pichlmeier U, Hartung H-P, Melms A, Kuker W, Weller M. Treatment of active secondary progressive MS with treosulfan: Open-label trial. J Neurol 2007;254(7):884-889.

150. Frohman EM, Brannon K, Racke MK, Hawker K: Mycophenolate mofetil in multiple sclerosis. Clin Neuropharmacol 2004;27:80-83.
151. Schneider-Gold C, Hartung HP, Gold R: Mycophenolate mofetil and tacrolimus: New therapeutic options in neuroimmunological diseases. Muscle Nerve 2006;34:284-291.
152. Ahrens N, Salama A, Haas J: Mycophenolate-mofetil in the treatment of refractory multiple sclerosis. J Neurol 2001;248:713-714.
153. Ducray F, Vukusic S, Gignoux L: Mycophenolate mofetil: An open-label study in 42 MS patients. Mult Scler 2004;10(Suppl):S263.
154. Vermersch P, Waucquier N, Bourteel H: Treatment of multiple sclerosis with a combination of interferon beta-1a (Avonex) and Mycophenolate mofetil (Cellcept): Results of a phase II clinical trial. Neurology 2004;62. A259.
155. Vermersch et al., 2007 Eur J Neurol. 14:85-89 Combination of IFN-beta-1a (Avonex(R)) and Mycophenolate mofetil (Cellcept(R)) in multiple sclerosis.
156. Gonsette RE, Dubois B: Pixantrone (BBR2778): A new immunosuppressant in multiple sclerosis with a low cardiotoxicity. J Neurol Sci 2004;223:81-86.
157. Beggiolin G, Crippa L, Menta E, et al: Bbr 2778, an aza-anthracenedione endowed with preclinical anticancer activity and lack of delayed cardiotoxicity. Tumori 2001;87:407-416.
158. Cavaletti G, Cavalletti E, Crippa L, et al: Pixantrone (BBR2778) reduces the severity of experimental allergic encephalomyelitis. J Neuroimmunol 2004;151:55-65.
159. Gonsette RE: New immunosuppressants with potential implication in multiple sclerosis. J Neurol Sci 2004;223:87-93.
160. Korn T, Magnus T, Toyka K, Jung S: Modulation of effector cell functions in experimental autoimmune encephalomyelitis by leflunomide: Mechanisms independent of pyrimidine depletion. J Leukoc Biol 2004;76:950-960.
161. Nakajima A, Yamanaka H, Kamatani N: [Leflunomide: Clinical effectiveness and mechanism of action.] Clin Calcium 2003;13:771-775.
162. Korn T, Toyka K, Hartung HP, Jung S: Suppression of experimental autoimmune neuritis by leflunomide. Brain 2001;124(Pt 9):1791-1802.
163. Smolen JS, Emery P, Kalden JR, et al: The efficacy of leflunomide monotherapy in rheumatoid arthritis: Towards the goals of disease modifying antirheumatic drug therapy. J Rheumatol Suppl 2004;71:13-20.
164. O'Connor PW, Li D, Freedman MS, et al: A Phase II study of the safety and efficacy of teriflunomide in multiple sclerosis with relapses. Neurology 2006;66:894-900.
165. Brunmark C, Runstrom A, Ohlsson L, et al: The new orally active immunoregulator laquinimod (ABR-215062) effectively inhibits development and relapses of experimental autoimmune encephalomyelitis. J Neuroimmunol 2002;130:163-172.
166. Jonsson S, Andersson G, Fex T, et al: Synthesis and biological evaluation of new 1,2-dihydro-4-hydroxy-2-oxo-3-quinolinecarboxamides for treatment of autoimmune disorders: Structure-activity relationship. J Med Chem 2004;47:2075-2088.
167. Runstrom A, Leanderson T, Ohlsson L, Axelsson B: Inhibition of the development of chronic experimental autoimmune encephalomyelitis by laquinimod (ABR-215062) in IFN-beta k.o. and wild type mice. J Neuroimmunol 2006;173:69-78.
168. Yang JS, Xu LY, Xiao BG, et al: Laquinimod (ABR-215062) suppresses the development of experimental autoimmune encephalomyelitis, modulates the Th1/Th2 balance and induces the Th3 cytokine TGF-beta in Lewis rats. J Neuroimmunol 2004;156:3-9.
169. Polman C, Barkhof F, Sandberg-Wollheim M, et al: Treatment with laquinimod reduces development of active MRI lesions in relapsing MS. Neurology 2005;64:987-991.
170. Brinkmann V, Davis MD, Heise CE, et al: The immune modulator FTY720 targets sphingosine 1-phosphate receptors. J Biol Chem 2002;277:21453-21457.
171. Chiba K: FTY720, a new class of immunomodulator, inhibits lymphocyte egress from secondary lymphoid tissues and thymus by agonistic activity at sphingosine 1-phosphate receptors. Pharmacol Ther 2005;108:308-319.
172. Matloubian M, Lo CG, Cinamon G, et al: Lymphocyte egress from thymus and peripheral lymphoid organs is dependent on S1P receptor 1. Nature 2004;427:355-360.
173. Cyster JG: Chemokines, sphingosine-1-phosphate, and cell migration in secondary lymphoid organs. Annu Rev Immunol 2005;23:127-159.
174. Yopp AC, Fu S, Honig SM, et al: FTY720-enhanced T cell homing is dependent on CCR2, CCR5, CCR7, and CXCR4: Evidence for distinct chemokine compartments. J Immunol 2004;173:855-865.

175. Mandala S, Hajdu R, Bergstrom J, et al: Alteration of lymphocyte trafficking by sphingosine-1-phosphate receptor agonists. Science 2002;296:346-349.
176. Rosen H, Goetzl EJ: Sphingosine 1-phosphate and its receptors: an Autocrine and paracrine network. Nat Rev Immunol 2005;5:560-570.
177. Fujino M, Funeshima N, Kitazawa Y, et al: Amelioration of experimental autoimmune encephalomyelitis in Lewis rats by FTY720 treatment. J Pharmacol Exp Ther 2003;305:70-77.
178. Webb M, Tham CS, Lin FF, et al: Sphingosine 1-phosphate receptor agonists attenuate relapsing-remitting experimental autoimmune encephalitis in SJL mice. J Neuroimmunol 2004;153: 108-121.
179. Kappos L, Radu EW, Antel J: Promising results with a novel oral immunomodulator-FTY720-in relapsing multiple sclerosis. Mult Scler 2005;11(Suppl):S13.
180. Schimrigk K, Brune N, Hellwig K, et al: Oral fumaric acid esters for the treatment of active multiple sclerosis: an open-label baseline-controlled pilot study. Eur J Neurol 2006;13(6):604-610.
181. Kappos L, Gold R, Miller DH, et al: Efficacy and safety of oral fumarate in patients with relapsing-remitting multiple sclerosis: A multicentre, randomised, double-blind, placebo-controlled phase IIb study. Lancet 2008;372(9648):1463-1472.
182. Gold R, Havrdova E, Kappos L, et al: Safety of a novel oral single-agent fumarate, BG00012, in patients with relapsing-remitting mutiple sclerosis: Results of a phase 2 study. J Neurol 2006;253(Suppl 2): 144.
183. Farrell R, Heaney D, Giovannoni G: Emerging therapies in multiple sclerosis. Expert Opin Emerg Drugs 2005;10:797-816.
184. Muraro PA, Cassiani-Ingoni R, Martin R: Using stem cells in multiple sclerosis therapies. Cytotherapy 2004;6:615-620.
185. Burt RK, Cohen B, Rose J, et al: Hematopoietic stem cell transplantation for multiple sclerosis. Arch Neurol 2005;62:860-864.
186. Blanco Y, Saiz A, Carreras E, Graus F: Autologous haematopoietic-stem-cell transplantation for multiple sclerosis. Lancet Neurol 2005;4:54-63.
187. Mancardi GL, Saccardi R, Filippi M, et al: Autologous hematopoietic stem cell transplantation suppresses Gd-enhanced MRI activity in MS. Neurology 2001;57:62-68.
188. Fassas A, Passweg JR, Anagnostopoulos A, et al: Hematopoietic stem cell transplantation for multiple sclerosis: A retrospective multicenter study. J Neurol 2002;249:1088-1097.
189. Saccardi R, Kozak T, Bocelli-Tyndall C, et al: Autologous stem cell transplantation for progressive multiple sclerosis: Update of the European Group for Blood and Marrow Transplantation autoimmune diseases working party database. Mult Scler 2006;12:814-823.
190. Nash RA, Bowen JD, McSweeney PA, et al: High-dose immunosuppressive therapy and autologous peripheral blood stem cell transplantation for severe multiple sclerosis. Blood 2003;102: 2364-2372.

21 Strategies to Promote Neuroprotection and Repair in Multiple Sclerosis

TAMIR BEN-HUR

Multiple sclerosis (MS) is the most common cause of neurologic disability in young adults. It is characterized by chronic inflammatory, demyelinating, multifocal lesions within the central nervous system (CNS)[1-4] and heterogeneous pathology.[5,6] A key issue in the treatment of neurologic diseases in general, and MS in particular, is that injurious processes are often considered irreversible, because neurons in the brain and spinal cord do not regenerate spontaneously in an efficient manner. The aims of current treatments are to relieve symptoms, reduce the frequency of relapses, and limit their lasting effects.[7,8] However, current conventional immunosuppressive and immunomodulating treatments in MS have only mild efficacy in terms of preventing long-term disability.[7] Therefore, it is clear that novel therapeutic approaches need to be developed to reduce tissue injury. Furthermore, when tissue injury has inevitably occurred, we need to develop ways to promote its repair. Traditional views regarded the CNS as a tissue that is not amenable to repair. This concept has gradually changed in reaction to the countless observations of mammalian and human CNS plasticity. Moreover, the emergence of stem cell biology has brought new insights into neural development and regeneration. This has raised hopes for therapeutic applications in regenerative medicine, either by transplanting cells to the CNS or by enhancing endogenous processes of repair. This chapter reviews current trends in neuroprotective and regenerative approaches to MS.

The Immunologic Basis of Central Nervous System Injury in Multiple Sclerosis and Its Relevance to Repair

MS etiology is multifactorial, including interplay between environmental factors and susceptibility genes. These factors trigger a cascade of events, involving engagement of the immune system, acute inflammatory injury to axons and glia, and demyelination.[9-13] In active MS lesions, there are activated microglia and macrophages containing myelin debris and reactive astrocytes. There is also infiltration of T cells and, to a lesser extent, B cells and plasma cells. This inflammatory process is associated with demyelinated axons and axonal destruction to varying degrees. CD4-positive T-cell responses against myelin basic protein (MBP), myelin oligodendrocyte protein (MOG), myelin-associated protein (MAG), and proteolipid protein (PLP) have been extensively studied in MS and its animal models.[14] These studies support a role for myelin-specific $CD4^+$ T cells in orchestrating the pathologic processes in most patients with MS. However, it is not entirely clear whether tissue injury in MS is a direct consequence of inflammation. In gray matter, for example, the inflammatory component is much less prominent, and the "degenerative" elements of demyelination and axonal loss are more pronounced. In some MS patients, there seems to be a primary degenerative disease with secondary-reactive inflammatory responses. This possibility is supported by observations from other diseases, and from traumatic and ischemic injuries, as well as amyotrophic lateral sclerosis (ALS), in which T-cell infiltrations may be found in the spinal cord.

The heterogeneity of MS in terms of variable disease course and response to therapy has long raised the notion of heterogeneity in the disease pathogenesis. More insight into this important issue was gained with the recent description of four pathologic patterns of white matter disease in MS.[6] T cells were present in all patterns, but demyelination seemed to be induced by macrophages in pattern I and by antibodies and complement in pattern II. In patterns III and IV, the demyelinating process displayed elements of a virus- or toxin-induced disease, rather than immune-mediated cytotoxicity. A therapeutic trial of plasma exchange, which is a rational therapy for antibody-mediated autoimmune diseases, was beneficial for all patients with pattern II but for none of the patients with other patterns.[15]

Clearly, the pathogenic processes that underlie tissue injury in MS are highly relevant to the design of any neuroprotective or regenerative approach. In cases of autoimmune-mediated demyelination and axonal loss, the immune system is a legitimate therapeutic target for neuroprotection. In cases where acute axonal injury is a major component of the pathology, enforcement of remyelination per se will not provide a sufficiently regenerative approach. Moreover, accumulating data has highlighted the important role of tissue support for the remyelinating response. Some pathologic specimens exhibited progressive loss of oligodendrocytes and myelin without reactive remyelination, whereas others exhibited strong T-cell and macrophage activity with robust remyelination.[16] Evidently, regeneration requires not only regenerative cells but also a permissive environment.

Animal Models of Myelin Diseases

There are various experimental models of genetic dysmyelinating diseases and of acquired demyelination in adult animals. The most commonly used experimental models of genetic deficiency in myelin include (1) the myelin-deficient (*md*) rat, which carries a point mutation in the gene encoding PLP that causes failure of myelination in the developing postnatal brain[17]; (2) the shaking (*sh*) pups,[18] a canine model of PLP gene deficiency, representing the human X-linked Pelizaeus-Merzbacher disease; and (3) the shiverer (*shi*) mouse, which lacks a functional MBP gene.[19] Experimental demyelination has been induced in the CNS of adult animals by a variety of means, including physical injury, toxins, and immune-mediated and viral-induced approaches. Injection of myelinotoxic chemicals, such as lysolecithin or ethidium bromide,[20-22] or of anti-galactocerebroside antibodies combined with complement[23] into normal animals causes a focal, persistent, demyelinating lesion in the white matter of the CNS. Demyelination occurs after injection, and all subsequent events are associated with the regenerative response, providing a useful means of separating demyelination from remyelination. To prevent host remyelination, focal X-irradiation of the lesion is performed to kill endogenous cells capable of reforming myelin. Therefore, remyelination after transplantation of myelin-forming cells into focally demyelinated, X-irradiated lesions is entirely by grafted cells, providing a useful model for the study of cell therapy. Widespread, disseminated demyelination has been achieved by providing cuprizone in the food or in drinking water.[24]

These models have proved very valuable in studies of remyelination by endogenous myelin-forming cells or by transplanted cells. However, they lack the inflammatory component that is central to the pathogenesis of MS. Clearly, for application in MS, neuroprotective or regenerative approaches should be studied in experimental models of demyelination that are mediated immunologically. Demyelination can also be induced by viral infection. Strains of Theiler's virus, a picornavirus, induce a biphasic disease in susceptible strains of mice: an early acute disease resembling encephalomyelitis is followed by late, chronic multifocal demyelinating disease.[25-27] The A-59[28] and JHM[29] strains of mouse hepatitis viruses also produce multifocal demyelination in mice.

The animal model that is considered to best represent human MS is experimental autoimmune encephalomyelitis (EAE). EAE is a T cell–mediated disease of the CNS that shares many clinical and pathologic features with MS and has proved to be especially useful in studies of the pathogenesis and treatment of MS.[30-32] The human relevance of EAE is also suggested by its spontaneous development in transgenic mice expressing human T-cell receptors specific for MBP, human leukocyte antigen (HLA)-DR molecules, and human CD4.[33] EAE can be induced in rodents by sensitizing the animals to myelin antigens, either actively by direct antigen exposure or passively by the adoptive transfer of myelin-specific T cells. This results in a Th1 cell response that orchestrates an attack on CNS myelin, causing demyelination and axonal damage.[34,35] Acute EAE is a transient, monophasic, paralytic disease from which most animals spontaneously recover. It is characterized pathologically by disseminated inflammatory foci throughout the CNS, with a minor component of demyelination.[36] Neurologic symptoms are believed to be the result of the inflammation and of reversible conduction blocks caused by edema. In most chronic EAE models, there is a persistent paralytic disease, characterized pathologically by inflammation, demyelination, and axonal damage.[27,37-39] These animals often do not recover, and they remain with permanent neurologic defects.

Several studies have indicated that the autoimmune inflammatory process is a direct cause of tissue injury and that axonal pathology is the best correlate of chronic neurologic impairment in EAE and MS.[40-46] Myelin regeneration can be achieved in patients and in EAE animals presenting with demyelinated lesions that are characterized by a small amount of axonal loss. If the neurologic disability is caused by large-scale axonal loss, the regenerative task of axonal growth and reconnection is different and significantly more complex. These points highlight the importance of choosing the most appropriate experimental model when studying neuroprotective or regenerative properties of novel therapies. Similarly important is the need to select the best candidate patients for regenerative treatments, in terms of the specific type of this heterogenous disease and the timing of therapy.

Does Immunomodulation Protect the Multiple Sclerosis Brain from Injury?

In patients with MS in whom long-lasting demyelination and axonal loss are the end results of the autoimmune process, effective immunomodulation and immunosuppression should slow down progression of the disease. This concept has been demonstrated in the EAE model, in which countless studies have shown that suppression of EAE protects animals from CNS tissue injury and from permanent neurologic disability. The mainstays of current immunomodulatory therapy, interferon (IFN)-beta and glatiramer acetate, have been approved for reducing relapse frequency.[7,8] However, more recent long-term follow-up studies have indicated that these therapies are also partially effective in delaying disability.[47] These studies, detailing up to 16 years of follow-up, showed that various forms of IFN-beta delayed or reduced the proportion of patients who advanced to a score of 6 or higher on the Enhanced Disability Status Scale (EDSS) or another clinical end point indicating sustained disability. The treatment also postponed conversion to secondary progressive MS.[48,49] Moreover, these results suggested that early treatment may be advantageous, because the cohort of patients initially assigned to placebo consistently lagged behind the treatment group, even if therapy was started after completion of the study period.

The neuroprotective effect of immunologic therapies provides the basic rationale for the use of immunosuppressive agents in MS. The most commonly used immunosuppressive agents in MS are azathioprine, cyclophosphamide, methotrexate, and mitoxantrone, which are usually used in patients who do not respond well to immunomodulatory medications. With the exception of mitoxantrone, which has been proven to slow disease progression,[50,51] the neuroprotective effect of immunosuppressive agents has not been subjected to double-blind, controlled studies. Accumulating data suggest that cyclophosphamide[52] and azathioprine[53] can provide neuroprotection, but immunologic therapies have a very modest protective effect in MS at best. Treatment may be limited by drug toxicity, leaving patients with insufficient immunomodulatory/suppressive properties. Alternatively, there may be degenerative processes that are independent of the immune pathogenesis of disease.

This issue has been partially addressed by trials of extreme immunosuppression. Complete ablation of the immune system, followed by autologous stem cell transplantation, was shown to be very effective in ameliorating EAE.[54] This procedure allows for a much more intensive chemotherapeutic regimen than in conventional immunosuppression. Accumulating data on intensive immunosuppressive chemotherapy with hematopoietic stem cell transplantation in MS patients show that, in some but not all patients, the disease ceased to progress.[55] In addition, immunosuppressive therapy failed to control the disease in its primary progressive form and in the late-degenerative phase. Therefore, although further studies are necessary to determine the extent to which immunomodulation can protect the brain from injury, it seems that other protective approaches should be implemented.

Novel Approaches for Neuroprotection in Multiple Sclerosis

The neurodegenerative process, whether directly induced by the inflammatory component of disease or by an autonomous process, is emerging as an important therapeutic target of its own. Several neurochemical systems or receptor-mediated signals have been implicated in this degenerative process (Fig. 21-1).

Recent work has highlighted the role of excess permeability of ion channels in axonal degeneration. Sodium (Na^+) channels may contribute to axonal degeneration, leading to permanent neurologic deficits. According to the proposed mechanism, the accumulation of Na^+ in the intra-axonal compartment induces reverse action of the sodium/calcium exchanger and, consequently, a lethal rise in intra-axonal calcium (Ca^{2+}). In the context of inflammatory induced neurodegeneration, Na^+ channels were shown to mediate nitric oxide (NO)-induced toxicity to electrically active axons. It was proposed that inhibition of mitochondrial

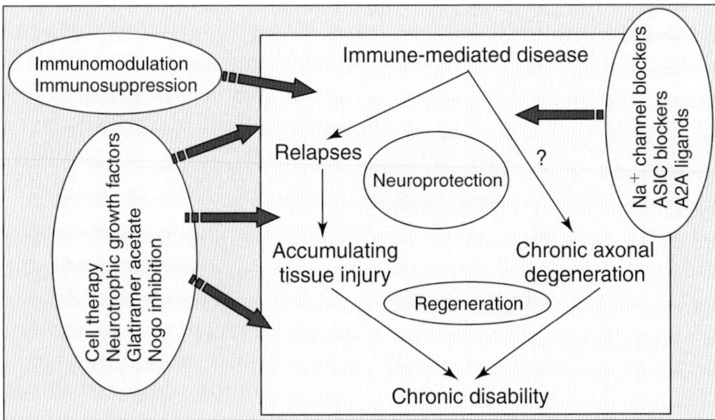

Figure 21–1 Potential therapeutic interventions and targets in multiple sclerosis. Chronic disability is the result of accumulating immune attacks and chronic neurodegeneration. Early interventions are mainly intended for neuroprotection, whereas later on there is need for regenerative processes. Some emerging therapies seem to target multiple mechanisms of injury, by ameliorating the autoimmune pathogenesis, protecting the tissue from injury, and improving endogenous repair mechanisms. A2A, adenosine receptors; ASIC, acid-sensing ion channels.

respiration by NO causes intra-axonal accumulation of Na^+ and Ca^{2+} ions. Axons could be protected from NO-mediated damage by low concentrations of Na^+ channel blockers.[56] Several different Na^+ channel blocking agents are effective in protecting axons from degeneration and improving the long-term neurologic function of the animals in chronic EAE models. These agents include flecainide,[57] lamotrigine,[58] and phenytoin.[59] The therapeutic target of Na^+ channel blockers may also include the injurious inflammatory process. One study demonstrated a marked increase in the expression of the voltage-gated sodium channel (Nav1.6) in activated microglia, which was associated with activation of phagocytic activity because tetrodotoxin reduced microglial phagocytic function. Moreover, phenytoin treatment ameliorated brain inflammatory infiltration in EAE, suggesting an anti-inflammatory effect in addition to its axonal protective effect.[60] Sodium channel blocking agents are currently being investigated in clinical trials with chronic MS patients.

The spectrum of ion channel–mediated neurodegeneration was recently extended by observations regarding the key role of acid-sensing ion channels (ASIC) in this process. It has long been appreciated that an acidic environment promotes neuronal cell death in ischemic conditions. The mechanism of this phenomenon was recently clarified by the demonstration that low extracellular pH activates inward ASIC currents. ASIC in neurons are permeable to Ca^{2+}, and their uncontrolled activation leads to toxic Ca^{2+} accumulation in the neurons, independent of glutamate receptor activation.[61] In models of brain ischemia, blockers of ASIC1 reduced neuronal injury and resulted in a prolonged therapeutic time window, compared with glutamate receptor antagonists.[61,62]

The specific role of ASIC1 in mediating axonal degeneration was recently examined in EAE as well. ASIC–/– mice exhibited significantly reduced axonal degeneration and markedly decreased clinical severity of EAE despite CNS inflammation comparable to that of control EAE mice. Likewise, administration of amiloride, which is a well-known blocker of ASIC1, had a protective effect against neurodegeneration in EAE in wild-type animals. This study supports the hypothesis that ASIC1 contributes to axonal degeneration in inflammatory lesions of the CNS and that ASIC1 blockers can provide neuroprotection in MS.[63]

Another neurochemical/receptor system that has been implicated in CNS injury is that of adenosine signaling, particularly through A2A adenosine receptors. Adenosinergic activity through activation of A2A receptors can modulate cellular processes that lead to cell death or survival. A2A receptor ligands have therefore been suggested as potential neuroprotective agents.[64]

Cannabinoid receptor agonists have immunomodulatory properties that downregulate myelin-specific T-cell responses, reduce inflammatory infiltrations in EAE, and attenuate the clinical severity of the experimental disease. These effects were mediated mainly by the cannabinoid receptor 1. In addition to the immunosuppressive effect that protected the CNS from immune-mediated injury, low doses of cannabinoids that were non-immunosuppressive exhibited a protective effect that attenuated axonal loss, suggesting a direct neuroprotective effect.[65]

Recombinant human erythropoietin is an emerging neurokine with versatile neuroprotective and neurotrophic effects. When administered intravenously in mice with MOG-induced EAE, it reduced axonal damage and demyelination and reduced the clinical severity of disease. This neuroprotective effect was associated with inhibition of inflammatory cell infiltration and microglial activation.[66] Recently, an open-label study (phase I/IIa) with recombinant human erythropoietin (rhEPO) in chronic progressive MS showed improvement in motor function and in cognitive performance, with a reduction in EDSS scores.[67]

Much work has been done in recent years on trophic and protective effects of glatiramer acetate in the CNS, in addition to its modulatory activity on immunologic responses toward myelin. In a MOG-EAE model, glatiramer acetate exhibited protective effects on retinal ganglion cells, preventing their death from the disease process of optic neuritis. This neuroprotective effect of glatiramer acetate was partially independent from its immunomodulatory effect.[68] Glatiramer acetate augmented and prolonged neurogenesis in EAE brains, as well as enhanced the migration and differentiation of newly generated precursor cells. This effect suggests that glatiramer acetate may enhance endogenous repair processes in the CNS in inflammatory diseases.[69] An additional mechanism by which glatiramer acetate might exert its effect is by enhancing "protective autoimmunity." It has been suggested that autoimmune T cells are not only the generators of the disease process but also are responsible for neuroprotection. The destructive versus beneficial sequelae of self-reactive T-cell actions are supposedly determined by the timing and force of their activity. In several immune-mediated models of disease, it was shown that glatiramer acetate may enhance protective autoimmunity without increasing the destructive arm of autoimmunity, possibly by its mild agonistic effect on such self-reactive T cells.[70] The immunomodulatory and neuroprotective effects of glatiramer acetate, as well as its effect on enhancing neurogenesis, might involve secretion of the brain-derived neurotrophic factor (BDNF) by T cells.[71,72] Indeed, BDNF has been found to enhance endogenous neurogenesis.[73-75]

In conclusion, the molecular mechanisms underlying neurodegeneration in MS are only beginning to unravel. This field still needs a unifying approach that will tie the various factors that have been described to play a role in this process, and will dictate the rationale for (combined) neuroprotective therapy.

Enhancing Repair Processes in Multiple Sclerosis

Experimental models of focal demyelination have an inherent advantage for studying the process of myelin repair, in that the demyelinating insult and consequent repair process are temporally separate. It has been shown in such models that endogenous cells in the adult rodent CNS have the potential for regenerating oligodendrocytes and myelin.[76,77] X-irradiation to kill proliferating cells in chemically induced demyelinated lesions prevents any spontaneous remyelination, suggesting that cell division is an absolute prerequisite for myelin regeneration.[78,79] Although differentiated oligodendrocytes may survive within such lesions, they are unable to rebuild myelin sheaths.[78,80,81] Unlike mature astrocytes that maintain the potential to react to injury and divide, fully differentiated oligodendrocytes are probably unable to revert into a proliferating state. Therefore, remyelination depends mainly on proliferating oligodendrocyte progenitor cells, which are identified by expression of neuron-glial antigen 2 (NG2) or platelet-derived growth factor receptor-α (PDGFRα) on their cell surface and are probably the major cycling cell population that reacts to demyelination.[76,77,82-86] The adult subventricular zone also contains multipotential neural precursor cells that express the embryonic polysialilated form of the neural cell adhesion molecule (PSA-NCAM). These precursors react to inflammation and demyelination by proliferation and differentiation, generating astrocytes and remyelinating oligodendrocytes.[76,87,88]

Bidirectional trophic interactions between oligodendrocytes and axons are necessary for their long-term survival. Compact myelin is vital for axonal endurance. For example, in PLP-deficient mice[89] and in cyclic nucleotide phosphodiesterase–deficient mice,[90] there is progressive axonal degeneration. Indeed, the chronic and supposedly irreversible neurologic disability in MS patients correlates best with the degree of axonal loss in the CNS.[42,44-46,91] Moreover, there is evidence that extensive axonal transection occurs in acute MS lesions.[13] In that sense, the importance of remyelination is not just to secure rapid saltatory conduction but also to protect axons from degeneration. Therefore, achieving early remyelination before the development of axonal damage is crucial to any therapeutic strategy. Attempts to regenerate myelin can be recognized pathologically in the brains of MS patients by the existence of shadow plaques, which are partially remyelinated lesions.[92-96] The importance of myelin sheaths for axon integrity in MS is indicated by the finding that areas of remyelination in MS brain are characterized by relative sparing of axons, compared with areas of demyelination.[9] Moreover, remyelination leading to structural repair is associated with recovery of function.[92-96]

However, much to our frustration, regenerative responses in MS are inadequate and eventually fail.[97,98] Failure of remyelination could stem either from insufficiency of endogenous remyelinating cells or from lack of environmental support for this process. In the adult rodent CNS, only progenitor cells that reside in proximity to the lesion margins migrate into the lesion core and remyelinate it; long-distance migration of progenitor cells does not occur.[76,99] In addition, only a subpopulation of local progenitor cells reacts to injury and generates new oligodendrocytes and myelin.[84] The limited recruitment of oligodendrocyte progenitors in the adult CNS may be related to their apparent dormant state. They have a considerably slower cell cycle than progenitor cells of the developing brain, and they require prolonged exposure to multiple growth factors before converting into rapidly proliferating cells.[100] It has long been appreciated that one of the roles of the inflammatory response is to set in motion endogenous repair processes. Accordingly, CNS remyelination is thought to be closely linked to the acute inflammatory phase of the disease,[101] whereas in the chronic stage regeneration does not occur.[102] The narrow time window defined by this association may underlie the limited recruitment of dormant progenitor cells, which are able to convert into remyelinating cells. Thus, although progenitor cells were demonstrable in acute and chronic MS lesions, they did not exhibit a reactive increase in cell number when compared with normal white matter.[103-105] Moreover, although progenitor cells decreased in number after experimental focal demyelination,[84,106] this was not observed in pathologic specimens of chronic MS lesions,[93,103,104] indicating again the lack of progenitor cell recruitment.

How can we augment the remyelinating process in the MS brain (see Fig. 21-1)? One option is to increase the number of cycling cells. PDGF,[107] glial growth factor 2,[108] and neurotrophin 3[109] act as mitogens for human and rodent oligodendrocyte progenitors. Sonic hedgehog signaling was found to maintain the stem cell niche and progenitor cells derived from there in the adult subventricular zone; stimulation of this pathway increased the production of progenitor cells.[110,111] Another option is to enhance oligodendrocyte differentiation, maturation, and survival. Various factors, including insulin growth factor-1,[112] lymphocyte inhibitory factor, and ciliary neurotrophic factor,[113,114] have been reported to enhance oligodendrocyte survival and myelination. However, their effects were related, in part, to modulation of the immune attack on the CNS.[112,113,115-119]

Gaining a deeper insight into the biology of remyelinating cells will further broaden our understanding of how to better recruit regenerating cells. For example, the expression of Olig1, a basic helix-loop-helix transcription factor in oligodendrocyte progenitors, was found to be essential for remyelination.[120] Also, selective overexpression of epidermal growth factor receptor in 2′,3′-cyclic nucleotide 3′-phosphodiesterase (CNP)-positive oligodendrocytes enhanced oligodendrocyte generation and remyelination.[121] These examples may represent valid therapeutic targets to increase the number and function of remyelinating cells in the CNS.

The demonstration of different pathologic patterns of demyelination in MS[6] has highlighted the fact that there are different patterns of remyelination. In some patients, there was progressive loss of oligodendrocytes and myelin without reactive remyelination; in others, who exhibited strong T-cell and macrophage activity, there was robust remyelination. These observations indicate the important role of tissue support in the remyelinating response[16] and the fact that a regenerative therapeutic approach will also require a permissive environment for remyelination. Moreover, in some MS brains there is a lack of response despite the presence of oligodendrocyte progenitors, leaving a sharp border of demyelination[103,104,122]. This suggests active inhibition of the remyelinating process. Re-expression of Notch1, a regulator of oligodendrocyte progenitor differentiation, has been suggested to inhibit remyelination in MS.[123] However, targeted ablation of Notch1 did not enhance remyelination in experimental animals.[124] Therapeutic targets to increase tissue permissiveness for repair processes may include the following:

1. *Integrins:* Integrins mediate growth factor induced oligodendrocyte differentiation and survival.[125,126]
2. *Activation of matrix metalloproteinases (MMPs):* These tissue enzymes remodel the extracellular matrix to facilitate cell migration and neurite growth. The remyelinating process is partially dependent on MMP-9 and MMP-12.[127,128] Caution is required, because a high concentration of MMPs in the brain results in tissue damage.[129,130]
3. *Inhibition of Nogo activity:* Nogo-A is a protein, expressed mainly on oligodendrocyte cell bodies and myelin sheaths, that causes collapse of axonal growth cones, thus inhibiting axonal regeneration.[131] It interacts with a receptor complex consisting of the Nogo receptor, the neurotrophin receptor $p75^{NTR}$, and another transmembrane protein termed LINGO-1.[132,133] Inhibition of Nogo activity by either anti-Nogo antibodies or T cells reactive to Nogo ameliorated both chronic EAE in C57BL/6 mice and relapsing EAE in SJL/J mice.[134,135] Interestingly, the beneficial effect was mediated in part by modulation of the autoimmune process. However, active immunization against Nogo is probably not a practical approach, because Nogo peptides can act also as encephalitogens in certain conditions.[136] Targeting of Nogo-induced signal transduction may be preferable. Indeed, it has been shown that LINGO-1 is an important negative regulator of myelination by oligodendrocytes,[137] and a LINGO-1 antagonist enhanced remyelination and axonal integrity and subsequent functional recovery in EAE.[138]
4. *Polysialic acid mimetic peptides:* These have been found to promote cell migration.[139]

5. *Immunoglobulins:* Immunoglobulins enhance viral-induced remyelination by an unknown mechanism,[140] although they have not shown any beneficial effect in clinical trials in MS.[141,142]

In conclusion, both environmental factors and basic properties of endogenous adult progenitor cells limit the degree of spontaneous remyelination. The apparent link between the acute inflammatory phase and myelin regeneration, and the necessity to remyelinate before axonal damage occurs, may define a narrow time window during which remyelination is feasible. In view of the great complexity of repair processes, it seems logical that enhancing and extending this window of opportunity will not be achieved by targeting one single factor or signaling pathway. A more rationale approach would be to search for nonredundant mediators of remyelination.[143]

Is Stem Cell Therapy a Rational Approach for Multiple Sclerosis?

Early studies have shown that a variety of cells are capable of remyelinating the CNS after transplantation. Transplanted myelin-forming cells remyelinated focal lesions in the optic nerve and spinal cord of experimental animals and restored normal conduction properties, indicating fully functional regenerated myelin.[144,145] Transplanted mammalian and human cells performed extensive myelination in genetic dysmyelinating models of disease.[145-152] MS, however, poses additional challenges for the cell therapy approach

MIGRATION OF TRANSPLANTED CELLS IN THE BRAIN

Because MS is a multifocal disease, the regenerative potential of transplanted cells depends on their ability to reach demyelinated lesions. Experimental models have shown that migration of endogenous remyelinating cells is limited, and therefore spontaneous remyelination in the lesioned CNS is a local event.[76,153] In the developing CNS, transplanted neural precursor cells migrate according to the developmental cues at that stage and integrate to adopt cellular identity according to local and temporal cues.[154-156] In contrast, the normal adult brain does not permit large-distance migration and does not support transplanted neural cell survival.[157]

Recent observations, however, have shown an association between the inflammatory process in the brain and induction of migration of endogenous and transplanted neural precursor cells. In EAE, brain inflammation attracted subventricular zone precursors expressing embryonic NCAM (PSA-NCAM),[88] as well as multipotential neural precursors that were introduced into the ventricles. Histopathologic sudies[158-160] and noninvasive high-resolution magnetic resonance imaging studies on magnetically labeled rodent and human cells[161,162] showed that the transplanted cells migrated along inflamed white matter tracts in response to induction of inflammation. These experiments highlight the dual, contrasting action of brain inflammation, which simultaneously inflicts brain injury and recruits components of the regenerative process. The combination of cell transplantation and immunomodulation for MS will therefore need to be developed as nonreciprocally antagonistic modes of treatment. To this end, it is important to analyze the pro-regenerative components involved in the inflammatory process and to target the immunomodulatory treatment without inhibiting regenerative processes.

Recent work has highlighted the role of chemokines in the migration of neural precursors in the developing brain. The chemokine stromal-derived factor 1 (SDF1) and its receptor CXCR4 were found to be important regulators of the migration of dentate granule cells,[163,164] sensory neurons,[165] and cortical interneurons[166] during development. Because CNS regeneration seems to be a recapitulation of developmental processes, this finding prompted studies on the role of chemokines in attracting neural precursor cells after injury. Both SDF1/CXCR4 and monocyte chemoattractant protein 1 (MCP-1) and its receptor CCR2 were shown to modulate neural precursor cell migration after cerebral ischemia.[167,168] Furthermore, neural precursors deficient in MCP-1 or CCR2 failed to migrate toward focal inflammatory sites.[169] The specific roles of these and other chemokines in attracting neural precursor cell migration in EAE and MS are still unknown.

ROUTE OF CELL DELIVERY

Because MS is a multifocal disease and in view of the limited capacity for cell migration, it is necessary to identify the optimal route of cell delivery that will promote efficient targeted migration of transplanted cells to multiple lesions for repair. Most white matter tracts that are involved in MS are in close proximity to ventricular and spinal subarachnoid spaces, so intraventricular and intrathecal transplantation may serve as an efficient route for delivery of remyelinating cells. After intracerebroventricular (ICV) injection, transplanted cells may disseminate throughout the neuroaxis without a separating barrier from the CNS white matter. As described earlier, the ICV route of transplantation has proved useful in obtaining widespread dissemination along inflamed white matter tracts of EAE rodents,[158,159,162,170] as well as widespread myelination in genetic dysmyelinating models of the *shi* mouse[171] and the *md* rat.[172]

An alternative route of cell delivery that has been proposed is the injection of multipotential neural precursor cells into the bloodstream intravenously.[173-175] It has been suggested that a small fraction of intravenously injected neural precursors can selectively home into the inflamed CNS. The specific homing of neural precursors to the brain is explained, in part, by the constitutive expression of a wide array of adhesion molecules (e.g., integrins, selectins) and chemokine receptors by the transplanted cells.[175-177] In particular, integrins may promote selective CNS homing through the interaction between transplanted cells and integrin receptor–expressing activated endothelial and ependymal cells surrounding inflamed brain tissues.[178,179] In EAE, such selective homing to the inflamed brain via membrane expression of CD44 and very late antigen-4 was permitted during a narrow time window. The significance of this observation is not yet clear, because in other studies neural precursors that were injected intravenously did not cross the blood–brain barrier but improved EAE symptoms via a peripheral effect.[180]

TIMING OF TRANSPLANTATION

In the developing brain, the targeted migration and lineage fate of transplanted cells are directed by the normal pattern of development occurring at the time of transplantation. Accordingly, human multipotential neural stem cells that were transplanted into embryonic rat brain during stages of neuroneogenesis generated mostly neurons,[154] but when they transplanted into the newborn brain, at a stage of gliogenesis, they generated mostly glia.[156] In contrast, the normal adult CNS does not support the survival of transplanted cells.[157] This may be due to the very small quantities of trophic factors in normal adult brain tissue that are necessary for maintaining the survival of resident cells but are insufficient for supporting the survival of transplanted cells. Because MS is a chronic, relapsing disease, transplanted cells would need to be able to survive for prolonged periods in the host CNS through phases of inflammation and remission. In view of the close link between inflammation and mobilization of regenerative cells, it is unclear whether transplanted neural precursors would be able to migrate extensively during the chronic phase of disease. Therefore, it may be best to introduce remyelinating cells early in the course of disease, in a form that will maintain their survival independent of tissue support, so that they will be ready for immediate mobilization upon tissue demand during relapses. To this end, neural precursors were introduced by ICV injection in the form of neurospheres in intact mice.[181] Such neurospheres created a trophic microenvironment sufficient to maintain the long-term survival of neural precursors without any support. Moreover, neurosphere cells retained their capacity to respond to brain inflammation by migration into inflamed white matter tracts.

MECHANISMS OF BENEFICIAL ACTION OF TRANSPLANTED CELLS

Making a rational choice regarding transplantable cells in MS depends on gaining insights as to the mechanisms by which they improve the clinical outcome of disease. This has been made possible by the observations that neural precursor cell transplantation ameliorates the clinical severity of acute[170] and chronic EAE.[159,175] Until recently, restorative neurotransplantation research focused mainly on the potential of the neural graft to replace damaged or missing cell populations. Early work demonstrated the remyelinating properties of various cell types, including oligodendrocyte progenitor cells,[151,182,183] Schwann cells,[184,185] olfactory nerve ensheathing cells,[186,187] and multipotential neural precursor and stem cells.[188-190] These properties have been extensively studied in focal demyelinated lesions and in genetic dysmyelinating animal models. However, to date, it has not been shown whether any of these cells are capable of remyelinating axons in EAE, a more clinically relevant disease model, mainly because the neuropathology in the most commonly used animal models, such as MOG peptide (residues 35-55)–induced EAE in C57BL/6 mice, does not permit remyelination. In this model, the acute phase manifests with extensive axonal injury, and there are very few naked axons that are amenable for remyelination.

Recent studies suggested that transplanted stem cells may also function by additional mechanisms. In Lewis rats with spinal cord homogenate–induced EAE, there is an acute, reversible paralytic disease that is the result of disseminated CNS inflammation without demyelination or axonal injury. The first indication of an anti-inflammatory effect of neural precursor cells was obtained when these cells were transplanted intraventricularly in acute EAE rats.[170] Cell transplantation attenuated the inflammatory brain process and clinical severity of disease. Follow-up studies examined the effect of neural precursor cell transplantation in MOG35-55 peptide–induced EAE in C57BL/6 mice. In this model, there is an acute paralytic disease caused by a T cell–mediated autoimmune process that results in severe axonal injury and demyelination. Subsequently, the mice remain with fixed neurologic sequela, the severity of which is correlated with the extent of axonal loss.[46] In MOG35-55 EAE, neural precursor cell transplantation attenuated the inflammatory process, reduced acute axonal injury, reduced chronic axonal loss and demyelination, and improved the clinical performance of the animals.[159,191] Therefore, the anti-inflammatory effect of neural precursor cells protected the CNS from immune-mediated tissue injury.

The exact mechanisms by which transplanted neural precursors attenuate brain inflammation are not yet clear. One school of thought suggests an immunomodulatory effect, by which neural precursors induce apoptosis of Th1 cells selectively.[191] This may cause a shift in the CNS inflammatory process toward a more favorable Th2-dominant environment. Alternatively, it has been suggested that neural precursors may inhibit T-cell activation and proliferation by a nonspecific, bystander immunosuppressive effect.[180] This notion emerged from coculture experiments that showed a striking inhibition of both EAE-derived and naïve T-cell activation and proliferation by neural precursors, after stimulation by various stimulants.[170,180] The suppressive effect of neural precursors on T cells was accompanied by a significant suppression of pro-inflammatory cytokines. The relevance of this neural precursor–T-cell interaction was demonstrated as intravenously administered neural precursor cells were transiently found in peripheral lymphoid organs, where they interacted with T cells to reduce their encephalitogenicity.[180] In this situation, the neural precursors did not cross the blood–brain barrier, and their entire effect was mediated by peripheral immunosuppression, resulting in reduced immune cell infiltration into the CNS and, consequently, milder CNS damage. Such a nonspecific, anti-inflammatory mechanism may be of major importance in the application of transplantation therapy in immune-mediated diseases, because it can protect both the host CNS and the graft from additional immune attacks. Recent studies have shown a similar beneficial immunosuppressive effect of bone marrow stromal cells (BMSCs) in attenuating EAE, adding another potential source of cells for therapy in MS.[192,193] BMSCs can be derived from the patient, expanded in vitro, and reintroduced intrathecally as an autologous graft.

Recent studies have also focused on the neuroprotective and neurotrophic properties of stem cells. Neural stem and precursor cells not only inhibit inflammation to protect the brain from deleterious consequences in models of immune-mediated disease but also may protect host neurons from degenerative processes and enhance the latent capacity of endogenous CNS progenitor cells for repair and of severed host axons for regeneration. The underlying molecular mechanisms are not fully understood but relate in part to the production of a myriad of growth factors[194] and to the modulation of the host environment into one more permissive for regeneration.

The neuroprotective effect of neural stem cells has been demonstrated in several models of neurodegeneration that have a limited inflammatory component. Transplanted neural stem cells could rescue dopaminergic neurons of the mesostriatal system in a Parkinson's disease model in rodents.[195] In models of ALS, neural stem cell transplantation has shown potential to prevent motor neurons from dying.[196-198] Transplantation of neural stem cells into mutant mice in which

Purkinje neurons die in postnatal week 4 or 5 did ameliorate the symptoms, not by replacing host Purkinje neurons but by supporting their mitochondrial function, dendritic growth, and synaptogenesis, subsequently leading to their rescue and restoration of motor coordination.[199] In a rat model of retinal degeneration, subretinal injection of human neural precursor cells provided almost full protection of visual functions.[200]

Both neuroprotective and trophic effects of neural stem cells were observed in an experimental model of spinal cord trauma. Neural stem cells seeded on a synthetic biodegradable scaffold and grafted into the hemi-sectioned adult rat spinal cord induced a significant improvement in animal movement through reduction of necrosis in the surrounding parenchyma and prevention of extensive secondary cell loss, inflammation, and formation of a glial scar.[201] Moreover, the graft induced a permissive environment for axonal regeneration. In a model of retinal degeneration, neural precursor cell transplantation promoted neurite growth in the optic nerve.[202] This effect was mediated by induction of MMPs that degrade inhibitory extracellular matrix and cell surface molecules, thus enabling axons to extend through the glial scar. Substantial endogenous reconstitution of the brain structural connectivity was found after administration of neural stem cells in biodegradable scaffolds into regions of extensive brain degeneration caused by hypoxia[203] or after intraventricular transplantation of newborn neural precursor cells in mice with ischemia/reperfusion injury.[204]

Moreover, recent work has indicated that transplanted neural precursors can enhance endogenous neurogenesis in pathologic conditions. Mice that were exposed prenatally to opioids display impaired learning, associated with reduced neurogenesis. Transplantation of neural precursors improved their learning functions. Interestingly, transplanted cells did not differentiate into neurons but enhanced host brain–derived neurogenesis in the hippocampus.[205] A similar neurotrophic effect was reported in physiologic conditions. Although neurogenesis in the dentate gyrus declines severely by middle age, transplantation of neural stem cells stimulated the endogenous neural stem cells in the subgranular zone to produce new dentate granule cells.[206] The trophic effects of stem cells may be mediated by release of neurotrophic growth factors,[159,194] promoting, for example, corticospinal axon growth in an organotypic co-culture system.[207] Therefore, transplanted neural stem and precursor cell therapy may enhance the adult CNS capacity to repair itself by restoring the ability of local neural progenitor cells to respond properly to disease states and replace damaged cells, as well as the ability of severed axons to regenerate. It is still unknown whether these trophic properties of stem cell are also relevant for EAE and MS.

In conclusion, stem cell therapy may be a rational approach for treating MS. Transplanted neural precursor cells can migrate extensively in the brain to the sites of disease; they integrate well into tissue and can potentially exert their therapeutic effects via different, interacting mechanisms, including their own myelinating qualities, their neurotrophic properties, and their immune regulatory functions. Each type of candidate cell, including neural stem/precursor cells, oligodendrocyte progenitors, olfactory ensheathing cells, and BMSCs, may have specific advantages and disadvantages (Table 21-1) and need to be directly evaluated and compared.

TABLE 21–1 Comparison of Candidate Cell Populations for Transplantation in Multiple Sclerosis

Cell Type	Source	Expansion	Autologous Graft	Myelinating Capability	Immuno-modulatory Properties	Trophic Properties
hESC-derived NPCs	IVF or other derived early embryos	Unlimited	No (except for partheno-genetic or iPS lines)	Yes	Yes	Unknown
Adult NSCs	Fetal brain	Good	No	Yes	Yes	Yes
OPCs	Fetal brain	Limited	No	Yes	Unknown	Unknown
OECs	Nasal mucosa	Limited	Yes	Yes	Unknown	Yes
Schwann cells	Peripheral nerve	Limited	Yes	Yes	Unknown	Unknown
BMSCs	Bone marrow	Good	Yes	No	Yes	Yes

BMSCs, bone marrow stromal cells; hESC, human embryonic stem cell; IVF, in vitro fertilization; iPS, inducible pluripotent stem cells; NPCs, neural precursor cells; NSCs, neural stem cells; OECs, olfactory ensheathing cells; OPCs, oligodendrocyte progenitor cells.

Conclusions

Gaining deeper insights into the immune-mediated and degenerative mechanisms of tissue injury in MS, as well as the regenerative process and its failure, is crucial for developing new treatments. Both cell therapy and targeting of endogenous repair mechanisms may be used to promote neuroprotection and repair in MS. These two therapeutic approaches are closely related, and progress in these areas is interlinked.

REFERENCES

1. Compston A, Coles A: Multiple sclerosis. Lancet 2002;359:1221-1231.
2. Dyment DA, Ebers GC: An array of sunshine in multiple sclerosis. N Engl J Med 2002;347:1445-1447.
3. Noseworthy JH, Lucchinetti C, Rodriguez M, Weinshenker BG: Multiple sclerosis. N Engl J Med 2000;343:938-952.
4. Wingerchuk DM, Lucchinetti CF, Noseworthy JH: Multiple sclerosis: Current pathophysiological concepts. Lab Invest 2001;81:263-281.
5. Lassmann H, Bruck W, Lucchinetti C: Heterogeneity of multiple sclerosis pathogenesis: Implications for diagnosis and therapy. Trends Mol Med 2000;7:115-121.
6. Lucchinetti C, Bruck W, Parisi J, et al: Heterogeneity of multiple sclerosis lesions: Implications for the pathogenesis of demyelination. Ann Neurol 2000;47:707-717.
7. Rudick RA, Cohen JA, Weinstock-Guttman B, et al: Management of multiple sclerosis. N Engl J Med 1997;337:1604-1611.
8. Tullman MJ, Lublin FD, Miller AE: Immunotherapy of multiple sclerosis: Current practice and future directions. J Rehabil Res Dev 2002;39:273-285.

9. Kornek B, Storch MK, Weissert R, et al: Multiple sclerosis and chronic autoimmune encephalomyelitis: A comparative quantitative study of axonal injury in active, inactive, and remyelinated lesions. Am J Pathol 2000;157:267-276.
10. Lassmann H: Neuropathology in multiple sclerosis: New concepts. Mult Scler 1998;4:93-98.
11. Lassmann H: Mechanisms of demyelination and tissue destruction in multiple sclerosis. Clin Neurol Neurosurg 2002;104:168-171.
12. Trapp BD, Bo L, Mork S, Chang A: Pathogenesis of tissue injury in MS lesions. J Neuroimmunol 1999;98:49-56.
13. Trapp BD, Peterson J, Ransohoff RM, et al: Axonal transection in the lesions of multiple sclerosis. N Engl J Med 1998;338:278-285.
14. Gold R, Linington C, Lassmann H: Understanding pathogenesis and therapy of multiple sclerosis via animal models: 70 Years of merits and culprits in experimental autoimmune encephalomyelitis research. Brain 2006;129:1953-1971.
15. Keegan M, Konig F, McClelland R, et al: Relation between humoral pathological changes in multiple sclerosis and response to therapeutic plasma exchange. Lancet 2005;366:579-582.
16. Lucchinetti C, Bruck W, Parisi J, et al: A quantitative analysis of oligodendrocytes in multiple sclerosis lesions: A study of 113 cases. Brain 1999;122:2279-2295.
17. Gordon MN, Kumar S, Espinosa de los Monteros A, et al: Developmental regulation of myelin-associated genes in the normal and the myelin deficient mutant rat. Adv Exp Med Biol 1990;265:11-22.
18. Griffiths IR, Duncan ID, McCulloch M: Shaking pups: A disorder of central myelination in the spaniel dog. II: Ultrastructural observations on the white matter of the cervical spinal cord. J Neurocytol 1981;10:847-858.
19. Readhead C, Hood L: The dysmyelinating mouse mutations shiverer (shi) and myelin deficient (shimld). Behav Genet 1990;20:213-234.
20. Blakemore WF: Ethidium bromide induced demyelination in the spinal cord of the cat. Neuropathol Appl Neurobiol 1982;8:365-375.
21. Ludwin SK: Central nervous system demyelination and remyelination in the mouse: An ultrastructural study of cuprizone toxicity. Lab Invest 1978;39:597-612.
22. Waxman SG, Kocsis JD, Nitta KC: Lysophosphatidyl choline-induced focal demyelination in the rabbit corpus callosum: Light-microscopic observations. J Neurol Sci 1979;44:45-53.
23. Carroll WM, Jennings AR, Mastaglia FL: Experimental demyelinating optic neuropathy induced by intra-neural injection of galactocerebroside antiserum. J Neurol Sci 1984;65:125-135.
24. Blakemore WF: Remyelination of the superior cerebellar peduncle in old mice following demyelination induced by cuprizone. J Neurol Sci 1974;22:121-126.
25. Oleszak EL, Chang JR, Friedman H, et al: Theiler's virus infection: A model for multiple sclerosis. Clin Microbiol Rev 2004;17:174-207.
26. Pirko I, Gamez J, Johnson AJ, et al: Dynamics of MRI lesion development in an animal model of viral-induced acute progressive CNS demyelination. Neuroimage 2004;21:576-582.
27. Tsunoda I, Iwasaki Y, Terunuma H, et al: A comparative study of acute and chronic diseases induced by two subgroups of Theiler's murine encephalomyelitis virus. Acta Neuropathol 1996;91:595-602.
28. Woyciechowska JL, Trapp BD, Patrick DH, et al: Acute and subacute demyelination induced by mouse hepatitis virus strain A59 in C3H mice. J Exp Pathol 1984;1:295-306.
29. Sorensen O, Perry D, Dales S: In vivo and in vitro models of demyelinating diseases: III. JHM virus infection of rats. Arch Neurol 1980;37:478-484.
30. Gold R, Hartung HP, Toyka KV: Animal models for autoimmune demyelinating disorders of the nervous system. Mol Med Today 2000;6:88-91.
31. Lassmann H: Chronic relapsing experimental allergic encephalomyelitis: Its value as an experimental model for multiple sclerosis. J Neurol 1983;229:207-220.
32. Swanborg RH: Experimental autoimmune encephalomyelitis in rodents as a model for human demyelinating disease. Clin Immunol Immunopathol 1995;77:4-13.
33. Ellmerich S, Takacs K, Mycko M, et al: Disease-related epitope spread in a humanized T cell receptor transgenic model of multiple sclerosis. Eur J Immunol 2004;34:1839-1848.
34. Izikson L, Klein RS, Luster AD, Weiner HL: Targeting monocyte recruitment in CNS autoimmune disease. Clin Immunol 2002;103:125-131.
35. Kuchroo VK, Anderson AC, Waldner H, et al: T cell response in experimental autoimmune encephalomyelitis (EAE): Role of self and cross-reactive antigens in shaping, tuning, and regulating the autopathogenic T cell repertoire. Annu Rev Immunol 2002;20:101-123.
36. Karussis DM, Lehmann D, Slavin S, et al: Inhibition of acute, experimental autoimmune encephalomyelitis by the synthetic immunomodulator linomide. Ann Neurol 1993;34:654-660.

37. Mendel I, Kerlero de Rosbo N, Ben-Nun A: A myelin oligodendrocyte glycoprotein peptide induces typical chronic experimental autoimmune encephalomyelitis in H-2b mice: Fine specificity and T cell receptor V beta expression of encephalitogenic T cells. Eur J Immunol 1995;25:1951-1959.
38. Oliver AR, Lyon GM, Ruddle NH: Rat and human myelin oligodendrocyte glycoproteins induce experimental autoimmune encephalomyelitis by different mechanisms in C57BL/6 mice. J Immunol 2003;171:462-468.
39. Slavin A, Ewing C, Liu J, et al: Induction of a multiple sclerosis-like disease in mice with an immunodominant epitope of myelin oligodendrocyte glycoprotein. Autoimmunity 1998;28:109-120.
40. Bjartmar C, Kidd G, Mork S, et al: Neurological disability correlates with spinal cord axonal loss and reduced N-acetyl aspartate in chronic multiple sclerosis patients. Ann Neurol 2000;48: 893-901.
41. Bjartmar C, Yin X, Trapp BD: Axonal pathology in myelin disorders. J Neurocytol 1999;28:383-395.
42. De Stefano N, Matthews PM, Fu L, et al: Axonal damage correlates with disability in patients with relapsing-remitting multiple sclerosis: Results of a longitudinal magnetic resonance spectroscopy study. Brain 1998;121:1469-1477.
43. Hemmer B, Archelos JJ, Hartung HP: New concepts in the immunopathogenesis of multiple sclerosis. Nat Rev Neurosci 2002;3:291-301.
44. Steinman L: Multiple sclerosis: A two-stage disease. Nat Immunol 2001;2:762-764.
45. Trapp BD, Ransohoff R, Rudick R: Axonal pathology in multiple sclerosis: Relationship to neurologic disability. Curr Opin Neurol 1999;12:295-302.
46. Wujek JR, Bjartmar C, Richer E, et al: Axon loss in the spinal cord determines permanent neurological disability in an animal model of multiple sclerosis. J Neuropathol Exp Neurol 2002;61:23-32.
47. Bermel RA, Rudick RA: Interferon-beta treatment for multiple sclerosis. Neurotherapeutics 2007;4:633-646.
48. Kappos L, Traboulsee A, Constantinescu C, et al: Long-term subcutaneous interferon beta-1a therapy in patients with relapsing-remitting MS. Neurology 2006;67:944-953.
49. Rudick RA, Cutter GR, Baier M, et al: Estimating long-term effects of disease-modifying drug therapy in multiple sclerosis patients. Mult Scler 2005;11:626-634.
50. Debouverie M, Taillandier L, Pittion-Vouyovitch S, et al: Clinical follow-up of 304 patients with multiple sclerosis three years after mitoxantrone treatment. Mult Scler 2007;13:626-631.
51. Hartung HP, Gonsette R, Konig N, et al: Mitoxantrone in progressive multiple sclerosis: A placebo-controlled, double-blind, randomised, multicentre trial. Lancet 2002;360:2018-2025.
52. Weiner HL: Immunosuppressive treatment in multiple sclerosis. J Neurol Sci 2004;223:1-11.
53. Casetta I, Iuliano G, Filippini G: Azathioprine for multiple sclerosis. Cochrane Database Syst Rev 2007. CD003982.
54. Karussis DM, Vourka-Karussis U, Lehmann D, et al: Prevention and reversal of adoptively transferred, chronic relapsing experimental autoimmune encephalomyelitis with a single high dose cytoreductive treatment followed by syngeneic bone marrow transplantation. J Clin Invest 1993;92:765-772.
55. Freedman MS: Bone marrow transplantation: Does it stop MS progression? J Neurol Sci 2007;259:85-89.
56. Kapoor R, Davies M, Blaker PA, et al: Blockers of sodium and calcium entry protect axons from nitric oxide-mediated degeneration. Ann Neurol 2003;53:174-180.
57. Bechtold DA, Kapoor R, Smith KJ: Axonal protection using flecainide in experimental autoimmune encephalomyelitis. Ann Neurol 2004;55:607-616.
58. Bechtold DA, Miller SJ, Dawson AC, et al: Axonal protection achieved in a model of multiple sclerosis using lamotrigine. J Neurol 2006;253:1542-1551.
59. Black JA, Liu S, Hains BC, et al: Long-term protection of central axons with phenytoin in monophasic and chronic-relapsing EAE. Brain 2006;129:3196-3208.
60. Craner MJ, Damarjian TG, Liu S, et al: Sodium channels contribute to microglia/macrophage activation and function in EAE and MS. Glia 2005;49:220-229.
61. Xiong ZG, Zhu XM, Chu XP, et al: Neuroprotection in ischemia: Blocking calcium-permeable acid-sensing ion channels. Cell 2004;118:687-698.
62. Pignataro G, Simon RP, Xiong ZG: Prolonged activation of ASIC1a and the time window for neuroprotection in cerebral ischaemia. Brain 2007;130(Pt 1):151-158.
63. Friese MA, Craner MJ, Etzensperger R, et al: Acid-sensing ion channel-1 contributes to axonal degeneration in autoimmune inflammation of the central nervous system. Nat Med 2007;13: 1483-1489.

64. Chen JF, Sonsalla PK, Pedata F, et al: Adenosine A2A receptors and brain injury: Broad spectrum of neuroprotection, multifaceted actions and "fine tuning" modulation. Prog Neurobiol 2007;83:310-331.
65. Croxford JL, Pryce G, Jackson SJ, et al: Cannabinoid-mediated neuroprotection, not immunosuppression, may be more relevant to multiple sclerosis. J Neuroimmunol 2008;193:120-129.
66. Li W, Maeda Y, Yuan RR, et al: Beneficial effect of erythropoietin on experimental allergic encephalomyelitis. Ann Neurol 2004;56:767-777.
67. Ehrenreich H, Fischer B, Norra C, et al: Exploring recombinant human erythropoietin in chronic progressive multiple sclerosis. Brain 2007;130:2577-2588.
68. Maier K, Kuhnert AV, Taheri N, et al: Effects of glatiramer acetate and interferon-beta on neurodegeneration in a model of multiple sclerosis: A comparative study. Am J Pathol 2006;169:1353-1364.
69. Aharoni R, Arnon R, Eilam R: Neurogenesis and neuroprotection induced by peripheral immunomodulatory treatment of experimental autoimmune encephalomyelitis. J Neurosci 2005;25:8217-8228.
70. Schwartz M, Kipnis J: Protective autoimmunity and neuroprotection in inflammatory and noninflammatory neurodegenerative diseases. J Neurol Sci 2005;233:163-166.
71. Aharoni R, Eilam R, Domev H, et al: The immunomodulator glatiramer acetate augments the expression of neurotrophic factors in brains of experimental autoimmune encephalomyelitis mice. Proc Natl Acad Sci U S A 2005;102:19045-19050.
72. Ziemssen T, Kumpfel T, Klinkert WE, et al: Glatiramer acetate-specific T-helper 1- and 2-type cell lines produce BDNF: Implications for multiple sclerosis therapy. Brain-derived neurotrophic factor. Brain 2002;125:2381-2391.
73. Benraiss A, Chmielnicki E, Lerner K, et al: Adenoviral brain-derived neurotrophic factor induces both neostriatal and olfactory neuronal recruitment from endogenous progenitor cells in the adult forebrain. J Neurosci 2001;21:6718-6731.
74. Sairanen M, Lucas G, Ernfors P, et al: Brain-derived neurotrophic factor and antidepressant drugs have different but coordinated effects on neuronal turnover, proliferation, and survival in the adult dentate gyrus. J Neurosci 2005;25:1089-1094.
75. Ziv Y, Ron N, Butovsky O, et al: Immune cells contribute to the maintenance of neurogenesis and spatial learning abilities in adulthood. Nat Neurosci 2006;9:268-275.
76. Gensert JM, Goldman JE: Endogenous progenitors remyelinate demyelinated axons in the adult CNS. Neuron 1997;19:197-203.
77. Redwine JM, Armstrong RC: In vivo proliferation of oligodendrocyte progenitors expressing PDGFalphaR during early remyelination. J Neurobiol 1998;37:413-428.
78. Keirstead HS, Blakemore WF: Identification of post-mitotic oligodendrocytes incapable of remyelination within the demyelinated adult spinal cord. J Neuropathol Exp Neurol 1997;56:1191-1201.
79. Targett MP, Sussman J, Scolding N, et al: Failure to achieve remyelination of demyelinated rat axons following transplantation of glial cells obtained from the adult human brain. Neuropathol Appl Neurobiol 1996;22:199-206.
80. Wolswijk G: Oligodendrocyte survival, loss and birth in lesions of chronic-stage multiple sclerosis. Brain 2000;123:105-115.
81. Wolswijk G: Oligodendrocyte precursor cells in the demyelinated multiple sclerosis spinal cord. Brain 2002;125:338-349.
82. Di Bello IC, Dawson MR, Levine JM, Reynolds R: Generation of oligodendroglial progenitors in acute inflammatory demyelinating lesions of the rat brain stem is associated with demyelination rather than inflammation. J Neurocytol 1999;28:365-381.
83. Frost EE, Nielsen JA, Le TQ: Armstrong RC PDGF and FGF2 regulate oligodendrocyte progenitor responses to demyelination. J Neurobiol 2003;54:457-472.
84. Keirstead HS, Levine JM, Blakemore WF: Response of the oligodendrocyte progenitor cell population (defined by NG2 labelling) to demyelination of the adult spinal cord. Glia 1998;22:161-170.
85. Levine JM, Reynolds R: Activation and proliferation of endogenous oligodendrocyte precursor cells during ethidium bromide-induced demyelination. Exp Neurol 1999;160:333-347.
86. Zhang SC, Ge B, Duncan ID: Adult brain retains the potential to generate oligodendroglial progenitors with extensive myelination capacity. Proc Natl Acad Sci U S A 1999;96:4089-4094.
87. Nait-Oumesmar B, Decker L, Lachapelle F, et al: Progenitor cells of the adult mouse subventricular zone proliferate, migrate and differentiate into oligodendrocytes after demyelination. Eur J Neurosci 1999;11:4357-4366.

88. Picard-Riera ND, Delarasse L, Goude C, et al: Experimental autoimmune encephalomyelitis mobilizes neural progenitors from the subventricular zone to undergo oligodendrogenesis in adult mice. Proc Nat Acad Sci U S A 2002;99:13211-13216.
89. Edgar JM, McLaughlin M, Yool D, et al: Oligodendroglial modulation of fast axonal transport in a mouse model of hereditary spastic paraplegia. J Cell Biol 2004;166:121-131.
90. Lappe-Siefke C, Goebbels S, Gravel M, et al: Disruption of Cnp1 uncouples oligodendroglial functions in axonal support and myelination. Nat Genet 2003;33:366-374.
91. Hemmer B, Cepok S, Nessler S, Sommer N: Pathogenesis of multiple sclerosis: An update on immunology. Curr Opin Neurol 2002;15:227-231.
92. Barkhof F, Bruck W, De Groot CJ, et al: Remyelinated lesions in multiple sclerosis: Magnetic resonance image appearance. Arch Neurol 2003;60:1073-1081.
93. Chang A, Tourtellotte WW, Rudick R, Trapp BD: Premyelinating oligodendrocytes in chronic lesions of multiple sclerosis. N Engl J Med 2002;346:165-173.
94. Compston A: Remyelination in multiple sclerosis: A challenge for therapy: The 1996 European Charcot Foundation Lecture. Mult Scler 1997;3:51-70.
95. Prineas JW, Barnard RO, Kwon EE, et al: Multiple sclerosis: Remyelination of nascent lesions. Ann Neurol 1993;33:137-151.
96. Raine CS, Wu E: Multiple sclerosis: Remyelination in acute lesions. J Neuropathol Exp Neurol 1993;52:199-204.
97. Chari DM, Blakemore WF: Efficient recolonisation of progenitor-depleted areas of the CNS by adult oligodendrocyte progenitor cells. Glia 2002;37:307-313.
98. Franklin RJ: Why does remyelination fail in multiple sclerosis? Nat Rev Neurosci 2002;3:705-714.
99. Franklin RJ, Blakemore WF: To what extent is oligodendrocyte progenitor migration a limiting factor in the remyelination of multiple sclerosis lesions?. Mult Scler 1997;3:84-87.
100. Wolswijk G, Noble M: Cooperation between PDGF and FGF converts slowly dividing Adult progenitor cells to rapidly dividing cells with characteristics of O-2A perinatal progenitor cells. J Cell Biol 1992;118:889-900.
101. Foote AK, Blakemore WF: Inflammation stimulates remyelination in areas of chronic demyelination. Brain 2005;128:528-539.
102. Sharief MK: Cytokines in multiple sclerosis: Pro-inflammation or pro-remyelination? Mult Scler 1998;4:169-173.
103. Chang A, Nishiyama A, Peterson J, et al: NG2-positive oligodendrocyte progenitor cells in adult human brain and multiple sclerosis lesions. J Neurosci 2000;20:6404-6412.
104. Scolding N, Franklin R, Stevens S, et al: Oligodendrocyte progenitors are present in the normal adult human CNS and in the lesions of multiple sclerosis. Brain 1998;121:2221-2228.
105. Wolswijk G: Oligodendrocyte regeneration in the adult rodent CNS and the failure of this process in multiple sclerosis. Prog Brain Res 1998;117:233-247.
106. Mason JL, Toews A, Hostettler JD, et al: Oligodendrocytes and progenitors become progressively depleted within chronically demyelinated lesions. Am J Pathol 2004;164:1673-1682.
107. Raff MC, Lillien LE, Richardson WD, et al: Platelet-derived growth factor from astrocytes drives the clock that times oligodendrocyte development in culture. Nature 1988;333:562-565.
108. Canoll PD, Musacchio JM, Hardy R, et al: GGF/neuregulin is a neuronal signal that promotes the proliferation and survival and inhibits the differentiation of oligodendrocyte progenitors. Neuron 1996;17:229-243.
109. Kumar S, Kahn MA, Dinh L, de Vellis J: NT-3-mediated TrkC receptor activation promotes proliferation and cell survival of rodent progenitor oligodendrocyte cells in vitro and in vivo. J Neurosci Res 1998;54:754-765.
110. Machold R, Hayashi S, Rutlin M, et al: Sonic hedgehog is required for progenitor cell maintenance in telencephalic stem cell niches. Neuron 2003;39:937-950.
111. Palma V, Lim DA, Dahmane N, et al: Sonic hedgehog controls stem cell behavior in the postnatal and adult brain. Development 2005;132:335-344.
112. Lovett-Racke AE, Bittner P, Cross AH, et al: Regulation of experimental autoimmune encephalomyelitis with insulin-like growth factor (IGF-1) and IGF-1/IGF-binding protein-3 complex (IGF- 1/IGFBP3). J Clin Invest 1998;101:1797-1804.
113. Butzkueven H, Zhang JG, Soilu-Hanninen M, et al: LIF receptor signaling limits immune-mediated demyelination by enhancing oligodendrocyte survival. Nat Med 2002;8:613-619.
114. Stankoff B, Aigrot MS, Noel F, et al: Ciliary neurotrophic factor (CNTF) enhances myelin formation: A novel role for CNTF and CNTF-related molecules. J Neurosci 2002;22:9221-9227.

115. Cannella B, Hoban CJ, Gao YL, et al: The neuregulin, glial growth factor 2, diminishes autoimmune demyelination and enhances remyelination in a chronic relapsing model for multiple sclerosis. Proc Natl Acad Sci U S A 1998;95:10100-10105.
116. Flugel A, Matsumuro K, Neumann H, et al: Anti-inflammatory activity of nerve growth factor in experimental autoimmune encephalomyelitis: Inhibition of monocyte transendothelial migration. Eur J Immunol 2001;31:11-22.
117. Linker RA, Maurer M, Gaupp S, et al: CNTF is a major protective factor in demyelinating CNS disease: A neurotrophic cytokine as modulator in neuroinflammation. Nat Med 2002;8: 620-624.
118. Ruffini F, Furlan R, Poliani PL, et al: Fibroblast growth factor-II gene therapy reverts the clinical course and the pathological signs of chronic experimental autoimmune encephalomyelitis in C57BL/6 mice. Gene Ther 2001;8:1207-1213.
119. Villoslada P, Hauser SL, Bartke I, et al: Human nerve growth factor protects common marmosets against autoimmune encephalomyelitis by switching the balance of T helper cell type 1 and 2 cytokines within the central nervous system. J Exp Med 2000;191:1799-1806.
120. Arnett HA, Fancy SP, Alberta JA, et al: bHLH transcription factor Olig1 is required to repair demyelinated lesions in the CNS. Science 2004;306:2111-2115.
121. Aguirre A, Dupree JL, Mangin JM, Gallo V: A functional role for EGFR signaling in myelination and remyelination. Nat Neurosci 2007;10:990-1002.
122. Wolswijk G: Chronic stage multiple sclerosis lesions contain a relatively quiescent population of oligodendrocyte precursor cells. J Neurosci 1998;18:601-609.
123. John GR, Shankar SL, Shafit-Zagardo B, et al: Multiple sclerosis: Re-expression of a developmental pathway that restricts oligodendrocyte maturation. Nat Med 2002;8:1115-1121.
124. Stidworthy MF, Genoud S, Li WW, et al: Notch1 and Jagged1 are expressed after CNS demyelination, but are not a major rate-determining factor during remyelination. Brain 2004;127:1928-1941.
125. Colognato H, Baron W, Avellana-Adalid V, et al: CNS integrins switch growth factor signalling to promote target-dependent survival. Nat Cell Biol 2002;4:833-841.
126. Ffrench-Constant C, Colognato H: Integrins: versatile integrators of extracellular signals. Trends Cell Biol 2004;14:678-686.
127. Larsen PH, DaSilva AG, Conant K, Yong VW: Myelin formation during development of the CNS is delayed in matrix metalloproteinase-9 and -12 null mice. J Neurosci 2006;26:2207-2214.
128. Larsen PH, Wells JE, Stallcup WB, et al: Matrix metalloproteinase-9 facilitates remyelination in part by processing the inhibitory NG2 proteoglycan. J Neurosci 2003;23:11127-11135.
129. Anthony DC, Miller KM, Fearn S, et al: Matrix metalloproteinase expression in an experimentally-induced DTH model of multiple sclerosis in the rat CNS. J Neuroimmunol 1998;87:62-72.
130. Newman TA, Woolley ST, Hughes PM, et al: T-cell- and macrophage-mediated axon damage in the absence of a CNS-specific immune response: Involvement of metalloproteinases. Brain 2001;124:2203-2214.
131. Chen MS, Huber AB, van der Haar ME, et al: Nogo-A is a myelin-associated neurite outgrowth inhibitor and an antigen for monoclonal antibody IN-1. Nature 2000;403:434-439.
132. Mi S, Lee X, Shao Z, et al: LINGO-1 is a component of the Nogo-66 receptor/p75 signaling complex. Nat Neurosci 2004;7:221-228.
133. Wong ST, Henley JR, Kanning KC, et al: A p75(NTR) and Nogo receptor complex mediates repulsive signaling by myelin-associated glycoprotein. Nat Neurosci 2002;5:1302-1308.
134. Fontoura P, Ho PP, DeVoss J, et al: Immunity to the extracellular domain of Nogo-A modulates experimental autoimmune encephalomyelitis. J Immunol 2004;173:6981-6992.
135. Karnezis T, Mandemakers W, McQualter JL, et al: The neurite outgrowth inhibitor Nogo A is involved in autoimmune-mediated demyelination. Nat Neurosci 2004;7:736-744.
136. Fontoura P, Steinman L: Nogo in multiple sclerosis: Growing roles of a growth inhibitor. J Neurol Sci 2006;245:201-210.
137. Mi S, Miller RH, Lee X, et al: LINGO-1 negatively regulates myelination by oligodendrocytes. Nat Neurosci 2005;8:745-751.
138. Mi S, Hu B, Hahm K, et al: LINGO-1 antagonist promotes spinal cord remyelination and axonal integrity in MOG-induced experimental autoimmune encephalomyelitis. Nat Med 2007;13: 1228-1233.
139. Torregrossa P, Buhl L, Bancila M, et al: Selection of poly-alpha 2,8-sialic acid mimotopes from a random phage peptide library and analysis of their bioactivity. J Biol Chem 2004;279:30707-30714.
140. Pirko I, Ciric B, Gamez J, et al: A human antibody that promotes remyelination enters the CNS and decreases lesion load as detected by T2-weighted spinal cord MRI in a virus-induced murine model of MS. FASEB J 2004;18:1577-1579.

141. Fazekas F, Sorensen PS, Filippi M, et al: MRI results from the European Study on Intravenous Immunoglobulin in Secondary Progressive Multiple Sclerosis (ESIMS). Mult Scler 2005;11:433-440.
142. Hommes OR, Sorensen PS, Fazekas F, et al: Intravenous immunoglobulin in secondary progressive multiple sclerosis: Randomised placebo-controlled trial. Lancet 2004;364:1149-1156.
143. Dubois-Dalcq M, Ffrench-Constant C, Franklin RJ: Enhancing central nervous system remyelination in multiple sclerosis. Neuron 2005;48:9-12.
144. Groves AK, Barnett SC, Franklin RJ, et al: Repair of demyelinated lesions by transplantation of purified O-2A progenitor cells. Nature 1993;362:453-455.
145. Kocsis JD: Restoration of function by glial cell transplantation into demyelinated spinal cord. J Neurotrauma 1999;16:695-703.
146. Akiyama Y, Radtke C, Kocsis JD: Remyelination of the rat spinal cord by transplantation of identified bone marrow stromal cells. J Neurosci 2002;22:6623-6630.
147. Blakemore WF, Gilson JM, Crang AJ: Transplanted glial cells migrate over a greater distance and remyelinate demyelinated lesions more rapidly than endogenous remyelinating cells. J Neurosci Res 2000;61:288-294.
148. Franklin RJ, Blakemore WF: Transplanting oligodendrocyte progenitors into the adult CNS. J Anat 1997;190;(Pt 1):23-33.
149. Halfpenny C, Benn T, Scolding N: Cell transplantation, myelin repair, and multiple sclerosis. Lancet Neurol 2002;1:31-40.
150. Warrington AE, Barbarese E, Pfeiffer SE: Differential myelinogenic capacity of specific developmental stages of the oligodendrocyte lineage upon transplantation into hypomyelinating hosts. J Neurosci Res 1993;34:1-13.
151. Windrem MS, Roy NS, Wang J, et al: Progenitor cells derived from the adult human subcortical white matter disperse and differentiate as oligodendrocytes within demyelinated lesions of the rat brain. J Neurosci Res 2002;69:966-975.
152. Zhang SC, Duncan ID: Remyelination and restoration of axonal function by glial cell transplantation. Prog Brain Res 2000;127:515-533.
153. Franklin RJ, Gilson JM, Blakemore WF: Local recruitment of remyelinating cells in the repair of demyelination in the central nervous system. J Neurosci Res 1997;50:337-344.
154. Brustle O, Choudhary K, Karram K, et al: Chimeric brains generated by intraventricular transplantation of fetal human brain cells into embryonic rats. Nat Biotechnol 1998;16:1040-1044.
155. Brustle O, Maskos U, McKay RD: Host-guided migration allows targeted introduction of neurons into the embryonic brain. Neuron 1995;15:1275-1285.
156. Flax JD, Aurora S, Yang C, et al: Engraftable human neural stem cells respond to developmental cues, replace neurons, and express foreign genes. Nat Biotechnol 1998;16:1033-1039.
157. O'Leary MT, Blakemore WF: Oligodendrocyte precursors survive poorly and do not migrate following transplantation into the normal adult central nervous system. J Neurosci Res 1997;48:159-167.
158. Ben-Hur T, Einstein O, Mizrachi-Kol R, et al: Transplanted multipotential neural precursor cells migrate into the inflamed white matter in response to experimental autoimmune encephalomyelitis. Glia 2003;41:73-80.
159. Einstein O, Grigoriadis N, Mizrachi-Kol R, et al: Transplanted neural precursor cells reduce brain inflammation to attenuate chronic experimental autoimmune encephalomyelitis. Exp Neurol 2006;198:275-284.
160. Tourbah A, Linnington C, Bachelin C, et al: Inflammation promotes survival and migration of the CG4 oligodendrocyte progenitors transplanted in the spinal cord of both inflammatory and demyelinated EAE rats. J Neurosci Res 1997;50:853-861.
161. Ben-Hur T, van Heeswijk RB, Einstein O, et al: Serial in vivo MR tracking of magnetically labeled neural spheres transplanted in chronic EAE mice. Magn Reson Med 2007;57:164-171.
162. Bulte JW, Ben-Hur T, Miller BR, et al: MR microscopy of magnetically labeled neurospheres transplanted into the Lewis EAE rat brain. Magn Reson Med 2003;50:201-205.
163. Bagri A, Gurney T, He X, et al: The chemokine SDF1 regulates migration of dentate granule cells. Development 2002;129:4249-4260.
164. Lu M, Grove EA, Miller RJ: Abnormal development of the hippocampal dentate gyrus in mice lacking the CXCR4 chemokine receptor. Proc Natl Acad Sci U S A 2002;99:7090-7095.
165. Belmadani A, Tran PB, Ren D, et al: The chemokine stromal cell-derived factor-1 regulates the migration of sensory neuron progenitors. J Neurosci 2005;25:3995-4003.
166. Stumm RK, Zhou C, Ara T, et al: CXCR4 regulates interneuron migration in the developing neocortex. J Neurosci 2003;23:5123-5130.

167. Imitola J, Raddassi K, Park KI, et al: Directed migration of neural stem cells to sites of CNS injury by the stromal cell-derived factor 1alpha/CXC chemokine receptor 4 pathway. Proc Natl Acad Sci U S A 2004;101:18117-18122.
168. Yan YP, Sailor KA, Lang BT, et al: Monocyte chemoattractant protein-1 plays a critical role in neuroblast migration after focal cerebral ischemia. J Cereb Blood Flow Metab 2007;27: 1213-1224.
169. Belmadani A, Tran PB, Ren D, Miller RJ: Chemokines regulate the migration of neural progenitors to sites of neuroinflammation. J Neurosci 2006;26:3182-3191.
170. Einstein O, Karussis D, Grigoriadis N, et al: Intraventricular transplantation of neural precursor cell spheres attenuates acute experimental allergic encephalomyelitis. Mol Cell Neurosci 2003;24:1074-1082.
171. Yandava BD, Billinghurst LL, Snyder EY: "Global" cell replacement is feasible via neural stem cell transplantation: Evidence from the dysmyelinated shiverer mouse brain. Proc Natl Acad Sci U S A 1999;96:7029-7034.
172. Learish RD, Brustle O, Zhang SC, Duncan ID: Intraventricular transplantation of oligodendrocyte progenitors into a fetal myelin mutant results in widespread formation of myelin. Ann Neurol 1999;46:716-722.
173. Inoue M, Honmou O, Oka S, et al: Comparative analysis of remyelinating potential of focal and intravenous administration of autologous bone marrow cells into the rat demyelinated spinal cord. Glia 2003;44:111-118.
174. Mahmood A, Lu D, Chopp M: Intravenous administration of marrow stromal cells (MSCs) increases the expression of growth factors in rat brain after traumatic brain injury. J Neurotrauma 2004;21:33-39.
175. Pluchino S, Quattrini A, Brambilla E, et al: Injection of adult neurospheres induces recovery in a chronic model of multiple sclerosis. Nature 2003;422:688-694.
176. Coulombel L, Auffray I, Gaugler MH, Rosemblatt M: Expression and function of integrins on hematopoietic progenitor cells. Acta Haematol 1997;97:13-21.
177. Tran PB, Ren D, Veldhouse TJ, Miller RJ: Chemokine receptors are expressed widely by embryonic and adult neural progenitor cells. J Neurosci Res 2004;76:20-34.
178. Brocke S, Piercy C, Steinman L, et al: Antibodies to CD44 and integrin alpha4, but not L-selectin, prevent central nervous system inflammation and experimental encephalomyelitis by blocking secondary leukocyte recruitment. Proc Natl Acad Sci U S A 1999;96:6896-6901.
179. Prestoz L, Relvas JB, Hopkins K, et al: Association between integrin-dependent migration capacity of neural stem cells in vitro and anatomical repair following transplantation. Mol Cell Neurosci 2001;18:473-484.
180. Einstein O, Fainstein N, Vaknin I, et al: Neural precursors attenuate autoimmune encephalomyelitis by peripheral immunosuppression. Ann Neurol 2007;61:209-218.
181. Einstein O, Ben-Menachem-Tzidon O, Mizrachi-Kol R, et al: Survival of neural precursor cells in growth factor-poor environment: Implications for transplantation in chronic disease. Glia 2006;53:449-455.
182. Archer DR, Cuddon PA, Lipsitz D, Duncan ID: Myelination of the canine central nervous system by glial cell transplantation: A model for repair of human myelin disease. Nat Med 1997;3:54-59.
183. Utzschneider DA, Archer DR, Kocsis JD, et al: Transplantation of glial cells enhances action potential conduction of amyelinated spinal cord axons in the myelin-deficient rat. Proc Natl Acad Sci U S A 1994;91:53-57.
184. Blakemore WF: Remyelination of CNS axons by Schwann cells transplanted from the sciatic nerve. Nature 1977;266:68-69.
185. Kohama I, Lankford KL, Preiningerova J, et al: Transplantation of cryopreserved adult human Schwann cells enhances axonal conduction in demyelinated spinal cord. J Neurosci 2001;21:944-950.
186. Barnett SC, Alexander CL, Iwashita Y, et al: Identification of a human olfactory ensheathing cell that can effect transplant-mediated remyelination of demyelinated CNS axons. Brain 2000;123 (Pt 8):1581-1588.
187. Imaizumi T, Lankford KL, Burton WV, et al: Xenotransplantation of transgenic pig olfactory ensheathing cells promotes axonal regeneration in rat spinal cord. Nat Biotechnol 2000;18:949-953.
188. Akiyama Y, Honmou O, Kato T, et al: Transplantation of clonal neural precursor cells derived from adult human brain establishes functional peripheral myelin in the rat spinal cord. Exp Neurol 2001;167:27-39.
189. Brustle O, Jones KN, Learish RD, et al: Embryonic stem cell-derived glial precursors: A source of myelinating transplants. Science 1999;285:754-756.

190. Liu S, Qu Y, Stewart TJ, et al: Embryonic stem cells differentiate into oligodendrocytes and myelinate in culture and after spinal cord transplantation. Proc Natl Acad Sci U S A 2000;97:6126-6131.
191. Pluchino S, Zanotti L, Rossi B, et al: Neurosphere-derived multipotent precursors promote neuroprotection by an immunomodulatory mechanism. Nature 2005;436:266-271.
192. Gerdoni E, Gallo B, Casazza S, et al: Mesenchymal stem cells effectively modulate pathogenic immune response in experimental autoimmune encephalomyelitis. Ann Neurol 2007;61:219-227.
193. Zappia E, Casazza S, Pedemonte E, et al: Mesenchymal stem cells ameliorate experimental autoimmune encephalomyelitis inducing T-cell anergy. Blood 2005;106:1755-1761.
194. Lu P, Jones LL, Snyder EY, Tuszynski MH: Neural stem cells constitutively secrete neurotrophic factors and promote extensive host axonal growth after spinal cord injury. Exp Neurol 2003;181:115-129.
195. Ourednik J, Ourednik V, Lynch WP, et al: Neural stem cells display an inherent mechanism for rescuing dysfunctional neurons. Nat Biotechnol 2002;20:1103-1110.
196. Ferrer-Alcon M, Winkler-Hirt C, Perrin FE, Kato AC: Grafted neural stem cells increase the life span and protect motoneurons in pmn mice. Neuroreport 2007;18:1463-1468.
197. Kerr DA, Llado J, Shamblott MJ, et al: Human embryonic germ cell derivatives facilitate motor recovery of rats with diffuse motor neuron injury. J Neurosci 2003;23:5131-5140.
198. Suzuki M, McHugh J, Tork C, et al: GDNF secreting human neural progenitor cells protect dying motor neurons, but not their projection to muscle, in a rat model of familial ALS. PLoS ONE 2007;2:e689.
199. Li J, Imitola J, Snyder EY, Sidman RL: Neural stem cells rescue nervous purkinje neurons by restoring molecular homeostasis of tissue plasminogen activator and downstream targets. J Neurosci 2006;26:7839-7848.
200. Gamm DM, Wang S, Lu B, et al: Protection of visual functions by human neural progenitors in a rat model of retinal disease. PLoS ONE 2007;2:e338.
201. Teng YD, Lavik EB, Qu X, et al: Functional recovery following traumatic spinal cord injury mediated by a unique polymer scaffold seeded with neural stem cells. Proc Natl Acad Sci U S A 2002;99:3024-3029.
202. Zhang Y, Klassen HJ, Tucker BA, et al: CNS progenitor cells promote a permissive environment for neurite outgrowth via a matrix metalloproteinase-2-dependent mechanism. J Neurosci 2007;27:4499-4506.
203. Park KI, Teng YD, Snyder EY: The injured brain interacts reciprocally with neural stem cells supported by scaffolds to reconstitute lost tissue. Nat Biotechnol 2002;20:1111-1117.
204. Capone C, Frigerio S, Fumagalli S, et al: Neurosphere-derived cells exert a neuroprotective action by changing the ischemic microenvironment. PLoS ONE 2007;2:e373.
205. Ben-Shaanan TL, Ben-Hur T, Yanai J: Transplantation of neural progenitors enhances production of endogenous cells in the impaired brain. Mol Psychiatry 2008;13:222-231.
206. Hattiangady B, Shuai B, Cai J, et al: Increased dentate neurogenesis after grafting of glial restricted progenitors or neural stem cells in the aging hippocampus. Stem Cells 2007;25:2104-2117.
207. Kamei N, Tanaka N, Oishi Y, et al: BDNF, NT-3, and NGF released from transplanted neural progenitor cells promote corticospinal axon growth in organotypic cocultures. Spine 2007;32:1272-1278.

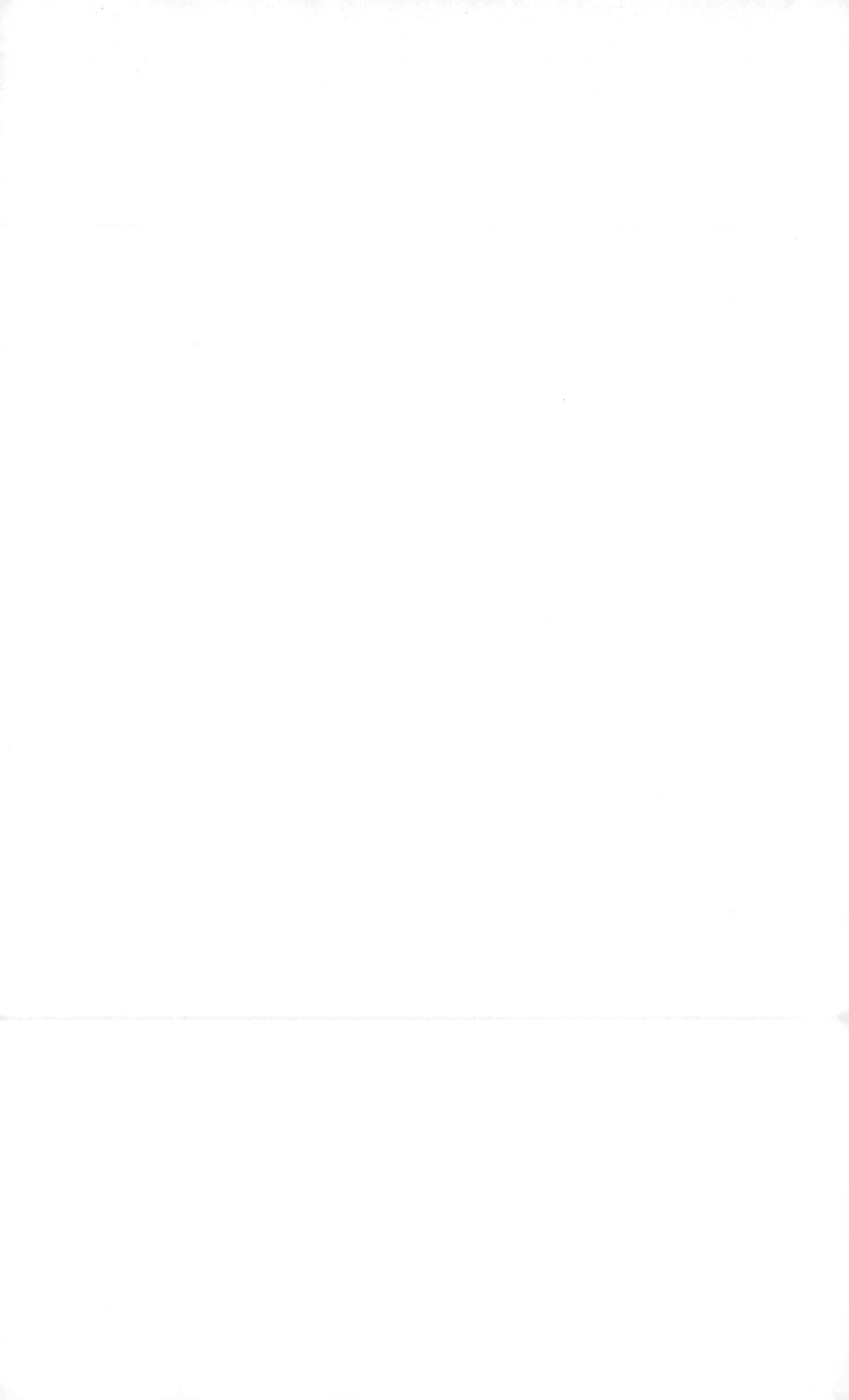

INDEX

D

E

H

I

K

L

M

N

O

P

W

X

Y

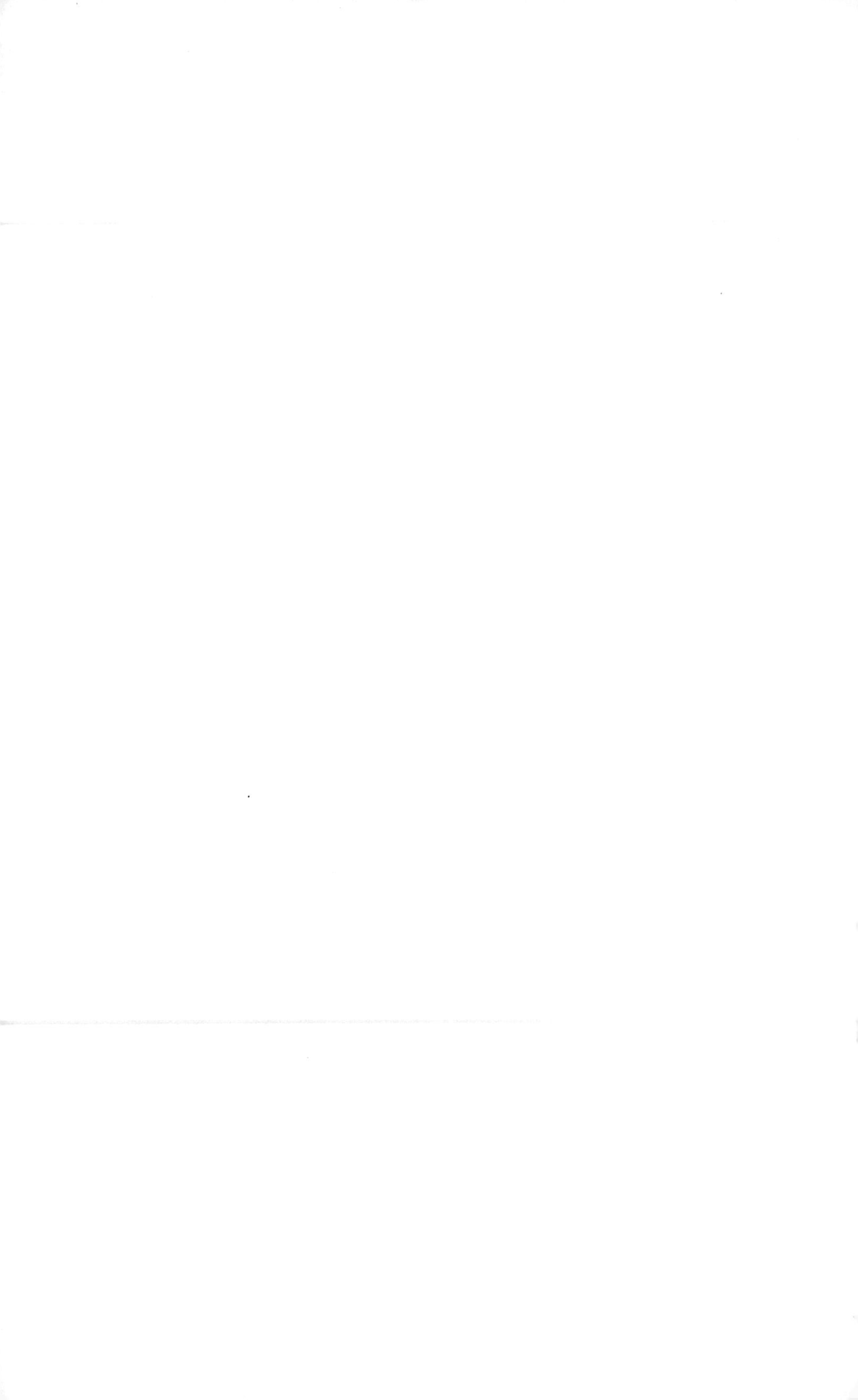

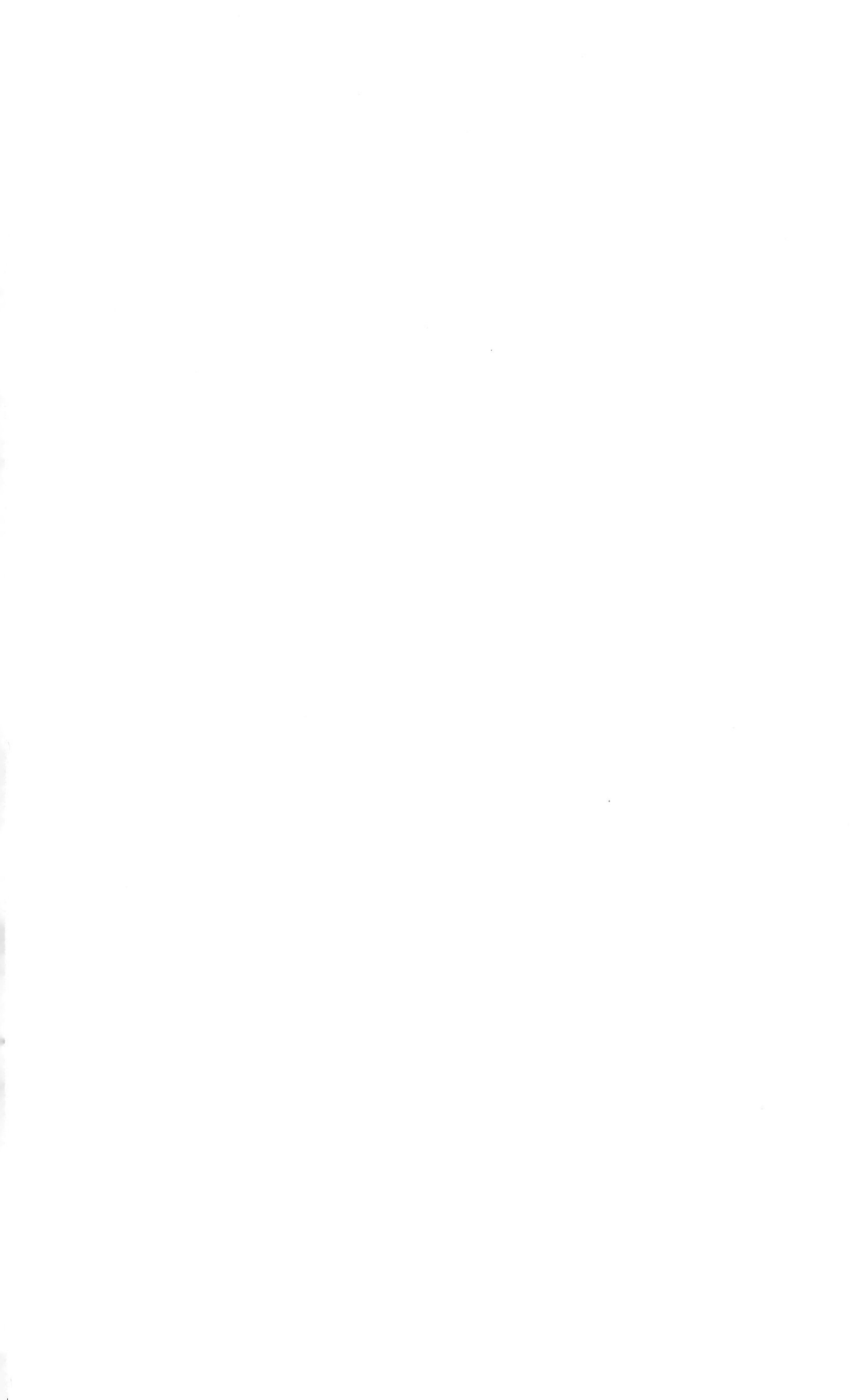

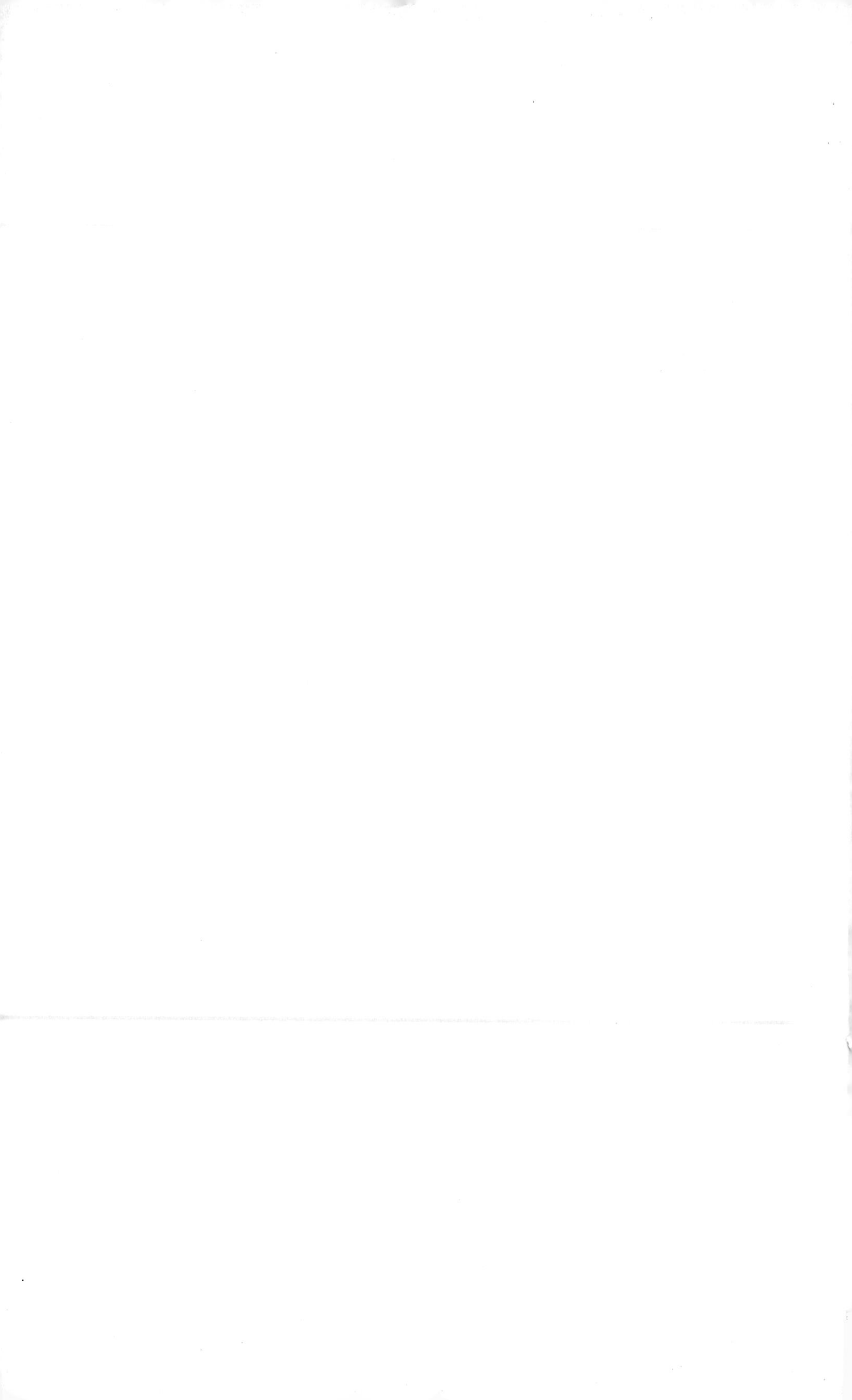